T0381246

PERSONALIZED MEDICINE
(BEYOND PET BIOMARKERS)

BIOTECHNOLOGY IN AGRICULTURE, INDUSTRY AND MEDICINE

Additional books in this series can be found on Nova's website
under the Series tab.

Additional e-books in this series can be found on Nova's website
under the eBooks tab.

BIOTECHNOLOGY IN AGRICULTURE, INDUSTRY AND MEDICINE

PERSONALIZED MEDICINE (BEYOND PET BIOMARKERS)

SUSHIL SHARMA

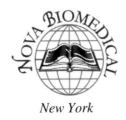

New York

Library of Congress Cataloging-in-Publication Data

Names: Sharma, Sushil, (Pharmacologist)
Title: Personalized medicine (beyond PET biomarkers) / editor, Sushil Sharma (Professor of Pharmacology & Course Director, Saint James School of Medicine, Cane Hall, St Vincent, St Vincent & Grenadines).
Description: Hauppauge, New York : Nova Science Publisher's, Inc., [2016] | Series: Biotechnology in agriculture, industry and medicine | Includes index.
Identifiers: LCCN 2016019043 (print) | LCCN 2016029900 (ebook) | ISBN 9781634853248 (hardcover) | ISBN 9781634853330 (ebook) | ISBN 9781634853330 ()
Subjects: LCSH: Personalized medicine. | Pharmacogenetics.
Classification: LCC RM301.3.G45 P347 2016 (print) | LCC RM301.3.G45 (ebook) | DDC 615.7--dc23
LC record available at https://lccn.loc.gov/2016019043

Published by Nova Science Publishers, Inc. † *New York*

DEDICATION

This book is dedicated *to author's late mother "Charnoly" and* to those patients who died because of lack of knowledge of physicians due to delayed, wrong, and futile therapeutic attempts.

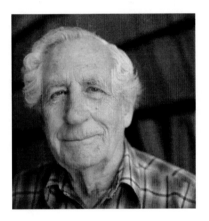

Professor Werner Kalow, MD (1917–2008).

Professor Werener Kalow, M.D (1917-2008) was one of the original founder and pioneer of Pharmacogenomics (*an essential discipline of personalized medicine*). Personalized medicine is a promising discipline of modern medicine that utilizes patient's genetic profile to make decisions regarding prevention, diagnosis, and treatment of diseases. Exact knowledge of a patient's genetic profile can help select the exact medication and the exact dose. Personalized medicine evolved primarily through the analyses of bioinformatics data from the human genome project, molecular imaging, and nanotheranostics.

CONTENTS

Words of Wisdom

It is important to know what person the disease has than what disease the person has.

(Hippocrates)

The real voyage of discovery consists not in seeking new landscapes, but in having new eyes.

Marcel Proust (1871–1922)

Personalized medicine (PM) is a clinical model that proposes the customization of healthcare - with medical decisions, practices, and/or products being tailored to the individual patient. In this model, diagnostic testing is used for selecting appropriate and optimal therapies based on the patient's genetic makeup or other molecular or cellular analysis. The use of genetic information plays a pivotal role in various aspects of PM (e.g., pharmacogenomics), and the term was first used in the context of genetics, though it has since broadened to cover all aspects of personalization measures.

(PM Caolition., 2014)

Doctors are doing a great job, but they can't be expected to know everything for every patient. As a patient, you shouldn't feel like you're imposing. You should feel like you're helping." In many cases, the current standard of care may be the safest, most sensible option, but it's also "one size fits all." Sometimes that's sufficient, but not always. It is in that "not always" category that personalized medicine (PM) is making the most headway.

(Randy Burkholder)

PM is defined as: "treatments targeted to the needs of individual patients on the basis of genetic, biomarker, phenotypic or psychosocial characteristics that distinguish a given patient from other patients with similar clinical presentations"

(Jameson and Longo, 2015).

The number of targeted therapies in the pipeline for all diseases is increasing dramatically. Personalized medicine (PM) in this era of genomic medicine means we're living in dynamic times. The big question is 'How do we take all this new information and use it for the benefit of the patient?

(J. Leonard Lichtenfeld)

Treatments targeted to the needs of individual patients on the basis of genetic, biomarker, phenotypic or psychosocial characteristics that distinguish a given patient from other patients with similar clinical presentations.

(Jameson and Longo, 2016)

Probably at no time in the history of medical research, going back to the time of William Harvey and the circulation of blood, in the 1600s, has there been more potential and promise for discovery that will benefit mankind in terms of the health of the species as where we are right now as a result of the Human Genome Project,

(Scott T. Weiss)

Biomarkers are biological parameters that can be measured to predict or monitor disease severity or treatment efficacy.

Moingeon (2016)

PM is based on genomic makeup of the patient and follows basic principle of prevention is better than cure. The promise of PM is "therapy with the right drug at the right dose in the right patient" Molecular imaging companion diagnostics can accomplish personalized theranostics of several chronic illnesses.

(Pharmacogenomics. The Promise of PM, 2000)

Representation of the trial-and-error or one-dose-fits-all approach versus PM, a situation in which everyone gets the same dose of a drug, regardless of genotype. In PM approach the dose of the drug is selected based upon genotypical, and hence phenotypical, variability of the metabolizing enzyme.

(Xie and Frueh, 2005)

"Currently patients are not yet asking the question 'Is this therapy going to work for me?' It will be very challenging to look forward to the day patients do ask that question." Usually "more complex and more heterogeneous the disease, more important is personalized treatment"

ABOUT THIS BOOK

Nova Science Publishers, New York, U.S.A has now released *Personalized Medicine (Beyond PET Biomarkers)*, which is an extension of the author's recently published book *Progress in PET Radiopharmaceuticals: Quality Control and Theranostics*. In addition to recently-developed clinically-significant PET-RPs as biomarkers, this book describes various other emerging biotechnologies including: genomic medicine, nanotechnology, novel molecular biomarkers, and noninvasive imaging biotechnologies for early theranostics and personalized patient care, with minimum or no adverse effects.

New therapeutic interventions including gene and cell therapies, pharmacogenomics, next generation sequencing, genome-wide association studies, proteomics, metabolomics, bioinformatics, systems biology complementing areas of pharmacokinetics and pharmacodynamics, human investigations and clinical trials, pharmacovigilance, pharmacoepidemiology, and population pharmacology are some of the most significant disciplines of predictive, precision, and personalized medicine (PM) as described in this book.

More specifically, different sub-specialties of omics biotechnology including: genomic, proteomic, glycomic, lipidomic, metabolomics, metalomic, and microRNA biomarkers are described to accomplish early and personalized theranostics of chronic illnesses with currently limited therapeutic options and success.

Recent advances in nanotechnology and novel biomarkers to accomplish personalized theranostics of chronic diseases including, but not limited to: cancer, fetal alcohol syndrome, Alzheimer's disease, Parkinson's disease, vascular dementia, amyotrophic lateral sclerosis, and multiple sclerosis. Usually, nanoparticles (NPs) are trapped in the reticuloendothelial system (RES) comprising the lungs, liver, and spleen. To prevent their entry into the RES system and enhance drug targeting, stealth property of polyethylene glycol (PEG) as a covalent linker is utilized. However, pegylation may reduce the biological activity of the antibody or other labile molecule attached to NPs. Therefore, positively-charged chitosans and negatively charged alginates have been developed. Liposomal encapsulated Doxorubicin (Adriamycin) was approved in the early seventies for the treatment of breast cancer. In addition, enhanced permeability and retention (EPR) property of newly synthesized micro vessels of a hyper proliferating tumor is utilized to selectively invade the cancer stem cells is intricately described.

Various noninvasive in-vivo imaging technologies including computerized tomography (CT), magnetic resonance imaging (MRI) along with magnetic-resonance spectroscopic (MRS) capability, single photon emission tomography (SPECT), positron emission tomography (PET), ultra sound alone or as hybrid images to obtain precise 5D anatomical landmarks, regional physiology, and biochemistry of the human body organs at cellular, molecular, and genetic level in health and disease are described. The book also describes in-vitro methods to acquire images of tissues and cells in culture employing digital infrared imaging, digital fluorescence microscopic, confocal microscopic, and fluorescence resonance transfer (FRET) resonance imaging for detecting apoptosis and/or necrosis at the cellular, molecular and genetic level.

This timely-released manuscript will attract basic scientists, researchers, and physicians interested in further developing the emerging concept of personalized medicine (PM), and will serve as a textbook for Masters, M.D., and Ph. D students, and a reference book for doctors, professors, basic researchers, scientists, and general public.

The author has explained recently-discovered novel biomarkers for the personalized diagnosis and treatment of cancer, cardiovascular diseases, neurodegenerative diseases, and other chronic inflammatory diseases such as asthma, COPD, cystic fibrosis, migraine, and rheumatoid arthritis to accomplish the long quested goal of evidence-based personalized theranostics (EBPT). Recently-discovered disease-specific biomarkers can be successfully employed alone or in combination for the personalized treatment of chronic multidrug-resistant illnesses. Particularly, progressive neurodegenerative diseases such as fetal alcohol syndrome, Parkinson's disease, drug addiction, Alzheimer's disease, vascular dementia, amyotrophic lateral sclerosis, and demyelinating relapse and remission multiple sclerosis (RRMS) are described in detail because personalized treatment of these devastating diseases is currently a significant challenge.

There are several other chronic drug resistant pro-inflammatory and infectious diseases, which could not be covered in sufficient detail owing to the lack of expertise, time, and limited space allocated to write this dedicated and clinically significant book. The author apologizes to the entire global scientific community for his own ignorance, and humbly requests readers to go through the book's interesting and most recent contents to enhance their basic knowledge regarding personalized medicine beyond PET biomarkers, which is one of the most demanding disciplines of modern medicine.

Sushil Sharma, Ph. D; D.M.R.I.T
Professor of Pharmacology &
Course Director
Saint James School of Medicine
Cane Hall, St Vincent
St Vincent & Grenadines
Tel: 784-456-7576
Email: Sharma@mail.sjsm.org

PREFACE

Although the concept of personalized medicine (PM) is not new, its exact clinical significance was recognized recently with the development of omics technology, nanotechnology, and in-vivo noninvasive imaging technology, as described in author's recent book *"Progress in PET Radiopharmaceuticals (Quality Control and Theranostics)* by Nova Science Publishers, New York. With the accomplishment of human genome project and next generation sequencing (NGS) the concept of personalized treatment has emerged a real therapeutic challenge for all chronic illnesses. There are several chronic proinflammatory illnesses particularly; multidrug-resistant malignancies and Alzheimer's disease, which require individualized therapy for successful clinical management and better quality of life.

This book describes primarily five major emerging disciplines including (i) omics (microarray) technology; (ii) nonobiotechnology; (iii) in-vivo imaging biotechnology; (iv) in-vitro imaging biotechnology; and (v) bioinformatics to accomplish the ultimate goal of evidence-based personalized theranostics (EBPT).

Particularly omics biotechnology include: *genomic, proteomic, glycomic, lipidomic, metabolomics*, and *metalomic* to successfully diagnose and treat a patient simultaneously utilizing recently-developed threanostic interventions. For instance, mouse avatars (*mice bearing tumors of a particular cancer patient*) can facilitate selecting the most appropriate therapeutic options for multidrug resistant malignancies. However heterogeneous and complex pharmacokinetics and pharmacodynamics of anticancer drugs in mouse avatars and humans provide a considerable biological variability in therapeutic response and prognosis. Hence a lot need to be explored, before the researchers could successfully accomplish EBPT.

One of the most important disciplines which has contributed significantly in accomplishing personalized treatment is nanotechnology. Several nanomedicines which can bypass the reticuloendothelial (RE) system by pegylation have enhanced tumor targeting to accomplish theranostic capability of drug-loaded nanoparticles (NPs). However the therapeutic potential of anti-tumor antibodies and other labile agents is considerably compromised by pegylation. The encapsulation of therapeutic drugs (*particularly labile proteins, enzymes, hormones, growth factors, RNA, DNA*) employing liposomes, chotosans, and alignates has revolutionized the basic concept of conventional therapeutic approaches. The chitosans are positively charged due to the presence of $-NH_3$ group on these macromolecules, whereas alginates are negatively changed due to the existence of $-COO^-$

moiety on their surface, which facilitates drug encapsulation in addition to providing their slow and steady release, in addition to excellent compatibility, and degradation in the biological system.

It is now well-recognized that angiogenesis is exceedingly essential for the tumor growth and development. Various integrins including; α5β3 have been implicated in tumor angiogenesis. Hence α5β3 antagonists are being developed. However these agents exhibit nonspecific inhibition of angiogenesis in various other tissues of the human body; hence are of limited therapeutic value at this moment. The microvessels in the hyper proliferating tumors are thin-walled and leaky and exhibit enhanced permeability and retention (EPR). Anticancer drugs are easily retained in the highly proliferating tumor cells, which facilitates their early irradiation. Hence EPR principle is being exploited to develop nanomedicines for the successful EBPT of multidrug-resistant malignancies and other chronic proinflammatory diseases including PD, AD, HD, MS, ALS, MDD, and drug addiction. In addition to the development of block co-polymers, disease-specific charnolomimetics, charnolicidals, and CB sequestration inhibiting agents have been proposed by the author to accomplish EBPT.

Recently metallic NPs (particularly gold nanoshells) for the remote ablation of deep-seated tumors have been developed. The gold nanoshells conjugated with PEG and encapsulated with anticancer drugs such as Doxorubicin exhibit enhance tumor to nontumor (T/NT) ratio due to EPR and can be heated from outside by infra red to achieve $60-80^0$C local body temperature. At this temperature the highly proliferating tumor cells are selectively destroyed. Although this novel approach provides enhanced drug targeting and minimum cardiotoxicity, the cancer patient feels uncomfortable during this personalized theranostics. Hence better therapeutic options are needed to combat the deleterious consequences of multidrug resistant malignancies and other chronic proinflammatory diseases. Recently superior metallic as well as nonmetallic NPs including: silica nanoparticles, carbon nano rods, nanotubes have been developed to accomplish early EBPT.

Novel nanotheranostic approaches are currently being developed to accomplish EBPT as described in detail in this book.

The another highly significant area of PM is bioimaging technology which includes: *(i) computerized tomography (CT); (ii) magnetic resonance imaging (MRI), (iii) magnetic resonance spectroscopy (MRS); (iv) single photon emission tomography (SPECT); (v) positron emission tomography (PET) imaging, and (vi) PET/SPECT/MRI/SPECT fusion imaging,* The researchers could reconstruct hybrid images to obtain anatomical, physiological, and pharmacological information at the cellular, molecular, and genetic levels regarding the disease process; however precise coregistration of these multimodality images is the most challenging area in in-vivo imaging technology, which has been resolved considerably to accomplish EBPT.

In addition, in-vitro imaging of cultured cells and cell-free systems have provided solution to several unresolved questions to accomplish EBPT. Particularly *(i) fluorescence microscopy, (ii) confocal microscopy; (iii) fluorescence activated\FACS analysis; (iv) fluorescence activated cell sorting (FACS); (v) fluorescence energy resonance (FRET) spectroscopy; (vi) fluorescence in-situ hybridization; microarray and microRNA, epigenetic technology, and (vi) autoradiography have provided valuable information regarding basic molecular mechanism(s) of diseases progression and regression (particularly apoptosis/antiapoptosis), beyond the scope of this book.*

The great Greek Philosopher and Physician, Aristotle described that diseases occurs due to the imbalance in primarily 4 major components in our body including: Vat, Pitt, cough, and blood as the researchers now have four DNA bases (*Adenine, Thymine, Cytosine, & Guanine*). At least cancer can be eradicated by prescribing specific structural analogs of these four bases of the DNA helix.

Currently-available drugs are associated with deleterious effects due to lack of specificity and targetability. Non-specific induction of CB formation during treatment of multidrug-resistant malignancies causes GIT disorders, myelosuppression, and alopecia. Hence anticancer drugs could be developed to enhance cancer stem-cell-specific CB formation to prevent the deleterious effects of anticancer drugs, whereas tissue-specific CB inhibitors could be developed for the clinical management of cardiovascular and neurodegenerative diseases. Furthermore, specific charnolophagy-inducers may be developed as intracellular detoxifiers to prevent CB sequestration, implicated in the release of caspase-3, cytochrome-C and apoptosis-inducing factor, in addition to Bax, involved in apoptotic signaling.

The author reported that inhibition of charnolophagy during zygote formation can induce craniofacial abnormalities in microbial (Zika virus) infections, metal ion (lead) toxicity, and fetal Alcohol syndrome victims. It is now realized that intrauterine exposure to neurotoxins including Ethanol can increase the genetic predisposition to drug abuse disorders during adolescence. In addition, lysosomal-resistant CB formation may induce zygote death and/or fetal mortality in chronic Ethanol abuse during pregnancy. CB aggregation in response to nutritional and/or environmental stress occurs primarily in the perinuclear space which may impair translational and transcriptional activity of genes, whereas antioxidants such as MTs, polyphenols, sirtuins, and resveratrol, inhibit CB formation by serving as free radical scavengers and are involved in zinc-mediated transcriptional regulation of genes involved in growth, proliferation, differentiation, and development. Accumulation of CB at the junction of axon hillock may hinder normal axoplasmic flow of various ions, neurotransmitter, hormones, growth factors, enzymes, and mitochondria to impair synaptic neurotransmission and cause cognitive impairment in various neurodegenerative disorders such as MDD, PD, MCI, AD, and drug addiction. Hence pharmacological or pharmacogenomic interventions to augment tissue-specific MTs and other antioxidants may provide protection in various neurodegenerative and cardiovascular disorders and facilitate personalized treatment of cancer and other chronic proinflammatory diseases as described in this timely-released interesting book.

Note: Although "Personalized Medicine" is the most commonly used term in clinical practice, the author has preferred to use "*Personalized Theranostics*" to be more specific and precise, because the ultimate goal of personalized medicine is to accomplish "*Evidence Based Personalized Theranostics*" by simultaneously diagnosing and treating the patient without losing crucial and precious time of the patient as well as health care providers. This unique theranostic approach avoids multi-drug-resistance and futile therapeutic attempts while laying primary emphasis on preventive and promotive aspects of healthcare. EBPT considers personalized genomics, pharmacogenomics, biomarkers, age, sex, nutritional status, race, and life-style profile of a patient during specifically designed personalized treatment. The other most important mission of EBPT is to avoid any invasive, painful interventions, and/or adverse effects of treatment as described in this timely-released book by Nova Science Publishers, New York, U.S.A.

ACKNOWLEDGMENTS

The author expresses sincere thanks to several international scientists, guides, and industries where he received advanced trainings and his friends and colleagues for the moral support and encouragement to write this interesting and timely released book by Nova Science Publishers on personalized medicine (PM) *to accomplish better, safe, and efficient therapeutic strategies for chronic illnesses.*

Recently innovative development of technologically-advanced cyclotrons, self-shielded hot cell designs, efficient remote-controlled synthesis modules, and sophisticated computers, equipped with efficient data acquisition and analyses capabilities has revolutionized the multidisciplinary field of evidence-based personalized medicine (EBPM). Several researchers, basic scientists, engineers, pharmacologists, pharmacists, nuclear physicists, and physicians have contributed remarkably in the development of novel PET biomarkers capable of providing *in vivo,* noninvasive 5D spatiotemporal information regarding the disease process of internal organs for early theranostics to accomplish the ultimate goal of EBPM. In addition to novel PET biomarkers, omic (*genomic, proteomic, glycomic, lipidomic, metabolomics, metallomic)* biomarkers and nanotechnology have evolved novel and unique concepts of personalized theranostics of chronic illnesses with currently limited therapeutic options and success.

Special thanks are due to President Nadya Columbus and her entire *Nova Science Publishers, Team* for the timely release of this book, which will serve as an essential guide for, doctors, medical students, nurses, and basic researchers globally to understand the basic concepts of PM for the successful treatment of multi-drug resistant cancer, cardiovascular diseases, neurological diseases (*particularly Alzheimer's disease, Parkinson's disease, and drug addiction*), and numerous other chronic proinflammatory illnesses. Several scientists have already contributed significantly and dedicated their entire life in this multidisciplinary area for which the author extends his heartiest appreciation and acknowledgement. Moral support and encouragement by Dr. Kallol Guha, President, Saint James Schools of Medicine, is gratefully acknowledged.

Several interesting topics on personalized medicine could not be covered due to limited expertise and space in this book. The author begs apologies and most humbly requests the entire global scientific community to go through the most interesting and thought-provoking contents of this technologically-advanced and clinically-significant book to augment their existing knowledge regarding EBPT, and ignore several limitations and/or deficiencies it may have. Any helpful criticism and/or suggestions for its improvement will be highly appreciated and gratefully acknowledged.

This manuscript promises to contribute further in the development of PM for improved patient care and will serve as a textbook for basic biomedical students and scientists, and reference book for physicians and other health care professionals.

Sushil Sharma, Ph.D.; D.M.R.I.T
Professor of Pharmacology & Course Director
Ex-Director Cyclotron & Positron Imaging Research Laboratory
University of North Dakota School of Medicine, Grand Forks, ND, USA
Saint James School of Medicine, Cane Hall, St Vincent Cane Hall, St Vincent & Grenadines. (West Indies) Email: Sharma@mail.sjsm.org

ABOUT THE AUTHOR

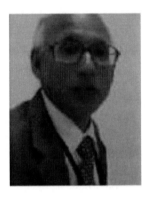

Sushil Sharma is currently professor of pharmacology & course director at the Saint James School of Medicine, St Vincent. Before joining this school, he served as a professor of pharmacology at the Saint James School of Medicine, Bonaire (Netherlands Antilles) and as a scientist in the University of Texas Health Sciences Center, Department of Neurology, at Houston, TX, and as an Associate Professor & Director of The Cyclotron & PET Radiopharmaceutical Laboratory of the Weil Cornell University Affiliated Methodist Hospital, Houston. TX. He also served as an Associated Professor & Director at the University of North Dakota, Center of Excellence in Neuroscience, Grand Forks in the Cyclotron & Positron Imaging Research Laboratory and as an Assistant Professor in the department of pharmacology, physiology, and therapeutics, Grand Forks, ND. He was invited to deliver a lecture on the *"Dopaminergic Neurotransmission In Drug Addiction"* in The Executive Office of The President, Washington DC On April 29, 2004. He received several advanced trainings on the synthesis and quality control of radiopharmaceuticals from Siemens Medical Solutions, Cardinal Health, Agilent Technologies, and General Electrics, U.S.A.

He served as a Research Scientist at the Saint Boniface Hospital Research Center, Department of Cardiovascular Pharmacology in Winnipeg, Canada and worked on hypertension, atherosclerosis, vascular neointimal hyperplasia, and cardiovascular remodeling. He served as a Senior Scientist in the Clinical Research Institute of Montreal in the Peptide Pharmacology Laboratory and in the McGill University on pain mechanisms and analgesia. As a Research Officer in the University of Montreal, Andre Viallet Clinical Research Center, Hospital St Luc in Montreal, he studied the deleterious effects of Vitamin-D deficiency and hypocalcemia.

He served as a research associate in the Department of Biochemistry & Molecular Biology on the "Neuropharmacology of Vitamin B_6 " and published several research papers on the influence of Vitamin B_6 deficiency and excess on the developing and adult rat brain and in human cultured cell lines. He was awarded MHRC post-doctoral fellowship in Canada. The primary objective of this study was to determine the therapeutic role of Vitamin B_6 as a coenzyme in GABA-ergic, dopaminergic, and serotonergic neurotransmission in relation to seizure susceptibility and hypertension. This research was extended to examine the deleterious effects of environmental neurotoxins including Kainic Acid, Domoic Acid, Picrotoxin, and Pentylene Tetrazole on B_6-deficient adult rats. Dr. Sharma discovered that intrauterine Kainic Acid, and Domoic Acid induce excito-neurotoxicity and selective neurodegeneration due to Charnoly Body (CB) formation in the hippocampal CA-3 and dentate gyrus regions resulting in loss of memory, as observed in AD patients. Brain regional GABA as well as 5-HT were significantly reduced in Vitamin B_6-deficient rats as observed in patients suffering from depression. Domoic acid-induced seizure discharge activity and thresholds were significantly reduced in Vitamin B_6-deficient animals and they exhibited seizure discharge activity of prolonged duration and delayed spontaneous or drug-induced neuronal recovery, as confirmed by computerized EEG and neurotransmitter analysis. In his book on "Beyond Diet and Depression" published by Nova Science Publishers, the author has described his own and other investigators original findings on Vitamin B_6 deficiency and excess and its effect on mood. Dr. Sharma was awarded the *Royal Society Fellowship* in the University of Sheffield U.K and as a Scientist E in the Defence Institute of Physiology & Allied Sciences, New Delhi (India).

As a scientific officer at the All India Institute of Medical Sciences (A.I.I.M.S), New Delhi he conducted his doctoral research on the neuropharmacology of the antiepileptic drugs in the developing normal and undernourished rat brain under the guidance of late Emeritus Professor, Dr. Baldev Singh (*Father Neuron*). He served at the A.I.I.M.S, New Delhi for 10 years from 1979-1989 where he discovered that protein undernourished developing postnatal rats are highly susceptible to Kainate neurotoxicity and exhibit electrocortical inhibition of prolonged duration in response to relatively reduced doses as compared to their normal litter mates. He discovered Charnoly Body (CB) as a pleomorphic, pre-apoptotic biomarker of compromised mitochondrial bioenergetics in the developing undernourished Purkinje cell dendrites and in the hippocampal neurons due to free radical-mediated lipid peroxidation of mitochondrial membranes. Recently he discovered α-Synuclein Index (SI) and IL-10 receptors on the cortical neurons as sensitive biomarker of various progressive neurodegenerative diseases.

He was selected in the Bio-Medical Group of The Bhabha Atomic Research Center (BARC), Trombay, Bombay to receive training on the synthesis of Medical Radiopharmaceuticals. He received Postgraduate Diploma in Medical Readiopharmaceutical Technology (D.M.R.I.T) from the Bombay University and served as a clinical research fellow in the Medical Radiopharmceutical Laboratory at the Postgraduate Institute of Medical Education & Research, Chandigarh (India).

Dr. Sharma has throughout first class academic career in his Undergraduate and Masters in Biophysics from The Panjab University Basic Medical School, Chandigarh. He was invited on several occasions to serve as a scientific consultant, chairperson, and speaker in the International and World Congresses. He is the recipient of 5 Gold Medals. He was awarded E. Merck (German) Gold Medal for the best doctoral research and a Gold Medal for his significant contributions in cardiovascular research on the basic molecular mechanism of vascular neointimal hyperplasia and the therapeutic potential of a specific 5-HT2A Receptor Antagonist, Sarpogrelate in Canada. He organized 5 International Conferences and has >241 publications and 120 research abstracts published in the international journals of high impact factor. He has written several books, published by Nova Science Publishers, New York. U.S.A.

He invented an electro-micro-injector for which he was invited in the *Invention & Innovation* session in the 3rd World Congress of Nuclear Medicine & Biology in Paris, France. He discovered *Charnoly Body* (CB) in the developing undernourished Purkinje neurons for which he was invited as a Chairperson in The 13th World Congress of Neurology, Hamburg, Germany, and as a guest speaker in the International Conference of Biometeorology in Calgary, Canada. Recently he was invited in the First and Second International Translational Conference in Nanomedicine, in Boston to deliver a lecture on "Charnoly body as a novel biomarker in Nanomdicine and was awarded the "*Certificate of Recognition*". Dr. Sharma has been invited as an international scientific consultant, chairperson, and invited speaker to deliver lectures in the area of his expertise in several biomedical institutes in several countries including; India, Japan, France, Australia, Germany, Canada, U.S.A, and China.

He conducted studies on the *mitochondrial genome knock out* (Rho$_{mgko}$) human dopaminergic neurons as an experimental model of aging to confirm that the mitochondrial bioenergetics is compromised in progressive neurodegenetative disorders and aging; hence agents that inhibit Charnoly Body (CB) formation such as antioxidants derived from the natural sources may provide better and safe therapeutic strategies for the clinical management of PD, AD, drug addiction, depression and several other chronic neurodegenerative diseases as described in this book. Recently he reported that Zn^{2+}-binding proteins metallothioneins (MTs) inhibit CB formation by serving as free radical scavengers. MTs are also induced in severe nutritional stress and following exposure to toxic environmental neurotoxins including NPs. CB formation occurs in the most vulnerable cells in response to severe undernutrition, neurotoxins exposure (such as Kainic Acid, Domoic Acid, & Acromelic Acid). Although MTs have been implicated in various neurodegenerative disorders, their exact pathophysiological significance is yet to be established. He discovered that CB formation triggers neurodegeneration, whereas MTs provide neuroprotection by serving as potent free radical scavengers and by inhibiting CB formation.

He developed several genetically-engineered mouse models of drug addiction, drug rehabilitation, and genetic resistance including *α-synuclein metalothionein triple knockout* (α-Syn-MT$_{tko}$) mice, *metallothiuoneins over-expressing weaver mutant mice* (wv/wv-MTs) mice and a sensitive method of CoQ$_{10}$ estimation from rare biological samples. He discovered α-Synuclein Index as an early and sensitive biomarker of progressive neurodegenerative α-synucleinopathies and proposed the involvement of CB formation in various neurodegenerative disorders including PD, AD, drug addiction, depression, and cancer. Recently he published a book on "*Monoamine Oxidase Inhibitors Clinical Pharmacology, Therapeutic Applications and Adverse Effects'* through Nova Science Publishers; where he has proposed monoamine oxidase-A and monoamine oxidase-B specific CB formation in the hippocampal, striatum, and hypothalamic regions to cause PD, AD, MDD, bulimia, anorexia nervosa, and several other neurodegenerative diseases of unknown etiopathogenesis. Hence therapeutic drugs may be developed to inhibit brain regional MAO-A or MAO-B-specific CB formation for the effective personalized treatment of various neurodegenerative disorders including PD, AD, and drug addiction.

While serving as a director of the cyclotron and PET imaging labs at the University of North Dakota School of Medicine, Grand Forks, N.D, U.S.A, he synthesized ^{18}FdG and ^{18}F-DOPA as biomarkers to evaluate the mitochondrial bioenergetics and dopaminergic neurotransmission in homozygous weaver (wv/wv) mice by employing microPET neuroimaging. He established that the striatal glucose metabolism as well as DA-ergic neurotransmission are significantly compromised in these experimental genotypes of progressive neurodegeneration. MTs over-expressing wv/wv mice exhibited attenuation of progressive loss of neurons, authenticating the therapeutic potential of MTs in PD, AD, and drug addiction. Dr. Sharma serves as an expert reviewer and consulting editor for several international journals of high impact factor. He also serves as an expert reviewer for the evaluation of research grants including: Michael Smith Foundation in Vancouver. Canada and National Foundation of Neurological Research, New Zeeland. He guided several MD and Ph. D students at the national and international level. He has served as a Co-Pi in several R01 NIH projects in U.S.A. Recently Dr. Sharma was awarded "*Certificate of Recognition*" in the 3rd International Translational Nanomedicine, in Boston, Mass, U.S.A.

ABBREVIATIONS

Ach: Acetyl Choline
AChEI: Acetylcholinesterase inhibitors:
AD: Alzheimer's disease
AD: Alzheimer's Disease
AD: Alzheimer's disease
ADEM: Acute disseminated encephalomyelitis:
ADNI: Alzheimer's Disease Imaging Initiative
AIDs: Acquired immunodeficiency disease
AIR: Autoimmune regulator
AIS: Acute ischemic stroke
ALS: Amyotrophic Lateral Sclerosis
ALS: Amyotrophic Lateral Sclerosis
ALS: Amyotrophic lateral sclerosis
ANG: Angiotensin
AOC: Area under the Curve
ApoA1: Apolipoprotein A1
Apo-E: Apolipoprotein-E
ApoE:Apolipoprotein-E
ARIA: Amyloid-related imaging abnormalities
ARND: Alcohol-related Neurodevelopment Disorders
AVAD: δ-Aminolevulinic acid Dehydratase
Aβ: Amyloid-β
Aβ: Amyloid-β:
BDDCS: Biopharmaceutics drug disposition classification system
BDNF: Brain Derived Growth Factor
Breg: Regulatory B cells
BSA: Bovine serum albumin
CAA-ri: Cerebral amyloid angiopathy-related inflammation:
CB: Charnoly Body
CB: Charnoly body (Multi lamellar stacks of electron
CCL21: Chemokine CC-ligand 21
CCR7: Chemokine CC-chemokine receptor
CDT: Carbohydrate-deficient transferrin

CDT: Carbohydrate-deficient transferrin
CFS: Chronic fatigue syndrome
CISs: Clinically isolated syndromes
CJD: Creutzfeldt-Jacob disease
CNS: Central Nervous System
CNS: Central Nervous System
COPD: Chronic obstructive pulmonary disease
CRP: C-Reactive Protein
CSF: Cerebrospinal Fluid
CSF: Cerebrospinal Fluid
CSF: Cerebrospinal fluid
CT: Computerized Tomography
CTE: Chronic traumatic encephalopathy
CTE: Chronic traumatic encephalopathy
DBP: DNA-binding protein,
dense degenerated mitochondrial membranes)
DKI: Diffusional kurtosis imaging
DLB: Dementia with Lewy body
DMS: Benign multiple sclerosis
DP: Disease prognosis
DTI: Diffusion tensor imaging
E.M: Electron Microscopy
EBPM: Evidence-based PM
ECM: Extracellular Matrix
EE: Environmental epidemiology
ELISA: Enzyme-linked Immunosorbent Assay
ELISA: Enzyme-linked immunosorbent assay
ER: Endoplasmic reticulum,
EtG: Ethyl glucuronide
EtS: Ethyl sulfate
FAEE: Fatty acid ethyl esters
fALS, familial ALS,
fALS: Familial ALS
FAS: Fetal Alcohol Syndrome
FASD: Fetal Alcohol Spectrum Disorders
FLASH: Fast low-angle shot
$[^{18}F]$-FdG: Fluorodeoxy glucose
FLC: Free light chain
fMRI: Functional magnetic resonance imaging
FTD: Frontotemporal Dementia
FTD: Frontotemporal dementia
FVC: Forced Vital capacity
GC-SF: granulocyte colony-stimulating factor
GFAP: Glial fibrillary acidic protein:
GGT: Gamma glutamyl transferase
GIF: Growth Inhibitory Factor

GSH: Glutathione
HBEC: Human brain microvascular endothelial cells
HCT: Hematopoietic cell transplantation:
HDL: High Density Lipoprotein
HDL: high-density lipoprotein,
HE: Hashimoto's encephalopathy
HNE: 4-hydroxy-2-nonenal,
IATM: Idiopathic acute transverse myelitis:
ICP-MS:Inductively coupled plasma mass spectrometry
IDE: Initial demyelinating event
IgG:Immunoglobulin gamma
IgMOB: IgM oligoclonal bands
IL-10: Interleukin-10
LDL: Low density Lipoprotein
LDL: Low-density lipoprotein,
LRP1: Low density lipoprotein receptor-related protein-1
MCI: Mild Cognitive Impairment
MCV: Mean corpuscular volume
MDA: Malondialdehyde
MDA: Manol dialdehyde
MEMS: Microelectromechanical systems
MGMT: O(6)-Methylguanine DNA methyltransferase
miRNA: MicroRNA
MME:Microcystic macular edema
MMPs: MMPss
MNCs: Mononcuclear cells
MND: Motoneuron Disease
MOGP: Myelin oligodendrocyte glycoprotein peptide
MRI: Magnetic Resonance Imaging
MRI: Magnetic Resonance Imaging
MRS: Magnetic Resonance Spectroscopy
MRS: Magnetic Resonance Spectroscopy
MS: Multiple sclerosis
MS-MLPA: Multiplex ligation-dependent probe amplification
MSP: Methylation-specific polymerase chain reaction
MT: Metallothionein
MTN: Motor neuron disease
MTR:Magnetization transfer ratio:
MTs: Metallothioneins
NAA/Cho: N-acetylaspartate/choline
NADP: Nicotinamide adenine dinucleotide phosphate
NADPH: Nicotinamide Dinucleotide Phosphate
NFkβ: Nuclear Factor kappa-B:
NFL: Neurofilament light protein
NFL:Light neurofilament subunits
NIND: Non-inflammatory neurological disease

Nm: Nanometer
NMO: Neuromyelitis optica
NOS: Nitric Oxide Synthase
3-NT, 3-nitrotyrosine
NPs: Nanoparticles
O.S: Oxidative stress
OCBs:Oligoclonal bands
OIND: Other Inflammatory neurological disorders
OIT: Oral Immunotherapy
OPC: Oligodendroglial progenitor cells:
OS: Oxidative stress
8-OxodG: 8-oxo-deoxyguanosine
PADs: Peptidylarginine deiminases
PBMCs: Peripheral blood mononuclear cells
PD: = Parkinson's disease
PDGFR-α: Platelet-derived growth factor receptor –α
PEG: Poly ethylene glycol
Pegylation: Covalent conjugation of drug with PEG
PET: Positron emission tomography
PEth: PhosphatidylEthanolamine
PGLA: Poly (lactic-co-glycolic) acid
PIB: Pittsburg Compound-B
PLN: Polymer lipid nanoparticle
PML: Progressive multifocal leukoencephalopathy
pMS: Pediatric-onset multiple sclerosis
PON: Peroxynitrite Ion
PTX: Paclitaxel
PUFA: Polyunsaturated fatty acids
QSPR: Quantitative structure–permeability relationships
RA: Rheumatoid arthritis
RES: Reticulo endothelial system
RNS: Reactive Nitrogen Specie
RNS: Reactive Nitrogen Species
ROC: Receiver operating characteristic
ROS: Reactive Oxygen Species
ROS: Reactive Oxygen Species
ROS: Reactive Oxygen Species
RP: Retinal periphlebitis
RRMS: Relapsing-remitting Multiple Sclerosis
SALS: Sporadic Amyotrophic Lateral Sclerosis
sAPP:Soluble Amyloid Precursor Protein
SI: α-Synuclein Index
SLE: System lupus erythromytosis
SMN: Survival Motor Neuron
SNP: Single Nucleotide Polymorphism
SNP: Single Nucleotide Polymorphism

SNP: Single-nucleotide polymorphism,
SNPs: Single nucleotide polymorphisms
SOD: Super oxide dismutase
SOD: Superoxide dismutase
SOD1: Superoxide Dismutase-1
SPECT: Single Photon Emission Computerized Tomography
SRM: Selected reaction monitoring
SS: Sjögren's syndrome
TBARS: Thiobarbituric acid reactive substances
TGFβ: Transforming growth factor β
TIMPs: Tissue Inhibitors of MMPss
TLFB: Timeline follow-back procedure to assess Alcohol exposure.
TRAPS:TNF receptor 1-associated periodic syndrome
Treg: Regulatory T cells
UCHL1: Ubiquitin C-terminal hydrolase-L1
VaD: Vascular Dement
VAP: Vesicle associated protein
VAPB: Vesicle associated protein-associated protein B
VCP: Valosin-containing protein
VEGF: Vascular endothelial growth factor
β-Tu: β-Tubulin

Chapter 1

FUNDAMENTAL OF EVIDENCE-BASED PERSONALIZED THERANOSTICS

ABSTRACT

Generally, two kinds of therapeutic strategies are implemented in clinical practice: (a) conventional and (b) personalized (*also named as stratified, predictive, precision, individualized, customized, and targeted*). The conventional therapeutic approach is based on trial *and error* and *one-size fit* all strategy, whereas the personalized medicine provides treatment tailored to the patient's cellular, molecular, and genetic profile, and considers pharmacogenomics and other disease-specific biomarkers to adopt theranostic approach. *The drug is selected based on genotypical, and hence phenotypical variability of the metabolizing enzyme(s).* The personalized medicine utilizes genomic, epigenomic, and other data (*including environmental exposure*) to define individual patterns of disease for the superior evidence based individualized diagnosis as well as treatment (EBPT). The stratification of patients to accomplish customized health care is accomplished based on a characteristic of some sort, who respond more favorably to a particular drug with significantly decreased risk of side effects in response to a particular treatment (*Customized Healthcare*). Pharmacogenomics is one of the most significant disciplines of PM. Usually *"more complex and more heterogeneous the disease, more significant is personalized treatment."* The primary objective of PM is to: direct *the emphasis in medicine from reaction to prevention, predict susceptibility to disease, improve disease detection, preempt disease progression, customize disease-prevention strategies, prescribe more effective drugs, avoid drugs with deleterious side effects, reduce the time, cost, and. failure rate of clinical trials, eliminate trial-and-error inefficiencies that increase health care costs and undermine patient care.* PM includes genes, environment, and life-style when treating a patient, because genetic profile and genetic makeup of a disease can improve the chance of survival and reduce the adverse effects of treatment. The most common chronic diseases with limited therapeutic success include depression, *asthma, cardiac arrhythmia, diabetes, migraine, arthritis, osteoporosis, Alzheimer's disease, and cancer.* Particularly, successful treatment of cancer and AD poses a significant challenge in >70% patients, as futile therapeutic attempts with polypharmacy, may cause deleterious side effects to cause early morbidity and morbidity; hence these patients require personalized treatment. In general, PM comprises five major disciplines including*: (a) biotechnology, (b) omics analyses, (c) novel biomarkers, (d) bioinformatics, and (e) theranostics (simultaneous diagnosis and treatment).* Recent developments in biotechnology have improved bio-informatics to discover novel disease-specific biomarkers. Omics analyses includes: *genomic, proteomic, metabolomic,* *lipidomic, glycomic, and metalomic.* Particularly, pharmacogenomics and next generation sequencing (NGS) to discover single nucleotide polymorphism (SNP) in chronic diseases including: cancer, mass SPECT imaging, LC/MS/MS analyses for the novel discovery of *in-vivo and invitro* biomarkers, companion diagnostics employing CT/SPECT/PET/ MRI/MRS are employed to accomplish EBPT. Furthermore, the most significant pharmacogenomic and pharmacodynamic genes are analyzed to evaluate the prognosis and therapeutic outcome of patients. Recently nanotheranostic approach employing ROS-scavenging antioxidant nanoparticles has emerged to accomplish EBPT. Thus, *PM promises to provide several benefits over conventional medical practice such as: (i) earlier therapeutic interventions, (ii) develop personalized theranostic decisions, (iii) increase probability of desired prognosis, (iv) improve targeted therapies, (v) reduce adverse effects, (vi) prevent and predict disease, and (vii) reduce healthcare costs*, as described in this chapter.

Keywords: precision medicine, personalized medicine, predictive medicine, customized medicine, individualized medicine, omics biotechnology, pharmacogenomics genes, pharmacodynamics genes, pharmacokinetic genes, nanotechnology, imaging technology, nanoparticles, nanotheranostics. bioinformatics

INTRODUCTION

In conventional clinical practice, it is ignored that the genetic makeup of each individual is different, which may significantly influence health and well-being of an individual. The conventional clinical practice is based primarily on the "*one size fit all*" concept. For instance, a patient being treated for high BP, might be placed on one of a number of BP medications. The physician makes a decision about what medication to prescribe based on only general information about what might actually work for that particular patient. *If the medication does not work after a few weeks, the patient is switched to another medication. This "trial-and-error" approach can lead to patient dissatisfaction, adverse drug responses, drug interactions, and poor compliance.*

Currently the researchers don't fully understand how different persons develop disease and respond to treatment. Each individual has a specific genetic makeup which may increase or decrease the propensity to acute or chronic illnesses. Designing health care based on each person's unique genetic makeup is the most promising strategy of personalized medicine (PM), also named *as individualized medicine, precision medicine, genomic medicine, predictive medicine, and generally as molecular medicine.* Thus PM promises to accomplish precise, predictable and robust health care system that is tailored to the individual patient. Improvement in our understanding of genetics and genomics, and how they influence health, disease, and drug responses in each person, is facilitating disease prevention, accurate diagnosis, avoid unnecessary drug prescriptions, and effective therapeutic options for several diseases.

The primary goal of PM is to maximize the likelihood of therapeutic efficacy and to minimize the risk of drug toxicity for a particular patient (Xie and Fruch, 2005). The ultimate goal of PM is to streamline clinical decision-making by distinguishing those patients most likely to benefit from a particularly treatment from those who will incur cost and suffer side effects without any benefit. One of the most significant contributors of this concept is pharmacogenomics (PGx) because individual genetic variations contribute significantly both to vulnerability to disease as well as response to drug. Although PGx is not a new science, the exact translation of PGx into clinical practice (*also named as personalized medicine, precision medicine, predictive medicine, and most recently as evidence based personalized theranostics: EBPT)* has not occurred at the same momentum as the modern science has been delivering novel concepts at a remarkable speed. It is currently believed that PGx will facilitate accomplishing safety and targetability of drugs by enhancing their margin of safety and therapeutic index with minimum or no adverse effects.

Recently Ghadimi and Jo (2016) reported that the revolution of genomic technologies, including gene expression profiling, high-resolution mapping of genomic imbalances, and next-generation sequencing (NGS), allows to establish molecular portraits of cancer cells with unprecedented precision, accuracy, and reproducibility to accomplish EBPT as described in this book. EBPT generates hope and justifies that disease diagnosis, prognosis, and the choice of treatment can be adapted to the individual needs of the patient based on his/her personalized molecular evidence. By analyzing *omics data, imaging data, and molecular diagnostic data, preoperative therapeutic strategies are now recommended for a variety of cancers.* Unfortunately, the response of individual tumors to treatment is heterogeneous, and varies from complete regression to resistance. This poses a significant challenge, as patients with resistant tumors could either be spared exposure to radiation or DNA-damaging drugs, i.e., could be referred to primary surgery, or dose-intensified protocols could be pursued. Because the response of an individual tumor as well as side effects represent the major limiting factors of current treatment strategies, identifying molecular biomarkers of response or for treatment toxicity has become extremely important. However, tumor responsiveness to multimodal treatments may not depend on the expression levels of just one or a few genes and/or proteins. Hence, interventions that allow comprehensive evaluation of genetic pathways and networks hold great promise in delivering tumor-specific signatures, since expression profile of thousands of genes can be monitored simultaneously employing modern omics technology.

Over the past several years, microarray technology has emerged as a promising approach in addressing specific clinical questions, the answers to which are critical for the successful accomplishment of EBPT, where patients will be treated based on the biology of their tumor and their genetic profile instead of conventional treatment based on clinical symptoms (For details, please refer: *Quackenbush, N Engl J Med 354: 2463-72, 2006; Jensen* et al., *Curr Opin Oncol 18:374-380, 2006; Bol and Ebner, Pharmacogenomics 7:227-235,2006; Nevins and Potti, Nat Rev Genet 8:601-609, 2007).* Jensen et al. (2006) reported that molecular profiling has proved invaluable tool in cancer research. Particularly, gene microarray technology has led to advances in exact tumor identification, staging and prediction of response. These investigators provided recent developments in microarrays technology as a novel strategy to advance the existing standard of treatment of patients with GIT cancers. Gene expression profiles can be used to identify, stage, and guide therapeutic interventions in many GIT cancers. In cases of unknown primary disease, genetic fingerprints can be used to define the origin of the tumor. Similarly, gene expression allows for accurate staging of patients with a variety of tumor types. The most exciting aspect of EBPT is the collection and analysis of data that guide therapeutic interventions by providing individualized gene fingerprints which correlate with sensitivity to specific chemotherapy, biologic therapy, or other cancer treatments. Hence gene microarray analysis has become a powerful resource in cancer EBPT. Thus personalized cancer treatment based on specific gene profiles is one of the most important strategies for patients with GIT and other cancers.

Although the basic concept of personalized medicine (PM) existed several years back, its real clinical significance was realized recently when several drug-resistant chronic diseases could not be cured successfully. Following the discovery of DNA recombinant technology and human genome sequencing, 3 most significant technologies which led to the evolution in PM are: *(i) omics technology, (ii) imaging technology, and (iii) nanotechnology.* The research and development on these three basic technologies is advancing to discover novel drugs and strategies for the successful treatment of cancer, cardiovascular, and neurodegenerative diseases with minimum or no adverse effects. There is a significant overlap between the terms *"Personalized Medicine, predictive medicine,* and *Precision Medicine."* The 21st century is an era of nano-theranostics and has developed a novel concept of PM; primarily for improving early diagnosis, treatment, and prognosis of multidrug-resistant chronic diseases including; malignancies, cardiovascular diseases, and neurodegenerative diseases. Indeed, PM warrants close collaboration from multi-disciplinary biomedical sciences.

According to the *National Research Council, "personalized medicine"* is a traditional term with a meaning similar to *"precision medicine."* However, the word "personalized" may be misinterpreted to imply that treatment is being developed uniquely for each individual. In *precision medicine*, the primary focus is laid on developing strategies which will be effective based on genetic, environmental, and lifestyle factors. Hence the term *"precision Medicine" may be preferred over "personalized or predictive medicine."* However, currently these terms are used interchangeably.

In this chapter, a brief overview and recent developments to accomplish the ultimate goal of EBPT are highlighted to educate healthcare professionals and public, as this emerging concept of interdisciplinary medicine has a great future promise to cure chronic multi-drug-resistant diseases with minimum or no adverse effects.

Definition of PM Although the concept of PM dates back many hundreds of years, it was not until the 19th century, that developments in chemistry, histochemistry and microscopy allowed scientists to begin to understand the underlying causes of disease. With the growth of the pharmaceutical and medical device industries emerged the evolution of *genetics, imaging, and data mining.* Observations of individual differences in response to drugs gave rise to research focused on identifying key enzymes that play a role in variation in drug metabolism and response and that served as the foundation for pharmacogenetics. Recently, sequencing of the human genome accelerated the transformation of PM from an idea to a practice. Developments in genomics, together with advances in computational biology, medical imaging, and regenerative medicine, created the possibility to develop tools to EBPT.

Early Examples of PM 1907: *Reuben Ottenberg discovered the first blood compatibility test for transfusion using blood typing techniques and cross-matching between donors and patients to prevent hemolytic transfusion reactions.* ***1956:*** *The genetic basis for the selective toxicity of fava beans ("favism") and the antimalarial drug Primaquine was discovered to be a deficiency in the metabolic enzyme, glucose-6-phosphate dehydrogenase (G6PD).* ***1977:*** *Cytochrome P450 2D6, a polymorphic metabolizing enzyme, was discovered for causing some patients to experience an "overdose" or exaggeration of the duration and intensity of the effects of Debrisoquine, a drug used for treating hypertension* or respond to treatment differently.

A 2013 survey by GfK, a global consumer research firm, found that just 27% of people interviewed had heard the term "PM." Of those, only 4% understood what the phrase most often implies: "medicine based on genomic makeup." PM should not to be confused with "*Genetic Medicine*." Genetics, a field more than 50 years old, is the study of heredity. It evaluates individual genes and their effects as they relate to biology and medicine. *"Single cell" genetic diseases include muscular dystrophy, cystic fibrosis, and sickle cell anemia. (However, even these "simple" hereditary disorders can be influenced by other genes, as well as by environmental factors such as diet and exposure to toxins).* Genomic and PM tackle more complex diseases, such as *cancer, heart disease, and diabetes*, influenced primarily by complex environmental factors and their interaction with the human genome. It is now known that because these diseases have multigene components—and in some cases might be caused by errors in the DNA between genes instead of within genes—they can be better understood using a genomic approach.

Because an individual's genome influences likelihood of developing (or not developing) a medical condition, PM focuses on wellness and disease prevention of an individual. For example, if a person's genomic information indicates a higher-than-average risk of developing diabetes or a particular form of cancer, that person may choose a lifestyle, or may be prescribed medications, to better regulate the health and wellness over which he or she has control. The person may benefit in the long run from making preventive lifestyle choices that will help counteract the biological risk. Genomic medicine may help determine a person's risk of developing specific clinical conditions including: *cancer, cardiovascular disease, neurodegenerative diseases, diabetes, obesity, and neuropsychiatric disorders*. Researchers are currently investigating the genomic and genetic mechanisms and developing predictive testing for various clinical conditions as: *Infectious diseases, from HIV/AIDS to the common cold, ovarian cancer, cardiovascular disease, diabetes, metabolic abnormalities, neuropsychiatric diseases, such as epilepsy, adverse drug reactions, and environmental exposure to toxins*.

The term PM was first used in the context of genetics, though it has now extended to cover all aspects of personalized measures (Lu et al., 2014). PM proposes the customization of healthcare - with medical decisions, practices, and/or products being tailored to the individual patient. In this model, diagnosis is used for selecting therapies based on the patient's genetic makeup or other molecular or cellular aspects. The use of genetic information has played a significant role in PM (e.g., *pharmacogenomics*). According to Dudley and Karczewski (2014), every person has a unique variation of the human genome. Although most of the individual variation has no effect on health, an individual's health originates from genetic variation with behaviors and influences from the environment. One way that biological variation makes itself clear, is responsiveness to drugs. For instance, ADHD medication works only for 10% of children, anticancer drugs are effective only for 25% of patients, and antidepressants are effective only with 60% of patients. Recent advances in PM rely on technology that evaluates a patient's biology, *DNA, RNA, or protein*, to confirm the disease. For example, PM techniques including: genome sequencing can detect mutations in DNA that influence diseases ranging from *cystic fibrosis to cancer*. Recently-developed technology called *RNA-seq*, can detect which RNA's are involved with specific diseases. Unlike DNA, RNA fluctuates frequently in response to the environmental alterations. Hence, sequencing RNA can confer a better understanding of individual health and well-being. Recent studies linked genetic differences to RNA (Battle et al., 2014), translation (Can et al., 2014), and protein levels (Wu et al., 2013). The PM can be applied to new and transformative strategies to health care based on the systems biology and predictive measures to evaluate health risks and design personalized health plans to help patients mitigate risks, prevent disease and to treat with precision. The basic concepts of PM received universal acceptance to personalized, proactive patient-driven treatment (Snyderman, 2012).

PM has been recognized interchangeably as precision medicine, individualized medicine, accurate medicine, molecular diagnostics, evidence-based medicine, targeted medicine, magic bullets, magic shotguns, molecular theranosics, multimodality diagnosis, companion diagnostics, theranostics, personalized theranostics, etc. PM is relatively new but rapidly developing field of healthcare that is informed by each person's unique clinical, genetic, genomic, and environmental information. Because these factors are different for every person, the nature of diseases—including their onset, course, and how they might respond to drugs or other interventions—is as individual as the people who have them. The primary goal of PM is to make the treatment as individualized as the disease. It involves identifying genetic, genomic, and clinical information that allows accurate predictions about a person's susceptibility of developing disease, the course of disease, and its response to treatment. In order for PM to be used effectively, these findings must be translated into *precise diagnostic tests and targeted therapies*. PM has already initiated in certain areas, such as testing patients genetic make up to determine their likelihood of having a serious adverse reaction to various anticancer drugs. Because the sequencing of the human genome provided insight into the biological workings behind numerous clinical conditions, the researchers are currently advancing PM vigorously. Although, it is not yet fully established in clinical practice, a number of top medical institutions now have PM programs, and many are actively conducting both basic research and clinical studies in genomic medicine to adopt this modern approach of patient care.

Genetic Predisposition to a Disease A genetic predisposition (*also called as genetic susceptibility or genetic propensity*) is an increased likelihood of developing a particular disease based on a person's genetic makeup. A genetic predisposition results from specific genetic variations that are inherited from a parent. These genetic changes contribute to the development of a disease but do not directly cause it. Some individuals with a predisposing genetic variation will never get the disease while others will, even within the same family. Genetic variations can have variable effects on the likelihood of developing a particular disease. For instance, certain mutations in the *BRCA1* or *BRCA2* genes increase the risk of developing breast cancer and ovarian cancer. Variations in other genes, such as *BARD1* and *BRIP1*, also increase breast cancer risk, but the contribution of these genetic changes to a person's overall risk is much smaller. Research is now focused on identifying genetic changes that have little effect on disease risk but are common in the general population. Although each of these variations increases a person's risk, having changes in several different genes may combine to increase disease risk significantly. Changes in genes may underlie susceptibility to diseases, including *cancer, obesity, diabetes, heart disease, and mental* illness. In people with a genetic predisposition, the risk of disease may depend on multiple factors in addition to genetic change. These include other genetic factors (also called modifiers) as well as lifestyle and environmental factors. Although a person's genetic makeup cannot be altered, some lifestyle and environmental modifications (*regular disease screenings* *and maintaining a healthy weight)* may be able to reduce disease risk in people with a genetic predisposition. The WHO provides information about genetic predisposition to several common diseases, including *cancer, diabetes, cardiovascular disease, and asthma.* Genetic Alliance UK offers a fact sheet on genetic predisposition to common diseases. The Genetic Science Learning Center at the University of Utah provides information about calculating the risk of genetic diseases and predicting disease based on family history. The Coriell PM Collaborative explains genetic and nongenetic risk factors for complex diseases. *(More detailed information about the genetics of breast and ovarian cancer is available from the National Cancer Institute).*

A particular disorder might be "running in a family" if more than one person has the condition. Some disorders that affect multiple family members are caused by gene mutations, which can be inherited. Other conditions that run in families are not caused by mutations in single genes. Instead, environmental factors such as dietary habits or a combination of genetic and environmental factors are responsible for these disorders. It is not always easy to determine whether a condition in a family is inherited. A physician can use a person's family history (health information about a person's immediate and extended family) to help determine whether a disorder has a genetic component.

Genome-Wide Association Studies in PM In order to discover whether a mutation is linked to a certain disease, a *"Genome-Wide Association Study"* (GWAS) is performed, which explores one disease, and sequence the genome of many patients with that particular disease to detect similar mutations in the genome. Mutations that are related to a disease by GWAS can be used to diagnose that disease, by following the genome sequence. For example, patients with age-related macular degeneration (ARMD) were evaluated by conducting GWAS, which detected two mutations, with a variation in one nucleotide (*Single Nucleotide Polymorphisms, or SNPs*) *(Haines, 2005).* Similar GWAS proved useful in identifying common genetic variations associated with other diseases. So far over 1300 GWAS have been accomplished (GWAS, 2014).

Disease Risk Assessment Generally, several genes can influence the likelihood of developing common and complex diseases, which can be used to predict risk for a particular disease, based on single or several genes (PM Coalition, 2014). This approach utilizes sequencing technology to evaluate disease risk to initiate treatment before the disease manifests in the patient. For example, if a specific DNA mutation increases the risk of developing type 2 diabetes in a particular patient, he/she may be instructed to adopt healthy lifestyle changes to minimize risks of developing type 2 diabetes later in life.

Applications of PM It is envisaged that improvements in PM will develop a unified therapeutic approach tailored to the individual and his/her genome. Hence PM may provide better theranostics with earlier intervention, efficient drug development, and better therapeutic options. The primary objective of PM is to: *direct the emphasis on medicine from reaction to prevention, predict susceptibility to disease, improve diagnosis, preempt disease progression, customize disease-prevention strategies, prescribe effective drugs, avoid drugs with undesirable side effects, reduce the time, cost, and failure of clinical trials, eliminate "trial-and-error" approach that increases health care costs and undermine patient care as described above.*

PHARMACOGENOMICS

Pharmacogenomics is one of the most important disciplines of PM. It is the study of how genes affect a person's response to particular drugs. This emerging field combines pharmacology and genomics to develop effective, safe medications and doses designed to genetic predisposition. Pharmacogenomics is a study of variations of DNA and RNA characteristics related to drug response, and is one of the most exciting areas of PM. The field arises from the convergence of advances in pharmacology and genomics. *Patients have variability in response to drugs that are currently available. It can be difficult to predict who will benefit from a medication, who will not respond at all, and who will experience adverse effects.* PGx seeks to understand how differences in genes and their expression affect the body's response to medications. PGx uses genetic information (*such as DNA sequence, gene expression, and copy number*) for explaining inter-individual differences in drug metabolism. *Advances in PGx have opened new possibilities in drug discovery and development as it* has allowed for more tailored treatment of a wide range of health problems, including cardiovascular disease (CVD), cancer, and HIV/AIDS. FDA's Center for Drug Evaluation and Research (CDER) has boosted pharmacogenomics by providing regulatory advice, reviewing applications, and developing policies and processes centered on genomics and individualized therapeutics. Stratification can be thought of as a core element of PM, which involves the use of two medical products – typically, *a diagnostic device and a therapeutic product* – to improve theranostic potential. A diagnostic device include both *in vitro* tests such as assays used in measurement of genetic factors and *in vivo* tests, such as *electroencephalography (EEG), electrocardiography (EKG), or imaging.* Many medical device therapies are now capable of being tailored to specific patient characteristics. *These include patient anatomy (e.g., size), physiology (e.g., nervous and cardiovascular systems, metabolism, reproduction) and environment (e.g., intensive care unit, home). Physiological sensors can be used to predict treatment responses for individual patients. The pharmacogenomics for discovery of genetic variants that predict adverse events to a specific drug is termed as "Toxgnostics" (Church et al., 2014).*

Original Discovery of Charnoly Body (CB) The author discovered CB as pleomorphic, multi-lamellar, electron-dense, stacks of degenerating mitochondrial membranes in the developing undernourished rat Purkinje neurons and in the hippocampal CA-3 and dentate gyrus regions of intrauterine environmental neurotoxins, Kainic acid and Domoic acid-exposed mice as noticed in the autopsy brain samples of AD patients (Sharma et al., 2013). CB formation occurs in the most susceptible cell due to ROS-mediated lipid peroxidation of mitochondrial membranes. The structural and functional breakdown of polyunsaturated fatty acids in the mitochondrial membranes occurs during CB formation due to free radical overproduction. The degenerated mitochondrial membrane fragments are aggregated to form electron-dense quasi-crystalline membrane stacks to form mature CBs. Cysteine-rich metal (Zn^{2+})-binding proteins, MTs inhibit CB formation by serving as free radical scavengers to provide neuroprotection in the developing and aging brain (Sharma and Ebadi, 2014), whereas brain regional reduction in MT3 causes AD in aging. Recently the researchers reported CB as universal biomarkers of cell injury in nanomedicine and drug addiction (Sharma and Ebadi, 2014; Sharma, 2015). Usually CB formation occurs following down-regulation of the mitochondrial genome in response to nutritional and/or environmental stress as the researchers discovered in mitochondrial genome knock out (RhO_{mgko}) cultured human dopaminergic (SK. N-SH) neurons as cellular model of aging due to inhibition of ubiquinone-NADH oxidoreductase (Complex-1) down-regulation. Complex-1 is a rate limiting enzyme complex in the electron transport chain for the ATP synthesis during oxidative phosphorylation. RhO_{mgko} neurons exhibited elliptical appearance with loss of neuritogenesis and synaptic connections. Transfection of aging RhO_{mgko} neurons with gene encoding ubiquinone-NADH oxidoreductase (complex-1) enhanced axonogensis, neuritogenesis, myelinogenesis, and synaptogenesis, confirming the physiological significance of mitochondrial bioenergetics in cognitive performance and general health and well-being (Sharma et al., 2004). *Nonspecific induction of CB causes adverse GIT symptoms, myelosuppression, alopecia, hepatotoxicity, cardiotoxicity, nephrotoxicity, and neurotoxicity in multidrug-resistant malignancies* (Sharma, 2014). Accumulation of CB at the junction of axon hillock, blocks normal axoplasmic flow of various ions, neurotransmitters, enzymes, neurotropic growth factors (BDNF, NGF), and mitochondria to cause impaired synaptic neurotransmission, leading to cognitive impairments as noticed in progressive neurodegenerative disorders including: PD, AD, chronic drug addiction, and major depressive disorders. Induction of CB in the endothelial and vascular smooth muscle cells during vascular neointimal hyperplasia triggers restenosis and atherosclerotic plaque formation to cause coronary artery diseases. Hence CB can be used as a novel and sensitive biomarker of cardiovascular diseases, neurodegenerative diseases, and cancer. Furthermore, the author has proposed two distinct types of CBs based on two types of monoamine oxidases (MAO-A, and MAO-B) on the outer mitochondrial membranes. Hence drugs may be developed to target specifically MAO-A or MAO-B-specific CB formation for the personalized treatment of various neurodegenerative diseases, cardiovascular diseases, and cancer (Sharma, 2016).

Therapeutic Strategies There are primarily two kinds of therapeutic strategies employed in the patient treatment. Conventional therapeutic approach is based on trial and error and one-size fit all strategy, whereas the modern PM provides medical treatment tailored to the patient's cellular, molecular, and genetic makeup and adopts pharmacogenomics and other sensitive disease-specific biomarkers to adopt theranostic approach to accomplish the ultimate goal of EBPT. *The drug is selected based upon genotypical, and hence phenotypical, variability of the metabolizing enzyme(s).* PM has been given various names including individualized, customized, precision, predictive, stratified, and targeted medicine (Figure 1). *PM* is defined as: "the use of genomic, epigenomic, exposure and other data to define individual patterns of disease, better individualized treatment. "Stratification" refers to the division of patients with a particular disease into subgroups, based on a characteristic of some sort, who respond favorably to a particular drug with significantly reduced risk of side effects in response to a particular treatment. (*Customized Healthcare*). Genomics (Pharmacogenomics) constitutes one of the most significant component of PM. Usually "*more complex and more heterogeneous the disease, more important is personalized treatment.*" PM includes genes, environment, and life-style choices when treating a patient, because genetic profile and genetic makeup of a tumor can improve the chances of survival and reduce the adverse effects of treatment. Hence PM has been assigned other names such as stratified medicine, targeted medicine, predictive medicine, and precision medicine as illustrated in Figure 2.

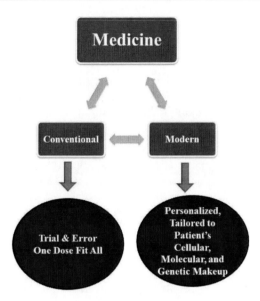

Figure 1. *Two Types of Therapy* A pictorial diagram illustrating primarily two kinds of therapeutic strategies, those are employed in the patient treatment. (i) Conventional therapeutic approach is based on trial and error and one-size fit all strategy, whereas the Modern personalized medicine (which is also named as precision medicine, predictive medicine, targeted medicine, and individualized medicine) provides medical treatment tailored to the patient's cellular, molecular, and genetic make up and adopts pharmacogenomic and other sensitive disease-specific biomarkers to adopt theranostic approach to accomplish the ultimate goal of evidence-based personalized medicine (EBPM). *The drug is selected based upon genotypical, and hence phenotypical, variability of the metabolizing enzyme(s).*

PERSONALIZED MEDICINE

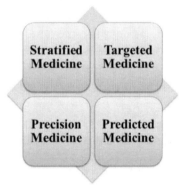

Figure 2. *Different Names of Persronalized Medicine* A pictorial diagram illustrating different names of personalized (individualized, customized) medicine, PM is sometimes used interchangeably with *"personalized medicine." "precision medicine", "predictive medicine, "stratified medicine, and "targeted medicine"* most synonymous to *"personalized medicine"* and is defined as: "the use of genomic, epigenomic, exposure and other data to define individual patterns of disease, eventually better individualized treatment." Stratification refers to the division of patients with a particular disease into subgroups, based on a characteristic of some sort, who respond more favorably to a particular drug with significantly decreased risk of side effects in response to a particular treatment. (*Customization of Healthcare*). Genomics (Phamracogenomics) constitutes one the most significant component of PM, Usually "more complex and more heterogenous the disease, more important is personalized treatment." PM includes genes, environment, and life-style when treating a patient, because genetic profile and genetic makeup of a tumor can improve the chance of survival and reduce the adverse effects of treatment.

Response Rates of Patients to Medications A 2001 study showed that the response rates of patients to medications from different therapeutic classes ranged from ~80% (*analgesics*) to ~25% (*oncology*). About 2.2 million adverse drug reactions occur each year in the US, including >100,000 deaths. By further elucidating why some patients respond or do not respond to a drug, and why some experience adverse reactions while others do not, the researchers may be in a position to use this information to design drug indications to certain populations, thus improving safety and efficacy of drugs by specifying the population(s) in which they should be used. *Percentage of patients for whom drugs are ineffective*: Depression: 38%; Asthma: 40%; Cardiac Arrhythmias: 40%; Diabetes: 43%; Migraine: 48%; Arthritis: 50%; Osteoporosis: 52%; Alzheimer's disease: 70%; Cancer: 75% as shown in Figure 3. (Source of data: Spear, B.B., Heath-Chiozzi, M., & Huff, J., 2001).

DRUG INEFFECTIVESSNESS

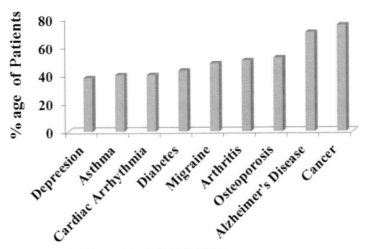

Source: Spear, B.B., Heath-Chiozzi, M., & Huff, J. (2001)

Figure 3. Drug *Ineffectiveness and Significance of PM* A histogram illustrating chronic diseases those are resistant to drug effectiveness These chronic diseases have limited therapeutic success. These include: depression, asthma, cardiac arrhythmia, diabetes, migraine, arthritis, osteoporosis, Alzheimer's disease, and cancer. Particularly, successful treatment of cancer and Alzheimer's disease poses a significant challenge as more than 70% patients remain refractory to treatment. Polypharmacy may cause undesirable side effective in these chronic patients. Obviously these patients require personalized treatment.

The distinct advantage of PM is that it utilizes information about a person's genes, proteins, and environment to prevent, diagnose, and treat disease. In PM approach, the dose of the drug is selected based upon genotypical, and hence phenotypical, variability of the metabolizing enzyme rather than a trial-and-error or one-dose-fits-all strategy as describe earlier (Xie and Frueh, 2005). *The term "PM" is described as providing "the right patient with the right drug at the right dose at the right time and may be thought of as the tailoring of medical treatment to the individual characteristics, needs and preferences of a patient during all stages of care, including prevention, diagnosis, treatment and follow-up.* Several terms, including *"PM" "stratified medicine," "targeted medicine," and "pharmacogenomics,"* are used interchangeably with "PM." *"Precision medicine" has been defined by the National Academy of Sciences (NAS) as "the use of genomic, epigenomic, exposure and other data to define individual patterns of disease, leading to better individual treatment.* "Stratification" refers to the division of patients with a particular disease into subgroups, based on a characteristic, who respond more frequently to a particular drug and are at decreased risk of side effects in response to a certain treatment. The primary objectives of PM are: • *"The use of new methods of molecular analysis to better manage a patient's disease or predisposition to disease."* • *"Providing the right treatment to the right patient, at the right dose at the right time."* • *"The tailoring of medical treatment to the individual characteristics of each patient."* • *"Health care that is informed by each person's unique clinical, genetic, and environmental background."*

The lack of efficacy in a given patient may reflect a complex interaction of factors and can also result from inadequate or inappropriate dosing regimens of a drug that would otherwise be effective, as well as lack of adequate patient compliance. PM also promises to enhance medical product development by improving the probability of success. For example, many drugs under development never reach the stage of being submitted to FDA in an application requesting approval for marketing. High attrition rates is due to failure of drugs to meet expected efficacy levels, to demonstrate improved outcomes over a comparator drug, or to demonstrate sufficient safety to justify their use. Improving our understanding of the underlying causes of variability in patient response should increase in the numbers of drugs that are safe and effective. There are several chronic diseases those are resistant to drug effectiveness. These chronic diseases have limited therapeutic success. These include: depression, asthma, cardiac arrhythmia, diabetes, migraine, arthritis, osteoporosis, AD, and cancer. Particularly, successful treatment of cancer and AD poses a significant challenge as >70% patients remain refractory to treatment, whereas polypharmacy may cause undesirable side effective in these chronic patients. Obviously these patients require personalized treatment. The most important key components of PM are (a) *biotechnology, (b) omics analyses, (c) novel biomarkers, (d) bioinformatics, and (e) theranostics (diagnosis and treatment simultaneously). Biotechnology has improved bio-informatics to discover novel disease-specific biomarkers to accomplish EBPT. Omics analyses includes: genomic, proteomic, metabolomic, lipidomic, and metalomic as* Figure 4 *illustrates.* Several biotechnologies have emerged to accomplish EBPT. These include but not limited to: Omics analyses (*genomics, proteomics, metabolomics, glycomics, lipidomics, metalomics*), particularly, phamacogenomics, next generation sequencing (NGS) to discover single nucleotide polymorphism (SNP) in certain chronic diseases including: cancer, mass spect imaging, LC/MS/MS analyses for the novel discovery of *in-vivo and in vitro* biomarkers, companion diagnostics employing CT/SPECT/PET/MRI/MRS, as illustrated in Figure 5. PM is primarily based on rigorous pharmacokinetic and pharmacodynamics principles. Several pharmacodynamics and pharmacogenomic genes have been discovered recently, which can influence the therapeutic response in a patient depending on his/her genomic profile. In general, clinically-significant genes can be subdivided as (i) pharmacodynamics genes as illustrated in the upper panel, and (b) pharmacogenomics genes in the lower panel of Figure 6.

Five Major Components of Personalized Medicine

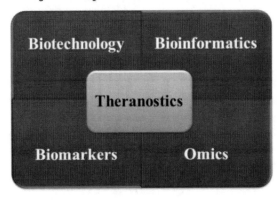

Figure 4. *Important Components of PM* A pictorial diagram illustrating important key components of personalized medicine. There are primarily 5 major components of PM, including: (a) *biotechnology, (b) omic analyses, (c) novel biomarkers, (d) bioinformatics, and (e) theranostics (diagnosis and treatment simultaneously).Biotechnology has improved bio-informatics to discover novel disease-specific biomarkers to accomplish EBPM. Omic analyses includes: genomic, proteomic, metabolomic, lipidomic, and metalomic).*

Emerging Biotechnologies in PM

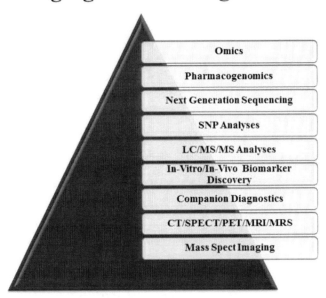

Figure 5. *Emerging Technologies in PM* A diagram illustrating emerging biotechnologies to accomplish PM. Numerous biotechnologies have emerged to fulfil the long-awaited dream of personalized treatment. These include but not limited to: Omics analyses (genomics, proteomics, metabolomics, glycomics, lipidomics, metalomics), particularly, phamacogenomics, next generation sequencing (NGS) to discover single nucleotide polymorphism (SNP) in crtain chronic diseases including cancer, mass spect imaging, LC/MS/MS analyses for the novel discovery of in-vivo and in-vitro biomarkers, and companion diagnostics employing CT/SPECT/PET/MRI/MRS to name a few.

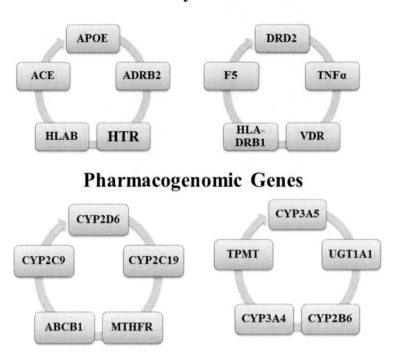

Pharmacodynamic Genes

APOE
ACE   ADRB2
HLAB   HTR

DRD2
F5   TNFα
HLA-DRB1   VDR

Pharmacogenomic Genes

CYP2D6
CYP2C9   CYP2C19
ABCB1   MTHFR

CYP3A5
TPMT   UGT1A1
CYP3A4   CYP2B6

Figure 6. *Pharmacodynamic and Pharmacogenomics Genes* A pictorial diagram illustrating pharmacodynamic and pharmacogenomics genes In general, clinically-significant genes can be subdivided as (i) pharmacodynamic genes as illustrated in the upper panel, and (b) pharmacogenomic genes as illustrated in the lower panel.

Personalized Diagnosis and Intervention Having the ability to look at a patient on an individual basis will permit accurate diagnosis and specific treatment strategies. Genotyping is performed to obtain an individual's DNA sequence by using bioassays (Human Genome Project, 2014). By having a detailed information of an individual's DNA sequence, their genome can be compared to a reference genome to assess the genetic variations that can account for possible diseases. Several companies including: *Navigenics, and Illumina*, have created *Direct-to-Consumer Genome Sequencing* accessible to the public to treat patients more effectively. An individual's genetic make-up also plays a significant role in how well they respond to a certain treatment, and therefore can change the course of treatment. Thus pharmacogenomics, utilizes an individual's genome to provide a more informed and tailored drug prescription to a patient *(What is pharmacogenomics, 2014)*.

Preventive and Promotive Aspects of PM In addition to specific treatment, PM can facilitate advancements of preventive care. For example, many women are being genotyped for mutations in the BRCA1 and BRCA2 gene if they are predisposed because of a family history of breast cancer or ovarian cancer (*BRCA1 and BRCA2: Cancer and Genetic Testing, 2014*). As more causes of diseases are mapped out according to mutations that exist within a genome, the easier they can be identified. Subsequently preventive and/or therapeutic measures can be adopted to prevent a disease from developing. The basic information of the DNA sequencing can reduce the impact or delay the onset of certain diseases and it will allow better decisions in determining the exact source of the disease and thus treating or preventing its progression, particularly for AD or cancers that are currently thought to be linked to mutations in the DNA (PM Coalition, 2014). A unique approach is to test efficacy and safety of a drug specific to a patient group/sub-group is companion diagnostics. This biotechnology is developed during or after a drug is available and is helpful in augmenting the therapeutic success based on the individual's genetic makeup (*Companion Diagnostics", 2014) and* have incorporated the pharmacogenomics related to the drug into their prescription label to assist in making the optimal treatment decision.

PM in Drug Development Having an individual's genomic information is exceedingly important in developing drugs as they await approval from the FDA for public use. Having a detailed information of an individual's genetic make-up can be an asset in deciding if a patient can be selected for inclusion or exclusion of a clinical trial. Being able to identify patients who will benefit most from a clinical trial will increase the safety from adverse effects caused by the product in testing, and will allow smaller and faster trials to lower overall costs (Paving the Way for PM, 2014). In addition, drugs that are deemed ineffective for the larger population can gain approval by the FDA by using personalized genomic data to qualify the effectiveness and need for that specific drug or therapy even though it may be needed by a small percentage of the population (The Path to PM, 2014).

Benefits of PM In general, the practice of medicine has primarily been reactive. The researchers may have to wait until the onset of clinical symptoms to treat or cure them. As the researchers don't exactly understand the genetic and environmental factors that cause chronic diseases such as cancer, AD, PD, and diabetes, our treatment criteria is inadequate, imprecise, unpredictable, uncertain, and ineffective. Generally therapeutic interventions are evaluated on diversified populations using statistical analyses. Consequently, they work for some patients but not for many others, due to individual genetic differences. Only 50% get the proper benefit and remaining may suffer from the deleterious adverse effects or multi-drug resistance. PM is based on each patient's unique genetic makeup, and attempts to eliminate the inherent limitations of traditional medicine. PM can have several benefits over conventional medicine as it promises to provide following benefits: (i) *earlier therapeutic interventions, (ii) make personalized theranostic decisions, (iii) increase probability of desired prognosis, (iv) improve targeted therapies, (v) reduce probability of adverse effects, (vi) prevention and prediction of disease rather than reaction to it, and (vii) reduce healthcare cost as illustrated in* Figure 7.

"Therapy with the right drug at the right dose in the right patient" is a description of how PM will affect the future of treatment (Pharmacogenomics. The Promise of PM, 2000). For instance, Tamoxifen is prescribed to women with ER+ breast cancer; but 65% of women developed resistance. Women with mutation in their *CYP2D6 gene* (a gene that encodes the metabolizing enzyme) were unable to efficiently metabolize Tamoxifen, making it ineffective for their cancer (Breast Cancer in the Personal Genomics Era, 2014). Hence women are now genotyped for those specific mutations, so that they can have the most effective personalized treatment. Identification of these mutations is carried out via high-throughput screening or phenotype screening. Several drug discovery and pharmaceutical companies including; *Persomics, Novartis, Foundation Medicine, and several others* are currently utilizing these technologies to not only advance the concept of PM, but also to amplify genetic research. Alternative multi-target approaches to the traditional approach of "forward" transfection library screening can entail reverse transfection orchemogenomics. Yet another application of

PM is pharmacy compounding. Though it may not utilize genetic information, the customized development of a drug whose properties (e.g., *dose level, ingredient selection, route of administration, etc.*) are selected and designed for an individual patient is also accepted as an area of PM (in contrast to mass-produced unit doses or fixed-dose combinations).

Oncogenomics in PM *Cancer Genomics, or "Oncogenomics," is the application of genomics and PM to cancer research and treatment, which* is one of the most promising branches of genomics because of its implications in drug therapy. Recently genetic variation was discovered in variety of cancers that appeared the same in traditional pathology. There was increasing awareness of tumor heterogeneity, or genetic diversity within a single tumor, which raise the possibility of finding that drugs that have not given good results to a general population may be successful for certain cases with particular genetic profiles. High-throughput sequencing is used to characterize genes associated with cancer to better understand disease pathology and improve drug-development. Trastuzumab (Herclon, Herceptin) is a monoclonal antibody that interferes with the HER2/neu receptor is used to treat certain breast cancers. This drug is used only if a patient's cancer is tested positive for over-expression of the HER2/neu receptor. Two tissue-typing tests are used to screen patients for benefit from Herceptin treatment. The tissue tests are *immunohistochemistry* (IHC) and *fluorescence in situ hybridization* (FISH) (Walter, 2006). Only Her2+ patients are treated with Herceptin therapy (Trastuzumab) (Telli et al. 2007). Similarly tyrosine kinase inhibitor such as *Imatinib* (Gleevec) was developed to treat chronic myeloid leukemia (CML), in which the BCR-ABL fusion gene (*the product of a reciprocal translocation between chromosome 9 and chromosome 22)* is present in >95% of cases and produces hyperactivated abl-driven protein signaling. These medications inhibit the Ableson tyrosine kinase (ABL) protein and are thus a typical example of "rational drug design" based on the disease pathophysiology (Saglio et al., 2004).

Benefits of Personalized Medicine

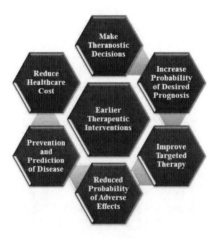

Figure 7. Benefits of PM A pictorial diagram illustrating benefits of PM. PM may provide (i) earlier therapeutic interventions, (ii) make personalized theranostic decisions, (iii) increase probability of desired prognosis, (iv) improve targeted therapies, (v) reduce probability of adverse effects, (vi) prevention and prediction of disease rather than reaction to it, and (vii) reduce healthcare cost.

Challenges in PM The current approaches to intellectual property rights, reimbursement policies, patient privacy and confidentiality as well as regulatory oversight will have to be redefined and restructured to accommodate the changes PM will bring to healthcare system (PM Coalition, 2014). Furthermore, the analysis and adoption of diagnostic data is a major challenge of PM *(*Huser et al., 2014). For example, genetic data obtained from NGS requires computer processing prior to its analysis (Analyze Genomes: Motivation, 2014). Hence, adequate technology will be required to accelerate the adoption of PM, which requires the interdisciplinary cooperation including: *medicine, oncology, biology, and software development.*

Regulatory oversight The FDA has taken initiatives to integrate PM into their regulatory policies. A report entitled *"Paving the Way for PM: FDA's role in a New Era of Medical Product Development,"* was developed which outlined steps to integrate genetic and biomarker information for clinical application and drug development. Specific regulatory science standards, research methods, reference material and other tools were developed to incorporate PM into their current regulatory practices. A *"genomic reference library"* was developed to compare the validity of various sequencing platforms to uphold reliability.

Intellectual Property Rights There is controversy regarding patent protection for *diagnostic tools, genes, and biomarkers.* In June 2013, the U.S Supreme Court ruled that natural occurring genes cannot be patented, while "synthetic DNA" that is edited or artificially-created can be patented. The Patent Office is reviewing issues related to patent laws for PM, such as whether "confirmatory" secondary genetic tests post initial diagnosis, can have full immunity from patent laws. Those who oppose patents argue that patents on DNA sequences are an impediment to ongoing research while proponents point to research exemption and stress that patents are necessary to protect the financial investments for commercial research and development.

Reimbursement Policies Reimbursement policies will have to be redefined to fit the changes that PM will bring to the healthcare system. Some of the factors that should be considered are the level of efficacy of various genetic tests in the general population, cost-effectiveness relative to benefits, how to deal with payment systems for rare conditions, and how to redefine the concept of "shared risk" to incorporate the effect of the newer concept of "individual risk factors"

Patient Privacy and Confidentiality One of the most important issues is the consequences for patients who are predisposed after genetic testing or found to be non-responsive towards certain treatments. This includes the psychological effects on patients due to genetic testing. The right of family members who do not consent is another issue, considering that genetic predispositions and risks are inheritable. The implications for certain ethnic groups and presence of a common allele would also have to be considered. In 2008, the *Genetic Information Nondiscrimination Act* (GINA) was passed to minimize the fear of patients participating in genetic research by ensuring that their genetic information will not be misused by employers or insurers. On February 19, 2015 FDA issued a press release*: "FDA permits marketing of first direct-to-consumer genetic carrier test for Bloom syndrome."*

The Role of FDA A significant information generated through NGS poses regulatory issues for FDA. FDA will encourage innovation while ensuring accuracy and has been issuing discussion papers, holding workshops, and collaborating with stakeholders. It has created precision FDA, a community research and development portal that allows for testing, piloting, and validating existing and new bioinformatics approaches to NGS processing.

FDA's Role in the PM Initiative PM *is an innovative approach to disease prevention and treatment that considers differences in people's genes, environment, and lifestyles. PM has led to new discoveries and several FDA-approved treatments that are tailored to specific characteristics of individuals, such as a person's genetic makeup, or the genetic profile of an individual's tumor. Patients with a variety of cancers now undergo molecular testing, to select treatments that improve chances of survival and reduce adverse effects. President Obama's PM Initiative identifies genetically-based drivers of disease to develop new, and more effective treatments. FDA's role is to ensure the accuracy of genetic tests derived from NGS, that collects data on a person's entire genome. Researchers are integrating segments of these data to detect genetic variants, meaningful differences that might eventually result in a treatment.* Over the past few years, a number of products that signal a new era of medical product development have entered the market. In just the last 2 years, the FDA approved 4 cancer drugs in patients whose tumors have specific genetic characteristics that are identified by a companion diagnostic test. Recently FDA approved a new therapy in cystic fibrosis patients with a specific genetic mutation. Furthermore, 3D printing was used to create a bioresorbable tracheal splint for treating a critically-ill infant, suggesting the promise of PM.

The patients with similar symptoms may have different illnesses, with different causes; and that interventions may work well in some patients but not in others with apparently the same disease. Advances in genomics to medical imaging to regenerative medicine, along with computational power of mobile and wireless capability and other technologies, are allowing patients to be treated precisely and effectively that better meet their personalized needs. FDA has made it a priority to evolve regulatory processes in response to—and in anticipation of—scientific developments that are critical for the development of EBPT.

PERSONALIZED TREATMENT

Personalized Treatment of Cystic Fibrosis and Cancer On January 31, 2012, the FDA approved therapy for cystic fibrosis (CF), a serious inherited disease that impairs the lungs and digestive system. The drug, Kalydeco™ (Ivacaftor), was approved for patients with the G551D mutation – a gene important for regulating the transport of water and electrolytes in the body. There are hundreds of known mutations that can lead to CF; the G551D mutation is responsible for only 4% of cases in the US (~ 1200 people). In these patients, Kalydeco worked by restoring the function of the protein that is made by the mutated gene. It allows a proper flow of salt and water on the surface of the lungs and helps prevent the buildup of sticky mucus that can lead to life-threatening lung infections and digestive problems. Kalydeco is the first drug to address the underlying cause rather than the symptoms of CF. Patients are experiencing improved lung function and weight gain. The approval of Kalydeco by FDA was patient-driven. The drug emerged out of a collaboration between the Cystic Fibrosis Foundation (CFF) and the Vertex Pharmaceuticals. Similarly, *cancer drugs – Crizotinib, Vemurafinib, Dabrafenib, and Tremetinib – were approved for patients whose tumors have specific genetic characteristics that are identified by a companion diagnostic test. Moreover, progress in regenerative medicine and stem cell research offers hope for the personalized products –the replacement or regeneration of missing or damaged tissues.*

3D Printed Tracheal Splint in PM 3D printing was used to create personalized medical devices based on imaging of a patient's anatomy. Physicians at the University of Michigan and Akron Children's Hospital utilized a CT imaging, computer-aided design, and 3D printing to create a bioresorbable airway splint to treat a critically-ill infant with *tracheobronchomalacia* – a life-threatening condition that occurs when the airway walls are weak and collapse during breathing or coughing. The tracheal splint was constructed based on CT images of the patient's airway and lungs. The device was "printed" by the 3D printer using Polycaprolactone (PCL) – a biodegradable material, allowing the body to heal and grow around it. The physicians implanted the tracheal splint overlying the patient's airway, creating a placeholder for the cells to grow around it. One year after surgery, imaging and bronchoscopy showed an open airway while full resorption of the bioresorbable stent is expected to take 3 years.

Personalized Treatment of HER-2 Positive Metastatic Breast Cancers Important discoveries about the role of cell growth and oncogenes in cancer resulted in the development and approval in 1998 of Trastuzumab (Herceptin®), the first genetically-guided therapy for the treatment of HER-2 positive metastatic breast cancers. A few years later, the *International Genome Sequencing Consortium* announced that it had completed the sequencing of the human genome. While there was considerable speculation about the pace at which this information might be applied in medical product development, there was no question that completion of the human genome project would unleash an explosion of genetic information related to complex diseases, pharmacogenomics important for drug development, and rapidly advancing sequencing and information technologies. Robert Weinberg discovered in 1979 "HER-2," a gene involved in multiple cancer pathways, which led to the development of Trastuzumab (Herceptin®, made by Genentech, Inc). UCLA researcher Dennis Slamon worked to understand the link between HER2 and specific types of cancer. He discovered that changes in the HER2 gene causes breast cancer cells to produce abnormally high amounts of HER2 protein. Overexpression of the HER2 protein occurred in ~20-25% of breast cancer patients, and resulted in an aggressive form of the disease, suggesting that HER2 overexpression could serve as both a biomarker of aggressive disease as well as a target for treatment for EBPT applications. It was the first molecularly targeted cancer therapy designed to "switch off" the HER2 gene, making the cancerous cells grow more slowly and without damaging normal tissue. This precision therapy also proved that patients on this new treatment suffered fewer severe side effects as compared with other cancer treatments. In September 1998, FDA approved Herceptin for the treatment of HER2 positive metastatic breast cancers and approved DAKO Corp HercepTest, an *in vitro* assay to detect HER2 protein overexpression in breast cancer cells. Currently, HER2 testing is performed for the clinical diagnosis of breast cancer patients.

Testing methods for HER2 evolved and FDA approved several tests for HER2 detection. Herceptin is not beneficial, and may cause harm, to patients with cancers that do not overexpress HER2, so the availability of a validated assay is critical for therapy. In 2012, Genentech was awarded approval by FDA for *Perjeta®*, a drug with a similar HER2 binding mechanism of action as Herceptin, that improved prognosis when used in combination with Herceptin and another chemotherapy medication, *Taxotere®*, in patients with HER2 positive breast cancers. *Perjeta* acts by targeting a different part of the HER-protein than *Herceptin*, resulting in further reduction in growth and survival of HER2-positive breast cancer cells. The molecular therapeutics of Herceptin also emphasized: *not all cancers are the same.*

Breast cancer – as well as other cancers – cannot be viewed as a single disease, but rather as a group of several subtypes, each with its distinct molecular signature.

Infrastructure to Support PM *Soon after the announcement of the completion of the human genome project, each of the FDA's medical product centers – the Center for Drug Evaluation and Research (CDER), the Center for Biologics Evaluation and Research (CBER), the Center for Devices and Radiological Health (CDRH) – as well as the National Center for Toxicological Research (NCTR)* put into place regulatory processes, policies, and infrastructure to meet the challenges of regulating these products. In 2002, CDER, in collaboration with the Drug Industry Association (DIA) and the pharmaceutical and biotechnology industries, organized workshops to discuss scientific developments in pharmacogenomics, which provided guidance and policy development, to build an infrastructure for regulatory review to provide pharmacogenomics principles in drug development. They also created the Voluntary Genomic Data Submission (VGDS) Program (later renamed the Voluntary Exploratory Data Submission Program (VXDS)), to discuss genetic information with the FDA. This program proved critical for encouraging scientific exchange between sponsors and the FDA about exploratory genomic data and in furthering successful integration of novel biomarker data in drug development. Likewise, leadership in FDA's CDRH recognized that biological insights from the completion of the human genome would give rise to a diagnostic revolution in medicine, including expansion of molecular testing and new molecular technologies. In 2002, CDRH created the *Office of In vitro Diagnostic Device Evaluation and Safety* (OIVD) as an organizational unit for comprehensive regulation of *in vitro* diagnostic devices (IVDs) and organized it into 3 divisions – (a) *Immunology and Hematology; (b) Chemistry and Toxicology; (c) and Microbiology*. In 2013, OIVD incorporated products related to radiological health and was renamed as the Office of *In vitro Diagnostics and Radiological Health (OIR)*. Combining the 3 key regulatory programs and radiological health (premarket review, compliance, and post-market safety monitoring) into a single geographic unit. The Genomics and Targeted Therapy Group in the Office of Clinical Pharmacology, Center for Drug Evaluation and Research (CDER) played a key role in establishing FDA on the leading-edge of PM and pharmacogenomics. This group works to advance the application of pharmacogenomics in the discovery, development, regulation, and use of medications. At its inception in 2004, the Group spearheaded CDER's hallmark Voluntary Genomic Data Submission (VGDS) Program and established review committee for the program. The group also worked to modernize the labeling of approved therapeutics with pharmacogenomic information and increased its capacity and become more integrated with drug product review divisions. Through pre-market review of therapeutics, policy development, regulatory research, and education, the group ensures that pharmacogenomic and targeted development strategies are promoted and applied in all phases of drug development ensures that all diagnostic device activity related to these products would spring from a common technical and regulatory base. In 2004, CDRH reorganized its Office of Science and Technology into the Office of Science and Engineering Laboratories (OSEL), which performs regulatory science research at FDA and collaborates with academia, healthcare providers, other government agencies, and industry, to integrate its organizational structure with its premarket review offices. Many of CBER's early efforts to expedite the development of innovative and complex biological products, such as *gene therapies, cell-based and tissue-engineered products, and new technologies to enhance the safety and availability of blood products, arose out of advances in genomics and proteomics.* CBER launched initiatives that seek to integrate genomics, proteomics, high sensitivity gene sequencing, and other scientific technologies into regulatory oversight. Stem cell-based treatments and new technologies involving the introduction of manipulated cells to fight disease, restore normal function, repair injuries, or regenerate failing organs present exciting possibilities, but also present challenges to facilitate the development of new products while helping to ensure their safety and effectiveness. To address these challenges, CBER has intramural research scientists who work with scientists at NIH, to develop new methods and knowledge for reducing uncertainty with regard to safety and efficacy of these new therapies. The National Center for Toxicological Research (NCTR) is a center that supports FDA's agency-wide needs. NCTR fosters national and international research collaborations and communications to promote rapid exchange of theories and emerging sciences with promise to inform FDA's regulatory decisions. NCTR's early research efforts towards PM included the identification of genetic polymorphisms that influence drug and carcinogen metabolism, individual cancer susceptibility and therapeutic drug efficacy; the epidemiological studies for post-market surveillance of chemical toxicants in foods, drugs, cosmetics, and medical devices; and the development and validation of DNA microarray technology for EBPT. In 2002, NCTR established the Centers of Excellence (*for Bioinformatics, Functional Genomics, and Structural Genomics*) in which studies related to PM are conducted, including the microarray quality control (MAQC) project. These centers of excellence were combined to form the division of systems biology to apply genomics, proteomics, and metabolomics to biomarker development. This division played a key role in the VGDS program by providing a database and analysis tools (ArrayTrack™) to manage the datasets provided by industry groups. In 2006, the previous division of PGx and molecular epidemiology was reorganized into the new vision of personalized nutrition and medicine for which the goals were to develop and implement research strategies that account for genetic, environmental, and cultural diversity that influence expression of genetic makeups and knowledge for improving personal and public health. FDA's office of special medical programs (OSMP), which serves as an agency focal point for special programs and initiatives that involve multiple medical product centers and are clinical, scientific, and/or regulatory in nature, also supports FDA's PM efforts. Within OSMP, the office of orphan products development (OOPD) implements incentives, including orphan drug and humanitarian use device and grant programs, to promote the development of products for rare diseases. In the case of drugs, rare disease is defined as condition affecting fewer than 200,000 people; in the case of devices, it is defined as that affects fewer than 4,000 people in the US.

Recent Studies Under the leadership of FDA Commissioner Margaret A. Hamburg, M.D., FDA has intensified its commitment to furthering PM. In 2011, Dr. Hamburg unveiled a restructuring of the commissioner's office and the agency's programs into four "directorates." As part of this effort, a new position of deputy commissioner for medical products and tobacco was established to provide leadership across the centers for *drugs, biologics, medical devices and tobacco products* and to oversee the office of special medical programs. The genomics and targeted therapy group in CDER has increased its capacity, and the offices of biostatistics, new drugs, and translational sciences have established for pharmacogenomics and biomarker development. In 2009, CDRH created a PM staff dedicated to addressing the opportunities and challenges associated with diagnostics used. In addition, CDRH's OSEL established a high-performance computer facility to support data- and computationally-intensive calculations and modeling. Other efforts are focused on identifying and characterizing biomarkers "*beyond genomics.*" For example, imaging technologies (e.g., *intravascular ultrasound, intravascular near infrared spectroscopy, magnetic resonance spectroscopy, magnetic resonance imaging, CT imaging, and PET imaging*) are being studied to evaluate atherosclerotic plaque characteristics to determine its vulnerability to rupture, and to identify the best stent to treat individual patients. Finally, CDRH's office of surveillance and biometrics (OSB) provides statistical support and epidemiological expertise for premarket and post-market issues associated with the design and evaluation of diagnostic studies in PM.

Whole Genome Sequencing Extensive DNA and RNA sequencing across multiple genes or the whole genome are already being used in clinical practice. Whole genome sequencing (WGS), in which the human genome can be sequenced at a reasonable cost in a reasonable amount of time, is expected to bring public health applications, yet WGS platforms are still evolving, and there are currently no agreed-upon approaches to assess their performance. FDA approval or clearance of diagnostic tests requires demonstration of their clinical validity. However, in the case of WGS, sequence-based assays, and extensive gene panels, tests will involve the analysis of many alleles *(3 billion base pairs in the case of WGS)*, so that demonstrating the validity of each variant may not be practical or feasible, since the clinical significance of these variants is unknown. Many variants are rare, so that it is difficult to find enough patients to run a clinical trial to determine whether they are significant. FDA has taken steps toward developing a new method for evaluating these tests. In June 2011, FDA sponsored a public workshop on evaluating the technical performance of NGS and on the bioinformatics data to interpret the data. It has started to assess sequence-based tests using a strategy that focuses on validating the performance of the sequencing platform –accurately, reliably, and precisely. The Agency is looking at possibilities for identifying a representative biomarkers that could be assessed to develop an understanding of the performance of the platform.

Companion Diagnostic for Co-Development In cases where a test is essential for the safe and effective use of a corresponding therapeutic product, it is termed a "companion diagnostic." *A companion diagnostic impacts the ability of a specific therapeutic product to achieve its established safety and effectiveness.* Companion diagnostics should be subject to oversight with appropriate controls, and a draft guidance has been issued that clarifies the definition and approval requirements that apply to the development and marketing of this particular category of diagnostic tests. If it is required for safe and effective use of a therapeutic product, then an FDA-approved or cleared test must be available at the time that the drug is approved. Companion diagnostics are often developed concurrently with a therapeutic, but can also be developed to optimize treatment with a therapeutic that has already been approved. The concept of co-development was first applied in 1998, when the approval of the therapeutic Trastuzumab (Herceptin), was paired with approval of an immunohistochemical IVD companion diagnostic device (HercepTest™) that measures expression levels of human epidermal growth factor receptor 2 (HER-2) in breast cancer tissue.

Personalized Cancer Treatment *In August 2011, FDA approved the drug Vemurafenib (Zelboraf) along with its companion diagnostic, the Cobas 4800 BRAF V600E mutation test, in treating metastatic or unresectable melanoma.* Metastatic melanoma is a highly aggressive skin cancer with a 5-year survival rate of only 15%. Vemurafenib inhibits the BRAF V600E mutation found in ~50% of melanoma patients. Melanomas that lack the mutation are not inhibited by the drug; therefore, using a test to identify the patients who would more likely benefit from the treatment accelerated development of the drug, facilitated a successful regulatory review, and led to an improved therapeutic profile.

Crizotinib/ALK testing In August 2011, FDA approved *Crizotinib* (Xalkori), a drug along with an ALK FISH probe companion diagnostic for the treatment of non-small cell lung cancer. Crizotinib targets tumors with an abnormal ALK gene, which occurs in ~5% of nonsmall cell lung cancer patients. Crizotinib's safety and effectiveness was established through a clinical trial involving only 255 patients, and the approval process for the drug and its associated test took only 4.9 months, well below average review times for priority drugs.

Tafinlar/Mekinist/THxID BRAF test In May 2013, FDA approved *Tafinlar* (Dabrafenib) and Mekinist (Trametinib) for patients with advanced or unresectable melanoma, the leading cause of death from skin disease. The FDA approved Tafinlar and Mekinist with a genetic test called the THxID BRAF test, a companion diagnostic that determines if a patient's melanoma cells have the V600E or V600K mutation in the BRAF gene. Approximately half of melanomas arising in the skin have a BRAF gene mutation. Tafinlar is intended for patients whose tumors express a single BRAF gene mutation, V600E. Mekinist is intended for patients who express that mutation or the V600K mutation.

Product Labeling Drug labeling is "intended to provide a summary of the scientific information needed for the safe and effective use of the drug. Labeling provides healthcare practitioners with information that is critical for treating patients. FDA requires product labeling to be balanced, scientifically accurate, and not misleading, and that clear instructions be communicated for drug prescribing and/or administration. PMs that may only be safe and effective in particular sub-populations, or must be administered in different doses in different sub-populations, must be labeled accordingly. In cases where a therapeutic product is approved together with a companion diagnostic device, the labeling of the two products must be consistent. In cases where an IVD companion diagnostic is developed with an already approved therapeutic product, it may be necessary to update the therapeutic product's labeling with appropriate test-related information if such information is essential to the safe and effective use of the product. Diagnostic tests may be developed that provide information that is helpful for determining whether a drug is appropriate for a patient or not, but is not essential for the safe and effective use of the therapeutic product. Pharmacogenomic information can appear in different sections of the labeling (*e.g., Therapeutic Indications, Warnings, and Precautions*). In 2009, FDA approved labeling changes to the drugs *Etuximab (Erbitux) and Panitumumab (Vectibix)* to advise against their use in patients with metastatic colorectal cancer whose tumors have certain mutations in the KRAS gene. The changes were based on the analysis of several clinical trials that revealed that the drugs provide no benefit to patients with those mutations. ~ 35 -40% of colorectal cancers contain a mutated KRAS gene by the companion diagnostic and associated with poor outcome. Using the companion diagnostic to stratify patients with respect to KRAS mutation spares some patients from an ineffective treatment, and not using either of these drugs as first-line treatments in inappropriate patients could save ~$600 million a year. In 2008, FDA approved labeling changes to *Abacavir-containing products* to recommend HLA testing prior to initiating Abacavir therapy. Abacavir is an antiviral used in the treatment of HIV infection and was first approved in 1998. Studies showed that patients who carry the HLA-B*5701 allele are at high risk for experiencing serious and sometimes fatal hypersensitivity reactions to the drug. The labeling was changed to recommend against its use in at-risk patients

Clinicians who were hesitant to prescribe Abacavir do so more readily as a result of the improved understanding of the risk associated with the drug and the availability of the test. The incidence of *Abacavir hypersensitivity reactions* has diminished worldwide and the drug has enjoyed a significant resurgence in sales in response to the adoption of HLA testing. In 2007, FDA approved *labeling changes to Warfarin*, an anticoagulant that is prescribed to people who are at high *risk for the formation of blood clots due to conditions such as deep vein thrombosis, heart valve disease or replacement, and irregular heart beat, or to prevent recurrence of pulmonary embolism, heart attack, and stroke. Warfarin has a narrow therapeutic window* and a wide range of *inter-individual variability* in response, requiring careful clinical dose adjustment for each patient. The "precautions" section of the labeling was updated to include information to alert physicians that people with variations in two genes, *CYP2C9 and VKORC1,* may require a lower initial dose of the drug. The labeling did not provide specific dosing recommendations. In 2010, FDA updated the *"Dosage and Administration"* section of the labeling, to include specific initial dosage recommendations for patients with different variant combinations testing would be most beneficial, and whether a clear clinical course of action exists once the PGx information is available.

Post-Market Surveillance One of the most exciting promises of PM is that it will allow for more focused clinical trials, the most expensive phase of drug development, by increasing the proportion of responders in the trial, increasing the average effect size, or both. While clinical trials for block-buster drugs enroll 7,000 patients, clinical trials for Crizotinib involved only 255 patients. For Kalydeco, the main trial involved only 161 patients; a second tested the drug in 52 children. Post-market surveillance is critical to the success of PM. FDA's ongoing efforts to refine methods for analysis of post-market data, including data mining of spontaneous reports and analysis of electronic health records from accessible, large healthcare databases, will benefit all medical products, including PM.

MicroArray and Sequencing Quality Control Project MAQC/SEQC Project with participation of hundreds of scientists from the genomics and bioinformatics communities, the project is expected to enhance our capacity to understand, predict, and eventually prevent idiosyncratic and serious adverse drug reactions by reliably utilizing patient-specific genomic information at the single-base resolution level. The project has been carried out in three phases. Phase I, evaluated the technical performance of multiple microarray platforms and the advantages and limitations of various bio-informatics data analysis methods in identifying differentially expressed genes (or biomarkers). The findings informed FDA's updated guidance on the submission of PGx data to the agency. Phase II evaluated methodologies for developing and validating classification models based on high-dimensional microarray data to predict clinical and toxicological endpoints, and also evaluated the technical performance of genome-wide association study platforms and different data-analysis methods. Phase III aims at assessing the technical performance of NGS platforms by generating large benchmark datasets with reference samples and evaluating advantages and limitations of various bioinformatics strategies in RNA and DNA analyses.

Genomic Reference Library for Evaluating Whole Genome Sequencing Whole genome sequencing (WGS) is widely used as a research tool and is becoming commercially available for other uses. Multiple sequencing instrumentation systems have been introduced, yet it is not clear how well sequencing works on an individual patient level, and there are no agreed measurement characteristics or the clinical application of results provided by these instruments. In partnership with the National Institute of Standards and Technology (NIST),

FDA's Office of *In vitro* Diagnostics and Radiological Health (OIR) in CDRH is developing genomic reference materials for evaluating WGS instrument systems. The reference materials will allow FDA to understand overall system performance, the variation between instrument types and uses, the types of errors each system may make, and specific measurement performance for individual sequences of interest. In addition, the project will generate products and testing methods that can be used with any technology or application. The reference materials will be available for purchase by industry and researchers and will serve as a national resource in understanding how WGS systems work.

Virtual Physiological Patient Advances in medical imaging and computational modeling have allowed incorporation of patient-specific simulations into clinical practice and medical device development. This can allow for personalized, custom-built medical devices designed for individual patient anatomic and physiological characteristics. CDRH is now developing a digital library of such models and simulations for evaluation, modification, sharing, and incorporation into medical device development. Source data will also be available to develop models de-novo. Allowing such precompetitive collaboration and sharing of modeling knowledge will likely help advance personalization of medical device development and use.

High-Performance Integrated Virtual Environment (HIVE) for NGS Analysis HIVE is a cloud-based environment optimized for the storage and analysis of extra-large data, primarily NGS data. This environment will provide secure web access for authorized users to deposit, retrieve, annotate, and compute High-Throughput Sequencing (HTS) data, and to analyze the outcomes using web-interface visual environments appropriately built in collaboration with research scientists and regulatory personnel. HIVE is a multicomponent cloud infrastructure where the distributed storage library and the distributed computational powerhouse are linked. The novel paradigm of moving computations to the data instead of moving data to computational nodes implemented in HIVE has significantly less taxing for hardware and network infrastructure. FDA's medical product centers are using HIVE for regulatory submissions. Development of High Resolution Human Leukocyte Antigen (HLA) Typing: The HLA system refers to a large number of genes and protein products that are related to immune system function. HLA typing is the process of testing patient or donor blood or other tissue samples for HLA antigens. The results can then be used to determine compatibility between the donor and patient (*HLA matching*). *More precise HLA matching through the application of molecular-based typing methods has been shown to improve transplant outcomes and is critical for bone marrow transplant outcomes, where poor matches can result in catastrophic health consequences.* However, ambiguous results occur even with the use of current "*gold standard*" DNA-based HLA typing methods, due to the variability and complexity of the HLA genes. CBER scientists, along with others in industry and academia, are working to apply technologies to develop a high resolution HLA typing method that achieves results without ambiguities.

Molecular Tools to Facilitate Blood Group Typing Blood group typing by molecular methods is of great interest in predicting highly specific RBC types and to enable the transfusion of compatible blood products. Molecular typing has benefits over traditional techniques and can increase the possibility of identifying suitable blood donors in complex patient cases. As RBC molecular typing kits are approved and become available, there will be a need for quality control standards. CBER's Division of Blood Applications is working to develop quality control DNA reference panels with coverage of ~90 genotypes from 17 blood groups that can be used in the evaluation, validation, and standardization of RBC molecular testing devices.

Clinical Trial Designs and Methodologies FDA is working to refine clinical trial design and statistical methods of analysis to address issues such as missing data, multiple endpoints, patient enrichment, and adaptive designs that arise in the development of targeted therapeutics. FDA is also looking specifically at clinical trials for oncology drug development. Development of cancer drugs is complicated because many cancers are heterogeneous, meaning that cancers in the same organ can have different origins and characteristics, each with their own specific genetic makeup. This heterogeneity is one reason why the availability of molecular typing has proved valuable in cases where patients require multiple transfusions throughout their lifetime, such as patients with sickle cell anemia. These patients develop immune antibodies to donor blood, making finding compatible blood for transfusion difficult. High-throughput, multiplex molecular typing create the possibility of large-scale donor screening for multiple antigens, including rare antigen combinations or genotypes. This will assist in providing well-matched RBCs for transfusion for these patients. Different people with cancer in the same organ respond differently to therapies. The I-SPY 2 trial, a highly collaborative initiative developed under a public-private partnership, involving the participation of >20 cancer centers, attempts to account for this heterogeneity and complexity of cancer at the outset. The "I-SPY 2 Trial," launched in March 2010, represents a new clinical trial model that will help scientists efficiently test promising drugs for women with higher risk, rapidly growing breast cancers. During the trial, drugs in development are individually targeted to the biology of each woman's tumor using specific genetic or other biomarkers. By applying an adaptive trial design, researchers will use data from one set of patients' treatments to treat other patients –quickly eliminating ineffective treatments and drugs.

Study Design Considerations for HLA Genotyping Devices The HLA region is the most variable part of the human genome. HLA typing is critical for tissue transplant matching, and sponsors face significant challenges developing and evaluating devices used to determine a patient's HLA type. CBER has created an HLA genotyping working group that is developing study design for both clinical and analytical performance, essential components of an HLA diagnostic device submission. Working with scientists at Booz Allen Hamilton and the FDA supercomputer center, the Genomics Evaluations Team for Safety (GETS) and the Office of Vaccines Research and Review (OVRR) in CBER are comparing different methods for analyzing genomic data for use in a predictive or prognostic fashion. By simulating full sized genomes for tens of thousands of humans and assigning medically-relevant phenotypes in a realistic manner, they have been able to determine which methods of the trial to be used to accomplish EBPT. The I-SPY 2 trial was developed under the Biomarkers Consortium, a public-private partnership that includes the FDA, the NIH, and major pharmaceutical companies, led by the Foundation for NIH.

Novel Device Diagnostics for Improving Drug Safety In the 1990s, multiple drugs were removed from the market because they increased the risk of a potentially fatal abnormal heart rhythm called *Torsade de Pointes*. Drugs that cause the abnormal heart rhythm also increase a measurement on the ECG called the "QT interval". However, not all drugs that prolong the QT interval cause Torsade de Pointes. Screening for drug-induced QT prolongation early in drug development may be preventing some effective new drugs (*benign QT prolonging drugs*) from reaching the market. An inter-center collaborative team from CDER and CDRH is assessing new device-based algorithms and biomarkers that can distinguish benign (*not harmful*) from malignant (*harmful)* drug-induced QT prolongation.

Medical Device Performance and Clinical Outcomes Through the Medical Device Epidemiology Network (MDEpiNet) Partnership, CDRH developed a Formal Evidence Synthesis Framework that combines existing data sources, including clinical trials, observational studies, patient registries, published literature, administrative claims data, and other known data sources. This framework will allow targeted, comprehensive, up-to-date benefit-risk profile for a specific medical device for subgroups of patients at any point of a life cycle to make optimally informed decisions and provide information that is more useful to practitioners, patients, and industry.

Biomarker Identification and Development Preventions and therapies can be chosen that maximize benefits while minimizing side effects and unnecessary treatments and tests. *The PM is focused on the development of biomarkers, technologies, and tools to classify individuals into subpopulations that differ in their susceptibility to a particular disease or their response to a specific treatment.* The classifications include: *genetics, sex, age, epigenetics, and life-style and environmental factors such as smoking and obesity.* NCTR's Division of Systems Biology works to identify important translational biomarkers and pathways of response that provide predictive, diagnostic, and prognostic value in both the preclinical testing of compounds and the management of patients.

Pharmacogenetics and Immunogenicity of Protein Therapeutics There has been a steady shift towards the use of recombinant human proteins in the treatment of human diseases, such as hemophilia. However, the safety and efficacy of these therapies are affected by proteins those can elicit an immune response by producing inhibitory antibodies. Genetic variability may lead some individuals, racial/ethnic groups, or other sub-populations to develop inhibitory antibodies at a higher frequency. Development of inhibitory antibodies to therapeutic proteins is a life-threatening adverse event, which requires expensive clinical intervention that can cost up to several million dollars per patient. Researchers at CBER are working to establish pharmacogenetic determinants of immunogenicity in patients with Hemophila A.

Effects of DNA Modifications on the Quality of Protein Products It has become apparent that SNPs are a significant cause for genetic variability in the population, including variation in individual response to prescribed medications. Evaluating the safety of protein-based therapeutics that mimic human proteins is complex, because several possible sequences of the protein exist in the normal population, anyone of which could be developed as a drug. In addition, there has recently been a surge in protein and DNA engineering that allow improved therapeutic product yields. Hemophilia A, also known as "Factor VIII deficiency" is the most common form of hemophilia and occurs in one of every 5,000 males in the US. In patients with this disease, the clotting factor (Factor VIII) is missing or nonfunctional, causing patients to have longer bleeding episodes after trauma or serious injury, or in more severe cases, episodes that occur spontaneously. In the treatment of hemophilia A, about 20% of patients develop inhibitory antibodies against life-saving therapies. In addition, the prevalence of this life-threatening reaction among patients of Black African descent is almost twice to that observed in patients of Caucasian descent. Researchers at CBER are working to establish the pharmacogenetic determinants of immunogenicity, using Factor VIII as a model system. The long-term goal of their research is to identify and utilize biomarkers to ensure the safety and efficacy of medications. They have developed an algorithm that considers 3 critical parameters – *mutations in Factor VIII, HLA type of the patients/recipients, and sequence of therapeutic Factor VIII agent* – to generate an immunogenicity score that predicts a patient's risk of immunological response to a given protein therapy and is consistent with clinical reports of immunogenicity. This approach is also useful in accessing the immunogenicity of bioengineered protein therapeutics, engineering the protein to achieve desirable therapeutic outcomes. All of these manipulations can affect the efficacy and safety of protein therapeutics but predicting how different manipulations can alter safety and efficacy remains a challenge. CBER initiated a research project to better understand the effects of DNA modifications on the quality of protein products. Using proteins that are involved in blood clotting as models, it has been demonstrated that while "synonymous" or "silent" mutations do not affect the protein sequence, they may affect protein levels as well as protein folding and function. The researchers are also trying to understand which mutations are deleterious and which may be safely employed in design of therapeutic protein products, and aim to develop methodologies to evaluate protein properties from gene sequence. This research could have wide implications for the development and evaluation of safe and effective protein therapeutics, including biosimilar products.

Identification of Genetic Risk Factors for Vaccine Reactions CBER's Office of Vaccines Research and Review (OVRR) together with the Genomics Evaluations Team for Safety (GETS) are involved in research collaborations that focus on identification of genetic risk factors associated with adverse reactions to vaccines. For example, a project with Harvard Pilgrim Healthcare and Georgia Kaiser Permanente attempts to identify genetic risk factors.

Understanding 'Silent' Mutations The genetic code governs how a cell translates DNA instructions, via RNA, into functional proteins. Inside the cell nucleus, DNA is transcribed into RNA and then edited to remove segments that do not code for amino acids. In the process of translation, RNA nucleotides spell out the sequence of amino acids in an encoded protein using 3-letter "codes" (called codons) each of which correspond to one of 20 amino acids. With an alphabet of 4 nucleotide bases, 64 codon triplets are possible, resulting in several codons that specify the same amino acid. Thus one can have a mutation in the DNA that does not result in an amino-acid change in the resulting protein. These single nucleotide changes that do not result in a change in the amino acid in the translated protein are referred to as "*synonymous mutations or "silent mutations.*" It was generally held that because synonymous mutations do not alter the sequence of the protein, they had no *functional or clinical consequences.* However, it is now understood that such changes may not be 'silent,' *and can impact protein expression, conformation, and function.* To date, >50 diseases have been shown to be caused entirely or in part by synonymous mutations. While only one synonymous mutation could cause disease, codon optimization more often than not results in the employment of synonymous mutations in more than half of the entire codon. Researchers at FDA's CBER are trying to understand the extent to which synonymous mutations occur genome-wide, the mechanisms by which they can affect protein function, and their global importance in human health and disease. Advancements in these areas could have applications in drug development as well as in the practice of clinical medicine. For example, synonymous mutations are introduced into protein therapeutics by way of genetic engineering as a strategy for increasing protein production. In recent years, new approaches, novel technologies and genomic data are helping us to elucidate the mechanisms by which synonymous codons affect *protein folding, structure and function that may have broad applicability:* *"Purpura"* – a condition of having an abnormally low platelet count – following measles-mumps-rubella (MMR) vaccination in children. A second study in collaboration with CDC and *Northern California Kaiser* looks at genetic risk factors of febrile seizures after MMR vaccination. Another study, in collaboration with the *Innovation Center for Biomedical Informatics (ICBI)* at Georgetown University, seeks to identify genes associated with vaccines, vaccine components, and several autoimmune diseases in order to assess plausibility of autoimmune diseases as adverse reactions to vaccines. Pathway models derived from this data may help predict autoimmune reactions to vaccines and other medical products in the future.

Evaluation of Personalized Cell-Based Products Mesenchymal or Multipotent Stem Cells (MSC): Stem cell-based treatments hold great promise to provide cells, tissues, and organs to treat a variety of clinical indications from cardiovascular disease to repairing or regenerating injured organs or limbs. However, these products are complex and raise a number of questions with regard to use in clinical trials, such as what are the critical product attributes to measure, will they form tumors in patients, and will they go to the wrong place in the body and cause harm? CBER has a consortium of scientists using a systems biology approach to identify the critical product characteristics that are measurable and correlated to desired clinical outcome using nonclinical functional assays. The outcome of these studies will be improved assays to characterize these cells as well as improved guidance to sponsors performing studies to evaluate MSC-based products, thus facilitating development of this new class of medical products.

Genetics of Drug Induced Hypersensitivity Reactions Understanding genetic susceptibilities to drug responses (i.e., *adverse reactions and efficacy*) is critical to the implementation of PM. Genetic variants have been associated with severe adverse reactions to Carbamazepine, a drug used in the treatment of epilepsy and trigeminal neuralgia. In particular, two HLA-related variants (HLA-B* 1502 in Asian populations and HLA-A* 3101 in Caucasian populations) have been associated with an increased risk of developing Stevens-Johnson (SJS) syndrome and toxic epidermal necrolysis (TEN), two forms of a life-threatening skin condition. However, these HLA variants predict only a portion of individuals who will develop these conditions, suggesting that other rare or non-HLA related variants may also play an important role. Scientists at NCTR, in collaboration with *scientists at the University of Liverpool (UK) and the Huashan Hospital (China)* are performing whole genome sequencing and genetic analysis to identify susceptibilities to Carbamazepine-induced SJS or TEN. By identifying additional factors that help to explain variation in patient response, they will be able to better predict in advance who will have an adverse reaction to the drug.

Genetics and Cardiovascular Risk In collaboration with researchers at the *University of Maryland,* scientists at NCTR are conducting research to identify genetic factors that interact with common lifestyle factors to contribute to heart disease. Research subjects were recruited from the Amish community in Lancaster, Pennsylvania. The volunteers were examined for metabolic responses to various diets and drugs that are associated with cardiovascular risk, specifically: *blood triglyceride response after a high fat meal, blood pressure response after a high salt meal, and platelet aggregation response after Aspirin or Clopidogrel administration.* The DNA from subjects who showed abnormal responses was sequenced using NGS technology and genetic association studies were conducted. This work is ongoing, and as candidate genetic markers are discovered, they are being validated in another cohort.

Identification of genetic factors that interact with dietary and drug exposures to increase risks of cardiovascular disease or efficacy of treatment will allow patients and their physicians to utilize PM to improve health.

Role of Genetics in Response to Clopidogrel Doses Clopidogrel (Plavix®) is a drug that inhibits aggregation of blood platelets, and is used in patients to prevent heart attacks or strokes caused by blood clots. Although Clopidogrel works in many individuals, some people do not respond well to the drug. This variation in treatment response may be linked to genetics. Clopidogrel is converted to an active drug in the human body through an enzyme encoded by the gene named CYP2C19. Individuals with genetically-impaired CYP2C19 metabolism have lower capacity to convert the drug to its active form. Consequently, these individuals have lower blood levels of the activated form of the drug, diminished antiplatelet responses, and higher rates of cardiovascular events and stent thrombosis. Researchers at FDA, in collaboration with the National Cancer Institute (NCI), the National Institute of General Medical Sciences (NIGMS) and the University of Maryland, are conducting a study to evaluate whether increasing the dose of Clopidogrel increases antiplatelet responses and active metabolite exposure in individuals with genetically reduced CYP2C19 metabolism relative to those with normal CYP2C19 metabolism.

PM for Heart Devices Researchers in the Office of Science and Engineering Laboratories at CDRH made advances in understanding the underlying biology of heart disease. They used new methods for analysis of the ECG to identify the underlying causes of heart disease and to predict which patients will benefit from cardiovascular therapies such as cardiac resynchronization therapy. This work has resulted in new methods to diagnose electrical conduction problems and to quantify scar tissue in the heart, with different criteria for women and men. These new methods are being used by outside research groups and are helping decipher why women benefit significantly more than men from cardiac resynchronization therapy. This example of PM diagnostics helps to explain why the efficacy and safety of medical products differs in patient subgroups and can be used to design more efficient clinical trials.

Role of Body Fluid Interaction Testing and Adaptive Optics in PM *The Office of Science and Engineering Laboratories at CDRH is collaborating with George Washington University* to develop a microfluidic, high-throughput microchip to test the interaction of tears with contact lenses, care products, and microbes. The goal is to guide patient prescription of lens materials and hygiene products. Moreover, in the area of personalized eye research, scientists are working on adaptive optics where a patient's ocular aberrations are measured to either provide custom photorefractive surgery (LASIK), a custom contact lens, a custom intraocular lens, or a super high resolution imaging to diagnose retinal disease down to the cellular level (*as well as other novel gene-based applications*). The first three enable a customized treatment; the last enables disease diagnosis and tailored treatment. Centers for Excellence in Regulatory Science and Innovation (CERSI): in support of their activities facilitating collaborative regulatory science research, FDA's Office of the Chief Scientist (OCS) established a program to fund academic Centers of Excellence in Regulatory Science and Innovation (CERSI). One of the major focuses of the Georgetown University CERSI is on PGx research – understanding what genetic variants predict response to therapy, building gene and protein based pathways models to understand adverse event mechanisms, and better understanding genetic variant information across ethnic groups to evaluate usefulness and thoroughness of clinical trial data.

Medical Product Development Of the new drugs approved since 2011, ~one-third had some type of genetic or other biomarker data included in the submission to characterize efficacy, safety, or PKs. Since 2010, CBER licensed *Provenge,* ® an autologous cancer vaccine, *Laviv,* ® an autologous fibroblast product, and 5 cord blood products for hematopoietic reconstitution, which require careful matching of donor and recipient. PM submissions to CDR H's Office of *In vitro* Diagnostics and Radiological Health (OIR) have increased since 2007. Review activity in CDER's Genomics and Targeted Therapy Group has steadily increased over the past 5 years. Recombinant protein therapeutics, which are particularly suited for EBPT, are the fastest growing segment of the pharmaceutical repertoire and are increasingly used to treat or manage some of the most complex medical conditions. Data from the last few years indicate that more and more drugs are being designed for small populations, a trend that is consistent with the increasing use of stratification in drug development. Multiple examples of targeted approaches to drug development have demonstrated that such approaches can shorten overall drug development and review times.

Common Conditions Involving Multiple Genes/Biomarkers Common conditions are often influenced by genetic, as well as environmental and social factors, in ways that are not yet well understood. Realization of the benefits of EBPT for common conditions affected by multiple genes will be a complex process that will depend on investment in clinical research well beyond the initial demonstration of gene-disease correlations. Currently used disease classification systems define diseases primarily on the basis of their signs and symptoms, those do not accommodate emerging information about disease mechanisms, particularly when it is at odds with traditional physical descriptions. As a result, many disease subtypes with distinct molecular causes are still classified as one disease, while multiple, different diseases that share a common molecular cause are not properly linked. The failure of our outdated disease classification systems to incorporate new biological insights serves as a barrier to progress in PM. The National Academy of Sciences has called for the creation of a "New Taxonomy" of disease that is designed to advance our understanding of pathogenesis and improve health that defines and describes diseases on the basis of their molecular biology in addition to traditional signs and symptoms. Although the costs of genetic sequencing have plummeted over the past decade, resulting in an explosion of information; the infrastructure to collect, analyze, integrate, share, and mine that information remains a significant challenge.

Clinical Implementation of New Diagnostics Many clinicians have been reluctant to use new diagnostics due to the ongoing controversy over clinical utility and the fact that biomarker clinical utility can often be a moving target. Clinicians also face the "information overload," making adoption of new tests difficult without decision support tools that could be accessed to identify, order, and interpret the appropriate tests. One of the disincentives to developing personalized therapies is the perceived lower return on investment that targeted drugs will provide because of smaller patient populations and therefore lower sales. While these concerns may be offset by the increased safety and effectiveness of these medicines that allows for smaller trial designs and leads to rapid uptake, premium pricing, and increased patient compliance, the relative costs and rewards of these investments will clearly vary from one product to the next, and uncertainties will remain for some time.

Access to EBPT Even though PM is bringing benefit to those who have disease with a diagnostic characteristic of interest, patients who do not have the characteristic are not benefitting. Additional work to target all subclassifications of a disease is needed to assure that many patients will not be "left out" of the sea change that PM brings. Moreover, the FDA will continue to facilitate the development of the PM by advancing the science and tools that will drive innovation, collaborating with scientists worldwide in important research activities, providing clarity and guidance to industry in order to help shepherd new products through regulatory review, and continuing to identify opportunities to streamline regulatory processes.

Selected PM Drugs and Relevant Genes Drug name (Brand name) Biomarker Indication Adjuvant therapy *Cevimeline* (Evoxac®) CYP2D6 Dry mouth: Cevimeline should be used with caution in individuals known or suspected to be deficient in CYP2D6 activity, based on previous experience, as they may be at a higher risk of adverse events.

Rasburicase (Elitek®) G6PD Hyperuricemia: Rasburicase administered to patients with glucose- 6-phosphate dehydrogenase (G6PD) deficiency can cause severe hemolysis. Do not administer the drug to patients with G6PD deficiency. Screen patients at higher risk for G6PD deficiency (*patients of African or Mediterranean ancestry*) prior to using the drug.

Sodium Phenylacetate & Sodium Benzoate (Ammonul®) Urea cycle disorders can result from decreased activity of any of the following enzymes: N-acetylglutamate synthetase (NAGS), carbamyl phosphate synthetase (CPS), argininosuccinate synthetase (ASS), ornithine transcarbamylase (OTC), argininosuccinate lyase (ASL), or arginase (ARG).Sodium Phenylacetate and Sodium Benzoate are metabolically active compounds that can serve as alternatives to urea for the excretion of waste nitrogen.

Sodium Phenylbutyrate (Buphenyl®) Indicated as adjunctive therapy in the chronic management of patients with urea cycle disorders involving deficiencies of carbamylphosphate synthetase (CPS), ornithine transcarbamylase (OTC), or argininosuccinate synthetase (ASS).

Analgesia & Anesthesiology Celecoxib (Celebrex®) CYP2C9 Pain: Patients who are known or suspected to be CYP2C9 poor metabolizers based on a previous history should be administered Celecoxib with caution as they may have abnormally high plasma levels due to reduced metabolic clearance.

Codeine CYP2D6 Pain: Some individuals may be rapid metabolizers because of a specific CYP2D6 genotype. These individuals convert Codeine into its active metabolite, Morphine, more rapidly and completely than other people, which results in higher than expected serum Morphine levels. Even at labeled dosage regimens, individuals who are ultra-rapid metabolizers may have life-threatening or fatal respiratory depression or experience signs of overdose (*such as extreme sleepiness, confusion, or shallow breathing*). Some individuals may be poor metabolizers because of a specific genotype. These individuals do not convert Codeine to Morphine sufficiently and may have no pain relief.

Mivacurium (Mivacron®) Cholinesterase gene Anesthesia adjunct: Is metabolized by plasma cholinesterase and should be used with great caution, if at all, in patients known to be or suspected of being homozygous for the atypical plasma cholinesterase gene.

Tramadol (Ultram®) CYP2D6 Pain: Based on a population PKs analysis of Phase 1 studies in healthy subjects, concentrations of Tramadol were ~20% higher in "poor metabolizers" versus "extensive metabolizers," while M1 concentrations were 40% lower.

Cardiovascular (CV) Carvedilol (Coreg®) CYP2D6 Retrospective analysis of side effects in clinical trials showed that poor CYP2D6 metabolizers had a higher rate of dizziness during up-titration, resulting from vasodilating effects of the higher concentrations of the α-blocking R(+)-enantiomer.

Medical Simulation Medical schools and residencies are currently facing a shift in their teaching paradigm. The increasing amount of medical information and research makes it difficult for medical education to stay current in its curriculum. As patients become concerned that students and residents are "practicing" on them, clinical medicine is becoming focused more on patient safety and quality than on bedside teaching and education. Educators have faced these challenges by restructuring curricula, developing small-group sessions, and increasing self-directed learning and independent research. Nevertheless, a disconnect still exists between the classroom and the clinical environment. *Many students feel that they are inadequately trained in history taking, physical examination, diagnosis, and management.* Medical simulation has been proposed as a technique to bridge this educational gap.

It has been emphasized that individual differences in drug efficacy, or susceptibility to adverse effects, collectively confer an important contribution to the burden of ill-health (Connor, 2003; Pirmohamed et al 2004). This can be reduced by studying the genetic basis and by clarifying pathways and mechanisms of drug action or metabolism to inform drug development, and by the development of genotype-based predictive tests of efficacy or toxicity (pharmacogenetics). Investigations to evaluate common disease susceptibility, reliable identification of genetic loci, and clinical application of this knowledge including: critical appraisal of the performance of genotype as a predictive test can accomplish ultimate the goal of PM. Hunter et al (2008) highlighted that while the extent of the clinical impact of research in both areas is uncertain, the reliable identification of loci involved in drug response (pharmacogenetics) appears to be less advanced than the identification of susceptibility loci for common disease. After two decades of research and expansion in the availability of drug therapies, and the promise of 'PM,' only four pharmacogenetic tests were mandated as part of the FDA drug approval in July 2009, while for another 10 tests FDA recommended no clinical utility (Roses 2000, Lemonick et al., 2001; Ioannidis et al., 2001; Goldstein et al., 2003; Pollack, 2005; FDA, 2006; Marr 2008; McClain et al 2008; Hynicka et al., 20008; Shurin and Nabel 2008; Goldstein 2009). It was realized that understanding the reasons for the blocks in development of PM could help improve efficiency of future research. Systematic reviews and field synopses previously exposed the obstacles to progress in complex disease genetics. These included: a focus on candidate genes rather than genome-wide analysis; inadequate sample size; suboptimal capture of genetic variation; chasing and reporting bias; all of which led to a failure to replicate and validate genetic associations (Ioannidis et al. 2001; Ioannidis et al. 2003; Colhoun et al. 2003). These overviews were followed by improvements in research design which made a significant contribution to the success in the identification in genes for common diseases (Ioannidis et al. 2006; Higgins et al. 2007; Ioannidis et al. 2008; Pennisi 2007). These considerations and the absence of a prior systematic, quantitative overview of pharmacogenetic research was the motivation for the studies related to drug PKs (*absorption/distribution/metabolism/ elimination*) and PDs (*the drug targets*).

Definition of Disease Category Disease categories are organ-specific with the exception of (i) cancer, which encompassed anybody site in which there was neoplasia, and (ii) anti-coagulation, classified as 'cardiovascular'. The cardiovascular disease category also included acute myocardial infarction and peripheral vascular disease; neurology/psychiatry included stroke, psychosis, and depression; endocrine disease included diabetes and hyperlipidemia (where the outcome assessed was a change in lipid level and not the effect on cardiovascular end-points).

Gene Nomenclature and Classification Genes were named according to HUGO (Human Genome Organization) Gene Nomenclature Committee (HGNC, Wellcome

Trust; http://www.genenames.org. The Pharmacogenetic Field Synopsis PLoS ONE | www.plosone.org classification of genes into dynamic or kinetic was checked with the Pharmacogenomics Knowledge database. Where it was not possible to precisely classify the specific gene according to HUGO nomenclature, an asterisk was placed after the initial characters (e.g., HTR* denotes serotonin receptor genes, of which HTR1B and HTR2A are specific examples).

A study in which the outcome investigated was the desired effect of the drug (e.g., pH lowering from use of a proton pump inhibitor) was defined as 'intended effect'; one in which the outcome was adverse was classified as an 'adverse effect' (both hypersensitivity and dose-dependent adverse reactions). For the 161 full-text papers, outcomes were classified as binary or continuous: examples of binary were death, disease recurrence, or an episode of bleeding; examples of continuous were changes in the plasma levels of a drug, gastric pH or international normalized ratio (INR, e.g., for the monitoring of Warfarin anticoagulation).

Continent of Correspondence The continent of correspondence was determined from the Medline citation and used as a marker for the geographic location of the study. The study design was categorized as: (i) prospective (including randomized clinical trials), (ii) case-control, (iii) cross-sectional, or (iv) meta-analysis. A primary pharmacogenetic study was defined as one in which the title of the study or the stated aims or purpose within the text of the abstract indicated that the primary intention of the study was to investigate the effect of genetic variation on drug response. If not explicitly stated, the study was classified as a secondary pharmacogenetic study.

Exclusions *These investigators excluded the following as 'drug' treatments: ionizing radiation, surgical procedures, non-drug-eluting stents, bone marrow transplantation, tobacco, Alcohol, environmental agents or pollutants (e.g., lead), herbal remedies, dietary or lifestyle interventions including acupuncture, massage, counseling, or exercise.* They analyzed the evidence-base behind the FDA list of approved pharmacogenetic tests. The articles cited in support of FDA labeling as 'test required' or 'test recommended' were reviewed (Document S1). Tests (gene and drug pairs) were cross-referenced with the generated database. FDA recommendations were contrasted with guidelines from authoritative medical bodies.

Statistical Analysis Statistical analyses were performed using SPSS for Windows version 17.0 and Stata 10. A value of $p < 0.001$ was taken as significant. Frequency distributions were analyzed for normality by 2-tailed Chi-Square. Impact factors were ranked by Mann Whitney U. Sample sizes were converted into logarithmic (loge) values and means compared with unpaired Student's t.test. Most pharmacogenetic studies were prospective in design (1496, 89.7%) with about one-half (852; 51.1%) set in Europe or Australasia and one-third in North America (511 studies; 30.7%). The most frequently investigated disease areas were cancer (456 studies; 27.3%), neurology/psychiatry (321; 19.2%) and cardiovascular disease (287; 17.2%) with a relative paucity of studies in infectious disease (106 studies, 6.4%) and respiratory medicine (49 studies, 2.9%). Most studies evaluated the effects of the drug under investigation (1190 studies; 71.6%); only one-eighth of studies (210, 12.6%) examined adverse drug effects, with PKs rather than PDs studies being more likely to do so.

Genes Investigated and Number of Participants There were in total 541 genes studied (176 somatic, 305 PDs and 70 PKs with some overlap for 10 genes). Seven genes included studies involving over 10,000 participants in aggregate: two somatic (TP53 and non-specified karyotype mutations), 2 PKs (MTHFR and CYP2C9) and 3 PDs genes (ACE, AGT and

APOE). About one-third (37.7%) of study participants were distributed among the 10 most frequently studied somatic genes; with the equivalent numbers in kinetic and dynamic studies being 68.5% and 41.8%, respectively. Thirteen of 70 (18.6%) kinetic genes, 22 of 305 (7.2%) dynamic genes and 12 of 176 (6.8%) somatic genes included more than 10 studies.

Most Frequently Studied Gene-Drug Combinations The 10 most studied cancer cell gene variants were *TP53 and Cisplatin/5-Fluorouracil/Paclitaxel response, ERBB2 (HER2/neu) and Anthracyclines/Trastuzumab response, EGFR and Gefitinib response, and RAS, FLT3, ABCB1, BCL2 and t (9; 22)* and other karyotype and cytogenetic mutations and response to a variety of combination chemotherapy regimens. The most studied germline PKs and PDs genes were ACE and cardiovascular drug response (n = 79), CYP2D6 and response to antidepressant therapy (n = 74), CYP2C19 and response to GIT drugs (mostly proton pump inhibitors, n = 52), MTHFR and response to nutritional drugs (predominantly Folate, n = 41), ADRB2 and response to respiratory medications (n = 34), CYP2C9 and cardiovascular drugs (mainly Warfarin, n = 33), APOE and response to drugs targeting the cardiovascular (n = 29) and CNS (n = 31), TPMT and response to chemotherapy/ immunosuppression (mostly Azathioprine, n = 29), and HTR* (n = 27) and DRD2 (n = 27) and response to CNS drugs. However with the exception of ERBB2(HER2/neu)/ Trastuzumab therapy, CYP2C9/Warfarin and TPMT/Azathioprine none of these genes are mandated or recommended by the FDA for pharmacogenetic testing. The 50 frequently studied genes and the aggregate number of participants per gene. (a) PDs genes (n = 305); (b) PKs genes (n = 70); and (c) somatic genes (n = 176)*refers to 1 gene and/or non-HUGO nomenclature.

PDs Genes Gastroentrology, Cardiovascular, Respiratory, CNS, Infections, Endocrine, Obstrectic/Gynecaology, Malignanat Immunosuppression, Nutrition/Blood, Muscle, Joint, ENT, Skin Vaccine, Anesthesia (*APOE, ACE, ADRB2, HLAB, HTR, DRD2, F5, TNF, HLA-DRB1, VDR*)

PKs Genes: (Gastrointestestinal, Cardiovascular, Respiratory, CNS, Infection, Endocrine, Obs/Gyn, Malignant/Immunosupprssion, Nutrition, Blood, Muscle, Joint, Eye, ENT, Skin, Vaccine, Anesthesia) [*CYP2D6, CYP2C9, CYP2C19, ABCB1, MTHFR, CYP3A5, TPMT, UGT1A1, CYP3A4, CYP2B6*]

A distinctive feature of the field of pharmacogenetics is the predominance of publications indexed as reviews, commentaries, letters and other opinion based pieces over primary research articles, whichever search strategy the researchers used to identify articles. This may have contributed to a high expectation of the delivery of PMs with modest realization of this goal (Marr, 2008; Pollack 2005; Roses 2000). Pharmacogenetic research currently centres mainly in cancer, cardiovascular and neurological/psychiatric disease with most studies being set in Europe and North America mainly among subjects of European ancestry. The relative dearth of research in other therapeutic areas (e.g., communicable disease) and among individuals of nonEuropean ancestry, among whom there is a considerable global disease burden, may be creating an imbalance that will require future work. Even if the relevant genetic variants and effect sizes are homogeneous across different ancestral groups (Ioannidis et al., 2004), differences in allele frequency can vary greatly (Limdi et al., 2008) and such variation means that the population impact of genetic variants influencing drug response will often differ by ethnicity even if effect sizes are similar. The major goal of pharmacogenetic research is development of genotype-based predictive tests of efficacy or toxicity. However, a prerequisite is the reliable identification of the relevant genetic loci. In genetic work, where many hundreds of thousands of hypotheses can be tested, research designs are needed that optimize the detection of true positive (while limiting the potential for false positive) association (Ioannidis et al., 2006; Higgins et al., 2007; Ioannidis et al., 2008). Despite some high quality studies, there are several features that suggest that only a proportion of the positive associations reported are genuine. These include: the small size of most studies coupled with the more frequent evaluation of common rather than rare variants (whose effect sizes would be small and which therefore requires large sample sizes for their reliable detection); use of surrogate outcome measures rather than more clinically relevant binary outcomes; and subgroup analyses with multiple hypothesis testing. Detailed data (information unlikely to be reported in abstracts) on outcome measures (binary/continuous), gene variants and reported p values were derived from the full text of a subset of 10%, which accurately reflected the span of studies in the database. Similar problems were recognized in the field of genetics of common disease a decade or so ago. What followed were efforts to systematically and comprehensively collate evidence from genetic association studies, large collaborative metaanalyses, larger primary studies, more comprehensive capture of genetic variation at any given locus, independent replication, and, whole genome association studies (Hindorff et al., 2009).

Somatic (12 meta-analyses, 7 genes) 30 503 (230–756) ABCB1 1 21 chr8 5 EGFR (4) 1 30 ERBB2 (2) 1 37 FLT3 1 11 RAS* 1 25 TP53 (2) 1 62

Dynamic (10 meta-analyses, 15 genes) 5 2,183 (751–6,638) ACE 1 72 APOA* 5 APOE 1 87 CETP 10 ESR* 4 F2 5 F5 1 20 HLA* 7 HTR2A 15 HTR2C 5 ITPA 1 MKRN2 2 NQO2 1 SLC6A4 3 TNF 1 20

Kinetic (9 meta-analyses, 7 genes) 52 1,450 (161–3,029) ABCB1 1 67 CYP* 2 CYP2C19 1 76 CYP2C9 (3) 1 52 CYP2D6 1 84 CYP3A4 1 23 CYP7A1 1

These developments have contributed to the discovery of many secure genetic associations that are providing new insights into disease pathogenesis, therapeutic targets and the possibility of developing predictive tests for disease. Several important efforts to collate and curate information on the genetic basis of drug response already exist, including those of the Pharmacogenetics Research Network (Pharmacogenetics Research Network. National, NIH, 2009). However, the challenge in identifying primary pharmacogenetics studies is illustrated by two alternative search strategies. The comprehensive Medline search was sensitive (yielding 100,000 articles) but nonspecific, with a large number of evaluated articles not satisfying definition of a pharmacogenetic study. These researchers knew of no previous attempts to systematically identify all published pharmacogenetic studies in this way but this analysis suggested that future attempts to do so should adopt an explicit, systematic and comprehensive search strategy such as the one they used. The terms "pharmacogenomic" and "pharmacogenetic" have both been used somewhat interchangeably in the literature.

Other developments that may be helpful include: a greater use of meta-analysis, particularly where four or more independent studies of the same gene have been conducted, perhaps with an online, continuously updated database similar to those established for AD, PD and Schizophrenia (Schizophrenia Gene, 2009; Bertram et al 2007; Frodsham and Higgins 2007; Tang et al., 2009). Other improvements might include: primary studies with larger sample sizes; wider use of haplotype tagging SNPs; studies of rare and structural genetic variants whose effects are predicted to be larger, and which may therefore be more suited for use as predictive tests; and a greater focus on genes influencing drug handling and adverse effects, to fill gaps in knowledge (Woodcock and Lesco, 2009).

Important studies with some of these features have been reported since the deadline for literature search. For example, the identification of a SNP in the SLCO1B1 gene, encoding the organic anion-transporting polypeptide OATP1B1, as a susceptibility factor for statin-induced myopathy involved GWAS of 85 individuals with definite or incipient statin myopathy (and 90 controls) from a trial involving over 12,000 subjects (Link et al. 2008). Here, the small size of the GWAS belied the large-scale effort to identify the few subjects who suffer extreme adverse effects. This study provided a paradigm for the identification of genetic loci underlying rare but serious adverse effects of a commonly used drug. Other examples which could be studied in a similar way include Heparin-induced thrombocytopenia (frequency 0.5–2%), oesteonecrosis of the jaw from bisphosphonate treatment (prevalence 4–7% in those receiving i.v bisphosphonates for hypercalcemia of malignancy), and angioedema from ACE inhibitors. Because of the large genetic effect sizes that might be detected with this approach (for example an odds ratio of 17 for statin myopathy in SLCO1B1 CC homozygotes), predictive tests may be more likely to emerge, though the rarity of the adverse effect means that rigorous assessment of the cost-effectiveness of the approach would first be required. Larger scale candidate gene studies are also providing evidence on loci influencing both drug response and adverse effects that might form the basis of predictive testing for dose adjustment or avoidance of toxic treatments (Colombo et al., 2008; Klien et al., 2009; Mega et al., 2009; Simon et al., 2009).

As more reliable information begins to emerge on alleles influencing drug response from larger, better designed whole genome and candidate gene studies, focus will need to shift to the evaluation of the predictive performance of genetic tests in clinical practice, including studies of cost-effectiveness. These evaluations will require use of different metrics to those conventionally reported in discovery-based genetic studies (such as odds ratios or proportion of variance (Jakobsdottir et al., 2009; Jannsens et al., 2006; Kraft et al., 2009). Instead, sensitivity and specificity, predictive values and the generation of multivariate models that include genotype will need evaluating (Klein et al., 2009; Bromley et al., 2009). In some cases, the most robust evaluation of the effectiveness of genetic tests may need to come from randomized trials comparing health outcomes among people randomized to pharmacogenetic testing or no testing, together with cost-effectiveness analyses when evaluating the usefulness of interventions. In concert, these efforts should help realize the promise of EBPT with resultant improvements in healthcare.

Recommendations for Future Research in Pharmacogenetics *Primary research in pharmacogenetics should emphasize both to adverse as well as intended effects of drugs, be appropriately powered, examine clinically-relevant end-points, be conducted among individuals of non-European as well as European ancestry, include studies of currently neglected drugs and disease areas, enhance the likelihood of identification of large effect sizes necessary for the generation of usefully predictive tests through the study of rare or structural genetic variants, and/or more extreme phenotypic differences in response or toxicity, ensure comprehensive SNP typing where candidate loci are studied, utilize whole genome analysis where mechanisms are uncertain, avoid post-hoc subgroup analysis, except where justified and powered, and report the findings with caution, include evidence of independent replication, exploit existing large randomized controlled trial datasets as a resource for pharmacogenetic evaluation (e.g., SLCO1B1 variants and statin-induced myopathy, based on the SEARCH trial involving 12,064 participants) (Link et al., 2008). Mechanisms should exist for: encouraging reporting null findings from high-quality studies,* *systematically and comprehensively collating, archiving and disseminating reports of pharmacogenetic research, to highlight continuing gaps in knowledge and promote successes, encouraging high quality updated systematic reviews and meta-analyses of pharmacogenetic research promising genotype-based predictive tests emerging from primary research should be: re-evaluated in independent prospective studies, assessed against clinically relevant outcomes, evaluated using the appropriate metrics for diagnostic, screening and predictive tests, tested where appropriate in randomized trials supporting information document S1 U.S. FDA.*

The Human Genome Project was completed by the U.S. Department of Energy and the NIH in 2003 after >10 years of continuous and dedicated research. The goals of this project were to learn the order of the 3 billion units of DNA that construct a human genome, as well as to identify the genes located in this huge data. By 2003, almost all of the pairs of chemicals that make up the units had been put in the correct sequence. The individual genes within the long strands of DNA, and the elements that control the genes, are still being explored. Current studies indicate that the human genome contains 22,000 to 23,000 genes. One of the early hopes of the genomic project was to pinpoint specific genes that caused common diseases. It is now realized that the answer is more complex, with many diseases the result of multiple genes interacting. Nevertheless, the information derived from the human genome project has the potential to completely transform healthcare system. It is now believed that genome-based medicine, frequently called PM, is the future of healthcare—the next logical step in which more is known about human genetics, disease, and wellness than ever before. Of all the scientific and social promises that stem from advances in our understanding of the human genome, genomic medicine may be the most eagerly awaited. The prospect of examining a person's almost entire genome, in order to make personalized risk predictions and treatment decisions seems quite promising.

The Human Genome The human genome is the blueprint for each person's body, influencing how the researchers look, our genetic predispositions for certain clinical conditions, how well our bodies fight disease or metabolize food, and which therapies our bodies do and do not respond to. The genome consists of an organism's total DNA, including its genes. DNA is composed of 4 chemicals, which are repeated in different sequences. (abbreviated as A, T, C, and G). That's why DNA is referred to as a code with a 4-letter alphabet. The sequence of the chemicals dictates the type of organism that develops, as well as other critical life functions. The human genome contains ~3 billion pairs of these chemicals. Genes are believed to make up only 2% of the human genome, with the rest consisting of "noncoding" regions, to regulate the function of genes and contribute to the structural integrity of chromosomes.

DEGREES OF RELATIONSHIP

First-degree relatives	Parents, children, brothers, and sisters
Second-degree relatives	Grandparents, aunts and uncles, nieces and nephews, and grandchildren
Third-degree relatives	First cousin

Some disorders are seen in more than one generation of a family. *For general information about disorders that run in families:* Genetics Home Reference provides summaries of genetic conditions. Each summary includes a brief description of the condition, an explanation of its genetic cause, and information about the condition's frequency and pattern of inheritance. The Coriell PM Collaborative provides a brief introduction to heritable diseases in the article *Heredity: It Runs in the Family.*

PM and Pharmacogenomics Pharmacogenomics holds the promise that drugs might one day be tailored to genetic makeup. Modern medications save millions of lives a year. Yet any one medication might not work, even if it works for other people. Or it might cause severe side effects but not for someone else. Age, lifestyle, and health can influence response to medications. PGx is the study of how a person's genetic makeup (genome) influences his or her response to medications. PGX is the most important part of a field called PM — also called individualized or precision medicine — that aims to customize health care, with decisions and treatments tailored to each individual patient in every possible manner. Although genomic testing is still a relatively new development in drug treatment, this field is expanding. Currently, >100 drugs have label information regarding PGx biomarkers that can be used to direct the use of a drug. Each gene provides the transcript for the production of a certain protein in the body. A particular protein may have an important role in drug treatment for one of several reasons, including the following:

- *The protein plays a significant role in breaking down the drug.*
- *It helps with the absorption or transport of the drug.*
- *The protein is the actual target of the drug.*
- *It has some role in a series of molecular events triggered by the drug.*

When researchers compare the genomes of people taking the same drug, they may discover that a set of people who share a certain genetic variation also share a common treatment response, such as:

- *A greater risk of side effects.*
- *Severe side effects at relatively low doses.*
- *The need for a higher dose to achieve a therapeutic effect.*
- *No benefit from the treatment.*
- *A greater or more likely benefit from the treatment.*
- *The optimal duration of treatment.*

This kind of treatment information is currently used to improve the selection and dosage of drugs to treat *cardiovascular disease, lung disease, HIV infection, cancer, arthritis, high cholesterol and depression.* In cancer treatments, there are two genomes that may influence prescribing decisions — the genome of the person with cancer and the genome of the cancerous (malignant) tumor. There are many causes of cancer, but most cancers are caused by damaged DNA that allows cells to grow unchecked. The "incorrect" genetic material of the unchecked growth — the malignant tumor — is really a separate genome that may provide clues for treatment. For example, the drug Trastuzumab (Herceptin) is most likely to be effective against breast cancer cells that have an extra copy of this gene and high levels of its protein. An example of PGx in treatment decisions is the use of a blood-thinning drug called Warfarin (Coumadin, Jantoven). If a patient has a blood clot, treatment may include a prescription for Warfarin to treat the current clot and to prevent additional blood clots from forming. The physcian's goal is to prescribe a dose that will be potent enough to prevent blood clotting but not potent enough to cause adverse reactions, such as internal bleeding (hemorrhage). The window for the effective and safe dose of this drug for any person is relatively narrow. Dosage has traditionally been based on such factors as weight, age, and kidney and liver function, as well as a laboratory test to assess the blood-thinning effect of the drug in each person. The dosing guidelines may have limited value in predicting the outcome for every person. In the early 2000s, studies comparing treatment outcomes with genomic data revealed that genetic variation was associated with either an increased risk of hemorrhage or with the need for a higher dose to be effective. Hence, the physcian may use the genomic information to help guide treatment decisions. A tissue sample swabbed from inside the cheek or a blood sample provides cells for a laboratory test to decipher personalized genome. Based on the results, the physician may judge more accurately what dose of Warfarin is likely to be safe and effective or whether Warfarin is even an appropriate treatment option. Although PGx has much promise and has made important strides in recent years, it's still in its infancy. Clinical trials are needed not only to identify links between genes and treatment outcomes but also to confirm initial findings, clarify the meaning of these associations and translate them into prescribing guidelines. Nonetheless, progress in this field points toward a time when PGx may be a part of routine EBPT of patients.

"*Currently patients are not yet asking the question 'Is this therapy going to work for me?' It will be challenging to look forward to the day patients do ask that question.*"

Wikipedia defines PM as "*a medical model that proposes the customization of healthcare* — with medical decisions, practices, and/or products tailored to the individual patient." But the definition preferred by the National Human Genome Research Institute is more specific, emphasizing that a personalized approach to medicine includes an "individual's genetic profile to guide decisions made in regard to the *prevention, diagnosis, and treatment of disease.*" Reaching that goal has been >20 years to sequence the first human genome. By 2003, scientists had done it; for the first time, they had complete sequence and map of all the genes in the human body. Advances in technology accelerated the pace of discovery and lowered the cost so much that scientists pushed on from that single reference genome to sequence the genomes of more than 1,000 individuals in all their variations. These days, individual patients — and sometimes healthy people, too — can have their personal genomes scanned or fully sequenced.

Prevention There have been recent, high-profile examples: Angelina Jolie made headlines with a proactive double mastectomy last year after tests showed she carried BRCA1, the same genetic marker for breast cancer that her mother, who died from the disease, carried. The National Cancer Institute puts the risk of breast cancer for those carrying a BRCA1 mutation at 65% and the risk of ovarian cancer at 39%. While it's important to remember that genes do provide information that can lead us to make more informed decisions about our health and healthcare, and, as in Jolie's case, that can change the future. If you get sick, knowing your genome or the molecular basis of your disease can be an important evidence for doctors seeking the most favorable treatment plan. In the case of cancer, genetic tests could lead to successful drug treatment rather than radical surgery. For instance, melanoma can be BRAF positive, meaning the tumor has a specific gene mutation that sets it apart from other melanomas. The lung cancer can be EGFR or ALK positive. Colon tumor may be KRAS positive The doctors will scan not just single genes or a handful, but also complete genomes. The challenge then will be figuring out what it all means and what to do next. Here are not yet enough products that have penetrated the consciousness of the average patient," says Edward Abrahams, president of the Washington, D.C.-based PM Coalition. *"Patients are not yet asking the question 'Is this therapy going to work for me?' I look forward to the day patients do ask that question. "I don't think anybody disagrees with the fact that patients are different and respond differently. But it's hard to make changes," You want to see evidence before you're willing to move away from one-size-fits-all traditional medicine. To change it, you have to show that what you're promising is an improvement."*

Testing In 2005, Stephanie Haney, now 45, had a pain on her right side that wouldn't go away. It hurt when she coughed or sneezed. She was pregnant, so she didn't investigate the cause, assuming perhaps she'd broken a rib. Two years later, she was diagnosed with stage 4 lung cancer. After undergoing chemotherapy, Haney began taking Tarceva (Erlotinib) in 2008. But 3 years later, the drug was no longer keeping the tumors at bay. Prompted by friends and a doctor, she had genetic testing on her tumors, which showed they were ALK (anaplastic lymphoma kinase) positive. This gave her doctor a major clue as to which drugs were most likely to work. Haney was able to start taking Xalkori (Crizotinib), designed specifically for ALK-positive lung cancer tumors. She joined a clinical trial for Xalkori in Philadelphia. Three years later, her tumors were barely visible. Researchers have discovered >1,800 disease genes since the Human Genome Project's completion. There are now >2,000 genetic tests for human conditions and 350 biotechnology-based products in clinical trials. Lung cancer treatment is one of the most advanced areas in terms of a PM approach, with several drugs approved by the FDA for different lung cancer biomarkers. Unfortunately, but not unexpectedly, Haney found out last October that the cancer had moved to her brain, one of several places lung cancer is prone to migrate. Because Xalkori will not break the blood-brain barrier, she just started another trial drug, LDK378, to treat the brain tumor. Caleb Nolan, 8, was diagnosed with cystic fibrosis when he was 3 weeks old, he has spent much of his childhood in hospitals, taking many rounds of medicines each day. Like other cystic fibrosis patients, Caleb has a mutation in a gene called CFTR that causes mucus to clog the lungs and obstruct the pancreas so the body can't absorb food. There are many different mutations of CFTR that lead to cystic fibrosis. Caleb, he has a mutation, G551D, found in 4 to 5% of cystic fibrosis patients, for which there is a treatment. Caleb is now on Kalydeco (Ivacaftor), a genetically targeted treatment approved by the FDA in 2012 and the first such drug that treats an underlying cause of cystic fibrosis. With Kalydeco, "Instead of the mucus building up, the medicine is thinning it," Shane says. "Now his body naturally does this. The medicine is preventing damage from the CF. Caleb hasn't been in the hospital since he's been on it [almost two years]. Usually, once kids reach their late teens or early 20s, they have to get a lung transplant. This should prevent that." The average lifespan of a person with cystic fibrosis is 37. Now, "Caleb could die of old age instead of CF,"If you have a family history that calls for it, insurance will pay for BRCA1 testing (in fact, the Affordable Care Act requires it). Patients with cancer are more likely to have their tests covered. "They have an interest in this because they don't want to prescribe drugs that won't work," "Insurance companies rightly want to see evidence that whatever they pay for works better than what we're used to paying for. But that's a barrier to innovation." When it comes to whole genome sequences, the uncertainties about outcomes are that much greater, but sequencing is getting cheaper now. In January, *Illumina*, a genetic-sequencing company based in San Diego, announced it had a new system that brought the cost for sequencing a human genome down to < $1,000. This doesn't put a sequencer in your local doctor's office — nor does it cover the cost of interpreting those results — but it does make it feasible for clinicians and researchers to gather the evidence needed to push PM over the tipping point. The D.C.-based PM Coalition has made defining levels of evidence that will be acceptable to the Centers for Medicare & Medicaid Services and private insurers a top priority. If a treatment or drug is outside medical guidelines, reimbursement is unlikely. "Medicine needs to be evidence-based," "Reimbursement is right up there with research in terms of priorities." Abrahams says.

With all this data come new questions and ethical and practical challenges about privacy, access, ownership, and more. In many cases, research or clinical trial participants aren't given their results at all. Companies like *Myriad Genetics*, the primary provider in the US of clinical BRCA1 testing, have returned individual results to doctors and patients, of course, but Myriad has kept the bulk of its data as a trade secret. Weiss, of Harvard Medical School, says patients will be the rightful owners of their personal genetic data. "This is confidential patient data," he says. "It can be used for medical research, but it's unlikely that your identity will be disclosed to some commercial third party in any identifiable way. Academic medical centers may partner with pharmaceutical companies, using their genomic data, but will do it in an anonymous way and only if the patient consents. The patient is going to be in control of what they do here, as they should be." Laws such as HIPPA (*Health Insurance Portability and Accountability Act*) and parts of the Affordable Care Act protect the privacy of personal health information. The passage of the *Genetic Information Nondiscrimination Ac*t (GINA) in 2008 was considered a major win, as it bars employers and health insurers from using genetic information or family history. Still, many people worry about such personal and sensitive information being out there. And genomic data is at the core of PM. *"You can't do PM when it comes to genomics without electronic medical records and without the ability to deliver genomic content to providers at their desktop,"* Weiss says. *"We're not really talking about the doctor-patient relationship here. We're talking about the mechanics of how you deliver huge amounts of data to clinicians in the office and at the bedside."*

The Obama administration began moving our healthcare system toward electronic records in the summer of 2009. Now >50% of medical records are available in electronic form. "We need to get to 100 %, and just having an electronic medical record isn't enough," "We still have to have software focused on the genomic content delivery to the caregiver." Ideally, doctors could tap into a single, large database filled with anonymous genetic information— biomarkers tied to patient demographics tied to specific drugs and treatments — to help make decisions about each individual's medical path. But getting there is sure to be a long and bumpy ride, with plenty of detours along the way. For Daryl Pritchard, director of policy research at the National Pharmaceutical Council, the end game is clear: "The use of that information — whether by a company or by a group of doctors or a provider group — is ultimately going to be advantageous to treating the condition." Starting with a good family history is a smart and simple way to begin a PM discussion with your doctor, says Geoffrey Ginsburg, director of the Center for Personalized and Precision Medicine at Duke University Medical Center, although it doesn't happen often enough, he suggests asking about whether any genetic tests are useful for regulating a dose of a drug, an approach known as PGx. Abrahams recommends asking your doctor the following question: *"Do you have the expectation that this drug will work for me?"* According to Randy Burkholder, the vice president of policy and research for Pharmaceutical Research and Manufacturers of America (PhRMA), a Washington, D.C.-based trade group representing American biopharmaceutical and biotechnology companies, the most important thing is not being afraid to ask your doctor questions. *"It can be a hard thing to do sometimes, especially when you're seeing a diagnosis,"*. *"Asking questions allows you to work with your doctor.* he says.

PM's greatest strides have been in cancer. Consider these statistics on the percent of tumors containing genetic mutations that could be targeted by drugs, as reported by the *Wall Street Journal* in 2011: *Melanoma: 73 %; Thyroid: 56 %; Colorectal: 51 %; Lung and pancreatic: 41 %; Breast: 32 %* "Cancer is a genetic disease," Ginsburg says. "In many ways, it is the poster child for a disease that has used PM strategies. It has used them in everything from risk assessment in healthy people — from screening, diagnosis, and prognosis — to selecting therapies based on genetics and the biology of the tumor. "HIV/AIDS is another area where PM has made great progress. "The virus mutates differently in each patient," "Now we can understand the viral load and analyze it, then prescribe the right cocktail of medicine to treat it". This is the progress the researchers seen taking AIDS from a death sentence to a chronic condition. But that's understanding the virus, not the person." Other diseases are clearly moving toward more comprehensive PM strategies, too, including heart disease, rheumatoid arthritis, multiple sclerosis, and infectious diseases. "Also, rare disease diagnosis is now becoming more amenable to PM strategies through genomics," Ginsburg says.

FUTURE PROSPECTS OF EBPT

Today, patients with breast, colorectal, and lung cancers, as well as melanoma and leukemia are offered a "molecular diagnosis," allowing to select treatments that are likely to improve their chances of survival. These cancers are no longer considered single diseases, but instead sub-classified on the basis of their genetics. *Advances in HLA genotyping are improving transplant outcomes and dramatically improving our ability to predict the potential for a patient to experience a severe hypersensitivity reaction to a drug, including drugs used to treat HIV, hemophilia, epilepsy, and bipolar disorder. The genotyping of drug-metabolizing enzymes has led to identify proper dosing schedules for drugs, and has helped patients avoid harmful side effects, drug interactions, and ineffective treatments. Similarly, "personalized" medical devices, tailored to individual and unique patient characteristics, are becoming common.* DNA sequencing and characterization of the human genome have unveiled several new drug targets. Translating new knowledge about PGx biomarkers into routine clinical practice has become a reality. As companies shift PGx investigations to early phase development, the researchers can expect to see the generation of more prospective biomarker applications and the development and approval of more drugs tailored by biomarker use. Currently >90% of pharmaceutical companies utilize at least some genomic-derived targets in their drug discovery program and PMs comprise 12-50% of company pipelines. While there is growing optimism, even the most ground-breaking personalized therapies are not "magic bullets," and significant scientific, medical, educational, business, regulatory, and policy challenges remain before PM can reach its potential and be fully integrated into patient care. A future where EBPT is a standard in medical practice and supported by continual learning systems that allows for adequate clinical decision support and the use of electronic medical records linked with personal genome sequences, while ever more plausible from a technical perspective, is still quite a far reaching goal. The most significant challenges include: limited understanding of the intrinsic biology of disease: the tools of the last two decades have left us with considerable amount of data, yet the researchers still have a limited knowlwdge of what it all means. Scientific understanding will remain the most important limiting factor for the momentum of EBPT. Recently Shungin et al. (2015) discovered genetic loci links of adipose tissue and the role of insulin biology to body fat distribution, whereas, Naci et al. (2015) described various factors which might fail to predict the clinical utility of treatment with a standard drug with a primary objective to accomplish EBPT. By taking coronary heart disease as a representative example, Goldstein, et al. (2014) provided evidence of incorporation of genetic risk into non-genetic risk prediction tools for complex traits. Furthermore, Murad et al. (2014) developed methods to evaluate a systematic review and meta-analysis and apply the results to patient care, whereas Dewey et al. (2014) described interpretation and implications of whole-genome sequencing in clinical practice. Lang et al. (2014) reported whole-exome sequencing to identify rare and low-frequency coding variants associated with LDL cholesterol. Ioanndis et al. (2014) emphasized the importance of reducing waste in research design and analysis to successfully accomplish EBPT. By employing type D personality as an example, he explained the concept of scientific inbreeding and same-team replication in EBPT. He also highlighted the expectations, validity and reality in omics analyses. By utilizing similar EBPT approach, Wong et al. (2009) described the reproducibility of computer-assisted joint alignment measurement in knee radiographs. Furthermore, Manarai et al. (2016) described novel methods to enhance reproducibility in PM to ultimately accomplish successful EBPT. All these recent and earlier discoveries suggest that EBPT can be accomplished by systematically conducting omics, imaging, and molecular diagnostic analyses simultaneously. Hence this multidisciplinary therapeutic approach has tremendous promise in future.

ACKNOWLEDGMENT

A significant portion of information provided in this chapter was derived from Dr. Margaret A. Hamburg's FDA report. The author acknowledge with thanks her contribution and leadership to advance EBPT for the health and well-beings of future generations. The author also acknowledges with thanks several other dedicated scientists for the information derived from Mr. Kendall Morgan's report).

REFERENCES

A Catalog of Published Genome-Wide Association Studies". Retrieved 28 June 2015.
Analyze Genomes: Motivation". Schapranow, Matthieu-P. Retrieved July 20, 2014.

Battle, A., S., Zhu, X., Potash, J. B., Weissman, M. M., McCormick, C., Haudenschild, C. D., Beckman, K. B., Shi, J., Mei, R., Urban, A. E., Montgomery, S. B., Levinson, D. F. & Koller, D. (2014). "Characterizing the genetic basis of transcriptome diversity through RNA-sequencing of 922 individuals". *Genome research, 24* (1), 14–24.

Bertram, L., McQueen, M. B., Mullin, K., Blacker, D. & Tanzi, R. E. (2007). Systematic meta-analyses of Alzheimer disease genetic association studies: the AlzGene database. *Nat Genet., 39*, 17–23

Bertram, H. C., Hoppe, C., Petersen, B. O., Duus, J. Ø., Mølgaard, C. & Michaelsen, K. F. (2007). An NMR-based metabonomic investigation on effects of milk and meat protein diets given to 8-year-old boys. *Br J Nutr., 97*, 758–763.

Biomarker Toolkit: Companion Diagnostics" (PDF). Amgen. Retrieved May 2, 2014.

Breast Cancer in the Personal Genomics Era". Current Genomics: Bentham Science. Retrieved April 28, 2014.

Bromley, C. M., Close, S., Cohen, N., Favis, R., Fijal, B., et al., (2009). Designing pharmacogenetic projects in industry: practical design perspectives from the Industry Pharmacogenomics Working Group. *Pharmacogenomics J., 9*, 14–22.

Can, C., Sarinay, C. E., Gun, B. W., Sophie, P. C., Spacek, Damek, S., Carlos L. A., Hua, T., Emiliano, R. & Michael, S. P. (2014). "Integrative analysis of RNA, translation, and protein levels reveals distinct regulatory variation across humans.". *Genome Research*. doi:10.1101/gr.193342.115. PMID 26297486.

Chabenne, A., Moon, C., Ojo, C., Khogali, A., Nepal, B. & Sharma, S. (2014). Biomarkers in Fetal Alcohol Syndrome (Recent Update) *Biomarkers and Genomic Medicine, 6*, 12-22.

Church, D., Kerr, R., Domingo, E., Rosmarin, D., Palles, C., Maskell, K., Tomlinson, I. & Kerr, D. (2014). "'Toxgnostics': an unmet need in cancer medicine". *Nat. Rev. Cancer, 6*, 440-445.

Colhoun, H. M., McKeigue, P. M. & Smith, D. G. (2003). Problems of reporting genetic associations with complex outcomes. *Lancet., 361*, 865–872.

Colombo, S., Rauch, A., Rotger, M., Fellay, J., Martinez, R., et al. (2008). The HCP5 single-nucleotide polymorphism: a simple screening tool for prediction of hypersensitivity reaction to abacavir. *J. Infect. Dis., 198*, 864–867.

Companion Diagnostics, (2014).

Connor, S. (2003). Glaxo chief: Our drugs do not work on most patients. The Independent. Available:http://www.independent.co.uk/news/science/glaxo-chief-our-drugs-do-not-work-on-most-patients-575942.html.

Dewey, F. E., Grove, M. E., Pan, C., Goldstein, B. A., Bernstein, J. A., Chaib, H., Merker, J. D., et al., (2014). Clinical interpretation and implications of whole-genome sequencing. *JAMA., 311*, 1035-1045.

Dudley, J. & Karczewski, K. (2014). Exploring Personal Genomics. Oxford: Oxford University Press.

Fact Sheet: BRCA1 and BRCA2: Cancer and Genetic Testing". National Cancer Institute (NCI). Retrieved April 28, 2014.

Frodsham, A. J. & Higgins, J. P. (2007). Online genetic databases informing human genome epidemiology. *BMC Med Res Methodol., 7*, 31.

Genetics Home Reference: What is pharmacogenomics?". National Institutes of Health (NIH). Retrieved April 28, 2014.

Goldstein, D. B., Tate, S. K. & Sisodiya, S. M. (2003). Pharmacogenetics goes genomic. *Nat Rev Genet., 4*, 937–947.

Goldstein, D. B. (2009). Common genetic variation and human traits. *N Engl J Med., 360*, 1696–1698.

Goldstein, B. A., Knowles, J. W., Salfati, E., Ioannidis, J. P. & Assimes, T. L. (2014). Simple, standardized incorporation of genetic risk into non-genetic risk prediction tools for complex traits: coronary heart disease as an example. *Front Genet., 5*, 254.

Genome Wide Association Studies, (2014).

Haines, J. L. (2005). "Complement Factor H Variant Increases the Risk of Age-Related Macular Degeneration". *Science, 308*, 419–421.

Higgins, J. P., Little, J., Ioannidis, J. P., Bray, M. S., Manolio, T. A., et al. (2007). Turning the pump handle: evolving methods for integrating the evidence on gene-disease association. *Am J Epidemiol., 166*, 863–866.

Hindorff, L. A., Mehta, J. P. & Manolio, T. A. (2009). A catalog of published genome-wide association studies. *National Human Genome Research Institute.,* (2009).

Holmes, M. V., Shah, T., Vickery, C., Smeeth, L., Hingorani, A. D. & Casas, J. P. (2009). Fulfilling the Promise of Personalized Medicine? Systematic Review and Field Synopsis of Pharmacogenetic Studies. *PLoS One., 2009, 4*(12), e7960.

Hunter, D. J., Altshuler, D. & Rader, D. J. (2008). From Darwin's finches to canaries in the coal mine–mining the genome for new biology. *N. Engl. J. Med., 358*, 2760–2763.

Huser, V., Sincan, M. & Cimino, J. J. (2014). "Developing genomic knowledge bases and databases to support clinical management: Current perspectives". *Pharmacogenomics and Personalized Medicine, 7*, 275–83.

Hynicka, L. M., Cahoon, W. D., Jr. & Bukaveckas, B. L. (2008). Genetic testing for warfarin therapy initiation. *Ann Pharmacother., 42*, 1298–1303.

Intellectual Property Issues Impacting the Future of PM". American Intellectual Property Law Association. Retrieved April 26, 2014.

Ioannidis, J. P., Boffetta, P., Little, J., O'Brien, T. R., Uitterlinden, A. G., et al. (2008). Assessment of cumulative evidence on genetic associations: interim guidelines. *Int. J. Epidemiol., 37*, 120–132.

Ioannidis, J. P., Gwinn, M., Little, J., Higgins, J. P., Bernstein, J. L., et al. (2006). A road map for efficient and reliable human genome epidemiology. *Nat Genet., 38*, 3–5.

Ioannidis, J. P., Ntzani, E. E., Trikalinos, T. A. & Contopoulos-Ioannidis, D. G. (2001). Replication validity of genetic association studies. *Nat Genet., 29*, 306–309.

Ioannidis, J. P., Ntzani, E. E. & Trikalinos, T. A. (2004). 'Racial' differences in genetic effects for complex diseases. *Nat Genet., 36*, 1312–1318.

Ioannidis, J. P., Trikalinos, T. A. & Khoury, M. J. (2006). Implications of small effect sizes of individual genetic variants on the design and interpretation of genetic association studies of complex diseases. *Am J Epidemiol., 164*, 609–614.

Ioannidis, J. P., Trikalinos, T. A., Ntzani, E. E. & Contopoulos-Ioannidis, D. G. (2003). Genetic associations in large versus small studies: an empirical assessment. *Lancet., 361*, 567–571.

Ioannidis, J. P. (2008). Effect of formal statistical significance on the credibility of observational associations. *Am. J. Epidemiol., 168*, 374–383.

Ioannidis, J. P. (2005). Why most published research findings are false. *PLoS Med., 2*, e124.

Ioannidis, J. P. (2010). Expectations, validity, and reality in omics. *J Clin Epidemiol.*, *63*(9), 945-949.

Ioannidis, J. P., Greenland, S., Hlatky, M. A., Khoury, M. J., Macleod, M. R., Moher, D., Schulz, K. F. & Tibshirani, R. (2014). Increasing value and reducing waste in research design, conduct, and analysis. *Lancet.*, *383*, 166-175.

Ioannidis, J. P. (2012). Scientific inbreeding and same-team replication: type D personality as an example. *J. Psychosom. Res.*, *73*(6), 408-410.

Jagtap, A., Gawande, S. & Sharma, S. (2015). Biomarkers in Vascular Dementia 6; (A Recent Update).

Jakobsdottir, J., Gorin, M. B., Conley, Y. P., Ferrell, R. E. & Weeks, D. E. (2009). Interpretation of genetic association studies: markers with replicated highly significant odds ratios may be poor classifiers. *PLoS Genet.*, *5*, e1000337.

Ghadimi, B. M. & Jo, P. (2016). Cancer Gene Profiling for Response Prediction. *Methods Mol Biol.*, *1381*, 163-179.

Jensen, E. H., McLoughlin, J. M. & Yeatman, T. J. (2006). Microarrays in gastrointestinal cancer: is personalized prediction of response to chemotherapy at hand? *Curr Opin Oncol.*, *18*(4), 374-380.

Klein, T. E., Altman, R. B., Eriksson, N., Gage, B. F., Kimmel, S. E., et al. (2009). Estimation of the warfarin dose with clinical and pharmacogenetic data. *N. Engl. J. Med.*, *360*, 753–764.

Kraft, P., Wacholder, S., Cornelis, M. C., Hu, F. B., Hayes, R. B., et al. (2009). Beyond odds ratios - communicating disease risk based on genetic profiles. *Nat Rev Genet.*

Lange, L. A., Hu, Y., Zhang, H., Xue, C., Schmidt, E. M. & Tang, Z. Z. (2014). Whole-exome sequencing identifies rare and low-frequency coding variants associated with LDL cholesterol. *Am J Hum Genet.*, *94*(2), 233-245.

Lemonick, M. D., Cray, D., Park, A., Thomas, C. B. & Thompson, D. (2009). Brave New Pharmacy. Time. 2001. Available: http:// www.time.com/ time/ magazine/ article/ 0,9171,998963-1,00.html Accessed 2009 November 10, URL: http:// www.webcitation. org/5lBD8FmTx.

Limdi, N. A., Arnett, D. K., Goldstein, J. A., Beasley, T. M., McGwin, G., et al. (2008). Influence of CYP2C9 and VKORC1 on warfarin dose, anticoagulation attainment and maintenance among European-Americans and African Americans. *Pharmacogenomics.*, *9*, 511–526.

Link, E., Parish, S., Armitage, J., Bowman, L., Heath, S., et al. (2008). SLCO1B1 variants and statin-induced myopathy–a genomewide study. *N. Engl. J. Med.*, *359*, 789–799.

Lu, Y. F., Goldstein, D. B., Angrist, M. & Cavalleri, G. (2014). "PM and human genetic diversity". *Cold Spring Harbor Perspectives in Medicine, 4* (9), a008581.

Manrai, A. K., Patel, C. J., Gehlenborg, N., Tatonetti, N. P., Ioannidis, J. P. & Kohane, I. S. (2016). Methods To Enhance The Reproducibility Of Precision Medicine. *Pac Symp Biocomput.*, *21*, 180-182.

McClain, M. R., Palomaki, G. E., Piper, M. & Haddow, J. E. (2008). A rapid-ACCE review of CYP2C9 and VKORC1 alleles testing to inform warfarin dosing in adults at elevated risk for thrombotic events to avoid serious bleeding. *Genet Med.*, *10*, 89–98

Mega, J. L., Close, S. L., Wiviott, S. D., Shen, L., Hockett, R. D., et al. (2009). Cytochrome p-450 polymorphisms and response to clopidogrel. *N. Engl. J. Med.*, *360*, 354–362.

Moher, D., Liberati, A., Tetzlaff, J. & Altman, D. G. (2009). Preferred reporting items for systematic reviews and meta-analyses: the PRISMA statement. *PLoS Med., 6*, e1000097.

Murad, M. H., Montori, V. M., Ioannidis, J. P., Jaeschke, R., Devereaux, P. J., Prasad, K., Neumann, I., Carrasco-Labra, A., Agoritsas, T., Hatala, R., Meade, M. O., Wyer, P., Cook, D. J. & Guyatt, G. (2014). How to read a systematic review and meta-analysis and apply the results to patient care: users' guides to the medical literature. *JAMA., 312*(2), 171-179.

Naci, H. & Ioannidis, J. P. (2015). How good is "evidence" from clinical studies of drug effects and why might such evidence fail in the prediction of the clinical utility of drugs? *Annu Rev Pharmacol Toxicol., 55*, 169-189.

Paving the Way for PM: FDA's Role in a New Era of Medical Product Development" (PDF). Federal Drug Administration (FDA). Retrieved April 28, 2014.

Pennisi, E. (2007). Breakthrough of the year. Human genetic variation. *Science., 318*, 1842–1843.

Pharmacogenomics. The Promise of PM" (PDF). *AAPS PharmSci*, 2000. January 28, 2000. Retrieved April 28, 2014.

Pirmohamed, M., James, S., Meakin, S., Green, C., Scott, A. K., et al. (2004). Adverse drug reactions as cause of admission to hospital: prospective analysis of 18 820 patients. *BMJ., 329*, 15–19.

PM 101: The Challenges". *PM Coalition.*, (2014).

Pollack, A. (2005). A Special Drug Just for You, At the End of a Long Pipeline. The New York Times.

Research Portfolio Online Reporting Tools: Human Genome Project". National Institutes of Health (NIH). Retrieved April 28, 2014.

Roses, A. D. (2000). Pharmacogenetics and the practice of medicine. *Nature.* 405, 857–865.

Saglio, G., Morotti, A., Mattioli, G., et al. (2004). "Rational approaches to the design of therapeutics targeting molecular markers: the case of chronic myelogenous leukemia". *Ann. N. Y. Acad. Sci., 1028*, 423–431.

Schizophrenia Gene (SZGene), Schizophrenia Research Forum. Accessed 2009 November 10, Available:http://www.schizophreniaforum.org/res/sczgene.

Sharma, S. (2014). Beyond Diet and Depression *(Volume-1)* Book Nova Sciences Publishers, New York, U.S.A.

Sharma, S. (2014). Beyond Diet and Depression *(Volume-2)* Book Nova Science Publishers, New York, U.S.A.

Sharma, S. (2015). Alleviating Stress of the Soldier & Civilian. Nova Science Publishers, New York. U.S.A.

Sharma, S. (2015). Monoamine Oxidase Inhibitors: Clinical Pharmacology, Benefits, & Adverse Effects. Nova Science Publishers, New York. U.S.A.

Sharma, S. & Ebadi, M. (2014). Charnoly body as a Universal Biomarker of Cell Injury. *Biomarkers and Genomic Medicine, 6.*

Sharma, S. & Ebadi, M. (2013). *In-Vivo* Molecular Imaging in Parkinson's Disease. In Parkinson's Disease. Eds. RF. Pfeiffer, ZK Wszolek, M. Ebadi. IInd Edition, Chapter 58, CRC Press Taylor & Francis Group. Boca Rotan, FL, USA. pp. 787-802.

Sharma, S. & Ebadi, M. (2014). Significance of Metallothioneins in Aging Brain. *Neurochemistry International., 65*, 40-48.

Sharma, S. & Ebadi, M. (2013). Antioxidant Targeting in Neurodegenerative Disorders. Ed. I. Laher, Springer Verlag. Germany. Chapter 85, p. 1-30.

Sharma, S., Gawande, S., Jagtap, A., Abeulela, R. & Salman, Z. (2014). Fetal Alcohol Syndrome; Prevention, Diagnosis, & Treatment. In Alcohol Abuse: Prevalence, Risk Factors. Nova Science Publishers, New York, U.S.A.

Sharma, S., Moon, C. S., Khogali, A., Haidous, A., Chabenne, A., Ojo, C., Jelebinkov, M., Kurdi, Y. & Ebadi, M. (2013). Biomarkers of Parkinson's Disease (Recent Update). *Neurochemistry International.*, *63*, 201-229.

Sharma, S., Nepal, B., Moon, C. S., Chabenne, A., Khogali, A., Ojo, C., Hong, E., Goudet, R., Sayed-Ahmad, A., Jacob, A., Murtaba, M. & Firlit, M. (2014). Psychology of Craving. Open Jr of *Medical Psychology.*, *3*, 120-125.

Sharma, S., Rais, A., Sandhu, R., Nel, W. & Ebadi, M. (2014). Clinical significance of metallothioneins in cell therapy and nanomedicine. *International Journal of Nanomedicine.*, *8*, 1477–1488.

Sharma, S. (2014). Molecular Pharmacology of Environmental Neurotoxins. In Kainic Acid: Neurotoxic Properties, Biological Sources, and Clinical Applications. Nova Science Publishers. New York. P1-47.

Sharma, S. (2014). Nanotheranostics in Evidence Based Personalized Medicine. *Current Drug Targets.*, *15*, 915-930.

Shungin, D., Winkler, T. W., Croteau-Chonka, D. C., Ferreira, T., et al., (2015). New genetic loci link adipose and insulin biology to body fat distribution. *Nature.*, *518*, 187-196.

Shurin, S. B. & Nabel, E. G. (2008). Pharmacogenomics–ready for prime time? *N. Engl. J. Med.*, *358*, 1061–1063.

Simon, T., Verstuyft, C., Mary-Krause, M., Quteineh, L., Drouet, E., et al., (2009). Genetic determinants of response to clopidogrel and cardiovascular events. *N Engl J Med.*, *360*, 363–375.

Snyderman, R. (2012). Personalized Health Care from Theory to Practice, *Biotechnology J.*, *7*.

Tang, S., Zhang, Z., Kavitha, G., Tan, E. K. & Ng, S. K. (2009). MDPD: an integrated genetic information resource for Parkinson's disease. *Nucleic Acids Res.*, *37*, D858–862.

Telli, M. L., Hunt, S. A., Carlson, R. W. & Guardino, A. E. (2007). "Trastuzumab-Related Cardiotoxicity: Calling Into Question the Concept of Reversibility". *Journal of Clinical Oncology, 25*, 3525–3533.

The Path to PM". *New England Journal of Medicine (NEJM).*, July 22, 2010.

Walter, C. (2006). "HER2/neu Status is an Important Biomarker in Guiding Personalized HER2/neu Therapy" (PDF). *Connection, 9*, 25–27.

What is Pharmacogenomics, (2014).

Wong, A. K., Inglis, D., Beattie, K. A., Doan, A., Ioannidis, G., Obeid, J., Adachi, J. D., Papaioannou, A., 2009. Reproducibility of computer-assisted joint alignment measurement in OA knee radiographs. *Osteoarthritis Cartilage.* 17(5), 579-585.

Woodcock, J. & Lesko, L. J. (2009). Pharmacogenetics–tailoring treatment for the outliers. *N. Engl. J. Med.*, *360*, 811–813.

Wu, L., Candille, S. I., Choi, Y., Xie, D., Jiang, L., Li-Pook-Than J., Tang, H. & Michael
Snyder, M. (2013). "Variation and genetic control of protein abundance in humans".
Nature, 499, 79–82.

Xie, H. G. & Fruch, F. W. (2005). Pharmacogenomics steps toward personalized medicine.
Personalized Medicine., 2, 325-337.

Chapter 2

PET BIOMARKERS IN EVIDENCE-BASED PERSONALIZED THERANOSTICS (RECENT UPDATE)

ABSTRACT

In general, PET imaging utilizes RPs labeled with positron-emitting radionuclides (^{11}C, ^{18}F, ^{64}Cu, ^{68}Ga) to visualize *in vivo* cellular metabolism, while SPECT imaging utilizes ^{99m}Tc or ^{123}I as γ-emitting radionuclides with high-spatial resolution, sensitivity, and specificity. Recently ^{18}FdG PET/CT in theranostic evaluation of pediatric malignancies and radiation exposure issues have been highlighted. In addition, ^{68}Ga-Aquibeprin and ^{68}Ga-Avebetrin as complementary biomarkers have been developed to target integrins $\alpha_5\beta_1$ and $\alpha_v\beta_3$ for the evaluation of tumor angiogenesis by PET imaging. In addition, *Azamacrocyclic Bifunctional Chelating Agents* (BCAs) have proved beneficial for PET imaging of multiple myeloma and ^{18}F-FPRGD2 PET/CT imaging for the early detection of musculoskeletal diseases. PET/MRI has emerged as an excellent approach for the clinical evaluation of upper abdomen malignancies to accomplish the ultimate goal of EBPT. ^{18}F-Fluoride PET imaging has emerged to determine vulnerable coronary plaques. Although PET imaging has superior quantitative capabilities, ^{123}I-MIBG SPECT is being utilized for the routine clinical evaluation of patients with heart failure and for the clinicl assessment of cardiac and coronary blood flow because it is economical, simple, and easily available to the patient in emergency. Recently an automated production of 6-[^{18}F]fluoro-L-DOPA and 2-[^{18}F]fluoro-L-tyrosine on a *GE FastLab Synthesizer* in conjuction with HPLC purification was developed for the clinical evaluation of PD and other neurological patients, in addition to PET imaging biomarkers for the therapeutic evaluation of brain tumors with radiolabeled amino acids. ^{11}C or ^{18}F-labelled Choline is preferred over ^{18}FdG to acquire better quality images with minimum BKg, particularly in the clinical management of malignant gliomas. The clinical utility of radiometals as PET imaging agents for drug delivery systems and the theranostic potential of ^{11}C-Choline in hepatocellular carcinoma, evaluating tumor metabolism by PET imaging, ^{18}FdG-PET/CT imaging of osteomyelitis, breast cancer and other gynecological cancers, integrated ^{18}FdG-PET/CT and MRI in oesophageal cancers, endoradiotherapy of prostate cancer using DOTA conjugated PSMA is highlighted in this chapter. Particularly, recent advances in ^{18}F or ^{64}Cu-Labeled Tenascin-C aptamer as an excellent personalized theranostic biomarker of cancer, and in multimodality fusion imaging (*including PET/MRI in AD diagnosis and cancer management*) and its impact on dose are discussed briefly. Furthermore combined ^{18}F-NaF/^{18}F-FDG PET/CT outperformed CT alone and was highly sensitive and specific for the early detection of osseous metastases. This chapter provides recent update on the comparative analyses of multimodality *in-vivo* imaging employing conventional as well as recently developed novel PET-RPs to accomplish EBPT.

Keywords: $\alpha_5\beta_1$ and $\alpha_v\beta_3$ integrins, ^{68}Ga-aquibeprin, ^{68}Ga-avebetrin, ^{18}F-FPRGD2 PET/CT imaging, multimodality fusion imaging, evidence based personalized theranostics (EBPT)

INTRODUCTION

It is now very well established that PET is an *in-vivo* functional imaging modality that measures pathophysiological status of disease noninvasively, and has become a key component for innovative drug delivery system (DDS) studies. PET is a molecular imaging technique that utilizes RPs labeled with positron-emitting radionuclides (^{11}C, ^{18}F, ^{64}Cu, ^{68}Ga) to visualize *in vivo* cellular metabolism, while SPECT utilizes ^{99m}Tc or ^{123}I as γ-emitting radionuclides with high-spatial resolution, sensitivity, and specificity. Besides being a powerful tool for diagnosis (*mostly in oncology with ^{18}FdG*), PET imaging can provide information about biochemical mechanisms in living tissues or interactions between neurotransmitter and brain receptors. In this chapter recent advances in PET imaging for personalized theranostics are described briefly. This multi-disciplinary field of nuclear medicine is now evolving to develop novel PET biomarkers as molecular probes for successful EBPT of various neurodegenerative disorders, cardiovascular disorders, and cancer. Particularly PET imaging has played a pivotal role in the early theranostics of Cancer and AD. Recently Deng and Wang (2015) highlighted that the development of multifunctional chelating agents is critical for developing PET RPs and therefore has become a demanding research topic. The optimal chelators should be readily attached to biomolecules covalently, able to form stable complexes with radiometals, and demonstrate good bio-distribution pattern *in vivo*. Indeed, the selection of suitable chelators can facilitate the development of an effective PET imaging probe by improving targeting properties and providing favorable *in vivo* PKs of radiolabeled probes.

This chapter focuses on the recent developments of multifunctional chelators that are suitable for both imaging and radiation therapy to accomplish theranostic capabilities. The chapter describes recent developments in the localization of tumor angiogenesis employing ^{68}Ga-Aquibeprin and ^{68}Ga-Avebetrin, ^{18}F-FPRGD2 PET/CT imaging to examine musculoskeltal lesions, and azamacrocyclic bifunctional chelating agents (BCAs) for PET imaging of multiple myeloma, and the clinical utility of radiometals as PET imaging and other agents to accomplish EBPT for the knowledge of a beginner and for the refreshment of experienced nuclear medicine experts.

^{68}Ga-Aquibeprin and ^{68}Ga-Avebetrin to Evaluate Tumor Angiogenesis Although in-vivo mapping of integrin $\alpha_v\beta_3$ expression was extensively investigated recently, its clinical significance still remains enigmatic. For imaging of angiogenesis, the integrin subtype $\alpha_5\beta_1$ is a promising target, for which Notni et al. (2015) developed [68]G-Aquibeprin as a PET radiopharmaceutical. These investigators synthesized Ga-Aquibeprin by click-chemistry (CuAAC) trimerization of a $\alpha_5\beta_1$ -integrin binding pseudopeptide on the TRAP chelator, followed by ^{68}Ga labeling. Integrin $\alpha_5\beta_1$ and $\alpha_v\beta_3$ affinities were determined by ELISA on immobilized integrins, using Fibronectin and Vitronectin, respectively, as competitors. Human melanoma bearing SCID mice (M21) were used for bio-distribution, PET imaging, and determination of *in-vivo* metabolism. Expression of α_5 and β_3 subunits was determined by immunohistochemistry (IHC) on paraffine embedded sections of M21 tumors. ^{68}Ga-Aquibeprin exhibited high selectivity for integrin $\alpha_5\beta_1$ over $\alpha_v\beta_3$, and hydrophilicity. SCID mice xenografted with M21 human melanoma were highly suitable for *in-vivo* evaluation, as M21 IHC showed not only an endothelial and cytoplasmatic expression of the β_3 integrin subunit, but also an expression of the α_5 integrin subunit in the endothelium of intratumoral microvessels. Ex-vivo bio-distribution (90 min p.i.) showed high uptake in M21 tumor, fast renal excretion, and reduced background; tumor-to-blood and -muscle ratios were 10.6 ± 2.5 and 20.9 ± 2.4. ^{68}Ga-Aquibeprin was stable *in vivo as* no metabolites were detected in mouse urine, blood serum, kidney and liver homogenate 30 min p.i. PET imaging was performed for ^{68}Ga-Aquibeprin and the structurally related c(RGDfK) trimer ^{68}Ga-Avebetrin, which revealed an inverse selectivity for integrin $\alpha_v\beta_3$ over $\alpha_5\beta_1$. *In-vivo* target specificity was confirmed by competition studies; tumor uptake of either tracer was not affected by co-administration of ~5 mg/kg of the respective other compound, indicating that ^{68}Ga-Aquibeprin and ^{68}Ga-Avebetrin may be recommended for complementary imaging of integrins $\alpha_5\beta_1$ and $\alpha_v\beta_3$ by PET, to evaluate their role in angiogenesis, tumor progression, metastasis, and myocardial infarct healing.

Azamacrocyclic Bifunctional Chelating Agents (BCAs) for PET Imaging of Multiple Myeloma Recently Azamacrocyclic bifunctional chelating agents (BCAs) proved essential for the development of PET RPs. Halime et al. (2015) established that their bioconjugation by a function on a carbon atom of the macrocyclic skeleton is suitable to maintain their *in vivo* inertness. By using a bisaminal template and selective N-alkylation approach, these investigators developed conjugable C-functionalized teta, te2a and cb-te2a as promising chelators for PET and radioimmunotherapy (RIT) because of their better complexation properties than DOTA or DOTA-like macrocycles, especially with ^{64}Cu or [67]Cu radionuclides. Chelators bear an isothiocyanate grafting function which is introduced by C-alkylation to avoid reduction in their chelating properties. These researchers reported that their synthesis is highly efficient and yields the targeted ligands, teta-Ph-NCS, te2a-Ph-NCS and cb-te2a-Ph-NCS and could be extended to other cyclam based-BCAs. The newly synthetized te2a-Ph-NCS was conjugated to an anti mCD138 monoclonal antibody (mAb) to evaluate its *in vivo* behavior as BCA and to explore PET-phenotypic imaging in multiple myeloma (MM). Mass spectrometric analysis of the immunoconjugate revealed that up to 4 chelates are conjugated per 9E7.4 mAb. The radiolabeling yield and specific activity of 9E7.4-CSN-Ph-te2a were 95 ± 2.8% and 188 ± 27 MBq mg(-1) respectively and the immunoreactivity of [64]Cu-9E7.4-CSN-Ph-te2a was 81 ± 7%. Animal experiments were carried out on 5T33-Luc(+) tumor bearing mice, either in s.c or orthotopic. For PET imaging, mice were injected with [64]Cu-9E7.4-CNS-Ph-te2a and acquisitions were made 2 and 20 h post-injection (PI). A bone uptake was localized in a sacroiliac of a MM orthotopic tumor. Nonspecific uptakes were observed at 2 h PI but a significant decrease was observed at 20 h PI which improved the contrast of the images.

18F-FPRGD2 PET*/CT for Musculosketal Diseases* A study was performed on musculoskeletal uptake of ^{18}F-FPRGD2, targeting the integrin αvβ3, in patients who had undergone ^{18}F-FPRGD2 PET and CT (PET/CT) for oncologic purposes (Withofs et al. 2015). These investigators reviewed whole-body ^{18}F-FPRGD2 PET/CT Images of 62 cancer patients to detect focal musculoskeletal ^{18}F-FPRGD2 uptake. A [18]FdG PET/CT was available for 37 patients. In each joint with an abnormal uptake, the SUV_{max} was estimated. In addition to 27 miscellaneous foci, a total of 260 musculoskeletal foci of ^{18}F-FPRGD2 uptake were detected in joints and discs (n = 160), entheses (osteotendinous and osteoligamentous junctions; n = 55) and recent fractures (n = 18). Out of the 146 lesions, 63% showed both ^{18}F-FPRGD2 and [18]FdG uptake, 33.6% did not show [18]FdG avidity and 3.4% showed only [18]FdG uptake. The uptake of the 92 lesions positive with ^{18}F-FPRGD2 and [18]FdG was similar with both RPs, but the blood pool or muscle ratios were significantly higher with ^{18}F-FPRGD2 than with [18]FdG, indicating that the ^{18}F-FPRGD2 uptake in joints, spine degenerative diseases and tendons was prevalent in their patients. One-third of ^{18}F-FPRGD2 foci showed no [18]FdG uptake suggesting that ^{18}F-FPRGD2 signal may not be exclusively related to inflammatory angiogenesis.

18F Dose Calibration As a result of a recent change in the National Institute of Standards and Technology (NIST) activity standard for ^{18}F, Zimmerman et al. (2015) determined new relative response ratios for a [68]Ge solid epoxy mock syringe source used in activity calibrators as a long-lived substitute for [18]F. New standardized solutions of each radionuclide were used to determine the response ratios while maintaining traceability to national standards, which updated published data from 2010. Following published methodology, solution-filled mock syringe sources, identical in geometry to the solid [68]Ge epoxy calibration source, were prepared using NIST-calibrated solutions of [68]$GeCl_4$ and [18]FdG and compared in several models of activity calibrators to determine the relative response ratios for these 2 radionuclides. The relative response ratios reflected the change in ^{18}F activity measurements from the recent -4% change in the NIST activity standard. The results allowed the [68]Ge activity of the mock syringe to be expressed in terms of equivalent ^{18}F activity, with uncertainty of about 0.8% for the activity calibrators, which revised previously derived relative response ratios for ^{18}F and [68]Ge by -3.7%, allowing commercial mock syringe surrogate source to calibrate their activity calibrators consistent with the recent change in the NIST ^{18}F standard.

PET Imaging in Drug Delivery Systems PET is a functional imaging modality that measures pathophysiology of disease noninvasively, and has become a key component for innovative drug delivery system (DDS) studies. Deng et al. (2015) highlighted that the development of multifunctional chelating agents is critical for developing PET RPs and has become a demanding research topic. The optimal chelators should be readily attached to biomolecules covalently, to form stable complexes with radiometals, and demonstrate good bio-distribution pattern *in vivo, which can be accomplished by* suitable chelators to develop an effective PET imaging probe by improving targeting properties and providing favorable PKs of radiolabeled probes. These investigators focused on the recent developments of multifunctional chelators that are suitable for both imaging and radiation therapy to accomplish EBPT.

18FdG PET/CT in Theranostic Evaluation of Pediateric Malignancies Uslu et al. (2015) reported that successful management of solid tumors in pediatric population requires noninvasive in-vivo imaging for accurate disease detection, characterization, and therapeutic monitoring. Technologic developments aim toward the creation of integrated imaging approaches that provide a comprehensive diagnosis in a single visit. These integrated diagnostic tests not only are convenient for young patients but also save direct and indirect health-care costs by streamlining procedures, minimizing hospitalizations and lost school or work time for children and their parents. [18]FdG PET/CT is a sensitive and specific imaging modality for whole-body evaluation of pediatric malignancies. However, concerns about ionizing radiation exposure have led to a search for alternative imaging modalities, such as whole-body MRI and PET/MRI. With the development of new approaches, it will be highly prudent to understand current benchmarks. These investigators attempted to synthesize literature on [18]FdG PET/CT for tumor staging in children, summarizing questions that have been solved and providing an outlook on unsolved issues.

PET & SPECT RPs for AD It is known that AD is a chronic neurodegenerative disorder and the most common cause of dementia among elderly population. The two main pathological hallmarks of AD are senile plaques (SPs) composed of Aβ peptides and neurofibrillary tangles (NFTs) of hyperphosphorylated tau protein, associated with a cholinergic deficit. While the process leading to the development of AD is complex and multifactorial, and the etiology of AD is not exactly known, this multifaceted illness requires combined therapeutic approach. Because definite diagnosis is achieved by postmortem examination of the brain, new noninvasive diagnostic imaging modalities for AD are in increasing demand, to detect and monitor the progression of this illness, and evaluate the efficacy of treatments. The good correlation of the density and neocortical spread of neurofibrillary tangles (NFTs) with disease progression offers an opportunity for the early diagnosis and staging using PET imaging (Ariza et al., 2015). Thus, PET imaging of NFTs not only holds promise as a diagnostic tool but also enables the development of disease modifying therapeutics for AD. These investigators highlighted on the structural diversity of tau PET tracers, the challenges related to the identification of high affinity and highly selective NFT ligands, and the development of tau PET radioligands. Oukoloff et al. (2015) highlighted the recent advances in PET and SPECT imaging of AD pathophysiology. Several RPs were developed for imaging the lesions in AD patients. Recently Ariza et al. (2015) reported on the past, present, and future of Tau PET imaging in the clinical management of AD. Tau aggregates and Aβ plaques can now be quantified by specific radioligands, leading to new FDA approved Pittsburgh's compound, ^{18}F-Florbitapir.

Automated Synthesis of ^{18}F-DOPA and ^{18}F-TYR on a GE FASTlab Synthesizer Lemaire et al. (2015) reported an efficient, fully automated, enantioselective synthesis of no-carrier-added (nca) 6-[([18])F]fluoro-L-dopa ([([18])F]FDOPA) and 2-[([18])F]fluoro-L-tyrosine ([([18])F]FTYR) on a GE FASTlab synthesizer in conjunction with HPLC purification. A PTC (phase-transfer catalyst) strategy was used to synthesize these PET RPs. The automation of the whole process was implemented in GE FASTlab module, with slight hardware modification using single use cassettes and HPLC. ^{18}F-DOPA and ^{18}F-TYR were produced in 36.3 ± 3.0% and 50.5 ± 2.7% radiochemical yield. The automated radiosynthesis required ~ 52 min. Total synthesis time including HPLC purification and formulation was ~62 min. Enantiomeric excesses for these two aromatic amino acids were >95%, and the specific activity was >740 GBq/μmol. This automated synthesis module provided high specific activity ^{18}F-DOPA and ^{18}F-TYR (>37 GBq EOS). GE FASTlab Synthesizer is fully adaptable for the production and could be implemented into a GMP environment.

^{123}I-MIBG SPECT for Patients with Heart Failure. Heart failure (HF) is characterized by activation of the sympathetic cardiac nerves. Recently Dimitriu-Leen et al. (2015) reported that the condition of cardiac sympathetic nerves can be evaluated by ^{123}I-Meta-iodobenzylguanidine [^{123}I-MIBG] imaging. Most cardiac ^{123}I-MIBG studies have relied on measurements from anterior planar images of the chest. However, it has become more common to include SPECT imaging in clinical and research protocols. These investigators examined recent trends in ^{123}I-MIBG SPECT imaging to provide the basis for its increased use in the clinical management of patients with HF. ^{123}I-MIBG SPECT proved complementary to planar imaging in patients with HF in studies of coronary artery disease after an acute myocardial infarction. Moreover, ^{123}I-MIBG SPECT was used to document regional denervation for arrhythmic event risk assessment. For better quantification of the size and severity of innervation abnormalities in ^{123}I-MIBG SPECT, protocols specifically for ^{123}I were developed. Furthermore, the introduction of new solid-state cameras created the potential for more rapid SPECT acquisitions or a reduction in RPs activity. Although PET imaging has superior quantitative capabilities, ^{123}I-MIBG SPECT is the widely available imaging method for assessing regional myocardial sympathetic innervation.

Assessment of Myocardial Blood Flow with SPECT It is realized that the quantitative assessment of myocardial blood flow (MBF) and coronary flow reserve (CFR) may be useful for the functional evaluation of coronary artery disease, allowing judgment of its severity, tracking of disease progression, and evaluation of the anti-ischemic efficacy of therapeutic strategies. Petretta et al. (2015) reported that quantitative estimates of myocardial perfusion and CFR can be derived from SPECT myocardial perfusion imaging. However, this method underestimates CFR, particularly at high flow rates. The recent introduction of cardiac-dedicated γ-cameras with solid-state detectors provides efficient perfusion imaging with improved resolution, allowing fast acquisition of dynamic functional images, holds great promise for MBF and CFR quantification with dynamic SPECT.

[18]F-Fluoride PET Imaging to Determine Vulnerable Coronary Plaques It is known that ischemic vascular events occur in relation to an underlying vulnerable plaque. The pathological hallmarks of high-risk plaques include inflammation and microcalcification. To date, non-invasive imaging have lacked the spatial resolution to detect these processes with precision to facilitate theranostic utility. PET imaging using targeted RPs confers a sensitive tool for identifying features of interest. Recent developments created hybrid imaging platforms which add the detailed spatial resolution of CT and imaging of individual coronary plaques feasible. In a study Adamson et al. (2015) compared the utility of PET-CT using ^{18}F-Fluoride and to detect high-risk or ruptured atherosclerotic plaques *in vivo*. ^{18}F-Fluoride localized to culprit and vulnerable plaques was determined by a combination of invasive imaging and histological tissue examination. However [18]FdG analysis was compromised by non-specific myocardial uptake that obscured the coronary arteries. These investigators discussed the limitations of this approach for vulnerable plaque assessment and current developments in cardiovascular imaging with [18]Fluoride.

Evaluation of Hepatocellular Carcinoma by Multimodality Imaging and ^{11}C-Choline-PET In recent decades, the use of RPs in the assessment of hepatocellular carcinoma (HCC) was established, and recent findings indicate that radiolabelled choline has considerable promise in this setting. Lopci et al. (2015) assessed the theranostic potential of ^{11}C-Choline PET (PET)/CT, compared with CT/MRI, in patients with HCC. The study comprised 45 patients (male to female ratio = 37:8, median age 70.5 years) referred owing to HCC: 27 at initial diagnosis and 18 for restaging after recurrence. In all cases whole-body ^{11}C-Choline PET/CT was performed and compared with contrast-enhanced CT or MRI or both for a total of 50 paired scans. The reference standard was either histological proof or a multidisciplinary consensus. Diagnostic accuracy was determined in a scan-based (SBA) and a lesion-based analysis (LBA). On SBA the sensitivity and specificity for PET were 88 and 90%, respectively, whereas for CT/MRI they were 90 and 73%, respectively. On LBA the sensitivity and specificity were 78 and 86%, respectively, for PET vs 65 and 55% for CT/MRI. Overall these researchers investigated 168 disease sites, of which 100 were in the liver and 68 were extrahepatic. When considering only liver lesions, ^{11}C-Choline PET and CT/MRI showed an accuracy of 66 and 85%, respectively, while for extrahepatic lesions PET showed an accuracy of 9 %, while the accuracy of CT/MRI was only 32%. In both cases, there was a significant difference in accuracy between the two modalities. Combination of the PET imaging with those of CT/MRI resulted in the highest diagnostic accuracy in both analyses, at 92% for SBA and 96% for LBA. In 11 patients the PET findings modified the therapeutic strategy, the modification proving appropriate in 10 of them, suggesting that ^{11}C-Choline PET shows good accuracy in investigating patients with HCC and prompts a change in treatment planning in one fourth of patients. The main strength of ^{11}C-choline PET/CT was in its ability to detect extrahepatic HCC localizations, but the combination with conventional imaging modalities allowed for the highest diagnostic accuracy.

PET/MRI of the Upper Abdomen Although PET/CT and contrast-enhanced CT were considered in the diagnosis of upper abdominal malignancies, it can be challenging in soft tissue delineation, especially in the upper abdomen. Gavra et al. (2015) reported recent development in PET/MRI with MRI providing superior soft tissue contrast and PET providing biochemical and metabolic information. These investigators emphasized that combined PET/MRI may allow simultaneous benefit in the assessment of patients in a single session, improving patient journey, lesion detectability, diagnostic performance, and prognostic information to accomplish the long quested goal of EBPT. PET/MRI also provides the ability for tissue characterization and reduces radiation exposure. The most powerful driver is PET, and the newer PET RPs with the addition of contrast-enhanced MRI, diffusion-weighted imaging, and MR spectroscopy increase the sensitivity and specificity of disease recognition. These investigators also highlighted the merits and limitations of PET/MRI in upper abdominal malignancies.

^{18}FdG-PET/CT Imaging of Differentiated Thyroid Carcinoma Recently ^{18}FdG-PET/CT has emerged as an important theranostic tool for the postoperative management of patients with differentiated thyroid cancer (DTC) and it is extensively used in selected clinical situations (Salvatori et al., 2015). Particularly, ^{18}FdG-PET/CT can be used to obtain prognostic information in patients with increased Thyroglobulin (Tg) levels and negative ^{131}I whole-body scan post-thyroidectomy and radioiodine (RAI) ablation. ^{18}FdG-PET/CT may also have promise in the initial staging and follow-up of high-risk patients with aggressive histological subtypes, in the identification of patients who are at the highest risk of disease-specific mortality, in the management of patients with RAI-refractory disease, in clinical trials of targeted therapies in patients with advanced metastatic disease, and in the evaluation of thyroid nodules with indeterminate fine-needle aspiration for cytology. However, several controversies including: the cutoff value of Tg in the selection of DTC patients for FDG-PET/CT, whether FDG-PET/CT imaging should be performed under thyrotropin stimulation or suppression, and the clinical significance of thyroid FDG-PET/CT incidentalomas yet remain to be resolved. These investigators provided an overview of the molecular basis,

clinical indications, and controversies regarding the use of ^{18}FdG-PET/CT in patients with DTC.

Endoradiotherapy of Prostate Cancer Using DOTA Conjugated PSMA Despite remarkable advances in the past years, the treatment of metastatic prostate cancer still remains challenging. In recent years, prostate-specific membrane antigen (PSMA) inhibitors were studied to develop low-molecular-weight ligands for imaging prostate cancer by PET or SPECT. However, the endoradiotherapeutic use of these compounds requires optimization with radionuclide-chelating agent and the linker moiety between chelator and pharmacophore, which influence the overall PKs of the resulting radioligand. In an effort to realize both detection and optimal treatment of prostate cancer, a tailor-made novel naphthyl-containing DOTA-conjugated PSMA inhibitor was developed. Benešová et al. (2015) synthesized the peptidomimetic structure by solid-phase peptide chemistry and characterized using reversed-phase HPLC and matrix-assisted laser desorption/ionization mass spectrometry. Subsequent $^{67/68}$Ga and ^{177}Lu labeling resulted in radiochemical yields of >97% or >99%, respectively. Competitive binding and internalization experiments were performed using the PSMA-positive LNCaP cell line. The *in vivo* biodistribution and dynamic small-animal PET imaging studies were investigated in BALB/c nu/nu mice bearing LNCaP xenografts. The chemically modified PSMA inhibitor PSMA-617 demonstrated radiolytic stability for 72 h. A high inhibition potency (equilibrium dissociation constant [K (i)] = 2.34 ± 2.94 nM on LNCaP; K (i) = 0.37 ± 0.21 nM) and highly efficient internalization into LNCaP cells were demonstrated. The microPET imaging demonstrated high tumor-to-background ratios as early as 1 h after injection. Organ distribution revealed specific uptake in LNCaP tumors and in the kidneys 1 h after injection. With regard to therapeutic use, the compound exhibited a rapid clearance from the kidneys from 113.3 ± 24.4 at 1 h to 2.13 ± 1.36 percentage injected dose per gram at 24 h. The favorable PKs of the molecule led to tumor-to-background ratios of 1,058 (tumor to blood) and 529 (tumor to muscle), respectively, 24 h after injection, suggesting that DOTA-conjugated PSMA inhibitor PSMA-617 is refined and advanced with respect to its tumor-targeting and PKs by systematic chemical modification of the linker region. Hence it is suitable for theranostic application and may help to improve the clinical management of prostate cancer in the future.

Evaluation of Tumor Metabolism by PET Imaging Lewis et al. (2015) reported that PET is a sensitive clinical imaging modality for evaluating tumor metabolism. Radiolabeled PET substrates can be traced at subphysiological concentrations, allowing noninvasive imaging of metabolism and intra-tumoral heterogeneity ranging from advanced cancer models to patients. Many PET radiotracers can be used to investigate carbohydrate, amino acid, and fatty acid metabolism of the tumor. These investigators discussed the more established metabolic tracers and recent studies on the development of new radiotracers. New technical developments, such as combined PET/MRI, could provide new imaging solutions to the diagnostic challenges in cancer medicine.

Multimodality Imaging and the Impact on Radiation Dose Mattson et al. (2015) reported that novel imaging technologies employing X-rays and RPs have developed tremendously. Indeed clinical application of CT has revolutionized medical imaging and plays an important role in medical care. Due to technical improvements, spatial, contrast and temporal resolutions have improved. In spite of significant reduction of CT doses, CT is still a dominating source of radiation exposure. Combinations with SPECT and PET and especially the use of SPECT/CT and PET/CT, provide additional information about physiology as well as cellular and molecular events and health and disease. However, significant dose contributions from SPECT and PET occur, making PET/CT and SPECT/CT high dose procedures. These investigators suggested more research to find optimal activities of RPs for various patients. Encouraged hydration, forced diuresis and use of optimized voiding intervals, laxatives, etc., can reduce the radiation exposure to the patients. The staff doses to fingers, hands and eye lenses indicated that finger doses could be a serious problem.

^{18}FdG-PET/CT Vs ^{99m}Tc-MIBI Imaging in the Evaluation of Cold Thyroid Nodules Recent studies reported that SUVs of ^{18}FdG-PET imaging might predict malignant thyroid nodules and can be used in the preoperative evaluation of thyroid lesions. Sager et al. (2015) evaluated ^{18}FdG-PET imaging in patients with cold thyroid nodules and compared the imaging findings with ^{99m}Tc -MIBI imaging and with post-op histopathology results. Twenty-three patients (18F, 5M) with 24 nodules that were suspicious in ultrasound and cold in ^{99m}Tc scan, were included in the study. Each nodule underwent sonographically guided fine-needle aspiration biopsy. ^{18}FdG-PET and MIBI imaging were performed with an interval of 3-5 days. All patients underwent thyroidectomy and their ^{18}FdG-PET, and MIBI thyroid imaging results were compared with post-thyroidectomy pathology results. Post-op histopathology results found 7 malignant and 17 benign nodules. Six of the seven malignant nodules had increased uptake, which were positive for malignancy in both PET and MIBI imaging. Each imaging method used different radiopharmaceuticals but showed one false-negative result in two different patients. ^{18}FdG-PET produced false positives in 8 nodules and MIBI images found false positives in 4 nodules. ^{18}FdG-PET imaging and MIBI imaging showed the same sensitivity in malignant nodule evaluation, but their specificity differed, suggesting that ^{18}FdG-PET imaging was not superior to MIBI imaging in differentiating malignant from benign thyroid nodules. Hence MIBI imaging should be the first choice in the preoperative evaluation of patients with cold thyroid nodules as an adjunct procedure to FNAB owing to its low cost and easy availability. Moreover this imaging can be performed routinely in patients who are hesitant to undergo FNAB.

PET/MRI Based AD Diagnosis Recent advances in neuroimaging technology and image analysis algorithms have significantly contributed to a better understanding of spatial and temporal aspects of brain change associated with AD. Unschuld (2015) demonstrated how functional (fMRI) and structural MRI may be used to identify distinct patterns of brain change associated with disease progression and increased risk for AD. Moreover, PET based measures of glucose metabolism (^{18}FdG) and Aβ plaque density (^{11}C-Pittsburgh Compound B, PiB and ^{18}F) have great theranostic potential for assessing personalized AD-pathology to complement the information provided by MRI and other clinical measures.

PET/MRI in Cancer Management The most recent multimodality technique, the hybrid PET/MRI combines two different technologies. The combined PET/MRI has significant potentials in clinical oncology providing new perspectives of functional and anatomical information. PET/MRI offers simultaneous estimates of multifunctional data such as PET mapping by specific radiotracers or MRI morphologic, MR molecular (MR spectroscopy, MRS), or MR functional (fMR) information *in vivo* as recently reported by Borbely (2015).

PET/CT Analyses of Cancer Recently Lu et al. (2015) reported that current cancer therapy strategy is generally population based, however, there are large differences in tumor response among patients. Hence it is important to know personalized tumor response. Many studies proposed the use of computerized PET/CT image analysis in the evaluation of tumor response. Computerized analysis has overcome limitations of qualitative and semiquantitative analysis and led to improved theransotic accuracy. These investigators summarized these studies in four steps: *(a) image registration, (b) tumor segmentation, (c) image feature extraction and (d) response evaluation*. They also proposed future works and possible challenges.

^{18}F or ^{64}Cu-Labeled Tenascin-C Aptamer as an EBPT Biomarker of Cancer It is known that Tenascin-C is an extracellular matrix glycoprotein that is expressed by injured tissues and by various cancers. Recent studies demonstrated that Tenascin-C expression by cancer lesions can predict tumor growth, metastasis, and angiogenesis, suggesting its significance as a potential therapeutic target. Currently there is no noninvasive method to determine tumoral Tenascin-C expression *in vivo*. To address the need for an agent to image and quantify Tenascin-C, Jacobson et al. (2015) reported the development of a radioactive PET tracer based on a Tenascin-C-specific single-stranded DNA aptamer (*Tenascin-C Aptamer*). These investigators radiolabeled Tenascin-C aptamer with ^{18}F and ^{64}Cu for PET imaging for the evaluation of tumor uptake. PKs of Tenascin-C aptamer was performed in comparison to a nonspecific scrambled aptamer (Sc aptamer). The labeled Tenascin-C aptamer provided clear visualization of Tenascin-C-positive but not Tenascin-C-negative tumors. The uptake of Tenascin-C aptamer was significantly higher than that of Sc aptamer in Tenascin-C-positive tumors. The labeled Tenascin-C aptamer had fast clearance from the blood and through the kidneys, resulting in high tumor contrast, suggesting that labeled Tenascin-C aptamer can be used as an excellent EBPT PET biomarker to image tumor expression of Tenascin-C with a high tumor-to-background ratio and might provide personalized medical data to determine appropriate tumor theranostics.

Molecular Targeting of Breast Cancer Humbert et al. (2015) described that the potential utility of PET RPs in the setting of response monitoring in breast cancer, with a special emphasis on glucose metabolic changes assessed with ^{18}FdG. In the neoadjuvant setting of breast cancer, the metabolic response can predict the final complete pathologic response after the first cycles of chemotherapy. Because tumor metabolic behavior depends on cancer subtype, studies are ongoing to define the optimal metabolic criteria of tumor response in each subtype. The recent multi-centric randomized AVATAXHER trial suggested, in the human epidermal growth factor 2-positive subtype, a clinical benefit of early tailoring the neoadjuvant treatment in women with poor metabolic response after the first course of treatment. In the bone-dominant metastatic setting, ^{18}FdG-PET/CT is the most accurate imaging modality for the assessment of tumor response to treatment when both metabolic information and morphologic information are considered. Nevertheless, there is a need to better define standardized metabolic criteria of response, including the heterogeneity of response, and to evaluate the costs and health outcome of ^{18}FdG-PET/CT compared with conventional imaging. New non-^{18}FdG radiotracers highlighting specific molecular biomarkers of breast cancer cells have emerged in the clinical evaluation of cancer, which can take into account the heterogeneity of tumor biology in metastatic lesions and may provide valuable information to select and monitor the effectiveness of novel therapeutics targeting specific molecular pathways of breast cancer.

PET Imaging Biomarkers for Theranostic Evaluation of Brain Tumors The researchers are getting used to referring to instrumentally detectable biological features as "*imaging biomarkers*". These two terms combined reflect the evolution of medical imaging during recent decades, and conceptually comprise the principle of noninvasive detection of internal molecular events that can become targets for therapeutic interventions. These targets include those biological pathways that are associated with tumor features including: *independence from growth and growth-inhibitory signals, avoidance of apoptosis and immune system control, unlimited potential for replication, self-sufficiency in vascular supply and neoangiogenesis, acquired tissue invasiveness and metastatic diffusion.* Recently Lopci et al. (2015) described relevant techniques and biomarkers for imaging primary brain tumors, and discussed future developments from the experimental context. There have been major improvements in neurosurgical techniques and radiotherapy planning of brain tumors, and developments of novel target drugs, thus increasing the need for reproducible, noninvasive, quantitative imaging biomarkers. However, conventional radiological criteria may be inappropriate to determine the best therapeutic option and to assess prognosis. Hence integration of molecular imaging for the evaluation of brain tumors has become necessary, and an important role is played by imaging biomarkers in PET and MRI.

PET Imaging of Brain Tumors with Radio-labelled Amino Acids. Routine diagnostics and treatment monitoring of brain tumors is usually based on contrast-enhanced MRI. However, the capacity of structural MRI to differentiate neoplastic tissue from non-specific treatment changes may be limited after therapeutic interventions such as neurosurgical resection, radio- and chemotherapy. Galldika and Langen (2015) reported that metabolic imaging using PET may provide additional information on tumor metabolism, which allows for more accurate diagnostics. In contrast to the widely used ^{18}FdG, which exhibits a poor tumor-to-background contrast within the brain, amino acid radiotracers provide high sensitivity to detect primary tumors, recurrent or residual gliomas, including low-grade gliomas. The method improves targeting of biopsy and provides additional information helpful for planning neurosurgery and radiotherapy. The amino acid PET neuroimaging allows a sensitive monitoring of therapeutic response, early detection of tumor recurrence, and an improved differentiation of tumor recurrence from treatment-related changes. In the past, the method had only limited availability due to the use of RPs with a short half-life. In recent years, however, novel amino acid tracers labeled with positron emitters with a longer half-life allow efficient and cost-effective application. These developments and the theranostic performance of PET using radiolabeled amino acids suggest that its application continues to spread and that the method may be available as a routine diagnostic tool for certain CNS tumors.

Radionuclide Imaging of Osteomyelitis Usually radionuclide procedures are performed as part of the diagnostic workup of osteomyelitis. Bone scintigraphy diagnoses osteomyelitis in bones not affected by underlying conditions. Degenerative joint disease, fracture, and orthopedic hardware decrease the specificity of the bone scan, making it less useful in these situations. Recently Palestro (2015) reported that ^{67}Ga scintigraphy was often used as an adjunct to bone scintigraphy for diagnosing osteomyelitis. However, now it is used primarily for spinal infections when ^{18}FdG imaging cannot be performed. Except for the spine, *in vitro*-labeled leukocyte imaging is chosen for diagnosing complicating osteomyelitis. Leukocytes accumulate in bone marrow as well as in infection. Performing complementary bone marrow imaging with ^{99m}Tc-sulfur colloid facilitates the differentiation between osteomyelitis and normal marrow and improves overall theranostic accuracy. Antigranulocyte antibodies and antibody fragments, such as ^{99m}Tc-Besilesomab and ^{99m}Tc-Sulesomab, were developed to eliminate the disadvantages associated with *in vitro*-labeled leukocytes. These agents, however, have their own shortcomings and are not widely available. As Biotin is used as a growth factor by certain bacteria, ^{111}In-Biotin is useful to diagnose spinal infections.

Radiolabeled synthetic fragments of Ubiquicidin, a naturally occurring human antimicrobial peptide that targets bacteria, can differentiate infection from sterile inflammation and may be useful to monitor response to treatment. [18]FdG is extremely useful in the theranostics of osteomyelitis. Sensitivity in excess of 95% and specificity ranging from 75%-99% have been reported. [18]FdG is the radiopharmaceutical of choice for spinal infection. The test is sensitive, with a highly negative predictive value, and differentiates degenerative from infectious vertebral body end-plate abnormalities. Data on the accuracy of [18]FdG for diagnosing diabetic pedal osteomyelitis are contradictory, and its role for this indication remains uncertain. Initial investigations suggested that [18]FdG accurately diagnoses prosthetic joint infection; more recent data indicate that it cannot differentiate infection from other causes of prosthetic failure. Preliminary data on the PET agents ^{68}Ga and [124]I-Fialuridine indicate that these agents may have a role in diagnosing osteomyelitis.

[18]FdG-PET/CT Imaging in Breast Cancer and Other Gynecological Cancers Hildebrandt et al. (2015) provided an update on the role of [18]FdG-PET/CT imaging in different clinical settings of the 4 most frequent female-specific cancer types: *breast, endometrial, ovarian, and cervical cancer*. The most recent knowledge regarding primary diagnosis, staging, response evaluation, prognostic and predictive values, recurrence detection, and radiotherapy planning was evaluated, including, when clinically relevant, considerations with respect to the epidemiology, treatment, and course of the diseases.

[11]C or ^{18}F-Labelled Choline for Malignant Brain Tumors It is well known that malignant gliomas and metastatic tumors are the most common forms of brain tumors. Neuroimaging plays a significant role, in diagnosis, treatment planning, and follow-up. To date MRI is considered the gold standard for imaging, however, despite providing superior structural detail it features poor specificity in identifying viable tumors in brain treated with surgery, radiation, or chemotherapy. Recently Giovannini et al. (2015) reported that in the last years functional neuroimaging has become widespread due to the use of molecular tracers employed in cellular metabolism which has improved the management of patients with brain tumors, especially during post-treatment phase. Despite the considerable progress of molecular imaging in oncology its use in the diagnosis of brain tumors is still limited by a few technical problems. Because ^{18}F-dG, the most common radiotracer used in oncology, is avidly accumulated by normal cortex, the low tumor/BKg ratio makes it difficult to distinguish the tumor from normal surrounding tissues. By contrast, radiotracers with higher specificity for the tumor are labeled with a short half-life isotopes which restricts their use to those centers equipped with a cyclotron and radiopharmacy facility. ^{11}C-Choline has been reported as a suitable tracer for neuroimaging malignant brain tumors. The recent availability of Choline labeled with a long half-life radioisotope as ^{18}F increases the possibility of studying its theranostic potential in the staging of brain tumors. These investigators provided clinical applications of PET/CT with Choline tracers in malignant brain tumors and brain metastases, with a special emphasis on malignant gliomas.

Integrated [18]FdG-PET/CT and MRI in Oesophageal Cancers van Rossum et al. (2015) reported that integrated [18]FdG-PET/CT and MRI with functional features of diffusion-weighted imaging (DWI) are advancing imaging technologies that have future potential to overcome limitations of conventional staging methods in the management of patients with oesophageal cancer. PET/CT has emerged as the standard procedure for patients with oesophageal cancer. Besides its important ability to detect unsuspected metastatic disease, it may be useful in the assessment of treatment response, radiation treatment planning, and detection of recurrent disease. In addition, high-resolution T_2-weighted MRI and DWI have potential complementary roles. Recent improvements in MRI protocols have resulted in better imaging quality with the potential improvement in staging, radiation treatment planning, and the assessment of treatment response. Optimal use and understanding of PET/CT and MRI in oesophageal cancer will contribute to the impact of these technologies in EBPT and achieving best possible outcomes. These investigators outlined the current and potential future roles of PET/CT and MRI in the multidisciplinary management of oesophageal cancer.

Combined ^{18}F-NaF/^{18}F-FDG PET/CT for the Early Detection of Osseous Metastases
Sodium fluoride PET (^{18}F-NaF) reemerged as a valuable radiopharmaceutical for the detection of osseous metastasis, highlighting the potential of co-administered ^{18}F-NaF and ^{18}FdG-PET/CT in a single imaging examination. Sampath et al. (2015) evaluated the potential of such combination by comparing dual tracer ^{18}F-NaF^{18}/FdG PET/CT with CT for the detection of osseous metastasis. Seventy-five participants with biopsy-proven malignancy were enrolled from a single center and underwent combined ^{18}F-NaF/^{18}FdG PET/CT and diagnostic CT scans. PET/CT as well as CT only images were reviewed and compared with the results of clinical, imaging, or histological follow-up. Sensitivity of the combined ^{18}F-NaF/^{18}FdG PET/CT was higher than that of CT alone (97.4% vs 66.7%). CT and ^{18}F-NaF/^{18}FdG PET/CT were concordant in 73% of studies. Of 20 discordant cases, ^{18}F-NaF/^{18}FdG PET/CT was correct in 19 (95%). Three cases were interpreted incorrectly, and all 3 were false positives. A single case of osseous metastasis was detected by CT alone, but not by ^{18}F-NaF/^{18}FdG PET/CT. Combined ^{18}F-NaF/^{18}FdG PET/CT outperformed CT alone and was highly sensitive and specific for the detection of osseous metastases. The concordantly interpreted false-positive cases demonstrated the difficulty of distinguishing degenerative from malignant disease, whereas the single case of metastasis seen on CT but not PET highlighted the need for careful review of CT images in multimodality studies.

REFERENCES

Adamson, P. D., Vesey, A. T., Joshi, N. V., Newby, D. E. & Dweck, M. R. (2015). Salt in the wound: ^{18}F-fluoride positron emission tomography for identification of vulnerable coronary plaques. *Cardiovasc Diagn Ther.*, 5(2), 150-155.

Ariza, M., Kolb, H. C., Moechars, D., Rombouts, F. & Andrés, J. I. (2015). Tau Positron Emission Tomography (PET) Imaging: Past, Present, and Future. *J Med Chem.*, 58(11), 4365-4382.

Benešová, M., Schäfer, M., Bauder-Wüst, U., Afshar-Oromieh, A., Kratochwil, C., Mier, W., Haberkorn, U., Kopka, K. & Eder, M. (2015). Preclinical Evaluation of a Tailor-Made DOTA-Conjugated PSMA Inhibitor with Optimized Linker Moiety for Imaging and Endoradiotherapy of Prostate Cancer. *J Nucl Med.*, 56(6), 914-920.

Borbély, K. (2015). [New trends and novel possibilities in the management of oncologic patients: clinical uses of PET/MRI]. *Magy Onkol.*, 59(1), 10-16.

Deng, H., Wang, H. & Li, Z. (2015). Matching Chelators to Radiometals for Positron Emission Tomography Imaging- Guided Targeted Drug Delivery. *Curr Drug Targets.*, 16(6), 610-624.

Dimitriu-Leen, A. C., Scholte, A. J. & Jacobson, A. F. (2015). ^{123}I-MIBG SPECT for Evaluation of Patients with Heart Failure. *J Nucl Med., 56* Suppl 4, 25S-30S.

Galldiks, N. & Langen, K. J. (2015). Applications of PET imaging of neurological tumors with radiolabeled amino acids. *Q J Nucl Med Mol Imaging., 59*(1), 70-82.

Gavra, M., Syed, R., Fraioli, F., Afaq, A. & Bomanji, J. (2015). PET/MRI in the Upper Abdomen. *Semin Nucl Med., 45*(4), 282-292.

Giovannini, E., Lazzeri, P., Milano, A., Gaeta, M. C. & Ciarmiello, A. (2015). Clinical applications of choline PET/CT in brain tumors. *Curr Pharm Des., 21*(1), 121-127.

Halime, Z., Frindel, M., Camus, N., Orain, P. Y., Lacombe, M., Chérel, M., Gestin, J. F., Faivre-Chauvet, A. & Tripier, R. (2015). New synthesis of phenyl-isothiocyanate C-functionalised cyclams. Bioconjugation and ^{64}Cu phenotypic PET imaging studies of multiple myeloma with the te2a derivative. *Org Biomol Chem., 13*(46), 11302-11314.

Hildebrandt, M. G., Kodahl, A. R., Teilmann-Jørgensen, D., Mogensen, O. & Jensen, P. T. (2015). [^{18}F]fluorodeoxyglucose PET/computed tomography in breast cancer and gynecologic cancers: a literature review. *PET Clin., 10*(1), 89-104.

Humbert, O., Cochet, A., Coudert, B., Berriolo-Riedinger, A., Kanoun, S., Brunotte, F. & Fumoleau, P. (2015). Role of positron emission tomography for the monitoring of response to therapy in breast cancer. *Oncologist., 20*(2), 94-104.

Jacobson, O., Yan, X., Niu, G., Weiss, I. D., Ma, Y., Szajek, L. P., Shen, B., Kiesewetter, D. O. & Chen, X. (2015). PET imaging of tenascin-C with a radiolabeled single-stranded DNA aptamer. *J Nucl Med.,* 2015 Apr, *56*(4), 616-621.

Lemaire, C., Libert, L., Franci, X., Genon, J. L., Kuci, S., Giacomelli, F. & Luxen, A. (2015). Automated production at the curie level of no-carrier-added 6-[(18) F] fluoro-L-dopa and 2-[(18) F] fluoro-L-tyrosine on a FAST lab synthesizer. *J. Labelled Comp. Radiopharm., 58*(7), 281-290.

Lewis, D. Y., Soloviev, D. & Brindle, K. M. (2015). Imaging tumor metabolism using positron emission tomography. *Cancer J., 21*(2), 129-136.

Lopci, E., Franzese, C., Grimaldi, M., Zucali, P. A., Navarria, P., Simonelli, M., Bello, L., Scorsetti, M. & Chiti, A. (2015). Imaging biomarkers in primary brain tumors. *Eur J Nucl Med Mol Imaging., 42*(4), 597-612.

Lopci, E., Torzilli, G., Poretti, D., de Neto, L. J., Donadon, M., Rimassa, L., Lanza, E., Sabongi, J. G., Ceriani, R., Personeni, N., Palmisano, A., Pedicini, V., Comito, T., Scorsetti, M. & Chiti, A. (2015). Diagnostic accuracy of ^{11}C-choline PET/CT in comparison with CT and/or MRI in patients with hepatocellular carcinoma. *Eur J Nucl Med Mol Imaging., 42*(9), 1399-1407.

Lu, W., Wan, J. & Zhang, H. H. (2015). Computerized PET/CT image analysis in the evaluation of tumor response to therapy. *Br J Radiol., 88*(1048), 20140625.

Mattsson, S., Andersson, M. & Söderberg, M. (2015). Technological advances in hybrid imaging and impact on dose. *Radiat Prot Dosimetry., 165*(1-4), 410-415.

Notni, J., Steiger, K., Hoffmann, F., Reich, D., Kapp, T. L., Rechenmacher, F., Neubauer, S., Kessler, H. & Wester, H. J. (2015). Complementary, Selective PET-Imaging of Integrin Subtypes $\alpha5\beta1$ and $\alpha v\beta3$ Using Ga-68-Aquibeprin and Ga-68-Avebetrin. *J Nucl Med.,* 2015.

Oukoloff, K., Cieslikiewicz-Bouet, M., Chao, S., Da Costa Branquinho, E., Bouteiller, C., Jean, L. & Renard, P. Y. (2015). PET and SPECT Radiotracers for Alzheimer's Disease. *Curr Med Chem., 22*(28), 3278-304.

Palestro, C. J. (2015). Radionuclide imaging of osteomyelitis. *Semin Nucl Med. 45*(1), 32-46.

Petretta, M., Storto, G., Pellegrino, T., Bonaduce, D. & Cuocolo, A. (2015). Quantitative Assessment of Myocardial Blood Flow with SPECT. *Prog. Cardiovasc. Dis., 57*(6), 607-614.

Sager, S., Vatankulu, B., Erdogan, E., Mut, S., Teksoz, S., Ozturk, T., Sonmezoglu, K. & Kanmaz, B. (2015). Comparison of F-18 FDG-PET/CT and Tc-99m MIBI in the preoperative evaluation of cold thyroid nodules in the same patient group. *Endocrine., 50*(1), 138-145.

Salvatori, M., Biondi, B. & Rufini, V. (2015). Imaging in endocrinology: 2-[18F]-fluoro-2-deoxy-D-glucose positron emission tomography/computed tomography in differentiated thyroid carcinoma: clinical indications and controversies in diagnosis and follow-up. *Eur J Endocrinol., 173*(3), R115-130.

Sampath, S. C., Sampath, S. C., Mosci, C., Lutz, A. M., Willmann, J. K., Mittra, E. S., Gambhir, S. S. & Iagaru, A. (2015). Detection of osseous metastasis by ^{18}F-NaF/^{18}F-FDG PET/CT versus CT alone. *Clin Nucl Med., 40*(3), e173-177.

Unschuld, P. G. (2015). Possibilities of modern imaging technologies in early diagnosis of Alzheimer disease]. *Ther Umsch., 72*(4), 261-269.

Uslu, L., Donig, J., Link, M., Rosenberg, J., Quon, A. & Daldrup-Link, H. E. (2015). Value of 18F-FDG PET and PET/CT for evaluation of pediatric malignancies. *J Nucl Med., 56*(2), 274-286.

van Rossum, P. S., van Lier, A. L., Lips, I. M., Meijer, G. J., Reerink, O., van Vulpen, M., Lam, M. G., van Hillegersberg, R. & Ruurda, J. P. (2015). Imaging of oesophageal cancer with FDG-PET/CT and MRI. *Clin Radiol., 70*(1), 81-95.

Withofs, N., Charlier, E., Simoni, P., Alvarez-Miezentseva, V., Mievis, F., Giacomelli, F., Mella, C., Gambhir, S. S., Malaise, O., de Seny, D., Malaise, M. & Hustinx, R. (2015). ^{18}F-FPRGD2 PET/CT imaging of musculoskeletal disorders. *Ann Nucl Med., 29*(10), 839-847.

Zimmerman, B. E., Bergeron, D. E. & Cessna, J. T. (2015). Impact of Recent Change in the National Institute of Standards and Technology Standard for ^{18}F on the Relative Response of ^{68}Ge-Based Mock Syringe Dose Calibrator Standards. *J Nucl Med., 56*(9), 1453-1457.

Chapter 3

HUMAN GENOMICS IN EVIDENCE-BASED PERSONALIZED THERANOSTICS (RECENT UPDATE)

ABSTRACT

Recently human genomics emerged as a promising approach to accomplish EBPT of multi-drug-resistant chronic diseases. In this chapter, clinical significance of human genomics in early detection of adrenocortial tumors, DMET Plus microarray, and genome-wide technologies to assess diseased population are highlighted. In additon, association of 5-hydroxymethylcytosine to gene hypermethylation in kidney cancer, genomics in healthcare and wellness, and data acquisition in oncology are described. Particularly, analysis of Illumina gene expression microarray data to build prediction models in oncology, cancer RNA-Seq nexus: transcriptome profiling, MutationAligner web resource to discover mutation in proteins of cancer patients, circulating APOL1 protein complexes in African Americans, and theranostic potential of next generation sequencing (NGS) are discussed. Furthermore, genomic correlates of prostate cancer grading, EBPT in oncology and improved patient care, skin biopsy and therapeutic potential of patient-specific stem cell-lines, progression of IgA nephropathy (IgAN) in end-stage kidney disease (ESKD), theranostic applications of microRNA biomarkers, and ethical issues in EBPT of cancer are explained.

Keywords: gene body hypermethylation, 5-hydroxymethylcytosine, illumina gene expression Mutationaligner, APOL1 protein complexes, IgA nephropathy (IgAN), end-stage kidney disease (ESKD), microRNA biomarkers

INTRODUCTION

Encompassing more than just DNA sequences, the definition of genomics includes *transcriptomics, proteomics, metabolomics, and epigenomics*, with integration of *genomic and environmental factors in systems biology*. While the researchers can learn a lot about cellular functions, integration of these diversified areas is far from enabling the prediction of theranostic outcomes. Only a limited specific biomarkers, genetic or otherwise, are 'actionable', *i.e.*, they can be used to guide therapy. *Recent pharmacogenetic studies revealed that polymorphisms of drug metabolizing enzymes, transporters and receptors contribute to variable drug response.* Owing to the complexity of drug actions, a genomics approach aims at finding novel drug targets and optimizing therapy to accomplish EBPT. However, PGx has made only a few achievements into clinical practice to date. Recently Sade'e and Daihum (2015) evaluated obstacles that need to be overcome to successfully accomplish EBPT. *These include the complexity of mechanisms underlying drug response, administered singly or in combination, uncertainty about the genetics of complex diseases, such as cancer, diabetes, cardiovascular, and mental disorders, and a lack of quantitative information regarding genetic variations, even for well-documented genes.* By resolving these important issues, PGx will yield significant therapeutic advances paving the way towards personalized health care.

In this chapter, clinical significance of genomics in early detection of cancers, DMET Plus microarray and genome-wide technologies to assess diseased population, association of 5-hydroxymethylcytosine to gene hypermethylation, and data acquisition to build prediction models in cancer are described. In addition, analysis of *Illumina* gene expression microarray to build prediction models, RNA-Seq nexus cancer transcriptome profiling, MutationAligner web resource to discover mutation in proteins, circulating APOL1 complexes in African Americans are discussed. Furthermore, genomic correlates of prostate cancer, skin biopsy and patient-specific stem cell lines, IgA nephropathy in end-stage kidney disease, clinical applications of microRNA biomarkers, and next generation sequencing (NGS) and ethical issues are described for the successful accomplishment of EBPT of cancer and other chronic multi-drug-resistnat diseases.

Clinical Significance of Genomics in PM It is now realized that despite the significant advances in drug therapy, some patients do not respond favorably or suffer severe adverse drug effects. Sadee (2011) reported that genomics in PM undergo profound changes with remarkable technological advances. Ability to sequence the entire human genome raised expectations that the researchers can use an individual's genomic blueprint to understand disease risk and predict therapeutic outcomes, thereby, optimizing drug therapy. Yet, there are concerns as to what extent genetic/genomic factors influence disease and treatment outcomes or whether predictive biomarkers could be successfully developed to accomplish EBPT.

Genomics of Adrenocortial Tumors The last decade witnessed the emergence of genomics, a set of high-throughput molecular measurements in biological samples. These pan-genomic and agnostic approaches revolutionized the molecular genetics of malignant and benign tumors. These techniques are now applied successfully to adrenocortical tumors. Recently Faillot and Assie (2016) reported exome sequencing whch identifies new drivers in all tumor types, including KCNJ5, ATP1A1, ATP2B3 and CACNA1D mutations in Aldosterone producing adenomas (APA), PRKACA mutations in Cortisol producing adenomas (CPA), ARMC5 mutations in primary bilateral macronodular adrenocortical hyperplasia (PBMAH), and ZNRF3 mutations in adrenocortical carcinomas (ACC). Moreover, various genomic approaches *-including exome sequencing, transcriptome, miRNome, genome, and methylome-,* converge into a single molecular classification of adrenocortical tumors. Particularly for ACC, two molecular groups have emerged, exhibiting major differences in outcomes. These ACC groups differ by their gene expression profiles, but also by recurrent mutations and specific DNA hypermethylation patterns in the subgroup of poor outcome. The dominant altered signaling pathways have now become therapeutic targets. The molecular groups of diseases individualize subtypes within diseases such as

APA, CPA, PBMAH and ACC. It has been emphasized that a revised nosology of adrenocortical tumors should impact the clinical research. Obvious consequences also include counseling for the new genetic diseases such as ARMC5 mutations in PBMAH, and a better prognostication of ACC based on targeted measurements of discriminant molecular alterations. Furthermore, identifying the main molecular groups of adrenocortical tumors by collecting the molecular variations is a significant step towards EBPT.

DMET Plus Microarray and Genome-wide Technologies The ability of the Affymetrix drug metabolism enzymes and transporters (DMET) Plus PGx genotyping chip to estimate population substructure and cryptic relatedness was evaluated by Jackson et al. (2016). The results were compared using genome-wide HapMap data for the same individuals. For 301 unrelated individuals, spanning 3 continental populations and one admixed population, genotypic data were collected using the *Affymetrix DMET Plus microarray*. Genome-wide data on these individuals were obtained from HapMap. Population substructure was assessed using *Eigenstrat and ADMIXTURE software* for both platforms. Cryptic relatedness was explored by inbreeding coefficient estimation. Nonparametric tests were used to determine correlations of the analytical results of the two genotyping platforms. Principal components analysis (PCA) identified population substructure for both datasets, with 15.8 and 16.6% of the total variance in the first two principal components for DMET Plus and HapMap data, respectively. ADMIXTURE results identified 4 subpopulations within each dataset. Nonparametric rank correlations indicated associations between analyses. Correlation coefficients indicated concordance between ADMIXTURE results. Inbreeding coefficients were slightly inflated using DMET Plus data and no cryptic relatedness was indicated using HapMap data. The inflated inbreeding estimates could be provided by DMET as a random sample of 1832 markers from HapMap also yielded inflated estimates of cryptic relatedness. Furthermore, use of SNPs in genes involved in metabolism and transport may have different allele frequencies in subpopulations than SNPs from the whole genome. The DMET Plus PGx genotyping chip was effective in quantifying population substructure across the 3 continental populations and inferring the presence of an admixed population. These microarrays offered sufficient knowledge for covariate adjustment of population substructure in genomic association studies.

Loss of 5-Hydroxymethylcytosine is Linked to Gene Hypermethylation in Kidney Cancer Both 5-methylcytosine (5mC) and its oxidized form 5-hydroxymethylcytosine (5hmC) have been proposed to be involved in tumorigenesis. Because the readout of the 5mC mapping method, bisulfite sequencing (BS-seq), is the sum of 5mC and 5hmC levels, the 5mC/5hmC patterns and relationship of these two modifications remain poorly understood. By profiling real 5mC (BS-seq corrected by Tet-assisted BS-seq, TAB-seq) and 5hmC (TAB-seq) levels simultaneously at single-nucleotide resolution, Chen et al. (2016) discovered that there is no loss of 5mC in kidney tumors compared with matched normal tissues. Conversely, 5hmC was lost in all kidney tumors. The 5hmC level was the prognostic biomarker for kidney cancer, with lower levels of 5hmC associated with reduced survival. The loss of 5hmC was linked to hypermethylation in tumors compared with normal tissues, particularly in gene regions. Gene hypermethylation was associated with silencing of the tumor-related genes. Downregulation of IDH1 was identified as a mechanism underlying 5hmC loss in kidney cancer. *Restoring 5hmC levels attenuated the invasion capacity of tumor cells and suppressed their growth in a xenograft model, suggesting that loss of 5hmC can be used as a prognostic biomarker as well as oncogenic event by remodeling the DNA methylation pattern in kidney cancer.*

Medical Genomics in Healthcare & Wellness Recent advances in genomics have led to the rapid and inexpensive collection of patient molecular data including omics data. The integration of these data with clinical measurements is able to impact on our understanding of the molecular basis of disease and on clinical management systems medicine is an approach to understanding disease through an integration of large patient datasets. It offers the possibility for personalized strategies for healthcare through the development of a new taxonomy of disease. In addition, advanced computing will be an important component in implementing systems medicine. Saqi et al. (2016) described 3 computational challenges associated with systems medicine: (a) *disease subtype discovery using integrated datasets, (b) obtaining a mechanistic understanding of disease, (c) and the development of an informatics platform for mining, analysis, and visualization of data from translational medicine to ultimately accomplish EBPT.*

Data Collection to Build Prediction Models in Oncology The advances in diagnostic and treatment *(Theranostic)* technology are responsible for a transformation in the internal medicine concept with the establishment of a new era of EBPT. Inter- and intra-patient tumor heterogeneity and the clinical outcome and/or treatment's toxicity's complexity, rationalize the effort to develop predictive models from decision support systems. *However, the variables from multiple disciplines: oncology, computer science, bioinformatics, statistics, genomics, imaging, among others could be extensive thus making traditional statistical analysis difficult to interpret.* Meldolesi e al (2016) emphasized that automated data-mining and machine learning approaches can organize these data, to unravel strategy to collect and analyze data for decision making, and introducing the concept of an *'umbrella protocol'* in the context of *'rapid learning healthcare'*.

Analysis of Illumina Gene Expression Microarray Data Generally, microarray profiling of gene expression is applied to studies in molecular biology and functional genomics. Experimental and technical variations make not only the statistical analysis of single studies but also meta-analyses of different studies challenging. Teumer et al. (2016) described the steps to reduce the variations of gene expression data without affecting true effect sizes. A software was established using gene expression data from 3358 whole blood cell and blood monocyte samples, from 3 German population-based cohorts, measured on the *Illumina HumanHT-12 v3 BeadChip* array. The adjustment for a few selected factors improved reliability of gene expression analyses. These adjustments were highly crucial for meta-analyses of different studies.

Cancer RNA-Seq Nexus: Transcriptome Cancer Profiling It is now well established that the genome-wide transcriptome profiling of cancerous and normal tissue samples can provide insights into the molecular mechanisms of cancer initiation and progression. Li et al. (2016) reported that RNA sequencing *(RNA-Seq)* has been used extensively in cancer research. However, no existing RNA-Seq database provides all of the following features: *(i) large-scale and comprehensive data archives and analyses, coding-transcript profiling, long non-coding RNA (lncRNA) profiling and coexpression networks; (ii) phenotype-oriented data organization and searching and (iii) the visualization of expression profiles, differential expression, and regulatory networks.* These researchers constructed the database that meets all these criteria, the *Cancer RNA-Seq Nexus* (CRN, http://syslab4.nchu.edu.tw/CRN). *CRN* has a user-friendly web interface to facilitate cancer research and EBPT. It is an open resource for data exploration, providing coding-transcript/lncRNA expression profiles to support researchers generating new hypotheses in cancer research and EBPT.

MutationAligner Web Resource in Cancer Patients The MutationAligner web resource, available at http://www.mutationaligner.org, enables discovery and exploration of somatic mutation hotspots in protein domains in >5000 cancer patient samples across 22 different tumor types. Using multiple sequence alignments of protein domains in the human genome, Gauthier et al. (2016) extended recurrence analysis by aggregating mutations in homologous positions across sets of paralogous genes. Protein domain analysis enhanced the statistical power to detect cancer-relevant mutations and linked mutations to the specific biological functions in domains. These authors described how the MutationAligner database and interactive web tool can be used to *analyze mutation hotspots in protein domains across genes and tumor types and* highlighted that MutationAligner will be an important resource for the cancer research by providing detailed clues for the functional importance of mutations, as well as for the design of *functional genomics experiments* and for *decision making in EBPT*. These investigators periodically update MutationAligner to incorporate additional analyses and new data from cancer genomics projects.

Circulating APOL1 Protein Complexes in African Americans It is now known that APOL1 gene renal-risk variants are associated with nephropathy and CVD in African Americans; however, little is known regarding the circulating APOL1 variant proteins which bind to HDL. Weckerle et al. (2016) examined whether APOL1 G1 and G2 renal-risk variant serum concentrations or lipoprotein differed from nonrisk G0 APOL1 in this population without nephropathy. Serum APOL1 protein levels were similar regardless of APOL1 genotype. In addition, serum APOL1 protein was bound to protein complexes in two nonoverlapping peaks, as APOL1 complex A and complex B. Neither of these protein complexes were associated with HDL or LDL. Complex A was composed of APOA1, haptoglobin-related protein (HPR), and complement C3, whereas complex B contained APOA1, HPR, IgM, and fibronectin as confirmed by proteomic analyses. Serum HPR was less abundant on complex B in individuals with G1 and G2 renal-risk variant genotypes, relative to G0, suggesting that these circulating complexes may play crucial roles in HDL metabolism and susceptibility to CVD.

APOL1 Genotype and Kidney Transplantation It has been noticed that two apolipoprotein L1 gene (APOL1) renal-risk variants in donors and African American (AA) recipients are associated with worse allograft survival in deceased-donor kidney transplantation (DDKT) from AA donors. To detect other factors influencing allograft survival from deceased AA kidney donors, APOL1 renal-risk variants were genotyped in AA kidney donors. Freedman et al. (2016) linked the APOL1 genotypes to outcomes in 478 newly analyzed DDKTs in the transplant recipients. *Multivariate analyses accounting for recipient age, sex, race, panel-reactive antibody level, HLA match, cold ischemia time, donor age, and expanded criteria donation were performed. The 478 transplantations and 675 DDKTs from a prior report were analyzed. Fully adjusted analyses limited to the new 478 DDKTs replicated shorter renal allograft survival in recipients of APOL1 2-renal-risk-variant kidneys. Analysis of 1153 DDKTs from AA donors revealed donor APOL1 high-risk genotype, older donor age, and younger recipient age adversely impacted allograft survival.* Although prolonged allograft survival was seen in many recipients of APOL1 2-renal-risk-variant kidneys, serum creatinine concentrations were higher than that in recipients of 0/1 APOL1 renal-risk-variant kidneys. A risk analysis revealed that APOL1 impacted renal allograft survival, but not recipient survival. Interactions between donor age and APOL1 genotype on renal allograft survival were insignificant. Shorter renal allograft survival was observed after DDKT from APOL1 2-renal-risk-variant donors. Younger recipient age and older donor age had adverse effects on renal allograft survival.

Progression of IgA Nephropathy (IgAN) to End-Stage Kidney Disease (ESKD) Generally the progression of IgA nephropathy (IgAN) to ESKD depends on several factors that are uncertain and hamper the risk assessment. Pesce et al. (2016) developed a clinical decision support system (CDSS) for a quantitative risk assessment of ESKD and its timing using data at the time of renal biopsy. They included 1040 biopsy-proven IgAN patients with long-term follow-up from Italy (N = 546), Norway (N = 441) and Japan (N = 53). Of these, 241 patients reached ESKD: 104 Italian [median time to ESKD = 5 (3-9) years], 134 Norwegian [median time to ESKD = 6 (2-11) years] and 3 Japanese [median time to ESKD = 3 (2-12) years]. They trained and validated two artificial neural networks (ANNs) for predicting first the ESKD status and then the time to ESKD (*as 3 categories: ≤3 years, between >3 and 8 years and over 8 years*). *The gender, age, histological grading, serum creatinine, 24-h proteinuria and hypertension at the time of renal biopsy were used as inputs.* The ANNs demonstrated high performance for both the prediction of ESKD and its timing. They embedded the two ANNs in a CDSS available online (www.igan.net). Entering the clinical parameters during renal biopsy, the CDSS returned as output the estimated risk and timing of ESKD for the patient. This CDSS provided useful information for identifying *'high-risk'* IgAN patients and helped stratify them in the context of EBPT.

Genomic Correlates of Prostate Cancer Grading The International Society of Urologic Pathology and 2016 WHO book proposed the use of a 5-tiered prostate cancer (PCa) grading system. The 5 prognostic grade groupings (PGGs) ranging from 1 to 5 were defined as Gleason grades ≤6, 3+4, 4+3, 8, and >8, respectively. Each group was associated with a distinct risk of biochemical PCa recurrence. In a study, Rubin et al. (2015) sought genomic support for PGGs using whole-exome and whole-genome sequencing data for 426 localized PCas treated by radical prostatectomy. After adjustment for tumor purity for the sequencing data, they observed increase in genomic amplifications and deletions and in nonsynonymous point mutations with increasing risk group. Interestingly, PGG1 (low risk) was haploid, whereas PGG2-5 exhibited increased polyploidy. Principal component analysis (PCA) of genomic profiles revealed that PGG1, PGG2, and PGG3 represent distinct classes, but PGG4 and PGG5 exhibit genomic similarity. These observations for the largest PCa genomic data set supported for increasing genomic alterations with increasing PGG, suggesting that future work is required to explore the clinical utility of PGGs in long-term follow-up. Gleason grading for prostate cancer provided information for guiding clinical care. A new proposal favored translating Gleason grades into 5 risk categories. This was a comprehensive analysis of the largest genomic data set on prostate cancer which demonstrated molecular support for new 5-tiered system.

Skin Biopsy and Theranostic Potential of Patient-Specific Stem Cell Lines It is now well established that the generation of patient-specific induced pluripotent stem (iPS) cells allows the development of next-generation patient-specific systems biology models reflecting personalized genomics profiles to better understand pathophysiology. Recently Li et al. (2016) described how to create a patient-specific iPS cell line. These researchers proposed 3 major steps: *(1) performing a skin biopsy on the patient; (2) extracting human fibroblasts* *from the skin biopsy tissue; and (3) reprogramming patient-specific fibroblasts into the pluripotent stem cell stage to accomplish EBPT.*

EBPT in Oncology and Improved Patient Care Aiming to advance PM in oncology and improve patient care, the American Association for Cancer Research launched an international initiative known as AACR Project: *Genomics, Evidence, Neoplasia, Information, Exchange* (GENIE). This venture will pool existing and future NGS data with clinical outcomes and related pathology reports from institutions in the US, Canada, and Europe, to find new mutations, assess potential biomarkers, and identify patients that might benefit from existing treatments

Theranostic Application of Genomic Biomarkers Recently Austin and Babiss (2016) highlighted that since the beginning of the human genome project there has been speculation about how this resource and the knowledge would change *therapeutic discovery, development, and drug delivery.* As the project neared completion, considerable claims and predictions were made about the changes that would be forthcoming. Many of these early predictions failed to materialize, however, leading to further speculation about the reasons, including the role of the pharmaceutical industry in realizing the promise of "*genomic medicine.*" Considerable strides were made in other areas of molecular biology and medicine, and in response scientific thinking evolved. *Researchers and regulators moved from a genotype-centric view to a view that all biomarkers are potential tools to improve drug development and therapeutic decision making.* Molecular biology is currently seen as encouraging more "PM"-the closer alignment of biological information (*derived from molecular diagnostics*) and therapy selection. *However, increasing expenditures in pharmaceutical research and development are not sustainable and not reaping sufficient gains for shareholders or society at large.* Thus, there is speculation about how biomarkers, PM, and the industry will interact and will be beneficial for patients. These authors explored the issues driving pharmaceutical productivity and the contribution of biomarkers in the future.

MicroRNAs as Biomarker(s) for EBPT of Cancer Recent studies established that microRNA, as a regulator of gene expression might be involved in various biological processes to distinguish between different cancer subtypes. Hence miRNAs can serve as potential biomarkers for the EBPT of cancer. However the exact role of cancer-associated miRNAs and their physiological significance remains enigmatic due to intricate relationship between differentially-expressed miRNAs and their precise targets. The researchers isolated small RNAs from FACs-sorted squamous cell carcinoma (SCCs) cells. Sequencing of miRNA detected 169 miRs as crucial drivers of malignant progression. Strand-specific screening revealed miR-21 passenger (miR*) strand to drive tumorigenesis independent of miR-21 guide strand with miR-21* expression levels being higher. Furthermore, Phactr4 was recognized as a direct miR-21* target, which results in phosphorylation of the Rb tumor suppressor and leads to increased cell proliferation. The intricate role of the tumor enhancing miR-21* emphasized the need for screening to discover the missing links between cancer and other uncharacterized miR passenger strands for the successful EBPT of cancer.

Next Generation Sequencing and Ethical Issues in EBPT In early 2015, NIH launched a new, Precision Medicine *Initiative* with the primary objective of improving the prevention, diagnosis, and treatment of cancers. The first-stage emphasis on oncology presented opportunities for clinical oncology to influence how the ethical challenges of precision medicine were articulated and addressed. Fiore and Goodman (2016) reviewed recent developments in the initiative on core ethical issues in clinical genomics. Unique ethical issues arose because of the extensive data generated by clinical whole-genome or whole-exome sequencing and the uncertainties with respect to data interpretations and disease associations. *Among the most ethically challenging issues were complicated informed consent processes, returning results - particularly secondary and incidental findings-and privacy and confidentiality.* It was realized that the first tests of PM ethics will be in clinical oncology, providing a unique opportunity to shape the agenda and integrate ethical considerations. These efforts can benefit from pre-existing research ethics analyses and recommendations from clinical and translational genetics research.

REFERENCES

Austin, F. M. J. & Babiss, L. (2016). Commentary: where and how could biomarkers be used in 2016? *AAPS J.*, *8*(1), E185-189.

Chen, K., Zhang, J., Guo, Z., Ma, Q., Xu, Z., Zhou, Y., Xu, Z., Li, Z., Liu, Y., Ye, X., Li, X., Yuan, B., Ke, Y., He, C., Zhou, L., Liu, J. & Ci, W. (2016). Loss of 5-hydroxymethylcytosine is linked to gene body hypermethylation in kidney cancer. *Cell Res.*, *26*(1), 103-118.

Faillot, S. & Assie, G. (2016). ENDOCRINE TUMOURS: The genomics of adrenocortical tumors. *Eur J Endocrinol.* Jan 6.

Fiore, R. N. & Goodman, K. W. (2016). Precision medicine ethics: selected issues and developments in next-generation sequencing, clinical oncology, and ethics. *Curr Opin Oncol.*, *28*(1), 83-87.

Freedman, B. I., Pastan, S. O., Israni, A. K., Schladt, D., Julian, B. A., Gautreaux, M. D., et al., (2016). APOL1 Genotype and Kidney Transplantation Outcomes From Deceased African American Donors. *Transplantation.*, *100*(1), 194-202.

Gauthier, N. P., Reznik, E., Gao, J., Sumer, S. O., Schultz, N., Sander, C. & Miller, M. L. (2016). Mutation Aligner: a resource of recurrent mutation hotspots in protein domains in cancer. *Nucleic Acids Res.*, *44*(D1), D986-91.

Huge Data-Sharing Project Launched. *Cancer Discov.*, 2016 Jan, 6(1), 4-5.

Jackson, J. N., Long, K. M., He, Y., Motsinger-Reif, A. A., McLeod, H. L. & Jack, J. (2016). A comparison of DMET Plus microarray and genome-wide technologies by assessing population substructure. *Pharmacogenet* Genomics., Jan 1.

Li, J. R., Sun, C. H., Li, W., Chao, R. F., Huang, C. C., Zhou, X. J. & Liu, C. C. (2016). Cancer RNA-Seq Nexus: a database of phenotype-specific transcriptome profiling in cancer cells. *Nucleic Acids Res.*, *44*(D1), D944-951.

Li, Y., Nguyen, H. V. & Tsang, S. H. (2016). Skin Biopsy and Patient-Specific Stem Cell Lines. *Methods Mol Biol.*, *1353*, 77-88.

Meldolesi, E., van Soest, J., Damiani, A., Dekker, A., Alitto, A. R., Campitelli, M., Dinapoli, N., Gatta, R., Gambacorta, M. A., Lanzotti, V., Lambin, P. & Valentini, V. (2016). Standardized data collection to build prediction models in oncology: a prototype for rectal cancer. *Future Oncol.*, *12*(1), 119-136.

Pesce, F., Diciolla, M., Binetti, G., Naso, D., Ostuni, V. C., Di Noia, T., Vågane. A. M., Bjørneklett. R., Suzuki, H., Tomino, Y., Di Sciascio, E. & Schena, F. P. (2016). Clinical decision support system for end-stage kidney disease risk estimation in IgA nephropathy patients. *Nephrol. Dial. Transplant.*, *31*(1), 80-86.

Rubin, M. A., Girelli, G. & Demichelis, F. (2015). Genomic Correlates to the Newly Proposed Grading Prognostic Groups for Prostate Cancer. *Eur Urol.*, Nov 9.

Sadee, W. (2011). Genomics and PM. *International Journal of Pharmaceutics.*, *415*, 2–4.

Sadee, W. & Zunyan DaiHum, Z. (2005). Pharmacogenetics/genomics and PM *Mol. Genet.*, *14* (suppl 2), R207-R214.

Saqi, M., Pellet, J., Roznovat, I., Mazein, A., Ballereau, S., De Meulder, B. & Auffray, C. (2016). Systems Medicine: The Future of Medical Genomics, Healthcare, and Wellness. *Methods Mol Biol.*, 1386, 43-60.

Teumer, A., Schurmann, C., Schillert, A., Schramm, K., Ziegler, A. & Prokisch, H. (2016). Analyzing Illumina Gene Expression Microarray Data Obtained From Human Whole Blood Cell and Blood Monocyte Samples. *Methods Mol Biol.*, *1368*, 85-97.

Weckerle, A., Snipes, J. A., Cheng, D., Gebre, A. K., Reisz, J. A., Murea, M., Shelness, G. S., Hawkins, G. A., Furdui, C. M., Freedman, B. I., Parks, J. S. & Ma, L. (2016). Characterization of circulating APOL1 protein complexes in African Americans. *J Lipid Res.*, *57*(1), 120-130.

Weiss, F. U., Schurmann, C., Teumer, A., Mayerle. J., Simon. P., Völzke. H., Greinacher, A., Kuehn. J. P., Zenker, M., Völker, U., Homuth, G. & Lerch, M. M. (2016). ABO blood type B and fucosyltransferase 2 non-secretor status as genetic risk factors for chronic pancreatitis. *Gut.*, *65*(2), 353-354.

Chapter 4

EVIDENCE-BASED PERSONALIZED THERANOSTICS (RECENT UPDATE-I)

ABSTRACT

In this chapter, recent knowledge regarding biomarker testing in cancer screening, biobanking, liquid biopsies for the early detection of solid tumors, and algorithms based on tumor molecular profiling are described for early prevention and treatment of cancer. Particularly, predictive value of KRAS mutation in colon cancer, differential diagnosis of plasmacytoid dendritic cell neoplasms, and molecular imaging as companion diagnostics are described for the personalized cancer theranostics. In addition, KCNT1 missense mutations have been detected in epileptic disorders. Personalized treatment of obstructive sleep apnea, combined multi-modality therapeutic approach, mass spectrometry, kinase-KCC2 coupling: Cl- rheostasis, disease susceptibility, therapeutic targets, determination of fluid responsiveness, and clinical utility of engineered heart tissue for drug screening are explained. Furthermore, PGx of Clopidogrel as an anticoagulant, clinical significance of online NMR/X-Ray structure pair data repository, and specific biomarkers are described to successfully accomplish EBPT of chronic obstructive pulmonary disease (COPD).

Keywords: plasmacytoid dendritic cell neoplasms, KCNT1 missense mutations, cancer screening, molecular imaging, biobanking, *KRAS* mutation, liquid biopsies, tumor molecular profiling, mass spectrometry, kinase-KCC2 coupling, Cl- rheostasis

INTRODUCTION

It is currently recognized that PM involves the prescription of specific therapeutics best suited for an individual based on his/her pharmacogenetic and pharmacogenomic information. *Several technologies including single nucleotide polymorphism genotyping. haplotyping, gene expression studies by biochip/microarrays, and proteomics are employed* to accomplish the final goal of EBPM. Novel theranostics strategy plays a crucial role in the development of PM, in which therapy and diagnosis can be integrated. Several examples of the PM include genotype-based selection of patients for effective cancer therapy to spare those who would not respond or would suffer undesirable side effects. Indeed, EBPT will reduce the costs of drugs by shortening the drug development cycle. The introduction of pharmacogenomics into clinical trials is minimizing the chances of futile therapeutic attempts and increasing the prospects of safer and more effective therapies for specific groups of patients. Hence, EBPT is anticipated to be an acceptable part of medical practice in near future (Jain 2002).

Recently biochip and microarray technologies have been developed to accomplish EBPT. Biochips (e.g., GeneChip, CYP450, electrochemical biochips, protein biochips, microfluidic biochips and nanotechnology-based biochips) have assumed a predominant role in molecular diagnostics, and their application in diagnosis is expected to facilitate the development of PM. Gene expression profiling by microarrays has advanced the progress of personalized cancer treatment based on the molecular classification of subtypes. Refinements in biochip miniaturization with the advent of nanotechnology will further contribute to molecular diagnostics and the development of PM (Jain., 2004). Therapies for patients with cancer have changed gradually over the past decade, moving away from the administration of broadly acting cytotoxic drugs towards the use of more-specific therapies that are targeted to each tumor. To facilitate this shift, tests need to be developed to identify those individuals who require therapy and those who are most likely to benefit from certain therapies. In particular, tests that predict the clinical outcome for patients on the basis of the genes expressed by their tumors are likely to impact patient management, heralding a new era of PM (Veer., 2008).

Common Molecular Classifiers of Colon Cancer It is well established that immune cells in the tumor microenvironment have an important role in regulating tumor progression. Therefore, stimulating immune reactions to tumors can be an attractive therapeutic and prevention strategy. Cancer cells and host cells interact with each other in the tumor microenvironment; thus, cancer immunology is an interdisciplinary area where integrated analyses of both host as well as tumor factors is needed. Cancer represents a heterogeneous group of diseases with different genetic and epigenetic alterations; therefore, its molecular classification (for example lung, prostate, and breast cancers) is an important component in clinical decision making. However, most studies on antitumor immunity and clinical outcome lack analysis of tumor molecular biomarkers. Ogino et al., (2011) discussed colorectal cancer as a prototypical example of cancer. Common molecular classifiers of colon cancer include: *KRAS*, *BRAF* and *PIK3CA* mutations, microsatellite instability, LINE-1 methylation, and CpG island methylator phenotype. Since tumor molecular features and immune reactions are inter-related, a comprehensive assessment of these factors is critical. Examining the effects of tumor–host interactions on clinical outcome and prognosis represents an evolving interdisciplinary field of molecular pathological epidemiology. Pathological immunity evaluation may provide information on prognosis and help identify patients who are more likely to benefit from immunotherapy.

Diagnosis of Plasmacytoid Dendritic Cell Neoplasms Facchetti et al. (2016) reported that plasmacytoid dendritic cell neoplasms manifest in two clinically and pathologically distinct forms. The first variant is represented by nodular aggregates of plasmacytoid dendritic cells found in lymph nodes, skin, and bone marrow (*'Mature plasmacytoid dendritic cells proliferation associated with myeloid neoplasms'*). This entity is rare, although underestimated in incidence, and affects predominantly males. It is associated with a myeloid neoplasm such as chronic myelomonocytic leukemia or other myeloid proliferations with monocytic differentiation. The concurrent myeloid neoplasm dominates the clinical pictures and guides treatment. The prognosis is usually dismal, but reflects the evolution of the associated myeloid leukemia rather than progressive expansion of plasmacytoid dendritic cells. A second form of plasmacytoid dendritic cells tumor has been described as 'blastic plasmacytoid dendritic cell neoplasm'. This tumor is characterized by cutaneous and bone marrow tropism, and proliferating cells derive from immediate $CD4^+CD56^+$ precursors of plasmacytoid dendritic cells. The diagnosis can be accomplished by immunohistochemistry, using plasmacytoid dendritic cell biomarkers. The clinical course of blastic plasmacytoid dendritic cell neoplasm is characterized by a rapid progression to systemic disease via hematogenous dissemination. The genomic landscape of this entity is currently under intense investigation. Recurrent somatic mutations have been discovered in different genes, a finding that may open important perspectives for EBPT for this rare, but highly aggressive leukemia.

Biomarker Tests in Cancer Screening Biomarker tests are being offered by laboratories and clinicians as self-pay health services to screen asymptomatic individuals. However, sufficient evidence may not be available to support this practice. Luzak et al. (2016) investigated the benefit-harm tradeoffs associated with 11 biomarkers currently offered in Germany as self-pay tests to screen for cancer. These investigators searched bibliographic databases for health technology assessments, systematic reviews and randomized-controlled trials (RCTs) through September 2015. They included publications that analyzed cancer screening biomarkers and reported patient-relevant outcomes (*mortality, morbidity, quality of life*), and potential harms of screening, among asymptomatic individuals in screening and non-screening arms. Six publications of secondary literature and four publications reporting results from two RCTs were included. For 10 cancer screening biomarkers, no direct evidence on patient-relevant outcomes was available. Only one trial, which assessed cancer antigen 125 (CA125) and vaginal ultrasound for ovarian cancer screening, provided the outcome of interest. Screening compared with usual care did not reduce ovarian cancer mortality. Although ovarian cancer screening with CA125 showed no benefit, false-positive tests, overdiagnosis and overtreatment were reported. These investigators emphasized that physicians and laboratories should provide patients with comprehensive information about the lack of evidence and potential harms caused by biomarker screening tests offered as a self-pay health service.

Molecular Imaging as Companion Diagnostics for Cancer Therapy The goal of individualized and targeted treatment and PM requires the assessment of potential therapeutic targets to direct treatment selection. The biomarkers used to direct precision medicine, often termed companion diagnostics, for highly targeted drugs have thus far been entirely based on *in vitro* assay of biopsy material. Molecular imaging companion diagnostics offer a number of features complementary to those from *in vitro* assay, including the ability to measure the heterogeneity of each patient's cancer across the entire disease burden and to measure early changes in response to treatment. Mankoff et al. (2016) discussed the use of molecular imaging methods as companion diagnostics for cancer therapy with a primary objective of predicting response to targeted therapy and measuring early (PDs) response as an indication of whether the treatment has "hit" the target. These investigators also discussed considerations for probe development for molecular imaging companion diagnostics, including small-molecule probes and larger molecules such as labeled antibodies and related constructs and described two examples where both predictive and pharmacodynamic molecular imaging biomarkers have been tested in humans: endocrine therapy for breast cancer and human epidermal growth factor receptor type 2-targeted therapy.

Biobanking: The Foundation of PM Biobanking was identified as a pivotal discipline to accelerate the discovery and future development of novel drugs. Robert (2011) described the recent developments in biobanking and biospecimen research, with special reference to tumor banks which are of primary interest in oncology. There is a significant deficiency of high-quality, well annotated cancer biospecimens. Biospecimens is a fast growing discipline that will improve biobanking methodology as it is becoming more professionally organized and increased attention to quality control. Biobank networks are growing rapidly to combine and share resources. This researcher suggested that biobanking must improve efficiently to serve the needs of EBPT and specimen research should be encouraged and supported at all levels from project funding to publication of results. Biobanking need to be run to high professional standards and the significance of adequate funding, training and certification must be emphasized. The emerging national and international biobank networks will permit biobanks to synergize. The development of biobanking community will facilitate teamwork to overcome common challenges and enhance communication among scientific community and general public.

Predictive Value of KRAS Mutation in Colon Cancer Patrick et al. (2010) described that in patients with metastatic colorectal cancer, the predictive value of *KRAS* mutational status in the selection of patients for treatment with anti–epidermal growth factor (EGFR) monoclonal antibodies has been established. In patients with non–small-cell lung cancer (NSCLC), the utility of determining *KRAS* mutational status to predict clinical benefit to anti-EGFR therapies remains unclear. This review has provided a brief description of Ras biology, an overview of aberrant Ras signaling in NSCLC, and summarized the clinical data for using *KRAS* mutational status as a negative predictive biomarker to anti-EGFR therapies. Retrospective investigations of *KRAS* mutational status as a negative predictor of clinical benefit from anti-EGFR therapies in NSCLC have been performed; however, small sample sizes as a result of low prevalence of *KRAS* mutations and the low rate of tumor sample collection have limited the strength of these analyses. Although an association between the presence of *KRAS* mutation and lack of response to EGFR tyrosine kinase inhibitors (TKIs) has been observed, it remains unclear whether there is an association between *KRAS* mutation and EGFR TKI progression-free and overall survival. Unlike colorectal cancer, *KRAS* mutations do not identify patients who do not benefit from anti-EGFR monoclonal antibodies in NSCLC. The future value of testing for *KRAS* mutational status may be to exclude the possibility of an *EGFR* mutation or anaplastic lymphoma kinase translocation or to identify a molecular subset of patients with NSCLC in whom to pursue a drug development strategy that targets the *KRAS* pathway.

Liquid Biopsies for Solid Tumors In the era of EBPT, detection of the molecular drivers of tumors and of specific DNA mutations predicting response or resistance to targeted agents has become routine practice in clinical oncology. Esposito et al., (2016) reported on the clinical applications of liquid biopsies and on the recent findings in EBPT. The tumor biopsy depicts only a single timeframe from a single site, and might be inadequate to characterize a tumor because of intratumoral and intermetastatic heterogeneity. Circulating tumor DNA offers a "real time" tool for monitoring tumor genomes in a non-invasive manner providing accessible genetic biomarkers for cancer diagnosis, prognosis, and response to therapy. The liquid biopsy can be used for a variety of clinical and investigational applications. Future development will have to provide a cost effective analysis mainly identifying the genes known to be mutated in each tumor. Therefore, developing standardized methodologies for DNA analyses and validation in large prospective clinical studies is mandatory to implement the 'liquid biopsy' approach in the clinical management of cancer patients.

Cancer Treatment Algorithms Based on Tumor Molecular Profiling With the advent of high-throughput molecular technologies, several EBPT studies include molecular screening programs and PM clinical trials. Molecular profiling programs establish the molecular profile of patients' tumors with the aim to guide therapy based on identified molecular alterations. Le Tourneau et al. (2015) assessed the clinical utility of tumor molecular profiling and determined whether treatment selection based on molecular alterations produces superior outcomes compared with unselected treatment. These trials use treatment algorithms to assign patients to specific targeted therapies based on tumor molecular alterations. These algorithms should be governed by fixed rules to ensure standardization and reproducibility. These rsearchers summarized key molecular, biological, and technical criteria that should be addressed when establishing treatment algorithms based on tumor molecular profiling for PM trials.

Cancer Prevention as an Important Component of PM It has been realized that cancer burden worldwide is projected to rise from 14 million new cases in 2012 to 24 million in 2035. Stewart et al. (2016) reported that although the greatest increases will be in developing countries, where cancer services are already hard pressed, even the richest nations will struggle to meet demands of increasing patient numbers and spiralling treatment costs. No country can treat its way out of the cancer problem. Consequently, cancer control must combine improvements in treatment with greater emphasis on prevention and early detection. Cancer prevention is founded on describing the burden of cancer, identifying the causes and evaluating and implementing preventive interventions. Around 40-50% of cancers could be prevented if current knowledge about risk factors is translated into effective public health strategies. The benefits of prevention are attested to by major successes *in: tobacco control, vaccination against oncogenic viruses, reduced exposure to environmental and occupational carcinogens, and screening. Progress is still needed in areas such as weight control and physical activity. Fresh impetus for prevention and early detection will come through interdisciplinary approaches, encompassing knowledge and tools from advances in cancer biology.* Examples include mutation profiles giving clues about etiology and biomarkers for early detection, to stratify individuals for screening or for prognosis. However, cancer prevention requires a broad perspective stretching from the submicroscopic to the macropolitical, recognizing the importance of molecular profiling and multisectoral engagement across urban planning, transport, environment, agriculture, economics, etc. and applying interventions that may just as easily rely on a legislative measure as on a molecule.

Treatment of Obstructive Sleep Apnea. Prospects for **Personalized Combined Modality Therapy**. Decon et al. (2016) reported that obstructive sleep apnea (OSA) is a common sleep disorder with serious associated morbidities. Although several treatment options are currently available, variable efficacy and adherence result in many patients either not being treated or receiving inadequate treatment long term. EBPT based on relevant patient characteristics may improve adherence to treatment and long-term clinical outcomes. Four key traits of upper airway anatomy and neuromuscular control interact to varying degrees within individuals to cause OSA. These are: (1) the pharyngeal critical closing pressure, (2) the stability of ventilator chemoreflex feedback control (loop gain), (3) the negative intraesophageal pressure that triggers arousal (arousal threshold), and (4) the level of stimulus required to activated upper airway dilator muscles (upper airway recruitment threshold). Simplified diagnostic methods are being developed to assess these pathophysiological traits, potentially allowing prediction of which treatment would best suit each patient. In contrast to current practice of using various treatment modes alone, model predictions and pilot clinical trials show improved outcomes by combining several therapeutic targeted to each patient's pathophysiological profile. These developments could improve efficacy and adherence to treatment and in turn reduce the social and economic health burden of OSA and the associated life-threatening morbidities. This article reviewed OSA pathophysiology and identified currently available and investigational treatments that may be combined to optimize therapy based on individual profiles of patient pathophysiological trait.

KCNT1 Missense Mutations in Epileptic Disorders Recently mutations in the sodium-gated potassium channel subunit gene KCNT1 have emerged as a cause of several different epileptic disorders. Lim et al. (2016) described the mutational and phenotypic spectrum associated with the gene and discussed the comorbidities found in patients, which included intellectual disability and psychiatric features. The gene may also be linked with cardiac disorders. KCNT1 missense mutations were detected in 39% of patients with the epileptic encephalopathy malignant migrating focal seizures of infancy (MMFSI), making it the most significant MMFSI disease-causing gene identified to date. Mutations in KCNT1 have also been described in 8 unrelated cases of sporadic and familial autosomal-dominant nocturnal frontal lobe epilepsy (ADNFLE). These patients have a high frequency of associated intellectual disability and psychiatric features. Two mutations in KCNT1 have been associated with both ADNFLE and MMFSI, suggesting that the genotype-phenotype relationship for KCNT1 mutations is not straight-forward. Mutations have also been detected in several patients with infantile epileptic encephalopathies other than MMFSI. All mutations in KCNT1 are missense mutations, and electrophysiological studies have shown that they result in increased potassium current. Together, these genetic and electrophysiological studies raise the possibility of delivering precision medicine by treating patients with KCNT1 mutations using drugs that alter the action of potassium channels to specifically target the biological effects of their disease-causing mutation. Better understanding of the mechanisms underlying KCNT1-related disease will produce further improvements in treatment of the associated severe seizure disorders.

Kinase-KCC2 Coupling: Cl- Rheostasis, Disease Susceptibility, Therapeutic Target Despite the importance of KCC2 for neurophysiology and its role in multiple neuropsychiatric diseases, our knowledge of the transporter's regulatory mechanisms is incomplete. The intracellular concentration of Cl (-) ([Cl (-)] i) in neurons is a highly regulated variable that is established and modulated by the finely tuned activity of the KCC2 cotransporter. Kahle, and Delpire (2016) reported that the phosphorylation state of KCC2 at specific residues in its cytoplasmic COOH terminus, such as Ser940 and Thr906/Thr1007, encodes discrete levels of transporter activity that elicit graded changes in neuronal Cl(-) extrusion to modulate the strength of synaptic inhibition via Cl(-)-permeable $GABA_A$ receptors. These researchers proposed that the functional and physical coupling of KCC2 to Cl (-)-sensitive kinase(s), such as the WNK1-SPAK kinase complex, constitutes a molecular "rheostat" that regulates [Cl (-)] i and thereby influences the functional plasticity of GABA. The rapid reversibility of (de)phosphorylation facilitates regulatory *precision*, and multisite phosphorylation allows for the control of KCC2 activity by different inputs via distinct or partially overlapping upstream signaling cascades that may become more or less important depending on the physiological context. While this adaptation mechanism is highly suited to maintaining homeostasis, its adjustable set points may render it vulnerable to perturbation and dysregulation. These researchers suggested that pharmacological modulation of this kinase-KCC2 rheostat might be an efficacious strategy to enhance Cl (-) extrusion and therapeutically restore GABA inhibition.

Determintion of Fluid Responsiveness Accurate assessment of intravascular fluid status and measurement of fluid responsiveness have become exceedingly important in peri-operative medicine and critical care. The objectives of this systematic review was to discuss current controversies surrounding fluid responsiveness and describe the merits and limitations of the cardiac output monitors in measuring fluid responsiveness. Ansari et al. (2016) searched the MEDLINE and EMBASE databases (2002-2015); inclusion criteria were: comparison with an established reference standard such as pulmonary artery catheter, transthoracic echocardiography and transoesophageal echocardiography. Examples of clinical measures included static (such as central venous pressure) and dynamic (such as stroke volume variation and pulse pressure variation) parameters. The static parameters measured were described as having little value; however, the dynamic parameters were shown to be good physiological determinants of fluid responsiveness. Due to heterogeneity of the methods and patient characteristics, these researchers did not perform a meta-analysis. In most studies, precision and limits of agreement between determinants of fluid responsiveness measured by different devices were not evaluated, and the definition of fluid responsiveness varied across studies, suggesting that future research should focus on the physiological principles that underlie the measurement of fluid responsiveness and the effect of different volume expansion strategies on outcomes.

Engineered Heart Tissue for Drug Screening. Recently Tzatzalos et al. (2016) reported that with the advent of induced pluripotent stem cell (iPSC) technology, patient-specific stem cells can be developed and expanded into an indefinite source of cells. Subsequent developments in cardiovascular biology have led to efficient differentiation of cardiomyocytes, the force-producing cells of the heart. iPSC-derived cardiomyocytes (iPSC-CMs) have provided well-characterized, healthy, and disease-specific CMs, which has enabled and driven the generation and scale-up of human physiological and disease-relevant engineered heart tissues. The combined technologies of engineered heart tissue and iPSC-CMs are being used to study diseases and to test drugs, and have advanced the field of cardiovascular tissue engineering into EBPT. These investigators discussed current developments in engineered heart tissue, including iPSC-CMs as a novel cell source and examined new research directions that have improved the function of engineered heart tissue by using mechanical or electrical conditioning or the incorporation of non-cardiomyocyte stromal cells. Furthermore, they discussed how engineered heart tissue can be used as a powerful tool for therapeutic drug testing.

Advantage of Online NMR/X-Ray Structure Pair Data Repository Everett et al. (2016) developed an online NMR/X-ray Structure Pair Data Repository. The NIGMS Protein Structure Initiative (PSI) provided many valuable reagents, 3D structures, and technologies for structural biology. The Northeast Structural Genomics Consortium was one of several PSI centers. NESG used both X-ray crystallography and NMR spectroscopy for protein structure determination. A key goal of the PSI was to provide experimental structures for at least one representative of each of hundreds of targeted protein domain families. In some cases, structures for identical constructs were determined by both NMR and X-ray crystallography. NMR spectroscopy and X-ray diffraction data for 41 of these "NMR/X-ray" structure pairs determined using conventional triple-resonance NMR methods with extensive side chain resonance assignments were organized in an online NMR/X-ray Structure Pair Data

Repository. In addition, several NMR data sets for perdeuterated, methyl-protonated protein samples were included in this repository. As an example of the utility of this repository, these data were used to address questions about the precision and accuracy of protein NMR structures outlined by Levy and coworkers several years ago (Andrec et al., Proteins 2007; 69:449-465). These results demonstrated that the agreement between NMR and X-ray crystal structures is improved using protein NMR spectroscopy. Furthermore, NMR / X-ray Structure Pair Data Repository will provide a valuable resource for new computational NMR methods development.

Genetic Component of Obesity That obesity has a genetic component is not surprising: researchers have known that it often runs in families. A recent study reported that among people who carried a single copy of the high-risk allele for the *FTO* gene, which is associated with fat mass and obesity, the risk of obesity increased by 30%. The risk of obesity increased by 67% among people who carried two alleles, and they gained 3.0 kg (6.6 lb) or more. Given that ~one sixth of the population of European descent is homozygous for this allele, this link between the *FTO* gene and obesity seems to be one of the strongest genotype–phenotype associations detected by modern genome-screening techniques. Christakis and Fowler (2007) suggested that friends have an even more important effect on a person's risk of obesity than genes do. These authors reconstructed a social network showing the ties between friends, neighbors, spouses, and family members of the Framingham Heart Study, making use of the fact that the participants had been asked to name their friends to facilitate follow-up in the study. The authors observed that when two persons perceived each other as friends, if one friend became obese, the other friend's chances of following suit increased by 171% during a given time interval. Among pairs of adult siblings, if one sibling became obese, the chance that the other would become obese increased by 40%. The results of this study indicated that obesity is clustered in communities. For example, the risk that the friend of a friend of an obese person would be obese was ~ 20% higher in the observed network than in a random network; this effect vanished only by the fourth degree of separation.

In the past 7 years, our understanding of networks has undergone a revolution because of the emergence of a new array of theoretical tools and techniques for mapping out real networks. These advances included some surprises indicating that most real networks in technological, social, and biologic systems have common designs that are governed by simple and quantifiable organizing principles. The growing interest in interconnectedness has brought into focus an often ignored issue: networks pervade all aspects of human health. One example of this trend involves social networks and their impact on the spread of obesity or pathogens — from influenza to the severe acute respiratory syndrome or the human immunodeficiency virus. The role of neural networks in various psychiatric and neurodegenerative diseases is another example. In fact, network analysis is poised to play the biggest role at the cellular level, since most cellular components are connected to each other through intricate regulatory, metabolic, and protein–protein interactions. Because of these many functional links, the defects of various genes spread throughout the intracellular network, affecting the activity of genes that otherwise carry no defects. To understand various disease mechanisms, it is not sufficient to know the precise list of "disease genes"; instead, the researchers should try to map out the detailed wiring diagram of the various cellular components that are influenced by these genes and gene products. Such network-based thinking has already provided insights into the pathogenesis of several diseases. For example, a recent study suggested that 18 of the 23 genes associated with ataxia are part of a highly interlinked subnetwork; in another example, a reverse-engineered subnetwork indicated that the androgen-receptor gene might be used to detect the aggressiveness of primary prostate cancer. The existence of intricate molecular links between subcellular components and disease genes raises another possibility: that is, diseases may not be as independent of each other as physicians currently consider them to be. For example, could a genetic origin account for the fact that obesity is a risk factor for diabetes? A quick look at the list of genes associated with these two diseases indicates that several genes, including ectoenzyme nucleotide pyrophosphate phosphodiesterase (*ENPP1*), peroxisome-proliferator–activated receptor γ (*PPARγ*), and *FTO,* may be implicated in both diseases. In addition to the well-known link between diabetes and obesity, the large number of genes shared by distinct disorders indicates that these diseases may have common genetic origins. Human diseases, therefore, themselves form a network in which two diseases are connected if they share at least one gene. In this disease network, obesity has links to several diseases, including asthma, lipodystrophy, and network-based thinking may account for the environmental and social influences on disease as well. In this context, the researchers must understand the human interactions encompassing social and family links, proximity-based contacts, and transportation networks. For example, recent advances in the study of sexual networks have led to new protocols for drug dispersion. These protocols are efficient in combating the AIDS in underdeveloped countries than current protocols that are based on social need. The Human Genome Project has revolutionized gene hunting, leading to an explosion in the detected associations between genes and disease phenotypes. The beauty of GWAS lies in their ability to quantify their own limitations. For instance, many of the disease-associated genetic mutations account for only a small fraction of disease occurrences. Networks, in this case those that pertain to social influence, may have just as strong an impact on the development of obesity as the otherwise strong genetic effects. In the past few years, the researchers learned that network effects increasingly affect all aspects of biologic and medical research, from disease mechanisms to drug discovery. It is only a matter of time until these advances will start to affect medical practice as well, marking the emergence of a new field that may be aptly called network medicine (Barabási 2007).

PGx of Clopidogrel The capacity of Clopidogrel to inhibit ADP-induced platelet aggregation shows wide inter-individual variability. To determine whether frequent functional variants of genes coding for candidate cytochrome P450 (CYP) isoenzymes involved in Clopidogrel metabolic activation (CYP2C19*2, CYP2B6*5, CYP1A2*1F, and CYP3A5*3 variants) influence the platelet responsiveness to Clopidogrel, Hulot et al. (2006) conducted a pharmacogenetic study in 28 healthy white male volunteers treated for 7 days with Clopidogrel 75mg/d. The pharmacodynamic response to Clopidogrel was associated with the CYP2C19 genotype. Twenty of the subjects were wild-type CYP2C19 (*1/*1) homozygotes, while the other 8 subjects were heterozygous for the loss-of-function polymorphism CYP2C19*2 (*1/*2). Baseline platelet activity was not influenced by the CYP2C19 genotype. In contrast, platelet aggregation in the presence of 10 M ADP decreased gradually during treatment with Clopidogrel 75 mg once daily in *1/*1 subjects, reaching 48.9% 14.9% on day 7, whereas it did not change in *1/*2 subjects. Similar results were observed with VASP phosphorylation. The CYP2C19*2 loss-of-function allele was associated with a marked decrease in platelet responsiveness to Clopidogrel in young healthy male volunteers and may therefore be an important genetic contributor to Clopidogrel resistance in the clinical setting. Clopidogrel, a thienopyridine derivative, inhibits platelet aggregation induced by adenosine diphosphate (ADP). Clopidogrel is a prodrug requiring several biotransformation steps, mediated mainly by cytochrome P-450 isoenzymes (CYP), in order to generate an active metabolite that binds irreversibly to the platelet ADP receptor P2Y12.

Several large clinical trials have shown that Clopidogrel effectively prevents thrombotic events in patients with atherosclerotic vascular disease. Clopidogrel, alone or combined with aspirin, is routinely used to treat patients with a variety of vascular disorders. The pharmacodynamic response to Clopidogrel varies widely from subject to subject, and about 25% of patients treated with standard Clopidogrel doses display low ex vivo inhibition of ADP-induced platelet aggregation. This poor response to Clopidogrel is associated with an increased risk of recurrent ischemic events. The mechanisms underlying Clopidogrel resistance are unclear. In addition to nonadherence to treatment, certain genetic factors may be involved in this phenomenon. A gain-of-function haplotype (H2) of the gene encoding the P2Y12 receptor has been described, but P2Y12 genetic variants are unlikely to have a marked effect on the response to Clopidogrel. On the other hand, several functional polymorphisms have been found in genes encoding cytochrome P-450 isoforms involved in Clopidogrel metabolic activation upstream of P2Y12 (eg, CYP 3A4/5, 2C19, 2B6, and 1A2), but their influence on the pharmacodynamic response to Clopidogrel has not been systematically investigated. This pharmacogenetic study determined whether the antiplatelet effect of standard-dose Clopidogrel in healthy white subjects is influenced by functional variants in genes encoding CYP isoenzymes involved in Clopidogrel metabolic activation. It was shown that the CYP2C19 genotype is a major determinant of the pharmacodynamic response to Clopidogrel in healthy volunteers. These authors did not determine the CYP2C19 activity phenotype, as several studies have established that CYP2C19 genotyping identifies >90% of poor metabolizers, indicating good genotype phenotype agreement. CYP2C19 catalytic efficiency is primarily influenced by the 681GA polymorphism in exon 5 (*CYP2C19*2, allelic frequency 15% in whites*), which creates an aberrant splice site and results in a truncated and nonfunctional enzyme. That Clopidogrel responsiveness is reduced in subjects carrying a single *2 allele is in keeping with previous reports of a "gene-dose effect" of the CYP2C19*2 allele on the PKs/PDs of proton pump inhibitors, which are also CYP2C19 substrates, suggesting that CYP2C19 *1/*2 subjects are not totally refractory to Clopidogrel but that they respond less well than CYP2C19 *1/*1 subjects.

It was found that VASP phosphorylation in response to Clopidogrel was reduced but not abolished in CYP2C19 *1/*2 subjects, compared with CYP2C19 *1/*1 subjects, suggesting that Clopidogrel is partly converted into the active metabolite in *1/*2 subjects as suggested also by Brandt et al (2007). It remains to be determined whether this is also the case in CYP2C19 *2/*2 homozygotes, or whether Clopidogrel responsiveness is totally abolished in these subjects. Of interest, 2 of the 7 subjects who had the weakest responses to Clopidogrel did not carry functional variants associated with CYP2C19 deficiency, suggesting that genetic or nongenetic factors other than loss-of-function CYP2C19 polymorphisms may also influence Clopidogrel responsiveness. These authors did not observe any effect of other tested polymorphisms on ADP-induced platelet response to Clopidogrel. However they observed low allelic frequencies for 2 of them, and the study was sufficiently powered to detect factors that only strongly affect Clopidogrel response (*as observed with CYP2C19*2 variant*). Thus the authors could not exclude a minor influence of these other polymorphisms on Clopidogrel response. This proof-of-concept PKs study took place in strictly controlled conditions and involved only a small number of healthy volunteers, thereby creating optimal conditions to investigate the influence of genetic factors on Clopidogrel responsiveness, notably because of normal baseline platelet function and a lack of potentially interfering treatments. Although the sample size of this study was small, it provided a 95% power to detect the observed difference of 22% in ADP-induced aggregation between genotype groups with an alpha risk of 5% and a standard deviation of 14.9%. This study showed that the CYP2C19*2 mutant allele is a major genetic determinant of the pharmacodynamic response to standard-dose Clopidogrel (75 mg/d) in healthy young white men. Further studies are required to investigate the influence of CYP2C19 functional polymorphisms on the response to Clopidogrel in the clinical setting, particularly following a loading dose or with doses higher than 75 mg/d, and especially on the risk of recurrent thrombotic events during Clopidogrel therapy.

Biomarkers for EBPT of COPD Chronic obstructive pulmonary disease (COPD) is a complex and heterogeneous disease, so its clinical management needs to be personalized. 'Complex' means that COPD has several components with non-linear dynamic interactions, whereas 'heterogeneous' indicates that not all these components are present in all patients or, in a given patient, at all time points. This complexity and heterogeneity explains and justifies the need for EBPT of patients with COPD. Agusti et al. (2016) proposed that the implementation of a 'control panel' will facilitate the EBPT of COPD in clinical practice. Such a control panel should provide complementary and relevant information on treatable clinical characteristics in a single patient at any given time. These authors considered these variables to be 'biomarkers'. Which treatable clinical characteristics should the COPD control panel include and which ones might be considered in the future and should be viewed as a working proposal has not been well work out till date.

REFERENCES

Agusti, A., Gea, J. & Faner, R. (2016). Biomarkers, the control panel and personalized COPD medicine. *Respirology.*, *21*(1), 24-33.

Ansari, B. M., Zochios, V., Falter, F. & Klein, A. A. (2016). Physiological controversies and methods used to determine fluid responsiveness: a qualitative systematic review. *Anaesthesia.*, *71*(1), 94-105.

Barabási, A. L. (2007). Network Medicine — From Obesity to the "Diseasome" *N. Engl. J. Med.*, *357*, 404-407.

Brandt, J.T., Close, S.L., Iturria, S.J., Payne, C.D., Farid, N.A., Ernest, C.S. 2nd, Lachno, D.R., Salazar, D., Winters, K.J. (2007). Common polymorphisms of CYP2C19 and CYP2C9 affect the pharmacokinetic and pharmacodynamic response to clopidogrel but not prasugrel. *J. Thromb. Haemost.* 5(12), 2429-2436.

Christakis, N.A., Fowler, J.H. (2007) The spread of obesity in large social network over 32 years. *New Eng. J. Med.* 357, 370-379.

Clarke, N. J. (2016). Mass Spectrometry in Precision Medicine: Phenotypic Measurements Alongside Pharmacogenomics. *Clin. Chem.*, *62*(1), 70-76.

Deacon, N. L., Jen, R., Li, Y. & Malhotra, A. (2016). Treatment of Obstructive Sleep Apnea. Prospects for Personalized Combined Modality Therapy. *Ann. Am. Thorac. Soc.*, *13*(1), 101-108.

Esposito, A., Criscitiello, C., Locatelli, M., Milano, M. & Curigliano, G. (2016). Liquid biopsies for solid tumors: Understanding tumor heterogeneity and real time monitoring of early resistance to targeted therapies. *Pharmacol Ther.*, *157*, 120-124.

Everett, J. K., Tejero, R., Murthy, S. B., Acton, T. B., Aramini, J. M., Baran, M. C., Benach, J., et al., (2016). A community resource of experimental data for NMR/X-ray crystal structure pairs.

Facchetti, F., Cigognetti, M., Fisogni, S., Rossi, G., Lonardi, S. & Vermi, W. (2016). Neoplasms derived from plasmacytoid dendritic cells. *Mod Pathol.* Jan 8.

Hulot, J. S., Bura, A., Villard, E., Azizi, M., Remones, V., Goyenvalle, C., Aiach, M., Lechat, P. & Gaussem, P. (2006). Cytochrome P450 2C19 loss-of-function polymorphism is a major determinant of Clopidogrel responsiveness in healthy subjects. *Blood.*, *108*, 2244-2247

Jain, K. K. (2002). PM, *Current Opinion in Molecular Therapeutics*, *4*(6), 548-558.

Jain, K. K. (2004). Applications of biochips: from diagnostics to PM. *Current Opinion in Drug Discovery & Development*, *7*(3), 285-289.

Kahle, K. T. & Delpire, E. (2016). Kinase-KCC2 coupling: Cl- rheostasis, disease susceptibility, therapeutic target. *J Neurophysiol.*, *115*(1), 8-18.

Le Tourneau, C., Kamal, M., Tsimberidou, A. M., Bedard, P., Pierron, G., Callens, C., Rouleau, E., Vincent-Salomon, A., Servant, N., Alt, M., Rouzier, R., Paoletti, X., Delattre, O. & Bièche, I. (2015). Treatment Algorithms Based on Tumor Molecular Profiling: The Essence of Precision Medicine Trials. *J Natl Cancer Inst.*, Nov 23, *108*(4).

Lim, C. X., Ricos, M. G., Dibbens, L. M. & Heron, S. E. (2016). KCNT1 mutations in seizure disorders: the phenotypic spectrum and functional effects. *J. Med. Genet.*, 2016 Jan 6.

Luzak, A., Schnell-Inderst, P., Bühn, S., Mayer-Zitarosa, A. & Siebert, U. (2016). Clinical effectiveness of cancer screening biomarker tests offered as self-pay health service: a systematic review. *Eur. J. Public. Health.*, pii: ckv227.

Mankoff, D. A., Edmonds, C. E., Farwell, M. D. & Pryma, D. A. (2016). Development of Companion Diagnostics. *Semin Nucl Med.*, *46*(1), 47-56.

Neuroimaging. *Clin N Am.*, 2016 Feb, *26*(1), 175-182.

Ogino, S., Galon, J., Fuchs C. S. & Dranoff, G. (2011). Cancer immunology—analysis of host and tumor factors for PM. *Nature Reviews Clinical Oncology*, *8*, 711-719.

Patrick, J., Roberts, P. J., Stinchcombe, T. E., Der, C. J. & Socinski, M. A. (2010). PM in Non–Small-Cell Lung Cancer: Is *KRAS* a Useful Marker in Selecting Patients for Epidermal Growth Factor Receptor–Targeted Therapy? *J. Clinical. Oncology.*, vol. *28*, 4769-4777.

Robert, E. H. (2011). Biobanking: the foundation of PM, *Current Opinion in Oncology*, Vol *23*, p 112-119.

Stewart, B. W., Bray, F., Forman, D., Ohgaki, H., Straif, K., Ullrich, A. & Wild, C. P. (2016). Cancer prevention as part of precision medicine: 'plenty to be done'. *Carcinogenesis.*, *37*(1), 2-9.

Tzatzalos, E., Abilez, O. J., Shukla, P. & Wu, J. C. (2016). Engineered heart tissues and induced pluripotent stem cells: Macro- and microstructures for disease modeling, drug screening, and translational studies. *Adv. Drug Deliv. Rev.*, *96*, 234-244.

Veer, L. J. & René, Bernards. (2008). Enabling personalized cancer medicine through analysis of gene-expression patterns. *Nature*, *452*, 564-570.

Chapter 5

EVIDENCE-BASED PERSONALIZED THERANOSTICS (RECENT UPDATE-II)

ABSTRACT

This chapter is divided in three main parts. Part-1 decribes recent trends in biotechnology; part-2 describes disease-specific biomarkers, and part-3 describes emerging strategies based on the pharmacogenomic profile of a patient to accomplish EBPT of cancer, neurodegenerative diseases, cardiovascular diseases, and various other chronic diseases.

Keywords: biotechnology, disese-specific biomarkers, pharmacogenomics, evidence-based personalized theranostics (EBPT)

INTRODUCTION

Recent developments to discover novel theranostic biomarkers has revolutionized the basic concept of personalized, predictive, and precision medicine (PPPM), which is also named as individualized medicine. A significant progress has been made based on the multidisciplinary and translational analysis of chronic diseases and on the exact landscape of system medicine. In general, 5 major disciplines have evolved to accomplish evidence based personalized theranostics (EBPT). These are: (a) *biotechnology, (b) genomic analyses, (c) novel biomarkers, (d) bioinformatics, and (e) theranostics (diagnosis and treatment simultaneously.* A remarkable progress in biotechnology has refined early and accurarate diagnosis as well as treatment (Theranostics) of chronic diseases. For example, LC-MS/MS is currently used for the precise determination of Teicoplanin in human plasma and the phosphatidylcholine-derived quaternary ammonium compounds from human blood plasma, serum, and urine samples. Quantitation of Tramadol and its metabolites in human blood can be performed using LC-MS/mapping feedback loops of major depressive disorders as described in this chapter. A microfluidic system has been developed for the automated monitoring of whole blood hemostasis and platelet function. In addition, gene profiling can be performed for response prediction and to determine single nucleotide polymorphism (SNP) in cancer.

Innovative methods have been developed for the successful transplantation of human pluripotent stem cells in liver using Gata6, and genome-wide association studies (GWAS) of lung cancer in Asian never-smoking women have been performed. The development in next generation sequencing (NGS) in lung cancer theranostics, functional respiratory imaging, carotid plaque imaging, and computer-assisted surgical navigation has made remarkable contribution in improving the current concept of EBPT. The identification of microRNA-29a in adult muscle stem cells and skeletal muscle regeneration, PGx genotyping chip to estimate population substructure and cryptic relatedness, visual open data analysis platform, and neuro-epigenetics of acute stress response have been developed. Furthermore, PKs of Harmane and its metabolites, PGx analysis of blood pressure and patient-centered assessment of cardiac events have further improved EBPT.

Technology-based treatment of schizophrenia, Dexamethasone therapy in childhood acute lymphoblastic leukemia, clinical management of thoracic aortic disease, mass spectrometric imaging of mouse brain lipids, determination of blood Alcohol concentration by ^{1}H NMR spectroscopy, genetic screening of gynecological cancer, miniturized and mobile drug manufacturing, diffusion analysis in neuronal tissue with MRI, functional MRI, confocal and super-resolution imaging by VividSTORM, companion diagnostics, 2D chromatographic analysis of complex herbal samples, nanocomposites for enrichment of Chloramphenicol and Thiamphenicol, localization of Radium-223 in naïve and mouse models of prostate cancer metastasis, PKs of 3,4-Divanillyltetrahydrofuran in rats by liquid chromatography/tandem mass spectrometry, chromatographic analyses of Doxorubcin associated with DNA in tumor and tissue, tyrosine kinase nonreceptor 2 (TNK2) point mutations in leukemia through kinase inhibitor screening and genomic analysis, quantitation of Teriflunomide in serum/plasma, genetically-manipulated pig model of neurodegeneration, engineered heart tissue and induced pulripotent stem cells, and *in-vitro* cardiac tissue models have been developed to accomplish EBPT. Medical genomics in health and immune diseases, multisystem physiological dysregulation, interferon-α signalling in melanoma, effect of cytochrome P450 2D6 variants in the Chinese population on Atomoxetine metabolism, functional characterization of CYP2D6 allelic variants, metabolomics in type 2 diabetes management, determination of genetics of metastatic head and neck squamous carcinoma, molecular phenotyping and multigene assays for the clinical management of breast cancer, genomics to guide weight management, transcriptional profiling of breast cancer, gene body hypermethylation in kidney cancer, blood transcriptomics and metabolomics, and companion molecular diagnosis have been developed to accomplish EBPT. Furthermore, NIR-Cyanine dye linker for isochronic fluorescence imaging in cancer theranostics, gastrin-releasing peptide receptor (GRPR) for prostate cancer theranostics, T53 dysfunction in diffuse B-cell lymphoma, transcutaneous measurement of PCO2 in the diagnosis of nocturnal hypercapnia, prenatal Cocaine exposure (PCE) and increased illicit-substance abuse in adolescence, multi-compartmental analyses for personalized diagnosis, NCI MATCH for gynecologic oncology, and detection and diagnosis of Ebola virus infection have improved the emerging concept of EBPT.

Recently soluble biomarkers to establish BIPED criteria, cancer screening, determine germline for cutaneous melanoma, and for the chemotherapy of gastric cancer were developed. However a poor association of serum biomarkers with brain metastasis was identified. Epigenetic disorders were detected with BRCAness in hereditary and sporadic breast cancer. Biomarkers for endometrial carcinoma and lung cancer are being explored for personalized treatment. In addition to salivary biomarkers, theranostics biomarkers for drug development in the treatment of COPD and allergen immunotherapy, and bladder cancer therapy are being invstigated. Recently behavioral intervention in adolescent sexual health, serum complement factors as inflammatory biomarkers in metabolic syndrome have been introduced.

The bioinformatics has emerged as a promising discipline to accomplish EBPT, immunology and bioinformatics for disease prediction and quantitation. For example, *ChainRank for contextualization of biological networks, CRISPR/Cas9-based genome engineering in human pluripotent stem cells, IGNITE Network for genomic medicine and research, EBPT of prostate cancer, patient-specific immune response profiles of breast cancer* have been developed. In addition, radiology informatics, and data collection to build prediction models in oncology have been introduced.

As a result of significant developments in biotechnology, human genomic analyses *(DNA sequencing, SNP analyses, and bioinformatics)* individualized treatment of several chronic diseases has become a reality. For instance: cell-based therapy for cystic fibrosis, immunotherapy of lung cancer, photodynamic therapy for personalized cancer immunotherapy, treatment of brain metastasis, novel multi-target Src and MEK kinase inhibitors as anticancer drugs, radiation planning for cervical cancer, precision treatment of obesity, blood transcriptomes analyses in prophylactic drug treatment of migraine, micro-dissected tumor tissues on chip for drug testing and treatment, antidotes for Cyanide poisoning, trace elements and Arsenic for a Realgar-containing traditional Chinese medicine Niuhuang Jiedu, anticancer effect of β-blockers, Siltuximab: for idiopathic multicentric castleman disease, ALK inhibitors in treatment of pancreatic ductal adenocarcinoma, RAS signaling and anti-RAS in cancer treatment. Molecular imaging of pancreatic cancer with antibodies for treatment and virtual reality intervention to improve weight gain, interdisciplinary approach to alleviate pain, treatment in ophthalmology, Nicotine addiction therapy, Oxytoxin in autism, and the use of smartphones for health and fitness have been developed.

This chapter describes briefly state of the art biotechnology, diseases-specific biomarkers, and EBPT of cancer, neurodegenerative diseases, cardiovascular diseases, and various other chronic diseases.

EBPT BIOTECHNOLOGY

Bioinformatics in Systems Medicine It is now well established that novel strategies to study human health and disease at a systems level can improve the overall health and well-being of patients by preventing, diagnosing, or curing disease. van Kampen and Moerland (2016) discussed how bioinformatics can contribute to systems medicine. These investigators explained the role of bioinformatics in the management and analysis of data, the importance of biological and clinical repositories to support systems medicine studies; how the integration and analysis of omics data through integrative bioinformatics may facilitate the determination of more predictive and robust disease signatures, lead to a better understanding of pathophysiological and molecular mechanisms to facilitate PM. They also focused on network analysis and discussed how gene networks can be constructed from omics data and how these networks can be merged into smaller modules. Furthermore, they discussed how these modules can be used to generate experimentally testable hypotheses, provide insight into disease mechanisms, and lead to predictive models. These investigators provided examples demonstrating how bioinformatics contributes to systems medicine and discussed future challenges that need to be addressed to enable the advancement in EBPT.

Multisystem Physiological Dysreulation Wiley et al. (2016) compared the relative fit of two alternative models of allostatic load (AL) and physiological systems to test factor invariance across age and sex. Data were from the *Midlife in the US II Biomarker Project*, a large (n = 1255) multisite study of adults aged 34 to 84 years (56.8% women). Specifically, 23 biomarkers were included, representing 7 physiological systems: *metabolic lipids, metabolic glucose, BP, parasympathetic nervous system, sympathetic nervous system, hypothalamic-pituitary-adrenal axis, and inflammation.* For factor invariance tests, age was categorized into 3 groups (≤45, 45-60, and >60 years). A bifactor model where biomarkers load onto a common AL factor and 7 unique system-specific factors provided the best fit to the biomarker data. Results from the bifactor model were consistent with invariance across age groups and sex. These results supported the theory that represents and operationalizes AL as multisystem physiological dysregulation and considering AL as the shared variance across biomarkers. These results also demonstrated that in addition to the variance in biomarkers accounted for by AL, individual physiological systems account for variance in system-specific biomarkers. A bifactor model allowed greater precision to examine both AL and the effects of specific systems.

Interferon-α Signalling in Melanoma Interferon-α (IFNα) is used for adjuvant systemic melanoma therapy. Understanding the molecular mechanism of IFNα effects and prediction of response in the IFNα therapy allows initiation and continuation of IFNα treatment for responder and exclusion of non-responder to *avoid therapy inefficacy and side-effects*. The transporter protein associated with antigen processing-1 (TAP1) is part of the MHC class I peptide-loading complex, and important for antigen presentation in tumor and antigen presenting cells. In the context of EBPT, Heise et al. (2016) addressed this potential biomarker TAP1 as a target of IFNα signalling. These investigators demonstrated that IFNα upregulates TAP1 expression in peripheral blood mononuclear cells (PBMCs) of patients with malignant melanoma receiving adjuvant high-dose immunotherapy. IFNα also induced TAP1 expression in mouse blood and tumor tissue and suppressed melanoma metastasis in an *in vivo* B16 tumor model. Besides its expression, TAP binding affinity and transport activity was induced by IFNα in monocytic THP1 cells. Furthermore, these data revealed that IFNα activates phosphorylation of STAT1 and STAT3 in THP1 and A375 melanoma cells. Inhibition of Janus kinases abrogated the IFNα-induced TAP1 expression, suggesting that the JAK/STAT pathway is a crucial mediator for TAP1 expression elicited by IFNα treatment, and that silencing of TAP1 expression provides tumor cells to escape cytotoxic T-lymphocyte recognition. The benefit of IFNα treatment could be mediated by the dual effect of TAP1 upregulation in antigen presenting cells on the one hand, and of TAP1 upregulation in 'silent' metastatic melanoma cells on the other hand. This work contributed to a better understanding of the mode of action of IFNα to identify biomarkers to predict, assess, and monitor therapeutic response of IFNα treatment.

Microfluidic System for Automated Monitoring of Whole Blood Hemostasis and Platelet Function. Accurate assessment of blood hemostasis is essential for the management of patients who use extracorporeal devices, receive anticoagulation therapy or experience coagulopathies. However, current monitoring devices do not measure effects of hemodynamic forces that contribute to platelet function and thrombus formation. Jain et al. (2016) described a microfluidic device that mimics a network of stenosed arteriolar vessels, permitting blood clotting within small sample volumes under pathophysiological flow. By applying a clotting time analysis based on a mathematical model of thrombus formation, coagulation and platelet function can be accurately measured *in vitro* in patient blood samples. When the device was integrated into an extracorporeal circuit in pig endotoxemia or heparin therapy models, it produced alterations in coagulation *ex vivo* that were more reliable than standard clotting assays, indicating that this disposable device may be useful for EBPT and for real-time surveillance of antithrombotic therapy.

Human Pluripotent Stem Cells into a Liver (Liver Bud-like Tissue Using Gata6) It is now known that human induced pluripotent stem cells (hiPSCs) have potential for EBPT and regenerative medicine. These cells are emerging as a powerful tool for biomedical discovery. While most of the methods using these cells have focused on deriving homogenous populations of specialized cells, there has been success in producing hiPSC-derived organotypic tissues or organoids. The researchers presented a novel approach for generating and then co-differentiating hiPSC-derived progenitors. With a genetically engineered pulse of GATA-binding protein 6 (GATA6) expression; they initiated rapid emergence of all three germ layers as a complex function of GATA6 expression levels and tissue context. Within 2 weeks a complex tissue was obtained that recapitulated early developmental processes and exhibited a liver bud-like phenotype, including hematopoietic and stromal cells as well as a neuronal niche. This novel approach demonstrated derivation of complex tissues from hiPSCs using a single autologous hiPSCs and generated a range of stromal cells that co-develop with parenchymal cells to form tissues with a potential for diversified functions.

CRISPR/Cas9-Based Genome Engineering in Human Pluripotent Stem Cells The advent of human induced pluripotent stem cells (hiPS cells) with human embryonic stem (hES)-cell-like properties has led to hPS cells with disease-specific genetic BKg for *in vitro* disease modeling and drug discovery as well as mechanistic and developmental studies. Kime et al. (2016) reported that to fully realize this potential, it will be necessary to modify the genome of hPS cells with precision and flexibility. Experiments utilizing site-specific double-strand break (DSB)-mediated genome engineering tools, including zinc finger nucleases (ZFNs) and transcription activator-like effector nucleases (TALENs), have paved the way to genome engineering in previously recalcitrant systems such as hPS cells. However, these methods are cumbersome and require lot of expertise. A major recent advance involving the clustered regularly interspaced short palindromic repeats (CRISPR) endonuclease has simplified the effort required for genome engineering and will be adopted as the rapid and flexible system for genome editing in hPS cells. These investigators described commonly practiced methods for CRISPR endonuclease genomic editing of hPS cells into cell lines containing genomes altered by insertion/deletion (indel) mutagenesis or insertion of recombinant genomic DNA to accomplish EBPT.

Computer-Assisted Surgical Navigation in PM Peters et al. (2016) performed a study to determine whether computer-assisted surgical navigation improves the accuracy of tibial component alignment in canine knee replacement (TKR). Retrospective radiographic review and prospective *ex vivo* study was performed on canine TKR radiographs (n = 17 sets) and canine cadaveric stifles (n = 12). Radiographs from TKR surgical workshops were reviewed to determine the incidence and magnitude of tibial component malalignment. Tibial component alignment was compared after either standard *("surgeon-guided")* component placement or computer-assisted *("navigation-guided")* placement. Results were compared against the current recommendations of a neutral *(0° varus-valgus)* ostectomy in the frontal plane and 6° of caudal slope in the sagittal plane. A prospective cadaveric study was then undertaken by performing TKR in 12 canine stifle joints. Malalignment of >3° in the frontal and sagittal planes was identified in 12% and 24% of the radiographs from the retrospective review, respectively. Surgical navigation reduced both the mean error and the variability in frontal plane alignment as compared with surgeon-guided procedures. The mean error in sagittal plane alignment was not different, but variability in alignment was significantly lower when navigation was used. Surgical navigation improved accuracy and decreased variability in tibial component alignment in canine TKR. These investigators suggested that clinical trials will be required to determine whether these improvements in surgical accuracy lead to better clinical outcomes in terms of joint function and a reduction in long-term implant.

Functional Respiratory Imaging Hjian et al., (2016) reported that functional imaging techniques offer improved visualization of anatomical structures such as; airways, lobe volumes and blood vessels. Computer-based flow simulations with a 3-D element add functionality to the images. By providing valuable detailed information about airway geometry, internal airflow distribution and inhalation profile, functional respiratory imaging can be used routinely in the clinic. Moreover, 3D visualization allows detailed follow-up of disease progression to assess effects of interventions. These authors explored the usefulness of functional respiratory imaging in different respiratory diseases. In patients with asthma and COPD, functional respiratory imaging was used for phenotyping these patients, to predict the responder and non-responder phenotype and to evaluate innovative therapeutic interventions to accomplish EBPT.

MicroRNA-29a of Muscle Stem Cells in Skeletal Muscle Regeneration The expansion of myogenic progenitors (MPs) in the adult muscle stem cell niche is critical for the regeneration of skeletal muscle. Activation of quiescent MPs depends on the dismantling of the basement membrane and increased access to growth factors such as fibroblast growth factor-2 (FGF2). Galimov et al. (2016) demonstrated using miRNA profiling in mouse and human myoblasts that the capacity of FGF2 to stimulate myoblast proliferation is mediated by miR-29a. FGF2 induced miR-29a expression and inhibition of miR-29a using pharmacological or genetic deletion decreased myoblast proliferation. Next generation RNA sequencing from miR-29a knockout myoblasts (Pax7$^{CE/+}$; miR-29a$^{flox/flox}$) identified members of the basement membrane as the most abundant miR-29a targets. These invetigators confirmd that miR-29a regulates Fbn1, Lamc1, Nid2, Col4a1, Hspg2 and Sparc in myoblasts *in vitro* and in MPs *in vivo*. Induction of FGF2 and miR-29a and downregulation of its target genes preceded muscle regeneration during cardiotoxin (CTX)-induced muscle injury. MP-specific Tamoxifen-induced deletion of miR-29a in adult skeletal muscle decreased the proliferation and formation of newly formed myofibers during both CTX-induced muscle injury and after a single bout of eccentric exercise. These results identified a novel miRNA-based checkpoint of the basement membrane in the muscle stem cell niche. Hence targeting miR-29a might provide useful therapeutic approaches to maintain muscle mass in disease states such as aging involving impaired FGF2 signaling.

Pharmacogenomics Genotyping Chip to Estimate Population Substructure and Cryptic Relatedness Jackon et al. (2016) evaluated the Affymetrix drug metabolism enzymes and transporters (DMET) Plus pharmacogenomics genotyping chip to estimate population substructure and cryptic relatedness. The results were compared using genome-wide HapMap data for the same individuals. For 301 unrelated individuals, spanning 3 continental populations and one admixed population, genotypic data were collected using the Affymetrix DMET Plus microarray. Genome-wide data on these individuals were obtained from HapMap release 3. Population substructure was assessed using Eigenstrat and ADMIXTURE software for both platforms. Cryptic relatedness was explored by inbreeding coefficient estimation. Nonparametric tests were used to determine correlations of the analytical results of the two genotyping platforms. Principal components analysis (PCA) identified population substructure for both datasets, with 15.8 and 16.6% of the total variance in the first two components for DMET Plus and HapMap data, respectively. ADMIXTURE results identified 4 subpopulations within each dataset. Nonparametric rank correlations indicated associations between analyses with an average across the 3 continental populations and for the admixed population. Concordance correlation coefficients indicated concordance between ADMIXTURE results. Inbreeding coefficients were slightly inflated using DMET Plus data and no cryptic relatedness was indicated using HapMap data. The inflated inbreeding estimation could be because of the limited number of markers provided by DMET as a random sample of 1832 markers from HapMap also yielded inflated estimates of cryptic relatedness. Furthermore, use of SNP located in genes involved in metabolism and transport may have different allele frequencies in subpopulations than SNPs sampled from the whole genome. The DMET Plus pharmacogenomics genotyping chip was successful in quantifying population substructure and inferring the presence of an admixed population. These microarrays offered sufficient insight for covariate adjustment of population substructure in genomic association studies.

Visual Open Data Analysis Platform in PM It is currently realized that with the accumulation of extensive health related data, predictive analytics could stimulate the transformation of reactive medicine towards *Predictive, Preventive, Precision, and Personalized* (PPPPM) Medicine, eventually affecting both cost and quality of health care. However, multi-dimensionality and multi-complexity, prevents data-driven methods from easy translation into clinically relevant models. Additionally, the application of predictive methods and data manipulation require extensive programming skills, limiting its direct exploitation by medical experts. This leaves a gap between potential and actual data usage. In this study, Poucke et al. (2016) addressed this problem by focusing on open, visual environments, applied by the medical community. These investigators reviewed code free applications of large-scale data technologies. A framework was developed for the meaningful use of data from critical care patients by integrating the MIMIC-II database in a data mining environment (RapidMiner) supporting scalable predictive analytics using visual tools (*RapidMiner's Radoop extension*). Guided by the Cross-Industry Standard Process for Data Mining (CRISP-DM), the ETL process (Extract, Transform, Load) was initiated by retrieving data from the MIMIC-II tables of interest. The correlation of platelet count and ICU survival was assessed. Using visual tools for ETL on Hadoop and predictive modeling in RapidMiner, 3 investigators developed processes for automatic building, parameter optimization and evaluation of predictive models, under different feature selection schemes. Because these processes can be easily adopted in other projects, this environment may be attractive for predictive analytics in health research.

Epigenetic Biomarkers of Acute Stress Response Stress research has become more integrative in nature, seeking to identify crucial relations between the different phenotypic levels of stress manifestations. Vaisvaser et al. (2016) investigated stress-induced variations in human microRNAs in peripheral blood mononuclear cells and assessed their relationship with neuronal and psychological indices. These researchers obtained blood samples from 49 healthy male participants before and 3 hrs after performing a social stress task, while undergoing fMRI. A seed-based functional connectivity (FC) analysis was conducted for the ventro-medial prefrontal cortex (vmPFC), a key area of stress regulation. A specific increase was identified in microRNA-29c (miR-29c) expression, corresponding with both the experience of sustained stress via self-reports, and alterations in vmPFC functional connectivity. miR-29c expression corresponded with increased connectivity of the vmPFC in the anterior insula (aIns), and decreased connectivity of the vmPFC in the left dorso-lateral prefrontal cortex (dlPFC), indicating that miR-29c mediates an indirect path linking enhanced vmPFC-aIns connectivity with subsequent sustained stress. The miR-29c expression and vmPFC FC, along with the effects on subjective stress and the localization of miR-29c in astrocytes, suggested that it may serve as a biomarker of stress-induced functional neural alterations reflecting regulatory processes. Such a model may be crucial for personalized intervention in stress psychopharmacology.

Poor Association of Serum Biomarkers with Brain Metastasis Lung cancers account for the majority of brain metastases, which pose major therapeutic challenges. Biomarkers for the development of brain metastases in patients with non-small cell lung cancers (NSCLC) may improve personalized care. In a study, 6 serum proteomic biomarkers were investigated but their associations with brain metastases were unknown. Li et al. (2016) collected serum NSE, CYFRA 21-1, ProGRP, SCC-Ag, TIMP1, and HE4 by ELISA-based proteomic assays from consecutive patients with stage IV NSCLC. Pre-treatment serum biomarker levels as well as age, histology, and epidermal growth factor receptor (EGFR) mutation status were evaluated for association with the presence of brain metastases using logistic regression and multivariable analysis. For patients without brain metastases at baseline, the incidence of brain metastases were compared according to baseline biomarkers and clinical factors using Gray's test in 118 patients who had brain metastases at baseline and a further 26 developed brain metastases subsequently. Pre-treatment serum biomarker levels were available in 104 patients. There was no association between the serum biomarkers and subsequent development of brain metastases. Age younger than 65 years was the only clinical factor associated with brain metastasis. A trend toward increased cumulative incidence of subsequent brain metastases was observed in patients with EGFR mutation, but this was not significant due to small sample size. This study revealed that serum NSE, CYFRA 21-1, Pro-GRP, SCC-Ag, TIMP1, and HE4 were not associated with brain metastases. However, this method may be applied to identify a patient cohort with a higher biologic propensity for developing brain metastases and may be useful for targeting the brain metastases.

PKs of Harmane and its Metabolites The β-carboline alkaloid Harmane is widely distributed in common foods, beverages and hallucinogenic plants. Harmane exerts potential in therapies for AD and depression. However, there is limited information on its metabolic profiles and PKs *in vivo*. Li et al. (2016) investigated the metabolic profiles and PKs of Harmane and its metabolites in rats *in vivo*. These scientists developed a selective, sensitive and rapid ultra-performance liquid chromatography combined with electrospray ionization tandem mass spectrometry (UPLC-ESI-MS/MS) and validated for the determination of Harmane and its endogenous metabolite Harmine, as well as 10 Harmane metabolites in rats after i.v. injection and oral administration at 1.0 and 30.0 mg/kg, respectively. The calibration curves of Harmane and Harmine revealed linearity within the range of 1-2000 ng/mL with accuracy, precision, selectivity, recovery, matrix effect and stability. Ten metabolites, including Harmane but not Harmine, were detected and identified after i.v. and oral administration. The bioavailability of Harmane following an oral dose was $19.41\pm 3.97\%$. According to the AUC_{0-t} values of all the metabolites, the levels of phase II metabolites were higher than those of phase I metabolites, and the sulphation pathways were the dominant metabolic routes for Harmane in both routes of administration. The PKs determined that sulphate conjugation was the predominant metabolic process of Harmane in rats.

Patient-Centered Assessment of Cardiac Events Collection of high-quality data from large populations is considered essential to generate knowledge that is critical in the era of EBPT. Cardiovascular disease (CVD) is a leading cause of mortality in China and is a focus biomarker discovery that would improve ability to assess and modify individual risk factors. Lu et al. (2016) conducted a Patient-centered Evaluative Assessment of Cardiac Events project during 2014-2015 in 4 provinces. *It was designed to screen 0.4 million community-dwelling residents aged 40-75 years with measurements of BP, height and weight, a lipid blood test, and a questionnaire on cardiovascular-related health status.* Participants at high risk of CVD were subjected to further health assessments, including *ECG, ultrasound scan, blood and urine analysis, and a questionnaire on lifestyle and medical history.* The blood and urine samples were used to establish a biobank. High-risk subjects were also suggested lifestyle changes and were followed-up either in a return clinic visit or by telephone interview, with measurement of BP, weight, ECG, and a questionnaire on survival status, hospitalizations, and lifestyle to accomplish EBPT.

Confocal and Super-Resolution Imaging by VividSTORM Single-molecule localization microscopy (SMLM) is gaining popularity as an efficient approach to visualize molecular distribution with nanoscale precision. However, it is challenging to obtain and analyze such data in tissue preparations. Barna et al. (2016) described a 5-D tissue processing and immunostaining procedure that is optimized for SMLM, and provided applications to fixed mouse brain, heart, and kidney tissues. These investigators described confocal and 3D-resolution imaging on these sections, which allowed the visualization of nanoscale protein within subcellular compartments of target cells within few minutes and described the use of *VividSTORM* (http://katonalab.hu/index.php/vividstorm), software for confocal and SMLM image analysis, which facilitates *the measurement of molecular abundance, clustering, internalization, surface density and intermolecular distances in a cell-specific and subcellular compartment-restricted manner* to accomplish EBPT.

ChainRank For Contextualization of Biological Networks Advances in high throughput technologies and biomedical knowledge have contributed to an exponential increase in associative data, which can be represented as complex networks of biological associations, suitable for systems analyses. However, these networks usually lack both, context specificity in time and space as well as the distinctive borders, usually assigned in the classical pathway of molecular events (*e.g., signal transduction*). This complex interaction calls for automated techniques that can identify targeted subnetworks specific to a given disease scenario. Tényi et al. (2016) introduced a method called, ChainRank, which finds relevant subnetworks by identifying and scoring chains of interactions that link specific network components. Scores can be generated from integrating multiple general and context specific measures (*e.g., experimental molecular data from expression to proteomics and metabolomics, literature evidence, network topology*). The performance of the novel ChainRank method was evaluated on creating selected signalling pathways from a human protein interaction network. These investigators recreated skeletal muscle specific signaling networks in healthy individuals and COPD patients. The ChainRank could identify main mediators of context specific molecular signalling. An improvement of up to factor 2.5 was revealed in the precision of finding proteins of the recreated pathways compared to random simulation. ChainRank could integrate user-defined scores and evaluate their effect on ranking interaction chains linking input data sets which can be used to contextualize networks, identify signaling and regulatory path amongst targeted genes or to analyze lethality in anticancer therapy.

PHARMACOGENOMICS

Cancer Pharmacology in PM Insel et al. (2015) collected reviews that emphasized current and emerging aspects in pharmacology and toxicology and that provided complementary insights regarding "*Cancer Pharmacology*," which included articles that emphasized fundamental aspects of pharmacology and toxicology and others that addressed translational and clinical features of cancer therapeutics. These investigators believed that these articles captured for readers the vitality and excitement of research in cancer biology and, especially, in the cancer therasnostics. Some of the articles were an extension of the theme, "Precision Medicine *and Prediction in Pharmacology*." The editors emphasized that cancer therapeutics is the area of clinical medicine that is moving toward personalized treatment (based on genetic features of tumors) in the US (via the Precision Medicine *Initiative introduced in 2015 by President Obama*) and abroad. The Editors chose 12 articles that fit into the "Cancer Pharmacology" Theme, but readers may identify others that are relevant to this area. The editors envisaged that this review will be of interest not only to readers who work in cancer pharmacology but also to those less familiar with discoveries related to cancer theranostics.

Genomics in Health and Wellness Recent advances in genomics have led to the rapid and relatively inexpensive collection of patient molecular data including multiple types of omics data. Saqi et al. (2016) highlighted that the integration of these data with clinical measurements has the potential to impact on our understanding of the molecular basis of disease and on disease management. Systems medicine is an approach to understanding disease through an integration of large patient datasets. It offers the possibility for personalized strategies for healthcare through the development of a new taxonomy of disease. Advanced computing will be an important component in effectively implementing systems medicine. These investgators described 3 computational challenges associated with systems medicine: (a) disease subtype discovery using integrated datasets, (b) obtaining a mechanistic understanding of disease, and (c) the development of an informatics platform for the mining, analysis, and visualization of data emerging from translational medicine studies.

Genomics to Guide Weight Management Precision medicine utilizes genomic and other data to optimize and personalize treatment. Although >2,500 genetic tests are currently available, for extreme and/or rare phenotypes, the question remains whether this approach can be used for the treatment of common, complex conditions like *obesity, inflammation, and insulin resistance*, which underlie a host of metabolic diseases. Bray et al. (2016) developed from a Trans-NIH Conference titled "*Genes, Behaviors, and Response to Weight Loss Interventions,*" provided an overview of the state of genetic and genomic research in the area of weight change and identified key areas for future research. Although many loci have been identified that are associated with cross-sectional measures of obesity/body size, relatively little is known regarding the genes/loci that influence dynamic measures of weight change over time. Although short-term weight loss has been achieved using different strategies, sustainable weight loss has proven elusive for many, and there are lacunae in the present knowledge regarding energy balance regulation. Elucidating the molecular basis of variability in weight change may improve treatment outcomes and develop innovative approaches that can take into account information from genomic and other sources in devising EBPT strategies.

Genomics of Immune Diseases Genomic DNA sequencing technologies have been one of the great advances of the 21st century, having decreased in cost and opening up new fields of investigation throughout research and clinical medicine. Genomics coupled with biochemical investigation has facilitated the molecular definition of new genetic diseases that reveal new concepts of immune regulation. Also, defining the genetic pathogenesis of these diseases has led to improved diagnosis, prognosis, genetic counseling, and new therapies. **Lenardo et al. (2015)** highlighted the patient phenotype to treatment using the newly defined XMEN disease, caused by the genetic loss of the MAGT1 magnesium transporter, which illustrates how genomics yields new immunoregulatory insights as well as how genomics is integrated into clinical immunology. These investigators also discussed PASLI (*PI3K dysregulation*) and CHAI/LATAIE (*CTLA-4 deficiency*), as additional examples of immunological diseases for personalized treatment using genomics.

Genomic Analyses of Blood Pressure African Americans suffer a higher prevalence of hypertension compared with other racial/ethnic groups. In a study, Gong et al., (2016) performed a genome-wide association study of blood pressure (BP) response to β-blockers in African Americans with uncomplicated hypertension. Genome-wide meta-analysis was performed in 318 African American hypertensive participants in the two Pharmacogenomic Evaluation of Antihypertensive Responses studies: 150 treated with Atenolol monotherapy and 168 treated with metoprolol monotherapy. The analysis adjusted for age, sex, baseline BP and principal components for ancestry. Genome-wide significant variants with $P<5\times10^{-8}$ and suggestive variants with $P < 5\times10^{-7}$ were evaluated in an additional cohort of 141 African Americans treated with the addition of Atenolol to Hydrochlorothiazide treatment. The validated variants were then meta-analyzed in these 3 groups of African Americans. Two variants discovered in the monotherapy meta-analysis were validated in the add-on therapy. African American participants heterozygous for SLC25A31 rs201279313 deletion versus wild-type genotype had better diastolic BP response to Atenolol monotherapy, Metoprolol monotherapy, and Atenolol add-on therapy. Similarly, LRRC15 rs11313667 was validated for systolic BP response to β-blocker therapy with 3-group meta-analysis. In this meta-analysis of BP response to β-blockers in African Americans, these investigators identified novel variants that may provide valuable information for personalized antihypertensive treatment in this group.

Sketching and Landscape of System Medicine Recently Kirschner (2016) reported that to understand the meaning of the term Systems Medicine and to distinguish it from other expressions currently in use, such as; precision, personalized, -omics, or big data medicine, its underlying history and development needs to be highlighted. Having this development in mind, it becomes evident that Systems Medicine is a genuine concept as well as a novel way of tackling the complexity that occurs in clinical medicine-and not just a rebranding of what has previously been done in the past. It seems that Systems Medicine has its origin in an integrative method to unravel biocomplexity, namely, *Systems Biology*. Scientist have gained useful experience that is on the verge toward implementation in clinical research and practice. Systems Medicine and Systems Biology have the same underlying theoretical principle in systems-based thinking-a methodology to understand complexity that can be traced back to ancient Greece. During the last decade due to a rapid methodological development in the life sciences and computing/IT technologies, Systems Biology has evolved from a scientific concept into an independent discipline most competent to tackle key questions of biocomplexity-with the potential to transform medicine and how it will be practiced in the future. To understand this process in more detail, the following section of this chapter will give a short summary of the foundation of systems-based thinking and the different developmental stages including systems theory, the development of modern Systems Biology, and its transition into clinical practice. These are the components to pave the way toward Systems Medicine to accomplish EBPT.

Immunology and Bioinformatics for Disease Prediction and Quantitation The understanding of the immune response is currently at the center of biomedical research. There are emerging expectations that immune-based interventions will provide new, personalized, and targeted therapeutic options for severe and highly prevalent diseases, from aggressive cancers to infectious and autoimmune diseases. Recently Eberhardt et al. (2016) repored that immunology should surpass its current descriptive and phenomenological nature, and become quantitative, and thereby predictive. Immunology is an ideal field for deploying the tools, methodologies, and philosophy of systems biology, an approach that combines quantitative experimental data, computational biology, and mathematical modeling. This is because, from an organism-wide perspective, the immunity is a biological system of systems, a paradigmatic instance of a multi-scale system. At the molecular scale, the critical phenotypic responses of immune cells are governed by biochemical networks, enriched in nested regulatory motifs such as feedback and feedforward loops. This network complexity confers the ability of highly nonlinear behavior, including examples of homeostasis, ultra-sensitivity, hysteresis, and biostability. Moving from the cellular level, different immune cell populations communicate with each other by direct physical contact or receiving and secreting signaling molecules such as cytokines. Moreover, the interaction of the immune system with its potential targets (e.g., *pathogens or tumor cells*) is complex, as it involves mechanisms that constitute regulated multi-feedback loop system. This leads to the consequence that today's immunologists are facing challenge of integrating massive quantities from multi-platforms. These investigators supported the idea that the analysis of the immune system demands the use of systems-level approaches to ensure the success for more effective and immune-based personalized theranostics.

Analyses of Blood Transcriptomes in PM Recently Li et al. (2016) reviewed the new methods and discussed how they can contribute to PM. These investigators emphasized that molecular analysis of blood samples is pivotal to clinical diagnosis. Recent developments have opened new opportunities to utilize transcriptomics and metabolomics for personalized and precision medicine. Efforts from human immunology have infused into this area exquisite characterizations of subpopulations of blood cells. It is now possible to infer from blood transcriptomics, the contribution of immune activation and of cell subpopulations. In parallel, high-resolution mass spectrometry has brought analytical capability, detecting >10,000 metabolites, together with environmental exposure, dietary intake, microbial activity, and pharmaceutical drugs. Transcriptomics and metabolomics can be integrated to provide a more comprehensive understanding of the human biological states to accomplish EBPT.

Companion Diagnostics The goal of individualized and targeted treatment and precision medicine requires the assessment of therapeutic targets to direct treatment strategies. The biomarkers used to direct precision medicine, often termed companion diagnostics, for targeted drugs have been based on *in vitro* assay of biopsy material. Molecular imaging companion diagnostics offer features complementary to those from *in vitro* assay, including the ability to measure the heterogeneity of each patient's cancer across the entire disease burden and to measure early changes in response to treatment. Mankoff et al. (2016) discussed the use of molecular imaging methods as companion diagnostics for cancer therapy with the goal of predicting response to targeted therapy and measuring early (*pharmacodynamic*) response as an indication of whether the treatment has "hit" the target. These investigators also discussed considerations for probe development for molecular imaging companion diagnostics, including both small-molecular probes and larger molecules such as labeled antibodies and related constructs. These investigators described two examples where both predictive and pharmacodynamic molecular imaging markers have been tested in humans: (a) endocrine therapy for breast cancer and (b) human epidermal growth factor receptor type 2-targeted therapy. They summarized the items needed to move molecular imaging companion diagnostics from early studies into multicenter trials and into the clinic for successful EBPT.

Nanocomposite for Enrichment of Chloramphenicol and Thiamphenicol Wu et al. (2016) reported in situ solvothermal growth method for immobilization of metal-organic framework-ionic liquid functionalized graphene (MOF-5/ILG) composite on etched stainless steel wire. The X-ray diffraction spectra, scanning electron microscopy and transmission electron microscopy images showed that the metal organic framework possessed good crystal shape and its structure is not disturbed by the introduction of ILG. The covalent bond established between the amino group of ILG and the carboxylic group of the metal organic framework improved the mechanical stability and structure uniformity of the microcrystals. This material combined the favorable attributes of both metal-organic framework and ILG, having high surface area (820m (2)/g) and good adsorption capability. Its adsorption properties were explored by preconcentrating chloramphenicol and thiamphenicol from aqueous solutions prior to gas chromatography-flame ionization detection. The MOF-5/ILG exhibited high enrichment capacity for the analytes as they could interact through π-π and H-bonding interaction. Under the optimum conditions, good linearity (r > 0.9981), low limits of detection (14.8-19.5ng/L), and good precision (S.D < 6.0%) were achieved. The method was applied to the determination of two antibiotics in milk, honey, urine and serum samples with relative recoveries of 82.3-103.2%.

Tyrosine Kinase Nonreceptor 2 (TNK2) Point Mutations in Leukemia through Integration of Kinase Inhibitor Screening and Genomic Analysis The amount of genomic information about leukemia cells currently far exceeds our overall understanding of the precise genetic events that ultimately drive disease development and progression. Effective implementation of PM will require tools to distinguish genetic alterations within the complex genetic landscape of leukemia. In a study, Maxson et al. (2016) performed kinase inhibitor screens to predict functional gene targets in primary specimens from patients with acute myeloid leukemia and chronic myelomonocytic leukemia. Deep sequencing of the same patient specimens identified genetic alterations that were subsequently integrated with the functionally important targets using the HitWalker algorithm to prioritize the mutant genes that explain the observed drug sensitivity patterns. Thee investigators identified tyrosine kinase nonreceptor 2 (TNK2) point mutations that exhibited oncogenic capacity. Particularly, the integration of functional and genomic data using HitWalker allowed prioritization of rare oncogenic mutations that may have been missed through genomic analysis alone. These mutations were sensitive to the multikinase inhibitor Dasatinib, which antagonizes TNK2 kinase activity, as well as novel TNK2 inhibitors, XMD8-87 and XMD16-5, with greater target specificity. They also identified activating truncation mutations in other tumor types that were sensitive to XMD8-87 and XMD16-5, exemplifying the potential utility of these compounds across tumor types dependent on TNK2. These findings highlighted a more sensitive approach for identifying genomic lesions that may be infrequently mutated or overlooked and provided a new method for the prioritization of candidate genetic mutations.

2D Chromatographic Analysis of Complex Herbal Samples Danshen is one of the most frequently used traditional Chinese herbs owing to its remarkable therapeutic effects. Phenolic acids and diterpenoids have proved to be the bioactive substance groups. To fully profile its chemical compositions and explore bioactive compounds, Cao et al. (2016) developed a comprehensive 2-D liquid chromatography system coupled to DAD detector and hybrid linear ion trap (LTQ) Orbitrap mass spectrometry (LC×LC-DAD-ESI/HRMS/MS(n)) based on the column combination of Hypersil gold CN (150mm×1mm, 3μm) and Accucore C18 (50mm×4.6mm, 2.6μm). Using the optimal segment gradient program, phenolic acids and diterpenoids were separated into two independent groups and a total of 328 peaks were detected on the contour plot of Danshen. By means of the accurate mass and reliable MS(n) data, 102 compounds were identified or tentatively identified and 7 of them were discovered from Danshen for the first time. Moreover, the LC×LC-DAD system was validated for the quantitative analysis of 14 bioactive analytes using the contour plot, exhibiting satisfactory linearity and high precision for both peak locating and peak volume calculating. This method could afford separation capability, reliable identification, and accurate quantitative results, suitable for analysis of complex herbal samples.

Chromatographic Analyses of Doxorubcin Associated with DNA in Tumor & Tissue Doxorubicin, a widely used anticancer agent, exhibits antitumor activity against a wide variety of malignancies. The drug exerts its cytotoxic effects by binding to and intercalating within the DNA of tumor and tissue cells. However, current assays are unable to accurately determine the concentration of the intracellular active form of Doxorubicin. Lucas et al. (2016) developed a sample processing and HPLC method to quantify Doxorubicin that is associated with DNA in tumors and tissues, which provided an intracellular cytotoxic measure of Doxorubicin after administration of small molecule and nanoparticle formulations of Doxorubicin. The assay used Daunorubicin as an internal standard; liquid-liquid phase extraction to isolate drug associated with DNA; a Shimadzu HPLC with fluorescence detection equipped with a Phenomenex Luna C18 (2μm, 2.0×100mm) analytical column and a gradient mobile phase of 0.1% formic acid in water or acetonitrile for separation and quantification. The assay had a lower limit of detection (LLOQ) of 10ng/mL and was linear up to 3000ng/mL. The intra- and inter-day precision of the assay expressed as a coefficient of variation (CV %) ranged from 4.01 to 8.81%. The suitability of this assay for measuring Doxorubicin associated with DNA was demonstrated by quantify the Doxorubicin concentration within tumor samples from SKOV3 and HEC1A mice obtained 72h after administration of PEGylated liposomal Doxorubicin (Doxil(®); PLD) at 6mg/kg IV x 1. The

HPLC assay allowed intracellular quantification of Doxorubicin and proved important tool for evaluating intracellular PKs of Doxorubicin and various nanoparticle formulations of Doxorubicin.

PKs of 3, 4-Divanillyltetrahydrofuran in Rats by Ultra-fast Liquid Chromatography/Tandem Mass Spectrometry. 3, 4-Divanillyltetrahydrofuran is the main active ingredient of nettle root which can increase steroid hormones in the bloodstream for many of body builders. To better understand its pharmacological activities, the researchers need to determine its PKs profiles. In this study, Shan et al. (2016) developed a rapid and sensitive ultra-fast liquid chromatography-tandem mass spectrometric (UFLC-MS/MS) method for the determination of 3, 4-Divanillyltetrahydrofuran in the plasma of rats. Chromatographic separation was performed on a C18 column at 40°C, with a gradient elution consisting of Methanol and water containing 0.3% (v/v) Formic acid at a flow rate of 0.8mL/min. The detection was performed using an electrospray triple-quadrupole MS/MS via positive ion multiple reaction monitoring mode. The lower limits-of-quantification were 0.5ng/mL. The intra- and inter-day precision (RSD %) was within 15% and the accuracy (RE %) ranged from 4.0% to 7.0%. This method could be successfully applied to study PKs of 3, 4-Divanillyltetrahydrofuran.

Analyses of Phosphatidylcholine-Derived Quaternary Ammonium Compounds by LC-MS/MS from Human Blood Plsama, Serum, and Urine Samples The determination of circulating Trimethylamine-N-oxide (TMAO), Choline, Betaine, l-Carnitine and O-Acetyl-l-carnitine concentration in different human matrices is of clinical interest. Recent results highlighted the prognostic value of TMAO and quaternary ammonium containing metabolites in cardiovascular and kidney diseases. Steuer et al. (2016) reported a method for the rapid and simultaneous measurement of closely related Phosphatidylcholine-derived metabolites in 3 different biological matrices by stable isotope dilution assay. Plasma, serum and urine samples were deproteinized and separated by HILIC-chromatography. Detection and quantification were performed using LC-MS/MS with electrospray ionization in positive mode. For accuracy and precision, calibration was performed covering more than the full reference range. Assay performance metrics included intra- and interday imprecision were below 10%. To exclude matrix effects standard addition methods were applied for all matrices. The calibration standards and quality control could be used instead of matrix-matched calibration and controls. Based on this study, these investigators highlighted that LC/MS/MS-based assay could improve future clinical studies evaluating TMAO and related substances as prognostic biomarkers for cardiovascular risk and all-cause mortality in different patients.

Mass Spectrometry in PM Recently Clarke (2016) reported that PM is becoming a major topic within the medical community and is gaining momentum as a standard approach in many disciplines. This approach involves the use of a patient's genetic makeup to allow the physician to choose the appropriate course of treatment. The genetic information directs the drug to be used to treat the patient. The genetic biomarkers associated with enzyme function may direct dosage recommendations. However therapeutic drug monitoring (TDM) is a second way in which PM can be practiced. A review of the use of mass spectrometry for TDM in the arena of precision medicine was undertaken. Because the measurement of a drug or its metabolites provides the physician with a snapshot of the therapeutic exposure, these concentrations can be thought of as an actual phenotype measurement based on the patient's genetics coupled with environmental, pharmacological, and nutritional variables. The TDM measurement by mass spectrometry provides the patient's current phenotype vs the phenotype imputed by the genetics. The mass spectrometry can provide an understanding of how a drug is interacting with the patient, and is orthoganol to the information provided by PGx assays. Moreover, the speed and relatively low expense of drug monitoring by mass spectrometry makes it highly suitable to accomplish EBPT.

Mass Spectrometric Imaging of Mouse Brain Lipids A comprehensive description of brain architecture at the molecular level is essential for understanding behavioral and cognitive processes in health and disease. Huang et al. (2016) highlighted that although fluorescent labeling of target proteins has been established to visualize a brain connectome, the molecular basis for various neurophysiological phenomena remains uncertain. These investigators reported a brain-wide, molecular-level, and microscale imaging of endogenous metabolites, in particular, lipids of mouse brain by using *laser activated electron tunneling* (LAET) and *mass spectrometry*. In this approach, *atomic electron emission* along with finely tuned laser beam size provides high resolution at sub-micrometer level to display spatial distribution of lipids in mouse brain slices. Electron-directed soft ionization has been achieved through exothermal capture of tunneling photoelectrons as well as unpaired electron-initiated chemical bond cleavages. Regionally specific lipids including saturated, mono-unsaturated, and poly-unsaturated fatty acids as well as other lipids may be implicated in neurological signaling pathways, have been discovered by using *LAET-MSI* technology.

LC-MS/MS Analyses of Teicoplanin in Human Plasma Kim et al. (2016) developed a direct injection-based, simple, accurate, LC-MS/MS method and validated for the determination of Teicoplanin in human plasma. Patient plasma samples were diluted in an aqueous buffer prior to injection into the LC-MS/MS system. Chromatographic separation was achieved using a Cadenza HS-C18 column and a gradient mixture of Acetonitrile-water (both containing 0.1% Formic acid) as the mobile phase at a flow rate of 0.5mL/min. The analytes were detected in multiple reaction monitoring mode with *positive ion electrospray ionization*. The concentration of Teicoplanin was determined as the sum of 6 components (A3-1, A2-1, A2-2, A2-3, A2-4, and A2-5). The calibration curve was linear over a concentration range of 1-50mg/L, which covered the clinically-accepted trough and therapeutic plasma levels. The intra-and inter-day precision and accuracy values were <15%. This method was applied to therapeutic drug monitoring of Teicoplanin in routine clinical practice with its usefulness for the determination of Teicoplanin concentration in human plasma.

Quantitation of Teriflunomide in Human Serum/Plasma Rule et al. (2016) reported that Leflunomide is a prodrug used for the treatment of rheumatoid arthritis. The active metabolite, Teriflunomide (A77 1726), inhibits the enzyme dihydroorotate dehydrogenase and thereby reduces the synthesis of Pyrimidine ribonucleotides. Teriflunomide is also administered directly and finds use in treating multiple sclerosis. Therapeutic concentrations are generally in the tens of μg/mL serum or plasma and, due to adverse effects and the time required to reach steady state, therapeutic drug monitoring is beneficial. The drug is also a potential teratogen. A method was developed to quantify Teriflunomide over a 40,000-fold concentration range of 5 ng/mL to 200 μg/mL in serum or plasma. This was accomplished by dividing the quantitative range into two separate but overlapping regions; a high curve and a low curve range. Samples were evaluated first against the high curve after a 100-fold dilution of the sample extract. Samples falling below the upper curve region were evaluated again without dilution and quantified, if possible, against the low curve calibration standards.

Appropriate choice of a concentration for the deuterated internal standard (D4-teriflunomide) allowed a single, identical, extraction procedure to be performed for both curve regions but with the dilution performed for high curve samples. This method was rugged and reliable with good accuracy and precision statistics.

ICP-MS Analyses of Trace Elements and Arsenic Species for a Realgar-Containing Chinese Medicine Niuhuang Jiedu Niuhuang Jiedu tablet (NHJDT) is a Realgar-containing traditional Chinese medicine. Jin et al. (2016) developed inductively coupled plasma-mass spectrometry (ICP-MS) method for the determination of 20 trace elements (Mg, K, Ca, Na, Fe, As, Zn, Sr, Ba, Cu, Mn, Ni, Pb, V, Cr, Se, Co, Mo, Cd, Hg) in NHJDT, as well as in water, gastric fluid, and intestinal fluid. A high performance liquid chromatography-inductively coupled plasma-mass spectrometry (HPLC-ICP-MS) method was also developed for the determination of arsenite (As (III)), arsenate (As (V)), monomethylarsonic acid (MMA), dimethylarsinic acid (DMA) and for arsenobetaine (AsB) and arsenocholine (AsC) in these extracts. Both methods were validated for linearity, sensitivity, precision, stability and accuracy. The reliability of the ICP-MS method was further evaluated using a standard reference material prepared from dried tomato leaves (NIST, SRM 1572a), which demonstrated that some manufacturers formulated lower amount of Realgar than required in the Chinese Pharmacopoeia in their preparations. In addition, almost same extraction profiles for total As and inorganic As were detected in water and in GIT fluids, while higher extraction rates for other 19 elements were observed in GIT fluids. These findings revealed that the toxicities of Hg, Cu, Cd and Pb in NHJDP are low, while As toxicity in NHJDT should be further investigated for cell-based therapy of cystic fibrosis.

Micro-dissected Tumor Tissues on Chip for Drug Testing and EBPT In cancer research and PM, new tissue culture models are needed to better predict the response of patients to therapies. With a concern for the small volume of tissue typically obtained through a biopsy, Astolfi et al. (2016) described a method to reproducibly section live tumor tissue to submillimeter sizes. These micro-dissected tissues (MDTs) shared with spheroids the advantages of being easily manipulated on-chip and kept alive for periods extending over one week, while being biologically relevant for numerous assays. At dimensions below ~420 μm in diameter, as suggested by a simple metabolite transport model and confirmed experimentally, continuous perfusion is not required to keep samples alive, simplifying the technical challenges. For the long-term culture of MDTs, a microfluidic platform was described that can trap samples in a low shear stress environment. These investigators reported the analysis of MDT viability for 8 different types of tissues (*4 mouse xenografts derived from human cancer cell lines, 3 from ovarian and prostate cancer patients, and 1 from a patient with benign prostatic hyperplasia*) analyzed by both confocal microscopy and flow cytometry over an 8-day incubation period. Finally, these researchers provided chemosensitivity testing of human tissue from a cancer patient using MDT chip method. This technology has the potential to improve EBPT success rates by identifying potential responders earlier during the course of treatment, providing opportunities for direct drug testing on patient tissues in early drug development stages.

Radium-223 (^{223}Ra) in Naïve and Mouse Models of Prostate Cancer Metastasis Bone-metastatic in castration-resistant prostate cancer (bmCRPC) represents a lethal stage of the most common noncutaneous cancer in men. The recent introduction of ^{223}Ra dichloride, a bone-seeking α-emitting radiopharmaceutical, demonstrates survival benefit and palliative effect for bmCRPC patients. Clinical results established safety and efficacy, yet questions remain regarding PDs and dosing for optimized patient benefit. Abou et al. (2016) determined the biodistribution of ^{223}Ra as well as interaction with the bone and tumor compartments in skeletally mature mice (C57Bl/6 and CD-1, n = 3-6) and metastasis models (LNCaP and PC3, n = 4). Differences in uptake were evaluated by μCT and histological investigation. Novel techniques were leveraged on whole-mount undecalcified cryosections to determine microdistribution of ^{223}Ra. All statistical tests were two-sided. ^{223}Ra uptake in the bones (>30% injected activity per gram) at 24 hrs was accompanied by remnant activity in the kidney (2.33% ± 0.36%), intestines (5.73% ± 2.04%), and spleen (10.5% ± 5.9%). Skeletal accumulation across strains did not correspond with bone volume or surface area but instead to local blood vessel density. Microdistribution analysis by autoradiography and α camera revealed targeting of the ossifying surfaces adjacent to the epiphyseal growth plate. In models of PCa metastasis, radioactivity did not localize directly within tumors but instead at the apposite bone surface. Osteoblastic and lytic lesions displayed similar intensity comparable with uptake at sites of normal bone remodeling. These investigators suggested that profiling the macro- and microdistribution of ^{223}Ra in healthy and diseased models has important implications to guide EBPT application of this emerging α-therapy approach for bmCRPC and other bone metastastic diseases.

Future of Radiology Informatics Rapid growth in the amount of electronically recorded data that is as part of routine clinical operations has generated significant interest in the use of *Big Data* methodologies to address clinical and research investigations. These methods can efficiently analyze and deliver insights from high-volume, high-variety, and high-growth rate datasets generated across the continuum of care, thereby forgoing the time, cost, and effort of more focused and controlled hypothesis-driven research. By virtue of an existing robust information technology infrastructure and years of archived digital data, radiology departments can take advantage of emerging *Big Data* techniques. Kansagra et al. (2016) described 4 areas in which *Big Data* is poised to have an immediate impact on radiology practice, research, and operations. In addition, they provided an overview of the *Big Data* adoption cycle and described how academic radiology departments can promote its development.

Next Generation Sequencing in Lung Cancer Theranostics It is now well established that cancer is a genetic disease characterized by uncontrolled growth of abnormal cells. Over time, somatic mutations accumulate in the cells due to replication errors, chromosome segregation errors, or DNA damage. When not caught by traditional mechanisms, these somatic mutations can lead to cellular proliferation, the hallmark of cancer. Kruglyak et al. (2016) reported that lung cancer is the leading cause of cancer-related mortality in the US, accounting for ~160,000 deaths annually. Five year survival rates for lung cancer remain low (<50%) for all stages, with worse prognosis (<15%) in late stage cases. Advances in NGS, offer the vision of EBPT or precision oncology, wherein an individual's treatment can be based on his or her individual molecular profile, rather than on historical population-based medicine. NGS has been used to identify new biomarker candidates for the early diagnosis of lung cancer and is used to guide EBPT. These investigators provided an overview of NGS technology and summarized its application to the EBPT of lung cancer. They also described how NGS can drive advances that bring us closer to precision oncology and discussed some of the technical challenges that will need to be resolved to accomplish the ultimate goal of EBPT.

GWAS of Lung Cancer in Asian Never-Smoking Women Genome-wide association studies (GWAS) of lung cancer in Asian never-smoking women identified six susceptibility loci associated with lung cancer risk. To further explore new susceptibility loci, Wang et al. **(2016)** acquired data from four GWAS of Asian non-smoking female lung cancer (6,877 cases and 6,277 controls) using the 1,000 Genomes Project (Phase 1 Release 3) data and genotyped additional samples (5,878 cases and 7,046 controls) for replication. In the meta-analysis, 3 new loci achieved genome-wide significance, marked by SNP rs7741164 at 6p21.1, rs72658409 at 9p21.3, and rs11610143 at 12q13.13. These findings identified new genetic susceptibility alleles for lung cancer in never-smoking women in Asia and highlighted the significance of follow-up to understand their biological significance.

Effect of Cytochrome P450 2D6 Variants in the Chinese Population on Atomoxetine Metabolism Linag et al. (2016) assessed the catalytic activities of 24 cytochrome P450 2D6 (CYP2D6) variants in the Chinese population toward Atomoxetine *in vitro* as well as CYP2D6.1. In this study, the co-expression enzyme of human recombinant CYPOR, CYPb5, and CYP2D6.1 or other CYP2D6 variants with the baculovirus-mediated insect cells (Sf21) was used to evaluate the catalytic activities of 24 CYP2D6 variants toward Atomoxetine metabolism. The metabolite of Atomoxetine (4-Hydroxy-Atomoxetine) was detected by ultra-high performance liquid chromatography-mass spectrometry. The intrinsic clearance (V_{max}/K_m) values of most variants were significantly altered when compared with CYP2D6.1. CYP2D6.94, CYP2D6.D336N, CYP2D6.R440C exhibited significantly increased values 172, 126, 121% respectively. CYP2D6.89 and CYP2D6.98 exhibited similar catalytic activity as the wild type, whereas 17 variants exhibited significantly decreased values due to increase K_m and/or decrease V_{max} values. However, CYP2D6.92 and CYP2D6.96 showed no or few activity because of producing nothing, suggesting that most of these newly found variants exhibit significantly altered catalytic activities compared with the wild type and these findings may provide valuable information for the growth and development of EBPT in China.

Functional Characterization of CYP2D6 Allelic Variants Xu et al. (2016) characterized 4 novel CYP2D6 alleles in Chinese Han population. CYP2D6 proteins of wild-type and the 4 novel variants along with CYP2D6.2 and CYP2D6.10 were heterologously expressed in yeast cells and their kinetic parameters were determined. *Compared with CYP2D6.1 (frequency in Chinese 24.65%), CYP2D6.X (1.63%), CYP2D6.Y (1.50%), CYP2D6.Z (0.81%), CYP2D6.10 (52.53%) and CYP2D6.75 (0.13%) exhibited low activity at different degrees, whereas the kinetic parameters of CYP2D6.2 (11.06%) were much the same with CYP2D6.1.* The novel allele CYP2D6.75 showed decreased enzyme activity. This was the first study to conduct functional analysis of four CYP2D6 novel alleles, which might be helpful for optimizing pharmacotherapy and designing EBPT.

Genetic Screening for Gynecological Cancer The landscape of cancer genetics in gynecological oncology is rapidly changing. The traditional family history-based approach has inherent limitations and misses >50% mutation carriers. This is now being replaced by population-based approaches. The need for changing the clinical paradigm from family history-based to population-based BRCA1/BRCA2 testing in Ashkenazi Jews is supported by data that demonstrate population-based BRCA1/BRCA2 testing does not cause psychological harm and is cost effective. Manchanda and Jacobs (2016) described various genetic testing strategies for gynecological cancers, including population-based approaches, panel and direct-to-consumer testing, as well as the need for genetic counseling. Advances in genetic testing technology and computational analytics facilitated an integrated systems medicine approach, providing promise for population-based genetic testing, risk stratification, and cancer prevention. Genomic information along-with biological/computational tools can be used to deliver predictive, preventive, personalized, participatory (P4) and precision medicine to accomplish EBPT in the future.

Ethnicity and Geography in Cancer Genomics It is currently realized that ethnic and geographic differences in cancer incidence, prognosis, and treatment outcomes can be attributed to diversity in the inherited (germline) and somatic genome. Although international large-scale sequencing efforts are beginning to unravel the genomic underpinnings of cancer traits, much remains to be known about the underlying mechanisms and determinants of genomic diversity. Carcinogenesis is a dynamic, complex phenomenon representing the interaction between genetic and environmental factors that results in divergent phenotypes across ethnicities and geography. For example, compared with whites, there is a higher incidence of prostate cancer among Africans and African Americans, and the disease is more aggressive and fatal. Genome-wide association studies identified germline susceptibility loci that may account for differences between the African and non-African patients, but the lack of availability of appropriate cohorts for replication studies and the incomplete understanding of genomic architecture across populations pose major limitations. Tan et al. (2016) discussed the transformative potential of routine diagnostic evaluation for somatic alterations, using lung cancer as an example, highlighting implications of population disparities, current hurdles in implementation, and the potential of clinical genomics in enhancing cancer prevention, diagnosis, and treatment. These investigators emphasized that as the researchers enter the era of precision cancer medicine, a concerted multinational effort is the key to addressing population and genomic diversity as well as overcoming barriers and geographical disparities in research and health care delivery.

Detection of SNP by NGS in Cancer Theranostics Shaw et al. (2016) emphasized that genetic heterogeneity explains variation in predisposition of cancer. Whole-genome analysis allows risk to be quantified, giving better targeted screening and quantification of the personalized risk posed by environmental factors. Array-based approaches to whole-genome analysis are being overtaken by NGS. The different platforms available for NGS are compared and the opportunities and risks of this approach were discussed: including the informatics required and the ethical issues. Methods applicable to the personal genome machine (PGM) were highlighted as an example of workflows.

Blood Transcriptomics & Metabolomics in PM Recent developments opened new opportunities to utilize transcriptomics and metabolomics for PM. Molecular analysis of blood samples is pivotal to clinical diagnosis and has been intensively investigated. Efforts from human immunology infused into this area exquisite characterizations of subpopulations of blood cells. Le et al. (2015) highlighted that it is now possible to infer from blood transcriptomics, with fine accuracy, the contribution of immune activation and of cell subpopulations. In parallel, high-resolution mass spectrometry brought analytical capability, detecting >10,000 metabolites, together with environmental exposure, dietary intake, microbial activity, and pharmaceutical drugs. Thus, the re-examination of blood chemicals by metabolomics is becoming exceedingly attractive area of EBPT. Furthermore, transcriptomics and metabolomics can be integrated to provide a more comprehensive understanding of the human biological states in health and disease.

Data Collection to Build Prediction Models in Oncology The advances in diagnostic and treatment technology are responsible for a remarkable transformation in the internal medicine with the establishment of a new idea of PM. Meldolesi et al. (2016) described the strategy to collect and analyze data properly for decision making and introduced the concept of an *'umbrella protocol' within the framework of 'rapid learning healthcare'*. Inter- and intra-patient tumor heterogeneity and the clinical outcome and/or treatment's toxicity's complexity, justify the effort to develop predictive models from decision support systems. *However, the number of evaluated variables coming from multiple disciplines: oncology, computer science, bioinformatics, statistics, genomics, imaging, among others could be very large thus making statistical analysis difficult to exploit.* Automated data-mining processes and machine learning approaches can be a solution to organize the massive amount of data, to elucidate important interaction relavent to accomplish EBPT.

IGNITE Network for Genomic Medicine and Research Patients, clinicians, researchers and payers are seeking to understand the value of using genomic information (*as reflected by genotyping, sequencing, family history or other data*) to inform clinical decision-making. However, challenges exist to widespread clinical implementation of genomic medicine, a prerequisite for developing evidence of its real-world utility. To address these challenges, the National Institutes of Health-funded IGNITE (*Implementing genomics in practice; www.ignite-genomics.org*) Network, comprised of 6 projects and a coordinating center, was established in 2013 to support the development, investigation and dissemination of genomic medicine practice models that integrate genomic data into the electronic health record and deploys tools for point of care decision making. IGNITE site projects are aligned in their purpose of testing these models, but individual projects vary in scope and design, including exploring genetic biomarkers for disease risk prediction and prevention, developing tools for using family history data, incorporating PGx data into clinical care, refining disease diagnosis using sequence-based mutation discovery, and creating novel educational approaches. Weitzel et al. (2016) described the IGNITE Network and member projects, including network structure, collaborative initiatives, clinical decision support strategies, methods for return of genomic test results, and educational initiatives for patients and providers. Clinical and outcomes data from individual sites and network-wide projects are anticipated to begin being published over the next few years. The IGNITE Network is an innovative series of projects and pilot demonstrations aiming to enhance translation of validated actionable genomic information into clinical settings and develop and use measures of outcome in response to genome-based clinical interventions using a pragmatic framework to provide early data and proofs of concept on the utility of these interventions. Through these efforts and collaboration with other stakeholders, IGNITE is poised to have a significant impact on the acceleration of genomic information into medical practice.

Genetics of Metastatic Head & Neck Squamous Carcinoma Recurrence and/or metastasis occurs in more than half of patients with head and neck squamous cell carcinoma (HNSCC), and these events pose threats to long-term survival. Hedberg et al. (2016) investigated genetic alterations that underlie recurrent/metastatic HNSCC. Whole-exome sequencing (WES) was performed on genomic DNA extracted from fresh-frozen whole blood and patient-matched tumor pairs from 13 HNSCC patients with synchronous lymph node metastases and 10 patients with metachronous recurrent tumors. Mutational concordance within and between tumor pairs was used to analyze the spatiotemporal evolution of HNSCC in individual patients and to identify potential therapeutic targets for functional evaluation.

Approximately 86% and 60% of single somatic nucleotide variants (SSNVs) identified in synchronous nodal metastases and metachronous recurrent tumors, respectively, were transmitted from the primary index tumor. Genes that were mutated in more than one metastatic or recurrent tumor, but not in the respective primary tumors, included C17orf104, inositol 1,4,5-trisphosphate receptor, type 3 (ITPR3), and discoidin domain receptor tyrosine kinase 2 (DDR2). A few DDR2 mutations confered enhanced sensitivity to SRC-family kinase (SFK) inhibitors in other malignancies. Similarly, HNSCC cell lines harboring endogenous and engineered DDR2 mutations were more sensitive to the SFK inhibitor Dasatinib than those with WT DDR2. In this WES study of patient-matched tumor pairs in HNSCC, these investigators found synchronous lymph node metastases to be genetically more similar to their paired index primary tumors than metachronous recurrent tumors. This study outlined a compendium of somatic mutations in primary, metastatic, and/or recurrent HNSCC cancers, with potential implications to accomplish EBPT.

DISEASE-SPECIFIC BIOMARKERS

Biomarkers for Drug Development and EBPT A study was performed to review and summarize biomarker data published from April 2014 to May 2015 and to provide insight to the ongoing work in osteoarthritis (OA). Bay-Jensen et al. (2016) used PubMed as searching machine, MeSH term [Biomarker] AND [Osteoarthritis] to summarize the BIPED criteria and set it in context of the medical needs of 2015. Only papers describing protein-based biomarkers measured in human body fluids from OA patients were included. Biomarkers of joint tissue turnover, cytokines, chemokines and peptide arrays were measured in different cohorts and studies. Amongst those were previously tested biomarkers such as Osteocalcin, Carboxy-terminal cross-linked fragment of type II Collagen (CTX-II) and cartilage oligomeric matrix protein (COMP). A majority of the biomarkers were classified as I, B or B according to the BIPED criteria. These researchers emphasized that there is still a huge, unmet need to identify, test, validate and qualify novel and well-known biomarkers. A pre-requisite for this is better characterization and classification of biomarkers to their needs, which may require better understanding of OA phenotypes. In addition, they provided references to recent guidelines from FDA and European Medicines Agency (EMA) on qualification and usage of biomarkers for drug development and PM.

Serum Complement Factors as Inflammatory Biomarkers in Metabolic Syndrome An epidemiological design, consisting of cross-sectional (n = 2376) and cohort (n = 976) studies, was adopted by Liu et al. (016) to investigate the association between complement factors 3 (C3) and 4, and the metabolic syndrome (MetS). In the cross-sectional study, the C3 and C4 concentrations in the MetS group were higher than those in the non-MetS group, and the levels of IgM, IgA, IgE, and IgG exhibited no significant differences between MetS and non-MetS. After multi-factor adjustment, the odds ratios (ORs) in the highest quartile of C3 and C4 concentrations were 7.047 and 1.961, respectively. After a 4 years follow-up, total 166 subjects were diagnosed with MetS, and the complement baseline levels from 2009 were used to predict the MetS risk in 2013. In the adjusted model, the relative risks (RRs) in the highest quartile of C3 and C4 levels were 4.779 and 2.590, respectively. Activation of complement factors may be an important part of inflammatory processes, and these results indicated that the elevated C3 and C4 levels were independent risk factors for MetS development. Molecular biology techniques are used to diagnose and monitor treatment in patients with chronic hepatitis B (CHB). These tools can detect and quantify viral genomes and analyze their sequences to determine genotype. The increasing use of these tools to monitor patients has improved the management of CHB infection by maximizing the potential for EBPT. HBV genotyping has become important and provides additional information to predict a response to therapy. More sensitive methods to determine HBV DNA levels are now available and the units of measurements have been standardized. HBsAg levels in serum reflect active covalently closed circular DNA (cccDNA) and to have additional value in EBPT decisions, especially as an on-treatment biomarker.

Personalized Clinical Management of Thoracic Aortic Disease Physicians and surgeons faced with patients with thoracic aortic disease (TAD) need to determine the diagnosis to facilitate decisions regarding appropriate investigations as well as which other specialists to involve, when to start medical therapy, when to refer for surgery, and how to plan follow-up and family screening. Increased understanding of conditions predisposing to thoracic aortic aneurysm (TAA) provides the opportunity for more personalized care. However, given advances in the genetics of TAD, clinicians are now faced with an expanded and often confusing list of associated differential diagnoses. Bradley et al. (2016) presented a practical guide to managing patients with TAD based on current knowledge and guidelines. Important "flags" on history taking and "tips" to diagnosis on physical examination along with what investigations to order and what referrals to request. Need for medical therapy, indications for surgical repair, and planning long-term follow-up of TAD can be determined by age, the underlying TAD diagnosis, previous vascular history in the patient or other family members (or both), aortic dimensions and growth rate, and any coexisting cardiovascular disease. Although medications may slow the progression of TAA, effective aortic surveillance and timely elective surgical repair remain the mainstays of prevention of acute aortic complications. Emergent repair of acute aortic dissection carries a far worse prognosis. Taking a practical approach to the management of TAD allows for standardized assessment and implementation of clinical guidelines. Ongoing discovery of new genes, better medical therapies, and innovative surgical techniques necessitate adapting knowledge and integrating it into everyday clinical practice.

Epigenetic Disorders with BRCAness in Hereditary and Sporadic Breast Cancer Murria Estal et al. (2016) identified the relevance of immunohistochemistry (IHC), copy number aberrations (CNA) and epigenetic disorders in BRCAness breast cancers (BCs). These Investigators studied 95 paraffin imbedded BCs, of which 41 carried BRCA1/BRCA2 germline mutations and 54 were non hereditary (BRCAX/Sporadic). Samples were assessed for BRCA1ness and CNAs by *Multiplex Ligation-dependent Probe Amplification* (MLPA); *Promoter Methylation* (PM) was assessed by methylation-specific-MLPA and the expression of miR-4417, miR-423-3p, miR-590-5p and miR-187-3p by quantitative RT-PCR. IHC biomarkers Ki67, ER, PR, HER2, CK5/6, EGFR and CK18 were detected with specific primary antibodies. BRCAness association with covariates was performed using multivariate binary logistic regression (stepwise backwards Wald option). BRCA1/2 mutational status, tumor size and histological grade among clinic-pathological variables; ER among IHC biomarkers; MYC among CNA; APC, ATM and RASSF1 among PM; and miR-590-5p, miR-4417 and miR-423 among microRNA expression, were the selected parameters related with the BRCAness status. The logistic regression performed with all these parameters selected ER+ as linked with the lack of BRCAness and MYC CNA, APC PM and miR-590-5p expression with BRCAness respectively). The ER, APC PM, MYC CNA and miR-590-5p expression, allowed detection of most BRCAness BC, suggesting that the identification of BRCAness can help establish EBPT to predict the response to specific treatments.

NIR-Cyanine Dye Linker for Isochronic Fluorescence Imaging in Cancer Theranostics Personalized anti-cancer medicine is boosted by the recent development of molecular diagnostics and targeted drugs requiring rapid and efficient ligation routes. Komljenovic et al. (2016) presented a novel approach to synthetize a conjugate to act simultaneously as an imaging as well as a chemotherapeutic agent by coupling functional peptides employing solid phase peptide synthesis. A fluorescent dye was developed with similarity in the polymethine part of the Cy7 molecule whose indolenine-N residues were substituted with a propylene linker. Methylating agent Temozolomide was functionalized with a Tetrazine as a diene component whereas Cy7-cell penetrating peptide conjugate acted as a dienophilic reaction partner for the inverse Diels-Alder click chemistry-mediated ligation route yielding a theranostic conjugate, *3-Mercapto-propionic-cyclohexenyl-Cy7-bis-temozolomide-bromide-cell penetrating peptide*. These researchers suggested that this synthesis route may facilitate delivery of the therapeutic compound to achieve sufficient concentrations at the target site or tissue. *Its versatility allowed a choice of adequate imaging tags applicable in PET, SPECT, CT, near-infrared imaging, and therapeutic substances including cytotoxic agents.* Imaging tags and therapeutics may be simultaneously bound to the conjugate applying click chemistry. This compound offered a basis for a further improvement in EBPT of cancer.

Miniturized and Mobile Drug Manufacturing Lewin et al. (2016) described developmental pharmaceutical manufacturing systems and techniques designed to overcome the shortcomings of traditional batch processing methods. Conventional pharmaceutical manufacturing processes do not adequately address the needs of military and civilian patient populations and healthcare providers. Recent advances within the *Defense Advanced Research Projects Agency* (DARPA) Battlefield Medicine program suggest that miniaturized, flexible platforms for end-to-end manufacturing of pharmaceuticals are possible. Advances in continuous-flow synthesis, chemistry, biological engineering, and downstream processing, along with online analytics, automation, and enhanced process control measures, pave the way for innovation to improve the pharmaceutical supply chain and drug manufacturing. These new technologies, along with current and ongoing advances in regulatory science, have the potential to *(a) permit "on demand" drug manufacturing on the battlefield and in other austere environments, (b) enhance preparedness for chemical, biological, radiological, and nuclear threats, (c) enhance health authorities' ability to respond to natural disasters and other catastrophic events, (d) minimize shortages of drugs, (e) address gaps in the orphan drug market, (f) support and enable the continued drive toward* precision medicine, *and (g) enhance access to needed medications in underserved areas across the globe. Hence, modular platforms under development by DARPA's Battlefield* Medicine *program may improve the safety, efficiency, and timeliness of drug manufacturing.*

EBPT OF CANCER

Patient-Specific Immune Response Profiles of Breast Cancer Transcriptional activity in hematopoietic cells regulate dedifferentiation, innate immunity and adaptive immunity. Understanding how these programs function in cancer can provide valuable insights into host immune response, cancer severity, and potential therapy response. Varn et al. (2016) utilized the transcriptomes of >200 murine hematopoietic cells, to infer the lineage-specific hematopoietic activity in human breast tumors. Correlating this activity with patient survival and tumor purity revealed that the transcriptional programs of many cell types influence patient prognosis and were found in environments of high lymphocytic infiltration. Collectively, these results allowed for a detailed and personalized assessment of the patient immune response to a tumor. When combined with patient biopsy genomic data, this method could enable a better understanding of the complex interplay between the host immune system and cancer.

Molecular Phenotype and Multigene Assays for Management of Breast Cancer Braunstein and Taghian (2016) highlighted that molecular profiling has revealed that breast cancer is not a single disease entity, but rather a class of heterogeneous subtypes, each with its own inherent biology and natural history. As a result, different treatment approaches have been optimized for various subtypes and, in turn, the ability to identify subtypes has become a critical component in the management of breast cancer. Comprehensive transcriptional profiling studies revealed at least 4 principal subtypes that are often distinguished by immunohistochemical staining of the *estrogen receptor (ER), progesterone receptor (PR), and HER2, along with a determination of histologic grade or Ki-67 staining: luminal A (ER+/HER2-/grade 1 or 2), luminal B (ER+/HER2-/grade 3), HER2 enriched (any HER2+ tumor), and basal like (ER-/PR-/HER2).* Although these subtypes show robust prognostic and predictive ability, there remain many cases that demand profiling that approximates the original transcriptionally-derived definitions of the intrinsic subtypes. The need for improved prognostication and risk stratification has led to the development of several multigene assays in breast cancer. Although there is little molecular overlap between current assays, they all rely heavily on quantifying the transcriptional output of ER signaling and proliferation-related genes. These data are then used in multivariate prediction models that incorporate other canonical risk factors such as the tumor size, lymph node involvement, and patient demographic parameters. Indeed, the advent of scalable molecular profiling technologies has introduced a number of assays for optimizing risk prediction and treatment assignment. In addition to the advances in transcriptional subtyping, recent reports characterized the most common genomic and epigenomic alterations that are likely to drive certain breast cancers. The identification of these "driver" lesions heralded an era of PM in which vulnerable oncogenic pathways may be targeted to disrupt the etiologic lesion(s) of a specific tumor. A number of such early targeted approaches yielded success in treating breast cancer, emphasizing the critical need for EBPT in this disease.

NCI MATCH for Gynecologic Oncology The Precision Medicine Initiative is an NCI driven program in cancer to generate the scientific evidence to move the concept of precision medicine into clinical practice. Moore and Manuel (2016) reported that the rapid development and widespread availability of NGS and other molecular diagnostics of tumors has heralded a new era of knowledge about each individual's tumor. This information has led to new therapeutic discoveries, and in most instances, it has been uninformative or of unclear significance. The NCI *Molecular Analysis for Therapy Choice* (MATCH) trial which screens for molecular features that may predict response to a drug with a given mechanism of action, is a multi-study, collaborative effort between the NCI and many pharmaceutical companies to clarify the significance of molecular alterations in tumors not previously studied. This trial design is in response to the recent appreciation that certain driver mutations which may be common in a particular tumor are mutated in other diseases at low frequency. In low frequency mutations, testing the utility of targeted therapy requires screening large numbers of patients. These researchers highlighted various types of novel trial designs that led to the development of the *NCI-MATCH*.

T53 Dysfunction in Diffuse B-Cell Lymphoma It is well-established that the aberrations of TP53 gene and dysregulation of the TP53 pathway are important in the pathogenesis of many cancers, including malignant lymphomas, especially diffuse large B cell lymphoma (DLBCL). Lu et al. (2016) reported that by regulating many downstream target genes or molecules, *TP53 governs major defenses against tumor growth and promotes cellular DNA repair, apoptosis, autophagy, cell cycle arrest, signaling, transcription, immune or inflammatory responses and metabolism.* Dysfunction of TP53, including microRNA regulations, copy number alterations of TP53 pathway and TP53 itself, dysregulation of TP53 regulators, and somatic mutations by abnormal TP53 function modes, play an important role in lymphoma generation, progression and invasion. The role of TP53 in DLBCL was explored recently. These investigators summarized recent advances on different mechanisms of TP53 in DLBCL and new therapeutic approaches to overcome TP53 inactivation.

Functional MRI In PM Benz et al. (2016) reported that DW and DCE MR imaging contribute to diagnosis, treatment planning, response assessment, and prognosis in personalized cancer medicine. Nevertheless, further standardization of these techniques needs to be addressed. Whole-body DW MR imaging is an exciting field; however, future studies need to investigate the biologic significance of these findings, their prognostic relevance, and cost-effectiveness in comparison with MDCT and PET/CT. New MR imaging probes, such as *targeted or activatable contrast agents and dynamic nuclear hyperpolarization*, offers great promise to further improve EBPT of cancer.

Personalized Cancer Screening Biomarkers Biomarker tests are being offered by laboratories and clinicians as self-pay health services to screen asymptomatic individuals; however, there is insufficient evidence to support this practice. Luzak et al. (2016) investigated the benefit-harm tradeoffs associated with 11 biomarkers currently offered in Germany as self-pay tests to screen for cancer. These investigators searched bibliographic databases for health technology assessments, systematic reviews and randomized-controlled trials (RCTs) by including publications that analyzed cancer screening biomarkers and reported patient-relevant outcomes (*mortality, morbidity, quality of life*), and potential harms of screening, among asymptomatic individuals in screening and non-screening arms. Six publications of secondary literature and four publications reporting results from two RCTs were included. For 10 cancer screening biomarkers, no direct evidence on patient-relevant outcomes was available. Only one trial, which assessed cancer antigen 125 (CA-125) and vaginal ultrasound for ovarian cancer screening, provided the outcome of interest. Screening compared with usual care did not reduce ovarian cancer mortality. Patient harms included overdiagnosis and false-positive results. Although ovarian cancer screening with CA-125 showed no benefit, false-positive tests, overdiagnosis and overtreatment were reported. Based on these findings these investigators suggested that physicians and researchers should provide patients with comprehensive information about the lack of evidence and potential harms caused by biomarker screening tests offered as a self-pay health service.

Personalized Biomarkers of Cutaneous Melanoma The identification of personalized germline biomarkers with biological relevance for the prediction of cutaneous melanoma (CM) prognosis is direly needed but it has been unsuccessful. As melanoma progression is controlled by host immunity, Vogelsang et al. (2016) presented a novel approach interrogating immunoregulatory pathways using the genome-wide maps of expression quantitative trait loci (eQTL) to expose biologically relevant germline variants modulating CM outcomes. Using whole genome eQTL data from a healthy population, these investigators identified 385 variants -significantly impacting the expression of 268 immune-relevant genes. The 40 most significant eQTLs were tested in a prospective cohort of 1,221 CM patients for their association with overall (OS) and recurrence-free survival using Cox regression analyses. A significant associations with better melanoma OS for rs6673928, impacting IL19 expression and rs6695772, controlling the expression of BATF3 was noticed. Both associations detected in the previously suspected melanoma prognostic locus at 1q32. Furthermore, they demonstrated that their combined effect on melanoma OS was enhanced reaching the level of clinical applicability. Their unique approach of interrogating lymphocyte-specific eQTLs revealed novel immunomodulatory eQTL predictors of CM prognosis that were independent of histopathological biomarkers. The enhanced effect of eQTLs suggested the personalized utilization of both SNPs and the promise of their design for the discovery of prognostic or risk germline biomarkers in other cancers.

Biomarkers in Endometrial Carcinoma Buhtoiarova et al. (2016) reported that type II and other high-grade endometrial carcinomas may challenge conventional treatment due to recurrence and metastatic spread, and hence are a persistent clinical dilemma. Effective targeted therapy for these is a goal for clinicians as well as researchers. An extensive review of the literature was performed for obtaining an in-depth understanding of the clinicopathological characteristics, etiologic factors, and molecular profile of these subsets of endometrial carcinoma. Progress made with current and emerging biomarkers for prognosis assessment and therapeutic targeting was summarized. There has been a significant increase in research on potential biomarkers of endometrial cancer, and beneficial targeted therapies have been identified. Clinical trials are now leading the charge for gains toward EBPT of aggressive endometrial carcinoma subtypes.

Biomarker-Based Therapy of Bladder Cancer The clinical management of bladder cancer experienced little change over the last 3 decades and there is compelling evidence to identify more effective treatments for advanced disease. Low clinical use of neoadjuvant therapies stems from historical limitations in the ability to predict patients most likely to respond to combination chemotherapies. Jones et al. (2016) focused on recent molecular and genetic studies, highlighting promising clinical trials and retrospective studies, and discussed emerging trials that use predictive biomarkers to match patients with therapies to which they are most likely to respond. These researchers highlighted that the implementation of predictive genomic and molecular biomarkers will revolutionize urologic oncology and the clinical management of bladder carcinoma.

Biomarkers in Personalized Lung Cancer Theranostics Cagle et a (2016) reported that two clinically validated and FDA-approved lung cancer predictive biomarkers (*epidermal growth factor receptor mutations and anaplastic lymphoma kinase (ALK) translocations*) occur in only about 20% of lung adenocarcinomas and acquired resistance develops to first generation drugs. Several other oncogenic drivers for lung adenocarcinoma have emerged as potentially druggable targets with new predictive biomarkers. Oncologists are requesting testing for ROS1 translocations, which predict susceptibility to Crizotinib, already approved for ALK positive lung cancers. Other potential biomarkers, which are currently undergoing clinical trials are RET, MET, HER2 and BRAF. Detection of these biomarkers includes fluorescent in situ hybridization and/or RT-PCR (*ROS1, RET, HER2*), mutation analysis (*BRAF*) and immunohistochemistry (*MET*). Screening by immunohistochemistry may be useful for some biomarkers (*ROS1, BRAF*). Targeted NGS may be useful as well. These 5 biomarkers are under consideration for inclusion in revised lung cancer biomarker guidelines.

ALK Inhibitors in Human Clinical Trials of Cancer Treatment The proto-oncogenic ALK is a druggable receptor tyrosine kinase for cancer treatment. Two inhibitors of ALK, Crizotinib and Ceritinib, were recently approved for the treatment of metastatic non-small-cell lung cancer, with marked improvement of progression-free survival of patients. Independent case reports also indicate their potential therapeutic activity in other ALK-rearranged cancers. Numerous single-agent and combination therapy trials are ongoing in lung and many other cancers. Chan et al. (2016) summarized current understanding of ALK signaling, genomic aberrations in cancer and emerging mechanisms of drug resistance. These investigators also provided a review on all ALK inhibitors and their current status of development in clinical setting.

Personalized Chemotherapy of Gastric Cancer Recently Kim et al. (2016) reported that gastric cancer (GC) is one of the most frequent malignant diseases in the elderly. Systemic chemotherapy showed an improvement of quality of life and survival benefit compared to supportive care alone in patients with advanced GC. Because comorbidities or age-related changes in PKs and PDs may lead to higher toxicity, however, many oncologists hesitate to recommend elderly patients to receive chemotherapy. Available data suggest that elderly patients with GC are able to tolerate and benefit from systemic chemotherapy to the same extent as younger patients. The age alone should not be the only criteria to preclude effective chemotherapy. However, proper patient selection is extremely important to deliver effective treatment safely. A *comprehensive geriatric assessment* (CGA) is useful to assess life expectancy and risk of morbidity in older patients and to guide optimal treatment. *Treatment should be personalized based on the nature of the disease, the life expectancy, the risk of complication, and the patient's preference.* Combination chemotherapy can be considered for older patients with metastatic GC who are classified as non-frail patients by CGA. For frail or vulnerable patients, monotherapy or only symptomatic treatment may be desirable. Targeted agents seem to be promising treatment options for elderly patients with GC considering their better efficacy and less toxicity.

Immunotherapy of Lung Cancer Lung cancer has long been considered an unsuitable target for immunotherapy due to its immunoresistant properties. However, recent evidence revealed that anti-tumor immune responses can occur in lung cancer patients, paving the way for lung cancer as a novel target for immunotherapy. In order to take full advantage of the potential of immunotherapy, research is focusing on the function of various immunological cell types in the tumor microenvironment. Immune cells, which facilitate or inhibit antitumor responses were identified and their prognostic value in lung cancer was established. Knowledge regarding these pro- and anti-tumor immune cells and their mechanisms of action has facilitated the identification of numerous immunotherapeutic strategies and opportunities for intervention. Immunotherapeutic approaches are now being developed and studied in lung cancer patients and phase 3 clinical trials are ongoing. These therapeutic approaches revealed promising clinical effects in patients with limited and advanced stage lung cancer, however, future studies will determine whether immunotherapy will earn its place in the EBPT of lung cancer.

RAS Signaling and Anti-RAS in EBPT of Cancer Usually activating mutations of oncogenic RAS genes are detected in human cancers. Fang et al. (2016) reported that the studies in genetically engineered mouse models (GEMMs) reveal that Kras-activating mutations predispose mice to early onset tumors in the *lung, pancreas, and GIT.* Nevertheless, most of these tumors do not have metastatic phenotypes. Metastasis occurs when tumors acquire additional genetic changes in other cancer driver genes. Studies on clinical specimens also demonstrated that KRAS mutations are present in premalignant tissues and that most of KRAS mutant human cancers have co-mutations in other cancer driver genes, *including TP53, STK11, CDKN2A, and KMT2C in lung cancer; APC, TP53, and PIK3CA in colon cancer; and TP53, CDKN2A, SMAD4, and MED12 in pancreatic cancer.* Extensive efforts have been made to develop therapeutic agents that target enzymes involved in RAS post-translational modifications, that inhibit downstream effectors of RAS signaling pathways that kill RAS mutant cancer cells through synthetic lethality. Recent clinical studies revealed that Sorafenib, a pan-RAF and VEGFR inhibitor, is beneficial for KRAS mutant lung cancer patients. Combination therapy of MEK inhibitors with either Docetaxel, AKT inhibitors, or PI3K inhibitors also improved clinical responses in some KRAS mutant cancer patients. These investigators discussed knowledge gained from GEMMs, human cancer cells, and patient-related studies on RAS-mediated tumorigenesis and anti-RAS therapy. Emerging evidence demonstrated that RAS mutant cancers are heterogeneous because of the presence of different mutant alleles and/or co-mutations in other cancer driver genes. Hence effective subclassifications of RAS mutant cancers may be necessary to improve patients' outcomes to accomplish EBPT.

Molecular Imaging with Antibodies for Personalized Treatment of Pancreatic Cancer Development of novel imaging probes for cancer diagnostics remains critical for early detection of disease, yet most imaging agents are hindered by suboptimal tumor accumulation. To overcome these limitations, researchers adapted antibodies for imaging purposes. Enagland et al. (2016) reported that as malignancies express atypical patterns of cell surface proteins in comparison to noncancerous tissues, novel antibody-based imaging agents can be constructed to target individual cancer cells or surrounding vasculature. Using molecular imaging techniques, these agents may be utilized for detection of malignancies and monitoring of therapeutic response. Currently, there are several imaging modalities employed for molecular imaging, including; *PET, SPECT, MRI, optical imaging (fluorescence and bioluminescence), and photoacoustic (PA) imaging.* While antibody-based imaging agents may be employed for a broad range of diseases, this report focused on the molecular imaging of pancreatic cancer, as there are limited resources for imaging and treatment of pancreatic malignancies. Moreover, pancreatic cancer remains the most lethal cancer with an overall 5-year survival rate of ~7%, despite significant advances in the imaging and treatment of many other cancers. These investigators discussed recent advances in molecular imaging of pancreatic cancer using antibody-based imaging agents by summarizing the current progress in each type of afore-described molecular imaging modality. Also, several considerations for designing and synthesizing novel antibody-based imaging agents were discussed, in addition to future directions of antibody-based imaging agents, emphasizing their potential applications for EBPT.

Personalized Treatment of Pancreatic Ductal Adenocarcinoma Generally, patients with pancreatic ductal adenocarcinoma (PDA) have a poor prognosis despite new treatments, ~7% survive for 5 years. Knudsen et al. (2016) reported that although there have been advances in systemic, primarily cytotoxic, therapies, it has been a challenge to treat patients with PDA using targeted therapies. Sequence analyses provided information about the genetic features of PDA and identified potential therapeutic targets. Preclinical and early-phase clinical studies found specific pathways could be rationally targeted; it might also be possible to take advantage of the genetic diversity of PDAs to develop therapeutic agents. The genetic diversity and instability of PDA cells were considered obstacles to treatment, but are now considered exploitable features. These researchers provided the latest findings in pancreatic cancer genetics and the promise of targeted therapy of PDA.

Radiatheray Planning for Cervical Cancer Mesko et al. (2016) reviewed the recent literature on advancements in external beam radiation therapy, brachytherapy, and stereotactic body radiation therapy (SBRT) in the treatment of cervical cancer. There is a growing transition from 3D-conformal radiation therapy to intensity modulated radiation therapy (IMRT), and from point A-based 2D- prescriptions to 3D volume-based prescriptions in image-guided brachytherapy (IGBT). These advances allow dose-escalation to at-risk regions while sparing normal tissues. Implementation of these techniques is resulting in improved local control and decreased toxicity in patients. With increased local control, the predominant pattern of recurrence is now distant failure, opening the door for SBRT as an emerging treatment option for select patients with limited numbers of metastases (*oligometastatic state*). The integration of IGBT, as well as dose sculpting with IMRT, is improving outcomes in women with locally advanced cervical cancer. The clinical evidence supports moving away from point A-based prescriptions and adopting IGBT techniques. The existing data supporting SBRT for gynecologic oligometastases are limited and require further investigations before widespread adoption; however, evidence from other disease sites is promising.

Novel Multi-Target Src and MEK Kinase Inhibitors as Anticancer Drugs Clinical studies have shown enhanced anticancer effects of combined inhibition of Src and MEK kinases. Development of multi-target drugs against Src and MEK is of potential therapeutic advantage against cancers. As a follow-up of previous studies, and by using molecular docking method, Cui et al. (2016) synthesized 9-anilinoacridines containing phenyl-urea moieties as potential novel dual Src and MEK inhibitors. The anti-proliferative assays against K562 and HepG-2 tumor cells showed that most of the derivatives displayed good cytotoxicity *in vitro*. In particular, kinase inhibition assays revealed that compound 8m inhibited Src (59.67%) and MEK (43.23%) at 10μM, and displayed moderate inhibitory activity against ERK and AKT, the downstream effectors of both Src and MEK. Moreover, compound 8m induced K562 cells apoptosis. Structure-activity relationships of these derivatives suggested that Acridine scaffold, particularly compound 8m, was of interest for developing novel multi-target Src and MEK kinase inhibitors.

β-Blockers as Anticancer Drugs Genetic variations β-ARs are distributed in different tissues of our body, which could be activated by neurotransmitters NE and EPI to mediate physiological activity and abnormal states, including cancer. He et al. (2016) reported that β-AR blockers could have significant implications in cancer therapy, but the precise molecular mechanisms remains unknown. These investigators suggested that by identifying the β-AR system signal pathways relevant to cancer, the researchers can understand the mechanisms of β-blockers for cancer treatment. Moreover, retrospective clinical data made β-blockers jump out of the traditional field of cardiovascular disease and strengthened confidence in cancer therapy. At last, genetic studies of β-adrenergic system offered crucial genes to analyze the effects of polymorphisms on cancer susceptibility, therapy response, and prognosis of cancer patients.

Companion Molecular Diagnosis for Personalized Therapeutics of Cancer The individualized targeted treatment and precision medicine requires the assessment of potential therapeutic targets for direct therapeutic selection. Mankoff et al. (2016) reported that the biomarkers used to direct precision medicine, often termed companion diagnostics, for highly targeted drugs are almost entirely based on *in vitro* assay of biopsy material. Molecular imaging companion diagnostics offer a number of features complementary to those from *in vitro* assay, including the ability to measure the heterogeneity of each patient's cancer across the entire disease burden and to measure early changes in response to treatment. These investigators discussed molecular imaging methods as companion diagnostics for cancer therapy with the goal of predicting response to targeted therapy and measuring early (PDs) response as an indication of whether the treatment has "hit" the target. They also discussed considerations for probe development for *molecular imaging companion diagnostics*, including both small-molecule probes and larger molecules such as labeled antibodies. Furthermore, they described two examples where both predictive and pharmacodynamic molecular imaging biomarkers have been tested: (a) *endocrine therapy for breast cancer and (b) human epidermal growth factor receptor type 2-targeted therapy*. They summarized the items needed to forward molecular imaging companion diagnostics from early studies into multicenter trials and into the clinics.

Photodynamic Therapy for Personalized Cancer Immunotherapy Photodynamic therapy (PDT), an approved cancer treatment can cause immunogenic apoptosis. Zheng et al. (2016) showed that PDT can cause the dysregulation of *"eat me" and "don't eat me"* signal by generating ROS-mediated ER stress. This dysregulation may contribute to the increased uptake of PDT-killed Lewis lung carcinoma (LLC) cells by homologous dendritic cells (DCs), accompanied by phenotypic maturation (CD80 (high), CD86 (high), and CD40 (high)) and functional stimulation (NO (high), IL-10(absent)) of dendritic cells as well as subsequent T-cell responses. C57BL/6 mice vaccinated with dendritic cells (DCs) pulsed with PDT-treated LLCs (PDT-DCs) or PDT-treated LLCs alone (PDT-LLCs) exhibited potent immunity against LLC tumors. In this study, the PDT-induced immune response was characterized as a process related to dysregulation of *"eat me" signal and "don't eat me"* signal, suggesting the possibility for developing PDT into an antitumor vaccination for personalized cancer immunotherapy.

Personalized Dexamethasone therapy in Childhood Acute Lymphoblastic Leukaemia (ALL) Jackson et al. (2016) reported that Dexamethasone is a key component in the treatment of childhood ALL. Despite playing a key role in the improved survival of ALL, Dexamethasone therapy has also contributed to the increased toxicity, which is now considered unacceptable given the favourable disease prognosis. Therefore the focus of treatment is now shifting towards reducing toxicity whilst maintaining current survival rates. As ~50% of patients were successfully treated on less intensive protocols of the 1980s, it was questioned whether therapy intensification is necessary in all patients. Furthermore, there remains a subset of children who are still not cured of their disease. New strategies are needed to identify patients who could benefit from dose reduction or intensification. However, adjusting a potentially life threatening therapy is a challenging task, particularly given the heterogeneous nature of ALL. These investigators focused on the patient stratification based on the Dexamethasone PKs, PDs and its action at the cellular level, and emphasized that a carefully designed, combined approach is needed to achieve improved personalization of Dexamethasone therapy.

Personalized Treatment of Prostate Cancer Noguchi et al. (2016) investigated the effect of Cyclophosphamide (CPA) in combination with personalized peptide vaccination (PPV) on regulatory T cells (Treg) and myeloid-derived suppressor cells (MDSC), and whether it could improve the antitumor effect of PPV. Seventy patients with metastatic castration-resistant prostate cancer received PPV plus oral low-dose CPA (50 mg/day), or PPV alone. PPV treatment used 4 peptides according to human leukocyte antigen types and antigen-specific humoral immune responses before PPV, for 8 s.c weekly injections. Peptide-specific cytotoxic T lymphocyte (CTL) and immunoglobulin G responses were measured before and after PPV. The incidence of grade 3 or 4 hematologic adverse events was higher in the PPV plus CPA arm than in the PPV alone arm. Decrease in Treg and increase in MDSC were more pronounced in PPV plus CPA treatment than in PPV alone. There was no correlation between the changes in Treg or MDSC and CTL response. There was no difference in positive immune responses between the two arms, although overall survival in patients with positive immune responses was longer than in those with negative immune responses. Significant differences in neither progression-free survival nor overall survival were observed between the two arms. Low-dose CPA revealed no change in the antitumor effect of PPV, due to the decrease in Treg and increase in MDSC, in patients under PPV.

Gastrin-Releasing Peptide Receptor (GRPR) for Prostate Cancer Theranostics It is now realized that a single tool for early detection, accurate staging, and personalized treatment of prostate cancer (PCa) would be a breakthrough. Gastrin-releasing peptide receptor (GRPR) targeting peptides could be promising probes for a theranostic approach for PCa overexpressing GRPR. However, the successful application of small peptides in a theranostic approach is hampered by their rapid *in vivo* degradation by proteolytic enzymes, such as neutral endopeptidase (NEP). Chatalic et al. (2016) demonstrated that co-injection of a NEP inhibitor (Phosphoramidon (PA) can lead to an enhancement of diagnostic sensitivity and therapeutic efficacy of the theranostic ^{68}Ga-/^{177}Lu-JMV4168 GRPR-antagonist. Co-injection of PA (300 µg) led to stabilization of ^{177}Lu-JMV4168 in murine peripheral blood. In PC-3 tumor-bearing mice, PA co-injection led to a 2-fold increase in tumor uptake of ^{68}Ga-/^{177}Lu-JMV4168, 1 hr after injection. In PET imaging with ^{68}Ga-JMV4168, PA co-injection enhanced PC-3 tumor signal intensity. Radionuclide therapy with ^{177}Lu-JMV4168 resulted in regression of PC-3 tumor size. The efficacy of the radionuclide therapy was confirmed by production of DNA double strand breaks, reduced cell proliferation, and increased apoptosis. Increased survival rates were observed in mice treated with ^{177}Lu-JMV4168 plus PA as compared to those without PA, indicting that co-injection of the enzyme inhibitor PA enhances the theranostic potential of GRPR-radioantagonists for PCa patients.

Multi-Compartmental Diffusion in Neuronal Tissue with MRI The ultimate goal of diffusion MRI (dMRI) models is specificity to neuronal microstructure, which may lead to specific clinical biomarkers using noninvasive imaging. While multi-compartment models are used to interpret water diffusion in the brain *in vivo*, the estimation of their parameters from the dMRI signal remains an unresolved problem. Practically, even when q space is highly oversampled, nonlinear fit outputs suffer from bias and poor precision, which has been alleviated by fixing some of the model parameters for improved precision at the expense of accuracy. Jelescu et al. (2016) used two-compartment model to show that fitting fails to determine the 5 model parameters from over 60 measurement points. The first reason was the existence of two local minima in the parameter space for the objective function of the fitting procedure. These minima correspond to qualitatively different sets of parameters, yet they both lie within biophysically plausible ranges. They showed that, at realistic signal-to-noise ratio values between the two minima based on the associated objective function values was impossible. Moreover, there was an ensemble of very low objective function values around each of these minima in the form of a pipe. The existence of such a direction in parameter space, along which the objective function profile was very flat, explained the bias and large uncertainty in parameter estimation, and the spurious parameter correlations: in the presence of noise, the minimum could be randomly displaced by a very large amount along each pipe suggesting that the biophysical interpretation of dMRI model parameters depends on establishing which of the minima is closer to the biophysical reality and the size of the uncertainty associated with each parameter.

EBPT OF NEURODEGENERATIVE DISORDERS

Genetically-Manipulated Pig Model of Neurodegeneration Increasing incidence of neurodegenerative disorders such as AD and PD has become one of the most challenging health issues in aging humans particularly in the US due to increasing life span. Holm et al. (2016) reported that one approach to combat this is to generate genetically modified animal models of neurodegenerative disorders for studying pathogenesis, prognosis, diagnosis, treatment, and prevention. Owing to the genetic, anatomic, physiologic, pathologic, and neurologic similarities between pigs and humans, genetically modified pig models of neurodegenerative disorders have been attractive large animal models to bridge the gap of preclinical investigations between rodents and humans. These researchers provided a neuroanatomical overview in pigs and discussed the generation of genetically modified pig models of AD, HD, PD, ALS, spinal muscular atrophy, and ataxia-telangiectasia. They also highlighted how non-invasive imaging including; PET, CT, and MRI, and behavioral analyses could be applied to characterize neurodegenerative pig models. Furthermore, they proposed a multiplex genome editing and preterm recloning (MAP) by using the precision genome editing CRISPR/Cas9 and somatic cell nuclear transfer (SCNT) technology. With this approach, it is expected to shorten the temporal requirement in generating multiple transgenic pigs, increase the survival rate of founder pigs, and generate genetically modified pigs that will resemble the disease-causing mutations and recapitulate pathological features of human illnesses.

Gene-Manipulated Mouse Models of Neurodegeneration The researchers raised several colonies of metallothionein transgenic (MT_{trans}), metallothioneins double gene knock out (MT_{dko}), α-Synuclein Knock out (α-Syn_{ko}), α-Synuclein-metallothionein triple knock out (α-Syn-MT_{tko}), weaver mutant (wv/wv), and metallothioneins-over-expressed weaver mutant (wv/wv-MTs) mice to establish our original hypothesis that *MTs provide ubiquinone (CoQ10)*

–mediated neuroprotection in PD, AD, and chronic drug addiction (Sharma and Ebadi, 2008); Sharma and Ebadi 2014). Chronic injections of a parkinsonian neurotoxin, 1-Methyl, 4-Phenyl, 1,2,3,6 Tetrahydropridine (MPTP: 10 mg/kg, i.p) for 7 days induced complete immobilization and typical Parkinsonism in MT_{dko} mice as compared to MT_{trans} mice which exhibited genetic resistant to MPTP Parkinsonism. MT_{trans} mice could still walk with their stiff legs and erect tail even after chronic MPTP (Neurotoxicity), indicating the neuroprotective role of MTs in PD (Sharma et al., 2004). MT_{dko} mice were mildely obese, overweight, and lethargic as compared to lean, thin, and agile MT_{trans} mice. α-Syn-MT_{tko} mice exhibited 40% mortality and reduced lifespan. Although MT_{dko} mice did not exhibit any overt clinical symptoms of PD, AD, or drug addiction, these genotypes were highly susceptible to 6-Hydroxy Dopamine (6-OH-DA), Salsolinol, 1-Benzyl Tetrahydroqunoline (1-Benzyl-TIQ), MPTP, and Cadmium toxicity. Homozygous wv/wv mice exhibited progressive neurodegeneration in the striatum, hippocampus, and cerebellar cortex. These three brain regions are primarily involved in PD, AD, and drug addiction respectively. Hence these experimental genotypes were used as animals models of multiple drug abuse. wv/wv mice exhibited typical Parkinsonism, early morbidity, and mortality as observed in chronic drug addiction and AD. MTs were significantly down-regulated in these genotypes. To establish the therapeutic potential of MTs in wv/wv mice, the researchers cross-bred the MT_{trans} males with wv/wv female mice to obtain a colony of MTs over-expressing wv/wv mice (wv/wv-MTs). The progeny was genotyped by performing tail PCR analysis. Progressive neurodegeneration as observed in wv/wv mice was significantly attenuated in wv/wv-MTs mice. Hence the researchers used these experimental genotypes as animal model of drug rehabilitation. These studies further authenticated free radical theory of neurodegeneration and confirmed the therapeutic potential of MTs in progressive neurodegenerative diseases such as PD, AD, and drug addiction. The researchers confirmed these finding *in vitro* using cultured human dopaminergic (SK-N-SH, SHS-Y5Y) cells and in mitochondrial genome knock out (RhOmgko) cells transfected with ubiquinone-NADH oxidoreductase (complex-1) gene. The researchers performed [18]FdG, and ^{18}F-DOPA microPE neuroimaging of these genotypes to establish that dopaminergic neurotransmission is governed by brain regional glucose metabolism. These studies further confirmed that MTs provide neuroprotection by acting as potent free radical scavengers and by inhibiting Charnoly Body (CB) formation involved in progressive neurodegeneration during nutritional stress and/or environmental neurotoxins (Kainic acid, Domoic acid, Acromelic acid, lead, PCB)-induced free radical overproduction and lipid peroxidation of highly vulnerable mitochondrial membranes. Furthermore, the researchers discovered α-Synuclein index (SI) as an early and sensitive biomarker of neurodegeneration (Sharma et al., 2003). Hence SI and CB can be used as central as well as peripheral biomarkers of neurodegenerative α-synucleinopathies and other neurodegenerative disorders of unknown etiopathogenesis.

Personalized Treatment of Brain Metastasis Haughton et al. (2016) reported that common and deadly complications of non-small cell lung cancer (NSCLC) are brain metastases (BM). These investigators presented treatment of BM in NSCLC in regards to targeted and immunotherapy. BM has a poorer prognosis with limited effective therapeutic options and current management strategies present several challenges from iatrogenic complications of supportive medications, optimal delivery of drug across the blood-brain barrier, and preservation of neurocognitive function. Long-term side effects and survivorship issues have become more significant in the era of targeted therapy where a systemic disease is much better controlled. Targeted therapies and immunotherapy are beginning to confer improvements in responses and survival rates. With further advancements, our knowledge in this era of EBPT will lead to improving the quality of life and overall survival of patients with BM from NSCLC.

Therapeutic Potential of Oxytoxin in Autism Guastella et al. (2016) recently reported that the impairment in reciprocal social interaction is a diagnostic hallmark of autism spectrum disorders. There is no effective medical treatment for these patients. Psychological treatments are costly, time intensive, and developmentally sensitive for efficacy. These investigators explored the potential of Oxytoxin-based therapies for social impairments in autism. Evidence suggested that acute Oxytoxin administration improves numerous biomarkers critical to the social circuitry underlying social deficits in autism. Oxytoxin may optimize these circuits and enhance reward, motivation, and learning to improve therapeutic outcomes. Despite this, the current evidence of therapeutic benefit from extended Oxytoxin treatment remains limited. They highlighted complexity in crossing from the laboratory to the autism clinical setting in evaluation of this treatment and discussed a clinical trial approach that provides opportunity for therapeutic response by using personalized strategies that better target specific circuitry to define who will obtain benefit, at what stage of development, and the optimal delivery approach for circuitry manipulation. For the autism field, the therapeutic challenges will be resolved by multiple treatment strategies, including major emphasis on specific interventions, such as Oxytoxin, that have a strong basis in the neurobiology of social behavior. More sophisticated and targeted clinical trials utilizing such approaches are now needed, placing Oxytoxin into the autism context.

Feedback Loops of Major Depressive Disorder Depression is a complex public health problem with considerable variation in treatment response. The systemic complexity of depression, or the feedback processes among diverse drivers of the disorder, contribute to the persistence of depression. Attempts were made to understand the complex causal feedback mechanisms that underlie depression by presenting the first broad boundary causal loop diagram of depression dynamics. Wittenborn et al. (2016) applied qualitative system dynamics methods to map the feedback mechanisms of depression. They used a structured approach to identify candidate causal mechanisms of depression and assessed the strength of empirical support for each mechanism and prioritized those with support from validation studies in the literature. Through an iterative process, these researchers synthesized the empirical literature and created a conceptual model of MDDs. The literature review and synthesis resulted in the development of the first causal loop diagram of reinforcing feedback processes of depression. It proposed candidate drivers of illness, or inertial factors, and their temporal functioning, as well as the interactions among drivers of depression. The final causal loop diagram defines 13 key reinforcing feedback loops that involved 9 candidate drivers of depression, indicating that future research is needed to expand this initial model of depression. Quantitative extensions may result in a better understanding of the systemic syndrome of depression and contribute to EBPT of depression.

Technology-Based Treatment of Schizophrenia Despite advances in schizophrenia treatment, symptom relapses and rehospitalizations impede recovery and are a principal driver of the high cost of care. Hence technology-delivered or technology-enhanced treatment may be a cost-effective to provide flexible EBPT to people in their homes and communities. However, evidence for the safety, acceptability, and efficacy of such interventions is only now being realized. Brunette et al. (2016) described a novel, technology-based approach to revent relapse after a hospitalization for psychosis, the *Health Technology Program (HTP)*. HTP provides in-person relapse prevention planning that directs use of tailored, technology-based treatment, based on cognitive-behavioral therapy (CBT) for psychosis, family psychoeducation for schizophrenia, and prescriber decision support through a Web-based program that solicits information from clients at every visit. Technology-based treatments are delivered through smartphones and computers.

Determination of Fluid Responsiveness Accurate assessment of intravascular fluid status and measurement of fluid responsiveness have become exceedingly important in peri-operative medicine and critical care. Ansari et al. (2016) discussed the current controversies surrounding fluid responsiveness and the merits and limitations of the major cardiac output monitors in clinical use in terms of usefulness in measuring fluid responsiveness. They searched the MEDLINE and EMBASE databases (2002-2015); inclusion criteria included comparison with an established reference standard such as pulmonary artery catheter, transthoracic echocardiography and transoesophageal echocardiography. Examples of clinical measures included static (*central venous pressure*) and dynamic (*stroke volume variation and pulse pressure variation*) parameters. The dynamic parameters were good physiological determinants of fluid responsiveness. Due to heterogeneity of the methods and patient characteristics, these investigators did not perform a meta-analysis. In most studies, precision and limits of agreement between determinants of fluid responsiveness were not evaluated, and the definition of fluid responsiveness varied across studies. These investigators emphasized that future research should focus on the physiological principles that underlie the measurement of fluid responsiveness and the effect of different volume expansion strategies on outcomes.

EBPT OF DRUG ADDICTION

Prenatal Cocaine Exposure (PCE) and Increased Illicit-Substance Abuse in Adolescence Prenatal Cocaine exposure (PCE) is associated with increased rates of illicit-substance use during adolescence. In addition, both PCE and illicit-substance use are associated with alterations in cortico-striato-limbic neurocircuitry, development of which is ongoing throughout adolescence. However, the relationship between illicit-substance use, PCE and functional neural responses has not been assessed. Yip et al. (2016) recruited 66 adolescents from a longitudinal study of childhood and adolescent development. The fMRI data were acquired during presentation of personalized stressful, favorite-food and neutral/relaxing imagery scripts and compared between 46 PCE and 22 non-prenatally-drug-exposed (NDE) adolescents with and without lifetime illicit-substance use initiation. Data were analyzed using multi-level ANOVAs. There was a significant interaction between illicit-substance use, PCE status and cue condition on neural responses within primarily cortical brain regions, including regions of the left and right insula. Among PCE versus NDE adolescents, illicit-substance use was associated with decreased subcortical and increased cortical activity during the favorite-food condition, whereas the opposite pattern of activation was observed during the neutral/relaxing condition. Among PCE versus NDE adolescents, illicit-substance use during stress processing was associated with decreased activity in cortical and subcortical regions including amygdala, hippocampus and prefrontal cortex. Neural activity within cortico-striato-limbic regions was negatively associated with subjective ratings of anxiety and craving among illicit-substance users, but not among non-users, suggesting different neural substrates of experimentation with illicit drugs between adolescents with and without in utero Cocaine exposure.

Determination of Blood Alcohol by ^1H NMR Spectroscopy. Zailer et al. (2016) *developed a* rapid, accurate and specific proton magnetic (^{1}H-NMR) spectroscopic procedure to determine Ethanol in blood, known as the *blood Alcohol concentration* (BAC). The limits of detection and quantification were 0.02g/L and 0.07g/L, respectively. The ^{1}H-NMR spectra showed linearity for blood and serum samples of a concentration range of 0.00-3.00g/L. This method was applied and validated for blood as the sample media. Driving under influence case samples were analyzed with the reference enzyme-based Alcohol dehydrogenase and gas chromatography techniques by the Forensic Medicine. The reference results were compared with the ^{1}H-NMR spectroscopic results. The validation and comparison indicated that ^{1}H-NMR was suitable for the quantification of BAC in blood. This technique had the advantages of automated analysis with good measurement precision and fast sample throughput. A drop of blood (V=20μL) was sufficient for an analysis leading to a possible simplification of the sample collection. Due to the non-destructive method, follow-up by ^{1}H NMR spectroscopy or DNA determinations by other techniques (*PCR, in situ hybridization*) are possible in resolving legal disputes.

Persoanlized Nicotine Addiction Therapy The tobacco addiction treatment is progressing through innovations in medication development, a focus on precision medicine, and application of new technologies for delivering support in real time and over time. Prochaska and Benowitz (2015) provided evidence for combined and extended cessation pharmacotherapy and behavioral strategies including; *provider advice, individual counseling, group programs, the national quitline, websites, social media, and incentives.* It is now realized that healthcare policies are changing to offer cessation treatment to the broad population of smokers. These investigators highlighted the horizon in the clinical and public health effort to address tobacco addiction.

Quantitation of Tramadol and its Metabolites in Human Blood Using LC-MS/MS The analgesic drug Tramadol and its metabolites are chiral compounds, with the (+)- and (-)-enantiomers showing different pharmacological and toxicological effects. Haage et al. (2016) developed a novel enantioselective method, based on LC-MS/MS in reversed phase mode which enabled measurement of the parent compound and its 3 main metabolites *(a) O-Desmethyltramadol, (b) N-Desmethyltramadol, and (c) N, O-Didesmethyltramadol simultaneously.* Whole blood samples of 0.5g were mixed with internal standards (Tramadol-(13) C-D3 and O-Desmethyl-cis-Tramadol-D6) and extracted under basic conditions (pH 11) by liquid-liquid extraction. Chromatography was performed on a chiral α-1-acid glycoprotein (AGP) column preceded by an AGP guard column. The mobile phase consisted of 0.8% Acetonitrile and 99.2% Ammonium acetate (20mM, pH 7.2). A post-column infusion with 0.05% Formic acid in Acetonitrile was used to enhance sensitivity. Quantitation as well as enantiomeric ratio measurements were covered by quality controls. Validation parameters for all 8 enantiomers included selectivity (high), matrix effects (*no ion suppression/ enhancement*), calibration model (linear, weight 1/X(2), in the range of 0.25-250ng/g), limit of quantitation (0.125-0.50ng/g), repeatability (2-6%) and intermediate precision (2-7%), accuracy (83-114%), dilution integrity (98-115%), carry over (not exceeding 0.07%) and stability (in blood and extract). This method was applied to blood samples from a healthy volunteer administrated a single 100mg dose and to a case sample concerning an impaired driver, which confirmed its applicability in human PKs studies as well as in toxicological and forensic investigations.

EBPT OF DIABETES

Personalized Diabetes Management Recently Kulzer et al. (2016) utilized structured self-monitoring of blood glucose (SMBG) data and data management software, within a 6-step cycle, which enables integrated Personalized *Diabetes Management* (PDM). The 2 PDM-ProValue studies were used to assess the effectiveness in improving patient outcomes and practice efficiencies in outpatient settings. The PDM-ProValue studies were 12-month, prospective, cluster-randomized, multicenter, trials to determine if use of integrated PDM in daily life improves glycemic control in insulin-treated type 2 diabetes patients. Fifty-four general medical practices (GPs) and 36 diabetes-specialized practices (DSPs) were recruited. The practices were assigned to the control groups (CNL) or the intervention groups (INT) via cluster-randomization. CNL practices were continued with their usual care; INT practices utilized integrated PDM. The sample size was 1,014 patients (n = 540 DSP patients, n = 474 GP patients). Each study was designed to detect difference in HbA1c change of at least 0.4% at 12 months with a power of 90% and 2-sided significance level of .05. Differences in timing and degree of treatment adaptions, treatment decisions, blood glucose target ranges, hypoglycemia, self-management behaviors, quality of life, patients attitudes, clinician satisfaction, practice processes, and resource consumption were assessed. Study endpoints were analyzed for the modified intent-to-treat and per protocol populations. These investigators proposed that effective and efficient strategies to optimize diabetes management are needed to determine if PDM is beneficial.

Metabolomics and Type 2 Diabetes It is now realized that type 2 diabetes (T2D) and its comorbidities have reached epidemic proportions, with more than half a billion cases expected by 2030. Metabolomics is a new approach for studying metabolic changes connected to disease development and progression and for finding predictive biomarkers to enable early interventions, which are most effective against T2D and its comorbidities. In metabolomics, the abundance of a comprehensive set of small biomolecules (metabolites) is measured, thus giving insight into disease-related metabolic alterations. Klein and Shearer (2016) provided an overview of basic metabolomics and highlighted current accomplishments in the prediction and diagnosis of T2D. These investigators summarized key metabolite fluctuations in response to T2D. Despite large variations in predictive biomarkers, many studies replicated elevated plasma levels of branched-chain amino acids and their derivatives, aromatic amino acids and α-hydroxybutyrate ahead of T2D manifestation. In contrast, glycine levels and lysophosphatidylcholine C18:2 were reduced in both predictive studies and with overt disease. These researchers highlighted that the use of metabolomics for predicting T2D comorbidities is gaining momentum, as are approaches for translating basic metabolomics research into clinical applications. As a result, metabolomics has the potential to enable decision-making in PM.

EBPT OF CARDIOVASCULAR DISEASES

In-vitro Cardiac Tissue Models It is well-known that cardiovascular disease is the leading cause of mortality worldwide. Mathur et al. (2016) emphasized that achieving the next phase of potential treatment strategies and better prognostic tools will require a concerted effort from interdisciplinary fields. Biomaterials-based cardiac tissue models are revolutionizing the area of preclinical research and translational applications. The goal of *in vitro* cardiac tissue modeling is to create functional models of the human myocardium, which is a challenging task due to the complex structure and function of the human heart. These investigators described the advances made in area of *in vitro* cardiac models using biomaterials. The field has progressed extensively in the past decade, and its applications is expected in drug screening, disease modeling, and EBPT.

Carotid Plaque Imaging in PM Currently, patients with carotid disease are selected for invasive recanalization therapies based on the degree of luminal narrowing and the presence or absence of recent ischemic symptoms. Bonati and Nederkoorn (2016) reported a risk model that takes into account other clinical variables, such as age, sex, and the type of recent symptoms, as well as presence of ulcerated plaque. A growing body of evidence indicates that noninvasive imaging of the carotid plaque by various methods identifies structural correlates of plaque vulnerability, which are associated with an increased risk of cerebrovascular event.

EBPT OF MISCELLANOUS DISEASES

Transcutaneous Measurement of PCO_2 in the Diagnosis of Nocturnal Hypercapnia It is now realized that measurement of PCO_2 is vital in determining effective alveolar ventilation. However, obtaining capillary PCO_2 by a skin prick of the earlobe is painful, and nocturnal measurements disturb sleep. End-expiratory measurement of PCO_2 is also well established, but there is a low precision in predicting arterial or capillary CO_2. Stieglitz et al. (2016) evaluated nocturnal measurement of noninvasive, transcutaneous PCO_2 ($PtcCO_2$) measurement in hypercapnic subjects. In this study, 31 subjects with chronic hypercapnic failure-in a stable phase of the underlying disease and a control group of 12 healthy volunteers were included. Transcutaneous measurements were recorded by the Tosca sensor (*Radiometer, Copenhagen, Denmark)* over a period of 6 hrs during night. A capillary blood gas was measured at midnight and 4:00 am. The mean nocturnal capillary PCO_2 ($PcapCO_2$) was 50.6 ± 10.2 mm Hg. In the 31 subjects with known hypercapnic respiratory failure, the correlation between $PtcCO_2$ and $PcapCO_2$ at midnight was 0.86 and at 4:00 am. The blood sampling caused no significant change in $PtcCO_2$. This study evaluated transcutaneous capnography as a continuous nocturnal measurement in hypercapnic subjects. Because CO_2 is not constant in patients with respiratory failure, but instead fluctuates, these investigators recommended the continuous transcutaneous measurement of PCO_2 as a method of choice for the diagnosis of nocturnal hypercapnia.

Biomarkers for Allergen Immunotherapy **Moingeon (2016)** reported that biomarkers are biological parameters that can be measured to predict or monitor disease severity or treatment efficacy. The induction of regulatory dendritic cells (DCs) with a downregulation of proallergic DC2s (ie, *DCs supporting the differentiation of T-helper lymphocyte type 2 cells*) in the blood of patients allergic to grass pollen was correlated with the early onset of allergen immunotherapy efficacy. The combined use of omics technologies to compare biological samples from clinical responders and nonresponders is being implemented in the context of nonhypothesis-driven approaches. Such comprehensive "panoromic" strategies help identify novel biomarkers, to be validated as companion diagnostics in large-scale clinical trials.

Salivary Biomarkers in PM Korte and Kinney (2016) provided a review of the robust salivary biomarkers, as well as combinatorial biomarkers and periodontal pathogens, that reveal high sensitivity and specificity for enhancing clinical decision-making in periodontal disease progression, risk and diagnosis. Periodontal diseases are complex and require an inflammatory response to bacterial pathogens in a susceptible host to stimulate tissue destruction. Traditional clinical assessments provide a diagnosis of periodontitis only after the biologic onset of the disease process, and are unable to substantiate disease activity or future risk. New technologies are capable of measuring combinations of inflammatory cytokines and proteinases for rapid testing. Utilizing saliva to identify and measure specific phenotypes and host-derived mediators will allow EBPT of periodontal diseases, which will strengthen the power of the clinical oral examination and medical history assessments, providing patients with evidence-based, targeted risk care.

Personalized Prophylactic Drug Treatment of Migraine Migraine is a highly disabling pain condition, which can influence the daily activities of those affected, including children and adolescents (Tajti et al., 2016). The pathomechanism of migraine is not fully understood, and the different types of prophylactic antimigraine drugs are unspecific for migraine. There is a need for preventive measures in the event of frequent migraine attacks, an impairment of the quality of life, severe accompanying or aura symptoms, and the failure of acute drug treatment. The following pharmacological classes have been recommended: *antidepressants, antiepileptics, antihistamines, β-adrenergic receptor blockers, and calcium ion channel antagonists, besides on a Botulinum toxin A and Nutraceuticals (Butterbur).* The most urgent goal as concerns pharmaceutical innovation is the development of pathomechanism-based antimigraine drugs and EBPT tailored to the children and adolescents.

Personalized Treatment of Hypertension-Induced Nephropathy It is known that unrelated disease processes occur in non-diabetic individuals with mild-to-moderate hypertension and low level or absent proteinuria who present with chronic kidney disease: primary glomerulosclerosis in those with recent African ancestry, and arteriolar nephrosclerosis with resultant glomerular ischemia related to hypertension and vascular disease risk factors in other cases. Recently Freedman and Cohen (2016) reported that nephrologists often apply a diagnosis of 'hypertensive nephrosclerosis' to patients, which implies that the hypertension is causative of their renal disease. Although nephropathies that are associated with variants in the apolipoprotein L1 gene (APOL1) cause secondarily elevated BP, they belong to the spectrum of focal segmental glomerulosclerosis and are not initiated by systemic hypertension. Because genetic testing for APOL1 variants and other glomerulosclerosis-associated gene variants is available and can provide a precise definition of disease pathogenesis, these investigators believed that the term 'hypertensive nephrosclerosis' should be abandoned and replaced with either gene-based (i.e., *APOL1-*

associated) glomerulosclerosis or arteriolar nephrosclerosis. In addition, EBPT will be highly significant to improve diagnostic accuracy as well as treatment in this field. Discrimination of these disparate disorders has the potential to eradicate primary forms of glomerulosclerosis that are associated with APOL1 renal-risk variants.

Siltuximab: For Idiopathic Multicentric Castleman Disease Human herpes virus-8 (HHV-8)-negative or idiopathic multicentric Castleman disease (iMCD) is a rare and fatal disorder as sits at the nexus of hematology/oncology, virology and immunology. Fajgenbaum and Kurzrock (2016) reported that management of iMCD has been challenging due to limited understanding of etiology and pathogenesis and few therapeutic options. The recent approvals in North America, Europe and Brazil of Siltuximab, a monoclonal antibody against IL-6, for iMCD provide a safe and effective therapy that targets a key aspect of pathogenesis. Siltuximab significantly reduced disease burden and symptoms in a large portion (34%) of patients. The optimal dose is 11 mg/kg i.v every 3 weeks. Presently, duration of treatment is often life-long or until treatment failure. Additional research is needed to recognize biomarkers that may assist with predicting treatment effectiveness in iMCD and to investigate the role of Siltuximab in HHV-8-positive MCD and pediatric iMCD patients.

Personalized Cell-Based Therapy for Cystic Fibrosis Cystic fibrsis (CF) is a recessive inherited disease associated with multiorgan failure that compromises epithelial and inflammatory cellular function. Suzuki et al. (2016) reported that induced pluripotent stem cells (iPSCs) have significantly advanced the potential of developing a personalized cell-based therapy for CF by generating patient-specific stem cells that can be differentiated into cells that repair tissues damaged by disease pathology. The F508del mutation in airway epithelial cell-derived CF-iPSCs was corrected with small/short DNA fragments (SDFs) and sequence-specific TALENs. An allele-specific PCR, cyclic enrichment strategy gave ~100-fold enrichment of the corrected CF-iPSCs after 6 enrichment cycles that facilitated isolation of corrected clones. The SDF-based gene modification to correct the CF-iPSCs resulted in pluripotent cells that, when differentiated into endoderm/airway-like epithelial cells, showed wild-type (wt) airway epithelial cell cAMP-dependent Cl ion transport or demonstrated the appropriate cell-type characteristics when differentiated along mesoderm/hematopoietic inflammatory cell lineage pathways.

Behavioral Intervention in Personalized Adolescent Sexual Health Although emergency department (ED) visits confer an opportunity to deliver behavioral interventions to improve health, provision of ED-based interventions targeting adolescent sexual health is rare. A study was conducted to evaluate the feasibility and preliminary effects of a novel sexual health service intervention for adolescents. Miller et al. (2016) recruited sexually active patients aged 14-19 years presenting to a Midwestern pediatric ED to receive an intervention to improve sexual health. Based on motivational interviewing (MI), including agenda setting, exploration of behaviors, a decisional balance exercise, tailored feedback, and provision of personalized health services (*including condoms, prescription for emergency contraception, urine testing for Chlamydia trachomatis and Neisseria gonorrheae, and referral to the hospital-affiliated adolescent clinic*). Data were collected before and after intervention and at a 3-month follow-up telephone interview. Surveys assessed sexual risk behaviors, satisfaction with the intervention, health care use, and demographics. Feasibility criteria were (1) subject-rated interventionist fidelity to MI principles (Likert scale 1 [strongly agree] to 4 [strongly disagree]), (2) subject satisfaction (Likert scale 1 [not at all] to 5 [very]), and (3) session duration (minutes, recorded by the interventionist). A secondary outcome was the proportion of subjects who completed at least 1 health service. Services provided at the adolescent clinic were determined by an electronic medical record review. Comparisons of responses between sex subgroups were analyzed using X test. A total of 69 adolescents were approached, 66 (96%) completed the screening survey, and 24 (37%) reported previous sexual activity. Of those, 20 (83%) agreed to participate. The mean (SD) age was 16.2 (1.4) years; 60% were female. Most (78%) reported that the interventionist maintained high fidelity to MI principles and most (80%) were very satisfied with the intervention. Most subjects (65%) accepted 1 or more health services, including 42% who completed clinic follow-up. *In the ED or the referral clinic, the following services were provided to the subjects: condoms, emergency contraception prescription, C. trachomatis/N. gonorrheae testing, hormonal birth control provision, and human immunodeficiency virus testing.* Fifteen subjects (75%) were reached for the 3-month follow-up, and condom use was maintained by 67% of those reporting sexual activity. This study demonstrated the utility of an MI-based service to connect youth with point-of-care services as well as resources for ongoing sexual health needs.

Virtual Reality Intervention to Improve Weight Gain Despite the plethora of weight loss programs available in the US, the prevalence of overweight and obesity (BMI$\geq$25kg/m^2) among US adults continues to rise due to the high probability of weight regain following weight loss. Thus, the development of novel interventions designed to improve weight maintenance are needed. Sullivan et al. (2016) virtual reality environments offer a promising platform for delivering weight maintenance interventions as they provide rapid feedback, learner experimentation, real-time personalized task selection and exploration. Utilizing virtual reality during weight maintenance allows to engage in repeated experiential learning, practice skills, and participate in real-life scenarios without real-life repercussions, which may diminish weight regain. These investigators conducted an 18-month trial (6 months weight loss, 12 months weight maintenance) in 202 overweight/obese adults (BMI 25-44.9 kg/m(2)). Participants who achieved $\geq$5% weight loss following a 6 month weight loss intervention delivered by phone conference call were randomized to weight maintenance interventions delivered by conference call or conducted in a virtual environment (Second Life®). The primary aim of the study was to compare weight change during maintenance between the phone conference call and virtual groups. In addition, potential mediators of weight change including; *energy and macronutrient intake, physical activity, consumption of fruits and vegetables, self-efficacy for both physical activity and diet, and attendance and completion of experiential learning assignments* was also assessed.

From Universal to Precision Treatment of Obesity Precision medicine utilizes genomic and other data to optimize and personalize treatment. Although >2,500 genetic tests are currently available, for extreme and/or rare phenotypes, the question remains whether this approach can be used for the treatment of common, complex conditions like *obesity, inflammation, and insulin resistance*, which underlie a host of metabolic diseases. Bray et al. (2016) developed a review from a Trans-NIH Conference titled "*Genes, Behaviors, and Response to Weight Loss Interventions,*"which confers the state of genetic and genomic research in the area of weight change and identifies key areas for future research. Although many loci were identified that are associated with cross-sectional measures of obesity/body size, relatively little is known regarding the genes/loci that influence dynamic measures of weight change over time. Although successful short-term weight loss has been achieved using many different strategies, sustainable weight loss proved elusive for many, and there are lacunae in our knowledge regarding energy balance regulation. Elucidating the molecular basis of variability in weight change has the potential to improve treatment outcomes and inform innovative approaches that can take into account information from genomic and other sources in devising EBPT of obesity.

Personalized Treatment in Ophthalmology PM is defined as: "*treatments targeted to the needs of individual patients on the basis of genetic, biomarker, phenotypic or psychosocial characteristics that distinguish a given patient from other patients with similar clinical presentations*" (Jameson and Longo, 2015). Rosenbaum et al. (2016) illustrated how molecular diagnosis can be applied to orbital inflammatory disease to achieve the ultimate goal of EBPT. The effort to subdivide diseases and to individualize therapies based on characteristics of the patient has been labeled PM.

Interdisciplinary Approach To Alleviate Pain According to the Institute of Medicine Relieving Pain in America Report and National Pain Strategy, pain affects over 100 million Americans and costs over $500 billion per year. Mackey (2016) emphasized that the researchers have now a greater appreciation for the complex nature of pain and that it can develop into a disease in itself. As such, the researchers need more efforts on prevention of chronic pain and interdisciplinary approaches. For precision pain medicine to be successful, the researchers need to link learning health systems with pain biomarkers (eg, *genomics, proteomics, patient reported outcomes, brain markers*) and its EBPT.

Antidotes for Cyanide Poisoning The FDA approved antidotes (i.e., Sodium nitrite, Sodium thiosulfate, and Hydroxocobalamin) are effective for treating Cyanide poisoning, but individually, each antidote has limitations (e.g., large effective dosage or delayed onset of action). To mitigate these limitations, next-generation Cyanide antidotes are being investigated, including 3-Mercaptopyruvate (3-MP) and Cobinamide (Cbi). Analytical methods capable of detecting these therapeutics individually and simultaneously (*for combination therapy*) are essential for the development of 3-MP and Cbi as potential Cyanide antidotes. Stutelberg et al (2016) developed a liquid chromatography-tandem mass-spectrometry method for the analysis of 3-MP and Cbi. Sample preparation of 3-MP consisted of spiking plasma with an internal standard ((13) C3-3-MP), precipitation of plasma proteins, and derivatizing 3-MP with Monobromobimane to produce 3-Mercaptopyruvate-bimane. Preparation of Cbi involved denaturing plasma proteins with simultaneous addition of Cyanide to convert each Cbi species to Dicyanocobinamide (Cbi (CN) 2). The limits of detection for 3-MP and Cbi were 0.5μM and 0.2μM, respectively. The accuracy and precision for 3-MP were 100 ± 9% and <8.3% relative standard deviation (RSD), respectively. For Cbi (CN) 2, the accuracy was 100 ± 13% and the precision was <9.5% RSD. This method was used to determine 3-MP and Cbi from treated animals which may facilitate FDA approval of these antidotes for the treatment of Cyanide poisoning.

Biomarkers for the Detection & Diagnosis of Ebola Virus Infection Ebola outbreak-2014 (*mainly Zaire strain related Ebola virus*) was declared most widely spread deadly persistent epidemic due to unavailability of rapid diagnostic, detection, and therapeutics. Recently Kaushik et al. (2016) reported that Ebola virus disease (EVD), a severe viral hemorrhagic fever syndrome is transmitted by direct contact with the body fluids of infected person and objects contaminated with virus or infected animals. WHO declared EVD epidemic as public health emergency of international concern with severe global economic burden. At fatal EBOV infection stage, patients usually die before the antibody response. Currently, rapid blood tests to diagnose EBOV infection include the antigen or antibodies capture using ELISA and RNA detection using RT/Q-PCR within 3-10 days after the onset of symptoms. Recently nanotechnology-based colorimetric and paper-based immunoassay methods have been developed to detect Ebola virus infection. Unfortunately, these methods are limited to lab only. As state-of-the art diagnostics time to confirm Ebola infection, varies from 6 hrs to about 3 days, it causes delay in therapeutic approaches. Thus developing a cost-effective, rapid, sensitive, and selective sensor to detect EVD at point-of-care (POC) is essential to establish rapid diagnostics to decide therapeutics. These researchers highlighted SoA of Ebola diagnostics to develop rapid, selective and sensitive POC detection of EBOV for global health care and proposed that *adopting miniaturized electrochemical EBOV immunosensing can detect virus titer at pM concentration within ~40 min compared to 3 days of ELISA test at nM levels.*

Smartphones for Personalized Health and Fitness Recently Higgins (2016) highlighted that healthcare providers are searching ways to monitor and improve patients' health and fitness, especially in between patient visits. Some insurance companies are using applications data as incentives to improve health and lower premiums. As more and more people use smartphones, they may improve patient's health and fitness. Specifically, fitness applications or "apps" on smartphones are programs that use data collected from a smartphone's inbuilt tools, such as the *Global Positioning System, accelerometer, microphone, speaker, and camera, to measure health and fitness parameters.* The apps then analyze these data and summarize them, as well as devise individualized plans based on users' goals, *provide frequent feedback,* personalized *coaching, and motivation by allowing milestones to be shared on social media.* The apps can help patients reach their health and fitness goals and discussed what features to look for, followed by an overview of popular health and fitness, in addition to patient scenarios with recommendations, limitations, and future research.

REFERENCES

Abou, D. S., Ulmert, D., Doucet, M., Hobbs, R. F., Riddle, R. C. & Thorek, D. L. (2015). Whole-Body and Microenvironmental Localization of Radium-223 in Naïve and Mouse Models of Prostate Cancer Metastasis. *J. Natl. Cancer Inst.*, *18*, 108(5).

Altshuler, D., Hirschhorn, J. N., Klannemark, M., Lindgren, C. M., Vohl, M. C., et al., (2000). The common PPARgamma Pro12Ala polymorphism is associated with decreased risk of type 2 diabetes. *Nat. Genet.*, *26*, 76–80.

Ansari, B. M., Zochios, V., Falter, F. & Klein, A. A. (2016). Physiological controversies and methods used to determine fluid responsiveness: a qualitative systematic review. *Anaesthesia.*, *71*, 94-105.

Astolfi, M., Péant, B., Lateef, M. A., Rousset, N., Kendall-Dupont, J., Carmona, E., Monet, F., Saad, F., Provencher, D., Mes-Masson, A. M. & Gervais, T. (2016). Micro-dissected tumor tissues on chip: an ex vivo method for drug testing and personalized therapy. *Lab Chip.*, *16*(2), 312-325.

Barna, L., Dudok, B., Miczán, V., Horváth, A., László, Z. I. & Katona, I. (2016). Correlated confocal and super-resolution imaging by VividSTORM. *Nat Protoc.*, *11*(1), 163-183.

Bay-Jensen, A. C., Reker, D., Kjelgaard-Petersen, C. F., Mobasheri, A., Karsdal, M. A., Ladel, C., Henrotin, Y. & Thudium, C. S. (2016). Osteoarthritis year in review 2015: soluble biomarkers and the BIPED criteria. *Osteoarthritis Cartilage.*, *24*(1), 9-20.

Benz, M. R., Vargas, H. A. & Sala, E. (2016). Functional MR Imaging Techniques in Oncology in the Era of PM. *Magn Reson Imaging Clin N Am.*, *24*(1), 1-10.

Bertram, L., McQueen, M. B., Mullin, K., Blacker, D. & Tanzi, R. E. (2007). Systematic meta-analyses of Alzheimer disease genetic association studies: the AlzGene database. *Nat. Genet.*, *39*, 17–23.

Bodmer, W. & Bonilla, C. (2008). Common and rare variants in multifactorial susceptibility to common diseases. *Nat. Genet.*, *40*, 695–701.

Bonati, L. H. & Nederkoorn, P. J. (2016). Clinical Perspective of Carotid Plaque Imaging. Neuroimaging *Clin. N. Am.*, *26*(1), 175-182.

Bradley, T. J., Alvarez, N. A. & Horne, S. G. (2016). A Practical Guide to Clinical Management of Thoracic Aortic Disease. *Can J Cardiol.*, *32*(1), 124-130.

Braunstein, L. Z. & Taghian, A. G. (2016). Molecular Phenotype, Multigene Assays, and the Locoregional Management of Breast Cancer. *Semin Radiat Oncol.*, *26*(1), 9-16.

Bray, M. S., Loos, R. J., McCaffery, J. M., Ling, C., Franks, P. W., Weinstock, G. M., Snyder, M. P., Vassy, J. L. & Agurs-Collins, T. (2016). Conference Working Group. NIH working group report-using genomic information to guide weight management: From universal to precision treatment. *Obesity (Silver Spring).*, *24*(1), 14-22.

Bray, M. S., Loos, R. J., McCaffery, J. M., Ling, C., Franks, P. W., Weinstock, G. M., Snyder, M. P., Vassy, J. L., Agurs-Collins, T. & Conference Working Group. (2016). NIH working group report-using genomic information to guide weight management: *From universal to* precision *treatment. Obesity (Silver Spring).*, *24*(1), 14-22.

Bromley, C. M., Close, S., Cohen, N., Favis, R., Fijal, B., et al. (2009). Designing pharmacogenetic projects in industry: practical design perspectives from the Industry Pharmacogenomics Working Group. *Pharmacogenomics J.*, *9*, 14–22.

Brunette, M. F., Rotondi, A. J., Ben-Zeev, D., Gottlieb, J. D., Mueser, K. T., Robinson, D. G., Achtyes, E. D., Gingerich, S., Marcy, P., Schooler, N. R., Meyer-Kalos, P. & Kane, J. M. (2016). Coordinated Technology-Delivered Treatment to Prevent Rehospitalization in Schizophrenia: A Novel Model of Care. *Psychiatr Serv.* 2016 Jan 4:appips201500257.

Buhtoiarova, T. N., Brenner, C. A. & Singh, M. (2016). Endometrial Carcinoma: Role of Current and Emerging Biomarkers in Resolving Persistent Clinical Dilemmas. *Am J Clin Pathol.*, *145*(1), 8-21.

Cagle, P. T., Raparia, K. & Portier, B. P. (2016). Emerging Biomarkers in Personalized Therapy of Lung Cancer. *Adv Exp Med Biol.*, *890*, 25-36.

Cao, J. L., Wei, J. C., Hu, Y. J., He, C. W., Chen, M. W., Wan, J. B. & Li, P. (2016). Qualitative and quantitative characterization of phenolic and diterpenoid constituents in Danshen (Salvia miltiorrhiza) by comprehensive two-dimensional liquid chromatography coupled with hybrid linear ion trap Orbitrap mass. *J. Chromatogr. A.*, *1427*, 79-89.

Chambers, D. C. (2016). Controlling Cytomegalovirus in the Age of PM. *Am J Respir Crit Care Med.*, *193*(1), 10-11.

Chan, E. L., Chin, C. H. & Lui, V. W. (2016). An update of ALK inhibitors in human clinical trials. *Future Oncol.*, *12*(1), 71-81.

Chatalic, K. L., Konijnenberg, M., Nonnekens, J., de Blois, E., Hoeben, S. & de Ridder, C. et al., (2016). *In vivo* Stabilization of a Gastrin-Releasing Peptide Receptor Antagonist

Enhances PET Imaging and Radionuclide Therapy of Prostate Cancer in Preclinical Studies. *Theranostics*, *6*(1), 104-117.

Chen, K., Zhang, J., Guo, Z., Ma, Q., Xu, Z., Zhou, Y., Xu, Z., et al., (2016). Loss of 5-hydroxymethylcytosine is linked to gene body hypermethylation in kidney cancer. *Cell Res.*, *26*(1), 103-118.

Colhoun, H. M., McKeigue, P. M. & Davey Smith, G. (2003). Problems of reporting genetic associations with complex outcomes. *Lancet*, *361*, 865–872.

Colombo, S., Rauch, A., Rotger, M., Fellay, J., Martinez, R., et al. (2008). The HCP5 single-nucleotide polymorphism: a simple screening tool for prediction of hypersensitivity reaction to abacavir. *J. Infect. Dis.*, *198*, 864–867.

Connor, S. (2003). Glaxo chief: Our drugs do not work on most patients. The Independent. Available: http://www.independent.co.uk/news/science/glaxochief-our-drugs-do-not-work-on-most-patients-575942.html Accessed 2009 November 10, Archived URL: http://www.webcitation.org/5lBCqy0gg.

Cui, Z., Li, X., Li, L., Zhang, B., Gao, C., Chen, Y., Tan, C., Liu, H., Xie, W., Yang, T. & Jiang, Y. (2016). Design, synthesis and evaluation of acridine derivatives as multi-target Src and MEK kinase inhibitors for anti-tumor treatment. *Bioorg Med Chem.*, *24*(2), 261-269.

Deng, H. & Wang, H., Li, Z. (2015). Matching Chelators to Radiometals for Positron Emission Tomography Imaging- Guided Targeted Drug Delivery. *Curr Drug Targets.*, *16*(6), 610-624.

Eberhardt, M., Lai, X., Tomar, N., Gupta, S., Schmeck, B., Steinkasserer, A., Schuler, G. & Vera, J. (2016). Third-Kind Encounters in Biomedicine: Immunology Meets Mathematics and Informatics to Become Quantitative and Predictive. *Methods Mol. Biol.*, *1386*, 135-179.

England, C. G., Hernandez, R., Eddine, S. B. & Cai, W. (2016). Molecular Imaging of Pancreatic Cancer with Antibodies. *Mol Pharm.*, *13*(1), 8-24.

Fajgenbaum, D. C. & Kurzrock, R. (2016). Siltuximab: a targeted therapy for idiopathic multicentric Castleman disease. *Immunotherapy.*, *8*(1), 17-26.

Fang, B. (2016). RAS signaling and anti-RAS therapy: lessons learned from genetically engineered mouse models, human cancer cells, and patient-related studies. *Acta Biochim Biophys Sin (Shanghai).*, *48*(1), 27-38.

Frank, B., Wiestler, M., Kropp, S., Hemminki, K., Spurdle, A. B., et al. (2008). Association of a common AKAP9 variant with breast cancer risk: a collaborative analysis. *J. Natl. Cancer Inst.*, *100*, 437–442. 30.

Freedman, B. I. & Cohen, A. H. (2016). Hypertension-attributed nephropathy: what's in a name? *Nat Rev Nephrol.*, *12*(1), 27-36.

Frodsham, A. J. & Higgins, J. P. (2007). Online genetic databases informing human genome epidemiology. *BMC Med. Res. Methodol.*, *7*, 31.

Galimov, A., Merry, T. L., Luca, E., Rushing, E. J., Mizbani, A., Turcekova, K., Hartung, A., Croce, C. M., Ristow, M. & Krützfeldt, J. (2016). microRNA-29a in adult muscle stem cells controls skeletal muscle regeneration during injury and exercise downstream of fibroblast growth factor-2. *Stem Cells.*, *34*(3), 768-780.

Goldstein, D. B. (2009). Common genetic variation and human traits. *N. Engl. J. Med.* 360, 1696–1698.

Goldstein, D. B., Tate, S. K. & Sisodiya, S. M. (2003). Pharmacogenetics goes genomic. *Nat. Rev. Genet.*, *4*, 937–947.

Gong, Y., Wang, Z., Beitelshees, A. L., McDonough, C. W., Langaee, T. Y., Hall, K., Schmidt, S. O., Curry, R. W., Jr. Gums, J. G., Bailey, K. R., Boerwinkle, E., Chapman, A. B., Turner, S. T., Cooper-DeHoff, R. M. & Johnson, J. A. (2016). Pharmacogenomic Genome-Wide Meta-Analysis of Blood Pressure Response to β-Blockers in Hypertensive African Americans. *Hypertension*. In press.

Guastella, A. J. & Hickie, I. B. (2016). Oxytoxin Treatment, Circuitry, and Autism: A Critical Review of the Literature Placing Oxytoxin into the Autism Context. *Biol Psychiatry.*, *79*(3), 234-242.

Guye, P., Ebrahimkhani, M. R., Kipniss, N., Velazquez, J. J., Schoenfeld, E., Kiani, S., Griffith, L. G. & Weiss, R. (2016). Genetically engineering self-organization of human pluripotent stem cells into a liver bud-like tissue using Gata6. *Nat Commun.*, *7*, 10243.

Haage, P., Kronstrand, R., Carlsson, B., Kugelberg, F. C. & Josefsson, M. (2016). Quantitation of the enantiomers of tramadol and its three main metabolites in human whole blood using LC-MS/MS. *J Pharm Biomed Anal.*, *119*, 1-9.

Hajian, B., Backer, J., Vos, W., Holsbeke, C. V., Clukers, J. & Backer, W. (2016). Functional respiratory imaging (FRI) for optimizing therapy development and patient care. *Expert Rev Respir Med.* In press.

Haughton, M. E., Chan, M. D., Watabe, K., Bonomi, M., Debinski, W., Lesser, G. J. & Ruiz, J. (2016). Treatment of brain metastases of lung cancer in the era of precision medicine. *Front Biosci (Elite Ed).*, *8*, 219-32.

He, R. H., He, Y. J., Tang, Y. J., Zhou, H. H., McLeod, H. L. & Liu, J. (2016). The potential anticancer effect of beta-blockers and the genetic variations involved in the interindividual difference. *Pharmacogenomics.*, *17*(1), 74-79.

Hedberg, M. L., Goh, G., Chiosea, S. I., Bauman, J. E., Freilino, M. L., Zeng, Y., Wang, L., Diergaarde, B. B., Gooding, W. E., Lui, V. W., Herbst, R. S., Lifton, R. P. & Grandis, J. R. (2016). Genetic landscape of metastatic and recurrent head and neck squamous cell carcinoma. *J. Clin. Invest.*, *126*(1), 169-180.

Heise, R., Amann, P. M., Ensslen, S., Marquardt, Y., Czaja, K., Joussen, S., Beer, D., Abele, R., Plewnia, G., Tampé, R., Merk, H. F., Hermanns, H. M. & Baron, J. M. Interferon Alpha Signalling and Its Relevance for the Upregulatory Effect of Transporter Proteins Associated with Antigen Processing (TAP) in Patients with Malignant Melanoma. *PLoS One.*, 2016 Jan 6, *11*(1), e0146325.

Herrmann, I. K. & Rösslein, M. (2016). PM: the enabling role of nanotechnology. *Nanomedicine (Lond).*, *11*(1), 1-3.

Higgins, J. P., Little, J., Ioannidis, J. P., Bray, M. S., Manolio, T. A., et al. (2007). Turning the pump handle: evolving methods for integrating the evidence on gene-disease association. *Am. J. Epidemiol.*, *166*, 863–866.

Higgins, J. P. (2016). Smartphone Applications for Patients' Health and Fitness. *Am. J Med.*, *129*(1), 11-19.

Hindorff, L. A., Mehta, J. P. & Manolio, T. A. (2009). A catalog of published genomewide association studies. National Human Genome Research Institute. Available: www.genome.gov/26525384 Archived URL: http://www.webcitation.org/5lBRp4wFx.

Holm, I. E., Alstrup, A. K. & Luo, Y. (2016). Genetically modified pig models for neurodegenerative disorders. *J Pathol.*, *238*(2), 267-287.

Holmes, M. V., Shah, T., Vickery, C., Smeeth, L., Hingorani, A. D., et al. (2009). Fulfilling the Promise of PM? Systematic Review and Field Synopsis of Pharmacogenetic Studies. *PLoS ONE, 4*(12), e7960.

Huang, L., Tang, X., Zhang, W., Jiang, R. & Zhong, H. (2016). Laser Activated Electron Tunneling Based Mass Spectrometric Imaging of Molecular Architectures of Mouse Brain Revealing Regional Specific Lipids. *Anal Chem., 88*, 732-739.

Hunter, D. J., Altshuler, D. & Rader, D. J. (2008). From Darwin's finches to canaries in the coal mine–mining the genome for new biology. *N. Engl. J. Med., 358*, 2760–2763.

Hynicka, L. M., Cahoon, W. D. Jr. & Bukaveckas, B. L. (2008). Genetic testing for warfarin therapy initiation. *Ann Pharmacother, 42*, 1298–1303.

Insel, P. A., Amara, S. G., Blaschke, T. F. & Meyer, U. A. (2015). Introduction to the Theme "Cancer Pharmacology".*Annu Rev Pharmacol Toxicol.*, 2015 Nov 9.

Ioannidis, J. P. (2005). Why most published research findings are false. *PLoS Med, 2*, e124.

Ioannidis, J. P. (2008). Effect of formal statistical significance on the credibility of observational associations. *Am. J. Epidemiol., 168*, 374–383.

Ioannidis, J. P., Boffetta, P., Little, J., O'Brien, T. R., Uitterlinden, A. G., et al. (2008). Assessment of cumulative evidence on genetic associations: interim guidelines. *Int J Epidemiol, 37*, 120–132.

Ioannidis, J. P., Gwinn, M., Little, J., Higgins, J. P., Bernstein, J. L., et al., (2006). A road map for efficient and reliable human genome epidemiology. *Nat. Genet., 38*, 3–5.

Ioannidis, J. P., Ntzani, E. E. & Trikalinos, T. A. (2004). 'Racial' differences in genetic effects for complex diseases. *Nat. Genet., 36*, 1312–1318.

Ioannidis, J. P., Ntzani, E. E., Trikalinos, T. A. & Contopoulos-Ioannidis, D. G. (2001). Replication validity of genetic association studies. *Nat. Genet., 29*, 306–309.

Ioannidis, J. P., Trikalinos, T. A. & Khoury, M. J. (2006). Implications of small effect sizes of individual genetic variants on the design and interpretation of genetic association studies of complex diseases. *Am.. J. Epidemiol., 164*, 609–614.

Ioannidis, J. P., Trikalinos, T. A., Ntzani, E. E. & Contopoulos-Ioannidis, D. G. (2003). Genetic associations in large versus small studies: an empirical assessment. *Lancet, 361*, 567–571.

Jackson, J. N., Long, K. M., He, Y., Motsinger-Reif, A. A., McLeod, H. L. & Jack, J. (2016). A comparison of DMET Plus microarray and genome-wide technologies by assessing population substructure. *Pharmacogenet Genomics.*, 2016 Jan 1.

Jackson, R. K., Irving, J. A. & Veal, G. J. (2016). Personalization of Dexamethasone therapy in childhood acute lymphoblastic leukaemia. *Br. J. Haematol.*, 2016 Jan 5.

Jain, A., Graveline, A., Waterhouse, A., Vernet, A., Flaumenhaft, R. & Ingber, D. E. (2016). A shear gradient-activated microfluidic device for automated monitoring of whole blood haemostasis and platelet function. *Nat Commun., 7*, 10176.

Jakobsdottir, J., Gorin, M. B., Conley, Y. P., Ferrell, R. E. & Weeks, D. E. (2009). Interpretation of genetic association studies: markers with replicated highly significant odds ratios may be poor classifiers. *PLoS Genet, 5*, e1000337.

Janssens, A. C., Aulchenko, Y. S., Elefante, S., Borsboom, G. J., Steyerberg, E. W., et al. 2006. Predictive testing for complex diseases using multiple genes: fact or fiction? *Genet. Med., 8*, 395–400.

Jelescu, I. O., Veraart, J., Fieremans, E. & Novikov, D. S. (2016). Degeneracy in model parameter estimation for multi-compartmental diffusion in neuronal tissue. *NMR Biomed.*, *29*(1), 33-47.

Jin, P., Liang, X., Xia, L., Jahouh, F., Wang, R., Kuang, Y. & Hu, X. (2016). Determination of 20 trace elements and arsenic species for a realgar-containing traditional Chinese medicine Niuhuang Jiedu tablets by direct inductively coupled plasma-mass spectrometry and high performance liquid chromatography-inductively coupled plasma-mass spectrometry. *J. Trace Elem. Med. Biol.*, *33*, 73-80.

Jones, R. T., Felsenstein, K. M. & Theodorescu, D. (2016). Pharmacogenomics: Biomarker-Directed Therapy for Bladder Cancer. *Urol. Clin. North Am.*, *43*(1), 77-86.

Kansagra, A. P., Yu, J. P., Chatterjee, A. R., Lenchik, L., Chow, D. S., Prater, A. B., Yeh, J., Doshi, A. M., Hawkins, C. M., Heilbrun, M. E., Smith, S. E., Oselkin, M., Gupta, P. & Ali, S. (2016). Big Data and the Future of Radiology Informatics. *Acad Radiol.*, *23*(1), 30-42.

Kaushik, A., Tiwari, S., Dev Jayant, R., Marty, A. & Nair, M. (2016). Towards detection and diagnosis of Ebola virus disease at point-of-care. *Biosens Bioelectron.*, *75*, 254-272.

Khoury, M. J., Little, J., Gwinn, M. & Ioannidis, J. P. (2007). On the synthesis and interpretation of consistent but weak gene-disease associations in the era of genome-wide association studies. *Int. J. Epidemiol.*, *36*, 439–445.

Kim, H. S., Kim, J. H., Kim, J. W. & Kim, B. C. (2016). Chemotherapy in Elderly Patients with Gastric Cancer. *J. Cancer.*, *7*(1), 88-94.

Kim, K. Y., Cho, S. H., Song, Y. H., Nam, M. S. & Kim, C. W. (2016). Direct injection LC-MS/MS method for the determination of teicoplanin in human plasma. *J. Chromatogr. B. Analyt. Technol. Biomed. Life Sc*i., *1008*, 125-31.

Kime, C., Mandegar, M. A., Srivastava, D, Yamanaka, S., Conklin, B. R. & Rand, T. A. (2016). Efficient CRISPR/Cas9-Based Genome Engineering in Human Pluripotent Stem Cells. *Cur.r Protoc. Hum. Genet.*, *88*, 21.4.1-21.4.23.

Kirschner, M. (2016). Systems Medicine: Sketching the Landscape. *Methods Mol Biol.*, *1386*, 3-15.

Klein, T. E., Altman, R. B., Eriksson, N., Gage, B. F., Kimmel, S. E., et al. 2009. Estimation of the warfarin dose with clinical and pharmacogenetic data. *N. Engl. J. Med.*, *360*, 753–764.

Klein, M. S. & Shearer, J. (2016). Metabolomics and Type 2 Diabetes: Translating Basic Research into Clinical Application. *J Diabetes Res.*, 2016, 3898502.

Knudsen, E. S., O'Reilly, E. M., Brody, J. R. & Witkiewicz, A. K. (2016). Genetic Diversity of Pancreatic Ductal Adenocarcinoma and Opportunities for Precision Medicine. *Gastroenterology.*, 2016 Jan, *150*(1), 48-63.

Komljenovic, D., Wiessler, M., Waldeck, W., Ehemann, V., Pipkorn, R., Schrenk, H.H., Debus, J. & Braun, K. (2016). NIR-Cyanine Dye Linker: a Promising Candidate for Isochronic Fluorescence Imaging in Molecular Cancer Diagnostics and Therapy Monitoring. *Theranostics.*, *6*(1), 131-141.

Korte, D. L. & Kinney, J. (2016). PM: an update of salivary biomarkers for periodontal diseases. *Periodontol*, 2000., *70*(1), 26-37.

Kraft, P., Wacholder, S., Cornelis, M. C., Hu, F. B., Hayes, R. B., et al. (2009). Beyond odds ratios - communicating disease risk based on genetic profiles. *Nat Rev Genet.*, *10*(4), 264-269.

Kruglyak, K. M., Lin, E. & Ong, F. S. (2016). Next-Generation Sequencing and Applications to the Diagnosis and Treatment of Lung Cancer. *Adv. Exp. Med. Biol.*, *890*, 123-136.

Kulzer, B., Daenschel, W., Daenschel, I., Siegel, E. G., Schramm, W., Parkin, C. G., Messinger, D., Weissmann, J., Djuric, Z., Mueller, A., Vesper, I. & Heinemann, L. (2015). Integrated Personalized Diabetes Management (PDM): Design of the ProValue Studies: Prospective, Cluster-Randomized, Controlled, Intervention Trials for Evaluation of the Effectiveness and Benefit of PDM in Patients With Insulin-Treated Type 2 Diabetes. *J. Diabetes Sci. Technol.*, 2015 Dec 7.

Lemonick, M. D., Cray, D., Park, A., Thomas, C. B. & Thompson, D. (2001). Brave New Pharmacy. Time. Available: http://www.time.com/time/magazine/article/ 0, 9171, 998963-1, 00.html Accessed 2009 November 10.

Lenardo, M., Lo, B. & Lucas, C. L. (2015). Genomics of Immune Diseases and New Therapies. *Annu Rev Immunol.*, Dec 23.

Lewin, J. J., 3rd., Choi, E. J. & Ling, G. (2016). Pharmacy on demand: New technologies to enable miniaturized and mobile drug manufacturing. *Am. J. Health Syst. Pharm.*, *73*(2), 45-54.

Li, B. T., Lou, E., Hsu, M., Yu, H. A., Naidoo, J., Zauderer, M. G., Sima, C., Johnson, M. L., Daras M., DeAngelis, L. M., Fleisher, M., Kris, M. G. & Azzoli, C. G. Serum Biomarkers Associated with Clinical Outcomes Fail to Predict Brain Metastases in Patients with Stage IV Non-Small Cell Lung Cancers. *PLoS One.*, 2016 Jan 5, 11(1), e0146063.

Li, S., Teng, L., Liu, W., Cheng, X., Jiang, B., Wang, Z. & Wang, C. H. (2016). Pharmacokinetic study of Harmane and its 10 metabolites in rat after intravenous and oral administration by UPLC-ESI-MS/MS. *Pharm Biol.*, Jan 5, 1-14.

Li, S., Todor, A. & Luo, R. (2015). Blood transcriptomics and metabolomics for PM. *Comput Struct Biotechnol J.*, *14*, 1-7.

Liang, B., Zhan, Y., Wang, Y., Gu, E., Dai, D., Cai, J. & Hu, G. (2016). Effect of 24 Cytochrome P450 2D6 Variants Found in the Chinese Population on Atomoxetine *Metabolism in vitro. Pharmacology.*, *97*(1-2), 78-83.

Lianos, G. D., Rausei, S., Dionigi, G. & Boni, L. (2016). Assessing safety and feasibility of minimally invasive surgical approaches for advanced gastric cancer. *Future Oncol.*, *12*(1), 5-8.

Lievense, L., Aerts, J. & Hegmans, J. (2016). Immune Therapy. *Adv Exp Med Biol.*, *893*, 59-90.

Limdi, N. A., Arnett, D. K., Goldstein, J. A., Beasley, T. M., McGwin, G., et al., (2008). Influence of CYP2C9 and VKORC1 on warfarin dose, anticoagulation attainment and maintenance among European-Americans and African-Americans. *Pharmacogenomics*, *9*, 511–526.

Link, E., Parish, S., Armitage, J., Bowman, L., Heath, S., et al. (2008). SLCO1B1 variants and statin-induced myopathy–a genomewide study. *N. Engl. J. Med.*, *359*, 789–799.

Liu, Z., Tang, Q., Wen, J., Tang, Y., Huang, D., Huang, Y., Xie, J., Luo, Y., Liang, M., Wu, C., Lu, Z., Tan, A., Gao, Y., Wang, Q., Jiang, Y., Yao, Z., Lin, X., Zhang, H., Mo, Z., Yang, X., 216. Elevated serum complement factors 3 and 4 are strong inflammatory markers of the metabolic syndrome development: a longitudinal cohort study. *Sci. Rep.*, *6*, 18713.

Liu, J., Konstantinopoulos, P. A. & Matulonis, U. A. (2016). Genomic testing and precision medicine - What does this mean for gynecologic oncology? *Gynecol Oncol.*, *140*(1), 3-5.

Lloyd, K. C., Khanna, C., Hendricks, W., Trent, J. & Kotlikoff, M. (2016). Precision medicine: an opportunity for a paradigm shift in veterinary medicine. *J. Am. Vet. Med. Assoc.*, *248*(1), 45-48.

Lu, J., Xuan, S., Downing, N. S., Wu, C., Li, L., Krumholz, H. M. & Jiang, L. (2016). Protocol for the China PEACE (Patient-centered Evaluative Assessment of Cardiac Events) Million Persons Project pilot. *BMJ Open.*, 2016 Jan 4, *6*(1), e010200.

Lu, T. X., Young, K. H., Xu, W. & Li, J. Y. (2016). TP53 dysfunction in diffuse large B-cell lymphoma. *Crit Rev Oncol. Hematol.*, *97*, 47-55.

Lucas, A. T., O'Neal, S. K., Santos, C. M., White, T. F., Zamboni, W. C. A sensitive high performance liquid chromatography assay for the quantification of Doxorubicin associated with DNA in tumor and tissues. *J Pharm Biomed Anal.*, *119*, 122-129.

Luzak, A., Schnell-Inderst, P., Bühn, S., Mayer-Zitarosa, A. & Siebert, U. (2016). Clinical effectiveness of cancer screening biomarker tests offered as self-pay health service: a systematic review. *Eur J Public Health.*, 2016 Jan 4.

Mackey, S. (2016). Future Directions for Pain Management: Lessons from the Institute of Medicine Pain Report and the National Pain Strategy. *Hand Clin.*, *32*(1), 91-98.

Manchanda R, Jacobs I. 2016. Genetic screening for gynecological cancer: where are we heading? *Future Oncol.*, *12*(2), 207-220.

Mankoff, D. A., Edmonds, C. E., Farwell, M. D. & Pryma, D. A. (2016). Development of Companion Diagnostics. *Semin. Nucl. Med.*, *46*(1), 47-56.

Marr, K. (2008). A Glimpse Into PM of the Future. The Washington Post. Available: http://www.washingtonpost.com/wp-dyn/content/ article/ 2008/09/28/ AR20080928024 82.html Accessed 2009 November 10.

Martinot-Peignoux, M. & Marcellin, P. (2016). Virological and serological tools to optimize the management of patients with chronic hepatitis B. *Liver Int.*, *36* Suppl 1, 78-84.

Mathur, A., Ma, Z., Loskill, P., Jeeawoody, S. & Healy, K. E. (2016). *In vitro* cardiac tissue models: Current status and future prospects. *Adv Drug Deliv Rev.*, *96*, 203-213.

Maxson, J. E., Abel, M. L., Wang, J., Deng, X., Reckel, S., Luty, S. B., et al. (2016). Identification and Characterization of Tyrosine Kinase Nonreceptor 2 Mutations in Leukemia through Integration of Kinase Inhibitor Screening and Genomic Analysis. *Cancer Res.*, *76*(1), 127-138.

McClain, M. R., Palomaki, G. E., Piper, M. & Haddow, J. E. (2008). A rapid-ACCE review of CYP2C9 and VKORC1 alleles testing to inform warfarin dosing in adults at elevated risk for thrombotic events to avoid serious bleeding. *Genet. Med.*, *10*, 89–98.

Mega, J. L., Close, S. L., Wiviott, S. D., Shen, L., Hockett, R. D., et al., (2009). Cytochrome p-450 polymorphisms and response to Clopidogrel. *N. Engl. J. Med.*, *360*, 354–362.

Meldolesi, E., van Soest, J., Damiani, A., Dekker, A., Alitto, A. R., Campitelli, M., Dinapoli, N., Gatta, R., Gambacorta, M. A., Lanzotti, V., Lambin, P. & Valentini, V. (2016). Standardized data collection to build prediction models in oncology: a prototype for rectal cancer. *Future Oncol.*, *12*(1), 119-136.

Mesko, S. & Kamrava, M. (2016). Moving from standardized to personalized boxes and pears in radiation planning for cervical cancer. *Curr. Opin. Obstet. Gynecol.*, *28*(1), 18-23.

Miller, M. K., Champassak, S., Goggin, K., Kelly, P., Dowd, M. D., Mollen, C. J., Humiston, S. G., Linebarger, J. & Apodaca, T. (2016). Brief Behavioral Intervention to Improve Adolescent Sexual Health: A Feasibility Study in the Emergency Department.

Moher, D., Liberati, A., Tetzlaff, J. & Altman, D. G. (2009). Preferred reporting items for systematic reviews and meta-analyses: the PRISMA statement. *PLoS Med*, *6*, e1000097.

Moingeon, P., 2016. Biomarkers for Allergen Immunotherapy: A "Panoromic" View.

Moore, K. N. & Mannel, R. S. (2016). Is the NCI MATCH trial a match for gynecologic oncology? *Gynecol Oncol.*, *140*(1), 161-166.

Estal, M. R., Suela, P. S., Jiménez de, J. I., Gonzalez, A C., Rojas, E. C., et al., (2016). Relationship of immunohistochemistry, copy number aberrations and epigenetic disorders with BRCAness pattern in hereditary and sporadic breast cancer. *Fam. Cancer.*, 2016 Jan 2.

Noguchi, M., Moriya, F., Koga, N., Matsueda, S., Sasada, T., Yamada, A., Kakuma, T. & Itoh, K. (2016). A randomized phase II clinical trial of personalized peptide vaccination with metronomic low-dose cyclophosphamide in patients with metastatic castration-resistant prostate cancer. *Cancer Immunol. Immunother.* In press.

Pennisi, E. (2007). Breakthrough of the year. Human genetic variation. *Science*, *318*, 1842–1843.

Peters, K. M., Hutter, E., Siston, R. A., Bertran, J. & Allen, M. J. (2016). Surgical Navigation Improves the Precision and Accuracy of Tibial Component Alignment in Canine Total Knee Replacement. *Vet. Surg.*, *45*(1), 52-59.

Pharmacogenetics Research Network. National Institute of General Medical Sciences, NIH. Available: http://www.nigms.nih.gov/Initiatives/PGRN Accessed 2009 November 10, Archived URL: http://www.webcitation.org/ 5lBSkNtMF.

Pollack, A. (2005). A Special Drug Just for You, At the End of a Long Pipeline. The New York Times. Available: http://www.nytimes.com/ 2005/11/08/health/08phar.html.

Poucke, S. V., Zhang, Z., Schmitz, M., Vukicevic, M., Laenen, M. V., Celi, L. A. & Deyne, C. D. (2016). Scalable Predictive Analysis in Critically Ill Patients Using a Visual Open Data Analysis Platform. *PLoS One.*, *11*(1), e0145791.

Prochaska, J. J. & Benowitz, N. L. (2016). The Past, Present, and Future of Nicotine Addiction Therapy. *Annu. Rev. Med.* (in press).

Roca, J., Cano, I., Gomez-Cabrero, D. & Tegnér, J. (2016). From Systems Understanding to PM: Lessons and Recommendations Based on a Multidisciplinary and Translational Analysis of COPD. *Methods Mol. Biol.*, *1386*, 283-303.

Rosenbaum, J. T., Sibley, C. H., Choi, D., Harrington, C. A. & Planck, S. R. (2016). Molecular diagnosis: Implications for ophthalmology. *Prog Retin Eye Res.*, *50*, 25-33.

Roses, A. D. (2000). Pharmacogenetics and the practice of medicine. *Nature* 405, 857–865.

Rule, G. S., Rockwood, A. L. & Johnson-Davis, K. L. (2016). Quantitation of Teriflunomide in Human Serum/Plasma Across a 40,000-Fold Concentration Range by LC/MS/MS. *Methods Mol Biol.*, *1383*, 195-203.

Sagoo, G. S., Tatt, I., Salanti, G., Butterworth, A. S., Sarwar, N., et al., (2008). Seven lipoprotein lipase gene polymorphisms, lipid fractions, and coronary disease: a HuGE association review and meta-analysis. *Am. J. Epidemiol.*, *168*, 1233–1246.

Saqi, M, Pellet, J., Roznovat, I., Mazein, A., Ballereau, S., De Meulder, B. & Auffray, C. (2016). Systems Medicine: The Future of Medical Genomics, Healthcare, and Wellness. *Methods Mol Biol.*, *1386*, 43-60.

Schizophrenia Gene (SZGene), Schizophrenia Research Forum. Available: http:// www. schizophreniaforum.org/res/sczgene Accessed 2009 November 10.

Scott, R. A. (2016). Unraveling the role for genetics in enabling precision prescription for weight loss-scaling up for success. *Obesity (Silver Spring).*, *24*(1), 12-13.

Shan, C. X., Cui, X. B., Yu, S., Chai, C., Wen, H. M., Wang, X. Z. & Sun, X. (2016). Study on pharmacokinetics of 3, 4-divanillyltetrahydrofuran in rats by ultra-fast liquid chromatography/tandem mass spectrometry. *J Chromatogr B Analyt Technol Biomed Life Sci.*, *1008*, 250-254.

Shaw, V., Bullock, K. & Greenhalf, W. (2016). Single-Nucleotide Polymorphism to Associate Cancer Risk. *Methods Mol. Biol.*, *1381*, 93-110.

Shurin, S. B. & Nabel, E. G. (2008). Pharmacogenomics–ready for prime time? *N. Engl. J. Med.*, *358*, 1061–1063.

Simon, T., Verstuyft, C., Mary-Krause, M., Quteineh, L., Drouet, E., et al. (2009). Genetic determinants of response to Clopidogrel and cardiovascular events. *N. Engl. J. Med.*, *360*, 363–375.

Steuer, C., Schütz, P., Bernasconi, L. & Huber, A. R. (2016). Simultaneous determination of phosphatidylcholine-derived quaternary ammonium compounds by a LC-MS/MS method in human blood plasma, serum and urine samples. *J Chromatogr B Analyt. Technol. Biomed. Life Sci.*, *1008*, 206-211.

Stieglitz, S., Matthes, S., Priegnitz, C., Hagmeyer, L. & Randerath, W. (2016). Comparison of Transcutaneous and Capillary Measurement of PCO2 in Hypercapnic Subjects. *Respir Care.*, *61*(1), 98-105.

Stutelberg, M. W., Dzisam, J. K., Monteil, A. R., Petrikovics, I., Boss, G. R., Patterson, S. E., Rockwood, G. A. & Logue, B. A. (2016). Simultaneous determination of 3-mercaptopyruvate and cobinamide in plasma by liquid chromatography-tandem mass spectrometry. *J Chromatogr B Analyt Technol Biomed Life Sci.*, *1008*, 181-188.

Sullivan, D. K., Goetz, J. R., Gibson, C. A., Mayo, M. S., Washburn, R. A., Lee, Y., Ptomey, L. T. & Donnelly, J. E. (2016). A virtual reality intervention (Second Life) to improve weight maintenance: Rationale and design for an 18-month randomized trial. *Contemp Clin Trials.*, *46*, 77-84.

Suzuki, S., Sargent, R. G., Illek, B., Fischer, H., Esmaeili-Shandiz, A., Yezzi, M. J., et al. (2016). TALENs Facilitate Single-step Seamless SDF Correction of F508del CFTR in Airway Epithelial Submucosal Gland Cell-derived CF-iPSCs. *Mol Ther Nucleic Acids.*, 2016 Jan 5, 5, e273.

Table of Valid Genomic Biomarkers in the Context of Approved Drug Labels. FDA (Created 2006 September 15, Updated 2008 September 10, Removed 2009 June). Accessed 2009 January 12, Archived URL: http://www. webcitation.org/5l6cpblur (older version). See Document S1 (recent version prior to removal of website).

Tajti, J., Szok, D., Csáti, A. & Vécsei, L. (2016). Prophylactic Drug Treatment of Migraine in Children and Adolescents: An Update. *Curr. Pain Headache. Rep.*, 2016 Jan, *20*(1), 1.

Tam, A. L., Lim, H. J., Wistuba, I. I., Tamrazi, A., Kuo, M. D., Ziv, E., Wong, S., Shih, A. J., Webster, R. J. 3rd, Fischer, G. S., Nagrath, S., Davis, S. E., White, S. B. & Ahrar, K. (2016). Image-Guided Biopsy in the Era of Personalized Cancer Care: Proceedings from the Society of Interventional Radiology Research Consensus Panel. *J. Vasc. Interv. Radiol.*, *27*(1), 8-19.

Tan, D. S., Mok, T. S. & Rebbeck, T. R. (2016). Cancer Genomics: Diversity and Disparity Across Ethnicity and Geography. *J. Clin. Oncol.*, *34*(1), 91-101.

Tang, S., Zhang, Z., Kavitha, G., Tan, E. K. & Ng, S. K. (2009). MDPD: an integrated genetic information resource for Parkinson's disease. *Nucleic Acids Res.*, *37*, D858–862.

Tényi, Á., de Atauri, P., Gomez-Cabrero, D., Cano, I., Clarke, K., Falciani, F., Cascante, M., Roca, J. & Maier, D. (2016). ChainRank, a chain prioritisation method for contextualisation of biological networks. *BMC Bioinformatics.*, *17*(1), 17.

Vaisvaser, S., Modai, S., Farberov, L., Lin, T., Sharon, H., Gilam, A., Volk, N., Admon, R., Edry, L., Fruchter, E., Wald, I., Bar-Haim, Y., Tarrasch, R.,Chen, A., Shomron, N. & Hendler, T. (2016). Neuro-Epigenetic Indications of Acute Stress Response in Humans: The Case of MicroRNA-29c. *PLoS One.*, *11*(1), e0146236.

van Kampen, A. H. & Moerland, P. D. (2016). Taking Bioinformatics to Systems Medicine. *Methods Mol Biol.* 1386, 17-41.

Varn, F. S., Andrews, E. H., Mullins, D. W. & Cheng, C. (2016). Integrative analysis of breast cancer reveals prognostic hematopoietic activity and patient-specific immune response profiles. *Nat Commun.*, *7*, 10248.

Vogelsang, M., Martinez, C. N., Rendleman, J., Bapodra, A. B., Malecek, K., Romanchuk, A., Kazlow, E., Shapiro, R. L., Berman, R. S., Krogsgaard, M., Osman, I. & Kirchhoff, T. (2016). The expression quantitative trait loci in immune pathways and their effect on cutaneous melanoma prognosis. *Clin. Cancer. Res.*, 2016 Jan 5.

Wang, Z., Seow, W. J., Shiraishi, K., Hsiung, C. A., Matsuo, K., et al., (2016). Modeling Multisystem Physiological Dysregulation. *Psychosom Med.* In press.

Wittenborn, A. K., Rahmandad, H., Rick, J. & Hosseinichimeh, N. (2016). Depression as a systemic syndrome: mapping the feedback loops of major depressive disorder. *Psychol. Med.*, *46*(3), 551-562.

Woodcock, J. & Lesko, L. J. (2009). Pharmacogenetics–tailoring treatment for the outliers. *N. Engl. J. Med.*, *360*, 811–813.

Wu, M., Ai, Y., Zeng, B. & Zhao, F. (2016). *In situ* solvothermal growth of metal-organic framework-ionic liquid functionalized graphene nanocomposite for highly efficient enrichment of chloramphenicol and thiamphenicol. *J Chromatogr A.*, *1427*, 1-7.

Xie, H. & Frueh, F. W. (2005). *Pharmacogenomics steps toward PM. PM*, *2*(4), 333.)

Xu, Q., Wu, Z., Yang, L., Zhang, X., Gai, Z., Chen, L., He, L. & Qin, S. (2016). Functional characterization of CYP2D6 novel allelic variants identified in the Chinese Han population. *Pharmacogenomics.*, *17*(2), 119-129.

Yip, S. W., Lacadie, C. M., Sinha, R., Mayes, L. C. & Potenza, M. N. (2016). Prenatal Cocaine exposure, illicit-substance use and stress and craving processes during adolescence. *Drug Alcohol. Depend.*, *158*, 76-85.

Zailer, E. & Diehl, B. W. (2016). Alternative determination of blood Alcohol concentration by (1)H NMR spectroscopy. *J Pharm Biomed Anal.*, *119*, 59-64.

Zehnbauer, B. A. & Buchman, T. G. (2016). Precision Diagnosis Is a Team Sport. *J. Mol. Diagn.*, *18*(1), 1-2.

Zehnbauer, B. A. & Buchman, T. G. (2016). Precision Diagnosis Is a Team Sport. *Crit. Care Med.*, *44*(1), 229-230.

Zheng, Y., Yin, G., Le, V., Zhang, A., Chen, S., Liang, X. & Liu, J. (2016). Photodynamic-therapy Activates Immune Response by disrupting Immunity Homeostasis of Tumor Cells, which Generates Vaccine for Cancer Therapy. *Int. J. Biol. Sci.*, *12*(1), 120-132.

Chapter 6

NANOTECHNOLOGY AND PHARMACOGENOMICS IN EVIDENCE-BASED PERSONALIZED THERANOSTICS (RECENT UPDATE)

ABSTRACT

Recently nanotechnology has contributed remarkably towards the development of EBPT. Nanotechnology is the manipulation of matter on an atomic, molecular, and supramolecular scale. The earliest, description of nanotechnology referred to the specific goal of precisely manipulating atoms and molecules for the construction of macroscale products, also referred to as *molecular nanotechnology*. Applications of pharmaceutical nanotools, cell based therapy, and molecular mechanisms are employed in nanotechnology and biotechnology. In addition, *the development of nanobioscience, nanopharmaceutical tools, omics, bioinformatics, and biosensors employing biomarker-targeted approaches has revolutionized the basic concept of EBPT. Nanoceramics composites, carbon nanotubes, nanofibers, micropatterned nanosheets, nanogels, liposomes, chitosans, alginates, block copolymers, biodegradable dendrimers, micelles, and metal NPs have been used in bone regeneration, lung repair, gene therapy, stem cell tissue engineering, regenerative medicine, brain and opthalamic treatments, cancer thernostics, biosensing, and bioimaging to accomplish EBPT as described briefly in the* chapter.

Keywords: nanopharmaceuticals, omics, biosensors, evidence based personalized theranostics (EBPT), pharmacogenomics

INTRODUCTION

Despite the marked advances in drug therapy, some patients do not respond favorably or suffer severe adverse drug effects. *Pharmacogenetic studies have shown that polymorphisms of drug metabolizing enzymes, transporters, and receptors contribute to variable drug response.* Owing to the complexity of drug actions, a broader genomics approach aims at finding new drug targets and optimizing therapy for the individual patient. However, PGx has made only a few advances into clinical practice to date. Sade'e and DaiHum (2016) evaluated obstacles that need to be overcome to accomplish EBPT. These include the complexity of mechanisms underlying drug response, given singly or in combination, uncertainty about the genetic underpinnings of complex diseases, such as cancer, diabetes, cardiovascular and mental disorders and a lack of understanding of the scope of genetic variations, even for well-studied genes. By resolving these hurdles, PGx will yield significant, but incremental, therapeutic advances paving the way towards personalized health care.

Pharmacogenetic studies have documented effects of genetic polymorphisms on drug response (Rosen., 2000; Lemonick et al., 2001; Connor, 2003; Goldstein et al., 2003; Pirmohamed et al., 2004; Polloack, 2005; Sade´e and DaiHum, 2005; Hunter et al., 2008; Marr, 2008; Goldstein, 2009). Recent availability of high-density genomic SNP maps, and expanding functional polymorphisms, have generated high expectations for applying pharmacogenetics to the optimization of therapies for individual patients. Because of increasing use of genomics and other -omics technologies, the term PGx has emerged to reflect this unique approach in drug discovery, development, and therapy. PGx is a harbinger of EBPT, a paradigm shift from the mindset of *'one-drug-fits-all'* to *'the right drug for the right patient at the right dose and time.'* This does not mean that each patient will be treated differentially from every other patient, an economically untenable proposition. Rather, patients are divided into groups based on genetic and other biomarkers that predict disease progression and therapeutic outcome. For drug therapy, one needs to avoid lack of response or toxicity. If the frequency of an adverse event can be reduced from 5 to 2%, by excluding 10% of the targeted population, a drug gains a more favorable risk/benefit ratio and could advance to first-choice treatment, thereby gaining market share. One can expect a growing trend to link the launch of new drugs with diagnostic biomarkers, often genetic, to improve treatment outcome for individual patients—the hallmark of EBPT. *Numerous factors contribute to variable drug response, including; age, sex, body weight, nutrition, organ function, infections, comedications, and genetic factors.* PGx is one of the several approaches in EBPT, with bioinformatics providing integration of relevant data. However, disease processes and drug therapies are complex, the behavior of which cannot be precisely predicted, limiting predictive power of PGx.

This chapter summarizes the current status of PGx and addresses challenges that need to be overcome to accomplish the long-quested goal of EBPT.

Genetic Causes of Interindividual Variability in Drug Response It is now realized that highly variable drug response and toxicity preclude clinical use of a drug. Even with some of the most current drugs, favorable response occurs in only 30–70% of patients, with a significant portion exhibiting adverse effects, yielding a poor risk/benefit ratio for a diverse patient population. PKs and PDs provide quantitative measures of drug exposure and effect, and therefore, are crucial disciplines for understanding variability. *PKs involves absorption, distribution, metabolism and excretion (ADME), whereas PDs concerns drug targets (receptors and enzymes), signaling events and pharmacological response.* Because ADME governs drug exposure, drug level monitoring yields phenotypic biomarkers useful for EBPT. Large inter-individual variability is usually associated *with mutations in cytochrome P450s* and in conjugating enzymes such as *glucuronyl transferases*. Whether severe adverse drug effects, a leading cause of death in the US (*Table of Valid Genomic Biomarkers in the Context of Approved Drug Labels, 2006*), are associated with polymorphic drug metabolizing enzymes, called 'unavoidable' because adverse drug effects occur upon proper drug treatment excluding medication errors, a high level of association between polymorphic CYP450 genes and the lead drugs causing adverse reactions has been observed, suggesting reducing the incidence of adverse effects with the use of genetic information (McClain et al., 2008). Drug transporters are encoded by several genes, playing a pivotal role in ADME and drug targeting (Hynicka et al., 2008). Numerous functional polymorphisms affect drug response (http://www.pharmgkb.org/), but their impact is poorly understood. Similarly, the effect of polymorphisms in genes encoding drug receptors is difficult to assess. Activating mutations are a possible exception, particularly those of tyrosine kinases, involved in cancer progression. For example, constitutive activity of the fusion protein BCR/ABL (*generated through chromosomal translocation in leukemi*a) conveys high sensitivity to Imatinib (Gleevec), whereas mutations of EGFR appear to correlate with responsiveness to Gefitinib (Iressa) (Ioannidis et al., 2001; Shurin and Nable, 2008). Furthermore, over-expression of ErbB2 is a prequisite for successful Herceptin treatment of breast cancer (Ioannidis et al., 2003).

Prospective Genotyping in Drug Therapy It has been realized that if a genetic factor is substantial and frequent, and failure to achieve optimal drug therapy has consequences, prospective genotyping may be indicated. However, in several cases, it may suffice to understand the genetic components affecting variable drug response to minimize the potential for adverse effects. Currently, under discussion for obligatory prospective genotyping is the potentially life-threatening toxicity of thiopurines in the treatment of childhood leukemias, in patients lacking functional thiopurine methyltransferase (TPMT) (Pirmohamed et al., 2004; Colhoun et al., 2003; Ioannidis et al., 2006; Higgins et al. 2007; Ioannidis et al., 2008). In homozygous carriers of TPMT null mutations, the dose of thiopurines has to be reduced at least 10-fold to avoid myelosuppression. However, only one in 300 subjects is homozygous, so that genotyping of 300 patients is needed for detecting a null carrier. The logistics of genotyping, and legal and economical considerations, have led to different options on prospective genotyping. Alternatively, careful monitoring of white blood cell count could suffice to avoid serious toxicity. Clearly, medical, legal, ethical and economic issues all play a significant role in the implementation of prospective genotyping at the bedside.

Multifactorial Drug Response Interindividual variability in drug response may be governed by mutations in a single gene, such as CYP2D6, with 5–10% poor metabolizers in a Caucasian population (*carriers of two null alleles*). However, most drugs interact with several CYP isozymes, conjugating enzymes such as glucuronyl transferase, UGT1A1, and transporters, each adding to genetic variability. The topoisomerase inhibitor Irinotecan (Camptothecin) serves to illustrate this point. Irinotecan has become a first-line defense against colon carcinomas, exhibiting enhanced efficacy over the use of 5-FU alone. However, leukopenia and diarrhea may become limiting and can be severe. Because UGT1A1 plays a major role in detoxifying the active metabolite of Irinotecan, prospective genotyping has been suggested to avoid undue toxicity in carriers of defective UGT1A1. However, Irinotecan interacts with several polymorphic drug metabolizing enzymes and transporters, being inactivated by CYP3A4 to APC, and requiring conversion by carboxyesterases to the active metabolite SN38. (Pennisi, 2007; Moher et al., 2009; Ioannidis 2005; Ioannidis, 2008; Ioannidis et al., 2006; Bodmer and Bonilla, 2008; Hindorff et al., 2009; Khoury et al., 2007; Altshuler, 2000). The latter is inactivated by UGT1A1 glucuronidation as the main degradation pathway. In addition, Irinotecan and its metabolites serve as substrates for transporters, including the ABC transporters (*ATP-drive extrusion pumps*) MDR1, MRP2 and BCRP. Each of these factors displays interindividual variability, with functional polymorphisms contributing to variable Irinotecan response. UGT1A1 is responsible for Bilirubin glucuronidation (Frank et al., 2008). Null mutations of UGT1A1 lead to Criggler–Najjar syndrome, whereas less complete defects are associated with Gilbert's syndrome. The most common functional polymorphism is a A (TA) 6TAA repeat in the promoter region of 1A1. The most common form carries six (TA) repeats (wt), whereas UGT1A128 carries 7 repeats, associated with lower UGT activity. However, additional polymorphisms (*in the Phenobarbital responsive enhancer module PBREM*) contribute to variable UGT expression. Haplotype analysis provided additional insight into the regulation of gene transcription, but a quantitative assessment of all factors is lacking (Pennisi, 2007; Ioannidis et al., 2006). As a consequence, use of TA repeat polymorphisms in predicting *in vivo* UGT activity and SN38 exposure after Irinotecan administration has been only partially successful. Hence, the value of prospective genotyping for UGT1A1 in Irinotecan therapy has to be determined empirically, in the target populations.

Interactions in Combination Drug Therapy Currently treatment with single drugs targeting a specific receptor is no longer considered optimal in the treatment of complex diseases, such as cancer and HIV/AIDS. With the administration of multiple drug simultaneously, however, possible drug–drug interactions multiply, leading to unexpected adverse effects that may be difficult to trace. For example, if drug A, metabolized by both CYP2D6 and CYP2C9, is administered together with a second drug acting as an inhibitor of CYP2C9, metabolism of drug A is significantly reduced in CYP2D6 poor metabolizers. For anti-HIV therapy, up to 3 antiviral drugs are given concomitantly, with Ritonavir serving as an antiviral 'boosting' agent (Sagoo et al., 2008). Ritonavir is a potent inhibitor of CYP3A4 and an inhibitor of membrane transporters such as Pgp (MDR1) [Table of Valid Genomic Biomarkers in the Context of Approved Drug Labels (2009)]. This permits the reduction of the dose of other antivirals that are also metabolized by CYP3A4 and transported by PGp; however, dose-titration becomes erratic. Moreover, *most patients are comedicated with antibiotics, antidepressants and statins to overcome lipodystrophic side effects of the antivirals.* This leads to a high rate of adverse effects, with polymorphisms in ADME-related genes determining frequency and severity. A causal relationship may be difficult to ascertain with a *one gene-one drug* approach, because effects distribute over a network of interactions. Rather, a systems approach is needed to integrate overall adverse effects with functional polymorphisms in multiple genes. A medical informatics approach involving large patient populations and assessment of all side effects in associations with the most prevalent pharmacogenetic biomarkers has been suggested.

Genetic Contribution to Phenotypic Variability It is now realized that even for well-studied genes, the overall genetic variability remains uncertain. Once a functional polymorphism has been experimentally validated, this biomarker is applied to clinical studies, without assessing its relative contribution to overall genetic variability. Most genes harbor multiple functional polymorphisms. For example, the serotonin transporter gene, SERT (SLC6A4), has been implicated in various mood and cognitive disorders. A polymorphism in the promoter region (LPR, long and short form) has been analyzed in association studies and affects SERT mRNA levels in lymphocytes and using a reporter gene assay (Ioannidis et al., 2004; Limdi et al., 2008). Yet, SERT is mainly transcribed in neurons located in the pontine area of brain stem, but there is controversial evidence that SERT levels differ between LPR genotypes in the CNS. Whereas non-synonymous polymorphisms in the SERT coding region are rare, further regulatory polymorphisms may contribute to disease susceptibility or treatment response. Hence a quantitative assessment is needed to evaluate the penetrance of SERT polymorphisms in mental disorders or in treatment with specific serotonin reuptake inhibitors, widely used antidepressants with efficacy in 60–70% of patients.

REFERENCES

Altshuler, D., Hirschhorn, J. N., Klannemark, M., Lindgren, C. M., Vohl, M. C., et al., (2000). The common PPARgamma Pro12Ala polymorphism is associated with decreased risk of type 2 diabetes. *Nat Genet*, *26*, 76–80.

Bertram, L., McQueen, M. B., Mullin, K., Blacker, D. & Tanzi, R. E. (2007). Systematic meta-analyses of Alzheimer disease genetic association studies: the AlzGene database. *Nat Genet*, *39*, 17–23.

Bodmer, W. & Bonilla, C. (2008). Common and rare variants in multifactorial susceptibility to common diseases. *Nat Genet*, *40*, 695–701.

Bromley, C. M., Close, S., Cohen, N., Favis, R., Fijal, B., et al., (2009). Designing pharmacogenetic projects in industry: practical design perspectives from the Industry Pharmacogenomics Working Group. *Pharmacogenomics J*, *9*, 14–22.

Colhoun, H. M., McKeigue, P. M. & Davey Smith, G. (2003). Problems of reporting genetic associations with complex outcomes. *Lancet*, *361*, 865–872.

Colombo, S., Rauch, A., Rotger, M., Fellay, J., Martinez, R., et al., (2008). The HCP5 single-nucleotide polymorphism: a simple screening tool for prediction of hypersensitivity reaction to abacavir. *J. Infect. Dis.*, *198*, 864–867.

Connor, S. (2003). Glaxo chief: Our drugs do not work on most patients. The Independent. Available:http://www.independent.co.uk/news/science/glaxochief-our-drugs-do-not-work-on-most-patients-575942.html Accessed 2009 November 10.

Frank, B., Wiestler, M., Kropp, S., Hemminki, K., Spurdle, A. B., et al., (2008). Association of a common AKAP9 variant with breast cancer risk: a collaborative analysis. *J. Natl. Cancer Inst.*, *100*, 437–442.

Frodsham, A. J. & Higgins, J. P. (2007). Online genetic databases informing human genome epidemiology. *BMC Med Res Methodol*, *7*, 31.

Goldstein, D. B. (2009). Common genetic variation and human traits. *N Engl J Med*, *360*, 1696–1698.

Goldstein, D. B., Tate, S. K. & Sisodiya, S. M. (2003). Pharmacogenetics goes genomic. *Nat Rev Genet*, *4*, 937–947.

Higgins, J. P., Little, J., Ioannidis, J. P., Bray, M. S., Manolio, T. A., et al., (2007). Turning the pump handle: evolving methods for integrating the evidence on gene-disease association. *Am. J. Epidemiol.*, *166*, 863–866.

Hindorff, L. A. J. H., Mehta, J. P. & Manolio, T. A. (2009). A catalog of published genomewide association studies. National Human Genome Research Institute. Available: www.genome.gov/26525384 Accessed 2009 November 10, Archived.

Holmes, M. V., Shah, T., Vickery, C., Smeeth, L., Hingorani, A. D., et al., (2009). Fulfilling the Promise of PM? Systematic Review and Field Synopsis of Pharmacogenetic Studies. *PLoS ONE*, *4*(12), e7960.

Hunter, D. J., Altshuler, D. & Rader, D. J. (2008). From Darwin's finches to canaries in the coal mine–mining the genome for new biology. *N. Engl. J. Med., 358*, 2760–2763.

Hynicka, L. M., Cahoon, W. D. Jr. & Bukaveckas, B. L. (2008). Genetic testing for warfarin therapy initiation. *Ann Pharmacother, 42*, 1298–1303.

Ioannidis, J. P. (2005). Why most published research findings are false. *PLoS Med, 2*, e124.

Ioannidis, J. P. (2008). Effect of formal statistical significance on the credibility of observational associations. *Am. J. Epidemiol., 168*, 374–383.

Ioannidis, J. P., Boffetta, P., Little, J., O'Brien, T. R., Uitterlinden, A. G., et al., (2008). Assessment of cumulative evidence on genetic associations: interim guidelines. *Int J Epidemiol, 37*, 120–132.

Ioannidis, J. P., Gwinn, M., Little, J., Higgins, J. P., Bernstein, J. L., et al., (2006). A road map for efficient and reliable human genome epidemiology. *Nat Genet, 38*, 3–5.

Ioannidis, J. P., Ntzani, E. E. & Trikalinos, T. A. (2004). 'Racial' differences in genetic effects for complex diseases. *Nat Genet, 36*, 1312–1318.

Ioannidis, J. P., Ntzani, E. E., Trikalinos, T. A. & Contopoulos-Ioannidis, D. G. (2001). Replication validity of genetic association studies. *Nat Genet, 29*, 306–309.

Ioannidis, J. P., Trikalinos, T. A. & Khoury, M. J. (2006). Implications of small effect sizes of individual genetic variants on the design and interpretation of genetic association studies ocomplex diseases. *Am J Epidemiol, 164*, 609–614.

Ioannidis, J. P., Trikalinos, T. A., Ntzani, E. E. & Contopoulos-Ioannidis, D. G. (2003). Genetic associations in large versus small studies: an empirical assessment. *Lancet, 361*, 567–571.

Jakobsdottir, J., Gorin, M. B., Conley, Y. P., Ferrell, R. E. & Weeks, D. E. (2009). Interpretation of genetic association studies: markers with replicated highly significant odds ratios may be poor classifiers. *PLoS Genet, 5*, e1000337.

Janssens, A. C., Aulchenko, Y. S., Elefante, S., Borsboom, G. J., Steyerberg, E. W., et al. 2006. Predictive testing for complex diseases using multiple genes: fact or fiction? *Genet. Med., 8*, 395–400.

Khoury, M. J., Little, J., Gwinn, M. & Ioannidis, J. P. (2007). On the synthesis and interpretation of consistent but weak gene-disease associations in the era of genome-wide association studies. *Int. J. Epidemiol., 36*, 439–445.

Klein, T. E., Altman, R. B., Eriksson, N., Gage, B. F., Kimmel, S. E., et al. (2009). Estimation of the warfarin dose with clinical and pharmacogenetic data. *N. Engl. J. Med., 360*, 753–764.

Kraft, P., Wacholder, S., Cornelis, M. C., Hu, F. B., Hayes, R. B., et al. (2009). Beyond odds ratios - communicating disease risk based on genetic profiles. *Nat Rev Genet., 10*, 264-269.

Lemonick, M. D., Cray, D., Park, A., Thomas, C. B. & Thompson, D. (2001). Brave New Pharmacy. Time. Available: http://www.time.com/time/magazine/article/ 0, 9171, 998963-1, 00.html Accessed 2009 November 10, Archived URL: http:// www. webcitation.org/5lBD8FmTx.

Limdi, N. A., Arnett, D. K., Goldstein, J. A., Beasley, T. M., McGwin, G., et al., (2008). Influence of CYP2C9 and VKORC1 on warfarin dose, anticoagulation attainment and maintenance among European-Americans and African-Americans. *Pharmacogenomics, 9*, 511–526.

Link, E., Parish, S., Armitage, J., Bowman, L., Heath, S., et al., (2008). SLCO1B1 variants and statin-induced myopathy–a genomewide study. *N. Engl. J. Med.*, *359*, 789–799.

Marr, K. (2008). A Glimpse Into PM of the Future. The Washington Post. Available: http://www.washingtonpost.com/wp-dyn/content/ article/2008/09/28/AR2008092802482.html Accessed 2009 November 10.

McClain, M. R., Palomaki, G. E., Piper, M. & Haddow, J. E. (2008). A rapid-ACCE review of CYP2C9 and VKORC1 alleles testing to inform warfarin dosing in adults at elevated risk for thrombotic events to avoid serious bleeding. *Genet Med.*, *10*, 89–98.

Mega, J. L., Close, S. L., Wiviott, S. D., Shen, L., Hockett, R. D., et al., (2009). Cytochrome p-450 polymorphisms and response to Clopidogrel. *N. Engl. J. Med.*, *360*, 354–362.

Moher, D., Liberati, A., Tetzlaff, J. & Altman, D. G. (2009). Preferred reporting items for systematic reviews and meta-analyses: the PRISMA statement. *PLoS Med*, *6*, e1000097.

Pennisi, E. (2007). Breakthrough of the year. Human genetic variation. *Science*, *318*, 1842–1843.

Pharmacogenetics Research Network. National Institute of General Medical Sciences, NIH. Available: http://www.nigms.nih.gov/Initiatives/PGRN Accessed 2009 November 10.

Pollack, A. (2005). A Special Drug Just for You, At the End of a Long Pipeline. The New York Times. Available: http://www.nytimes.com/ 2005/11/08/health/08phar.html Accessed 2009 November 10.

Roses, A. D. (2000). Pharmacogenetics and the practice of medicine. *Nature*, *405*, 857–865.

Sade´e, W. & DaiHum, Z. (2005). Pharmacogenetics/genomics and PM *Mol. Genet.*, *14* (suppl 2), R207-R214.

Sagoo, G. S., Tatt, I., Salanti, G., Butterworth, A. S., Sarwar, N., et al., (2008). Seven lipoprotein lipase gene polymorphisms, lipid fractions, and coronary disease: a HuGE association review and meta-analysis. *Am. J. Epidemiol.*, *168*, 1233–1246.

Schizophrenia Gene (SZGene), Schizophrenia Research Forum. Available: http:// www.schizophreniaforum.org/res/sczgene Accessed 2009 November 10.

Shurin, S. B. & Nabel, E. G. (2008). Pharmacogenomics–ready for prime time? *N. Engl. J. Med.*, *358*, 1061–1063.

Simon, T., Verstuyft, C., Mary-Krause, M., Quteineh, L., Drouet, E., et al., (2009). Genetic determinants of response to Clopidogrel and cardiovascular events. *N. Engl. J. Med.*, *360*, 363–375.

Table of Valid Genomic Biomarkers in the Context of Approved Drug Labels. FDA (Created 2006 September 15, Updated 2008 September 10, Removed 2009 June). Accessed 2009 January 12, Archived URL: http://www. webcitation.org/5l6cpblur (older version). See Document S1 (recent version prior to removal of website).

Tang, S., Zhang, Z., Kavitha, G., Tan, E. K. & Ng, S. K. (2009). MDPD: an integrated genetic information resource for Parkinson's disease. *Nucleic Acids Res*, *37*, D858–862.

Woodcock, J. & Lesko, L. J. (2009). Pharmacogenetics–tailoring treatment for the outliers. *N Engl. J. Med.*, *360*, 811–813.

Chapter 7

NANOTECHNOLOGY IN EVIDENCE-BASED PERSONALIZED THERANOSTICS (RECENT UPDATE)

ABSTRACT

It is now well established that efficient drug delivery systems are exceedingly important for novel drug discovery. The evidence-based personalized theranostics (EBPT) promise to deliver the right drug at the right time to a right patient as it covers clinically-significant genetic predisposition and chronopharmacological aspects of nanotheranostics. Recently nanotechnology has confered clinically-significant knowledge at the cellular, molecular, and genetic level to accomplish the long quested goal of EBPT. Particularly drug encapsulation in pegylated liposomes has improved pharmacokinetics (PKs) as well as pharmacodynamics (PDs) of cancer, cardiovascular diseases, and neurodegenerative diseases. Particularly, long-circulating liposomes and block copolymers concentrate slowly via enhanced permeability and retention (EPR) effect in the solid tumors and are highly significant for the drug delivery in successful EBPT of cancer. Selective targeting of siRNA and oligonucleotides to tumor cells to inhibit multi-drug resistant (MDR) malignancies has also shown great promise. In addition, implantable drug delivery devices have improved EBPT of several chronic diseases. Recently, microRNA, metallothioneins (MTs), α-synuclein index, and Charnoly Body (CB) emerged as novel drug discovery biomarkers. Hence CB antagonists-loaded ROS scavenging targeted nanoparticles (NPs) may be developed for the successful EBPT of neurodegenerative and cardiovascular diseases. Nonspecific induction of CBs in the hyper-proliferative cells may cause alopecia, gastrointestinal tract (GIT) symptoms, myelosuppression, neurotoxicity, and infertility in multi-drug-resistant malignancies. Therefore selective CB agonists may be developed to augment cancer stem cell specific CB formation to eliminate MDR malignancies with minimum or no adverse effects. This chapter highlights recent advances on safe, economical, and effective clinical management of neurodegenerative diseases, cardiovascular diseases, and cancer by adopting emerging nanotheranostic strategies to accomplish EBPT.

Keywords: nanotheranostics, pegylation, Charnolybody, charnolophagy, charnolopathy, chronopharmacology, metallothioneins, MicroRNA, α-synuclein index

INTRODUCTION

Indeed nanotechnology has significant impact on environment and health related issues as it is now utilized in nanomedicine, green nanotechnology, energy, and industrial applications. Most of these applications are limited to passive NPs such as: titanium oxide and zinc oxide NPs used in sun screens, cosmetics, and food products; Silver NPs for food packaging, clothing, disinfectants, and house hold appliances; Carbon nanotubes for stain-resistant textiles; and Cerium oxide as a fuel catalyst in commercial products (Sanvicens and Marco, 2008; Swami et al., 2012). Currently, over 1300 nanotechnology products are now commercially available. In developing countries nanotechnology is being utilized to treat infectious diseases and in environmental purification processes (*ground water treatment, waste water treatment, desalination of water, water filtration, and nanoremediation*) to prevent global health-related deleterious consequences (Nanotechnology Information Center, 2011). Industrial applications of nanotechnology include building construction materials, ceramics, military items, nanowires, nanorods, and graphene layers beyond the scope of this chapter (Jayasena and Subbiah, 2011).

Recently nanotechnology emerged as a promising approach by performing diagnosis as well as treatment simultaneously on a single platform (*also named as Nanotheranostics*). Nanotheranostics covers a wide range of *in vitro* diagnostics and prognostics, *in vivo* molecular imaging, molecular therapeutics, image-guided therapy, biosensors, system biology and translational medicine, PM, and biomedical research. This chapter is focused primarily on the novel strategies of drug discovery and drug delivery for better, safe, economical, early, and effective treatment of chronic diseases by adopting nanotheranostics strategies to accomplish the ultimate goal of EBPT. Particularly magnetic NPs provide an excellent platform for theranostic applications because of their biocompatibility, responses to the external magnetic field, and sizes comparable to that of functional biomolecules (Ho et al., 2011). *Magnetic NPs have control over size, surface functionalization, magnetic properties, and specific binding capabilities.* Moreover, the combination of the deep tissue penetration of the magnetic field enhances MRI sensitivity and heating makes them highly suitable for theranostic applications. Recently magnetic NPs for MRI and magnetic fluid hyperthermia (MFH), particularly Iron oxide (Fe_3O_4), gold-Iron oxide (Au- Fe_3O_4), metallic Iron (Fe), and Fe-based alloy, such as Iron-Cobalt (FeCo) and Iron-Platinum (FePt) NPs were developed. Because of the ease of fabrication and FDA approval, Fe_3O_4 NPs with controlled sizes and surface properties are being investigated for MRI and MFH applications. Porous hollow Fe_3O_4 NPs have similar magnetic, chemical, and biological properties as the Fe_3O_4 NPs, and their structure provides targeted drug delivery. Moreover, multiomdal theranostics can be accomplished by Au-Fe_3O_4 NPs which combine both magnetically active Fe_3O_4 and optically active Au. Metallic Fe and FeCo NPs can be used to develop nanoprobes with even higher magnetization. The primary limitation of metallic NPs is that these are highly reactive and are oxidized in biological fluids. However upon coating with Fe_3O_4 or a graphitic shell, they become stable to provide better contrast for MRI and effective heating for MFH. Indeed FePt NPs are more stable than Fe and FeCo NPs and can be utilized as contrast agents for both MRI as well as CT; in addition to controlled heating with MFH for theranostic applications. A recent study focused on the basic nanotheranostic approach, nanomaterials used, and future directions (Ahmed et al., 2011). More specifically, application of the magnetic NPs for diagnosis, drug delivery, gene delivery, bioseparation, hyperthermia, phototherapy, chemotherapy, and dynamic functional imaging for the treatment of cancer was described in addition to multifunctional NPs with surface modification for intracellular drug delivery. In addition, mesoporous silica nanoparticles (MSNs) and organic/inorganic-MSN hybrids were developed for theranostic applications (Chen et al., 2013). These NPs with their large and easily functionalized surface areas and pore volumes are highly suitable for targeted delivery of therapeutic agents. When combined with other organic/inorganic nanomaterials, the organic/inorganic-MSN hybrids exhibit synergies and increased versatility. In general, nanotheranostics covers diversified aspects of *in vitro* diagnostics and prognostics, *in vivo* molecular imaging, molecular therapeutics, image-guided therapy, biosensors, system biology and translational medicine, PM and several desciplines of biomedical research that can be applied to diagnosis as well as treatment to accomplish EBPT as the author has decribed in one his recent publications (Sharma, 2014).

Nanotheranostics has recently shown great promise in: (a) improved molecular imaging for tracking tumor-specific cytotoxic T lymphocytes (Lin et al., 2014); (b) bio-distribution of fluorescent nanoprobes employing hybrid fluorescence-mediated tomography (Gremse et al., 2014); (c) India ink incorporated multifunctional phase-transition nanodroplets for photo-acoustic/ultrasound imaging and tumor therapy (Jian et al., 2014); (d) contrast-enhanced imaging for the detection of focused ultrasound-induced blood brain barrier opening (Fan et al., 2014); (e) stem cell grafts monitoring with MRI using Maga as a reporter gene (Cho et al., 2014); (f) tumor imaging using stable oligonucleotide aptamer probes (Zeng et al. 21014); (g) drug delivery vehicles for cancer targeting (Zhu et al., 2014); (h) immuno NPs-integrated control of cancer cells using bioelectronics device (Hondroulis et al. 2014). NPs-mediated systemic delivery of siRNA for the treatment of cancers and viral Infections (Draz et al. 2014); self-assembly of gold NPs for CT imaging and NIR photothermal therapy (Deng et al. 2014); Mn-Porphyrin conjugated Au nanoshells encapsulated Doxorubicin for MRI and photothermal therapy of cancer (Jing et al., 2014); MRI of breast tumor initiating cells using fibronectin targeting NPs (Sun et al., 2014); and NPs with magnetic hyperthermia and remote-control drug release for cancer treatment (Hayashi et al., 2014). In addition, an EGFR targeted PET Imaging probe was developed for the detection of colonic adenocarcinomas (Turker et al., 2014); hair metabolomics for the identification of fetal compromise for biomarker discovery (Sulek et al., 2014); and FMN-coated fluorescent USPIO for cell labeling and non-invasive MR imaging (Mertens et al., 2014). These advances were intended to improve the conventional treatment protocols and further develop nanotheranostics to accomplish successful EBPT. In general, EBPT takes advantage of the genetic information along with phenotypic and environmental factors for healthcare designed specifically to a particular individual and eliminates the limitations of conventional *"one size fits all"* therapeutic approach. EBPT provides excellent platform to translate scientific knowledge from the lab to clinic to diagnose and predict disease to improve patient-specific treatment based on the characteristic (genomic) features of the disease and facilitates developing novel theranostic strategies (Kim et al. 2013). Furthermore, EBPT adopts chronopharmacological aspects for clinical applications (Clairambault et al., 2009; Ohdo et al., 2010). Owing to limited studies and experimental protocols as yet available for the risk assessment; these studies also raised serious concerns of toxicity of some NPs and their negative impact on the environment (Gajewicz et al., 2012). *Above all nanotechnology has gained considerable interest as a versatile approach for novel drug discovery, drug delivery, clinical diagnosis and treatment simultaneously to accomplish EBPT* (Mura et al., 2013). Hence nanotheranostics hold great promise because it provides excellent opportunity to monitor *in-vivo PKs* for validating the prognosis.

Further efforts to practice nanotheranostics for EBPM will optimize treatment as it covers *individual variability, early detection, economical therapeutic approach, and prognosis, allowing screening of patients who respond better to treatment.* These extraordinary properties make nanotheranostics attractive to accomplish EBPT by achieving minimum discomfort, safety, and maximum clinical benefits. It is envisaged that solution of several unresolved problems of modern medicine may be accomplished by further development of nanotheranostics. A recent report provided an inventory of nanomedicines currently available to accomplish EBPT (Etheridge et al., 2013). Currently FDA has approved >247 nanomedicines and several others are at various stages of clinical trials and approval. Hence innovations in nanotechnology will augment novel drug discovery and efficient drug delivery in future. In this chapter recently-developed drugs delivery systems including: covalent conjugation of drugs with polyethylene glycol (pegylation), block copolymers, dendrimers and aptamers, radiolabeled liposomes, chitosans and alginates, gellan/ xanthan gels, drug delivery nanodevices, quantum dots (Q-Dots) for cell tracking, siRNA, microRNA, metallothioneins (MTs), and Charnoly Body (CB) as novel drug discovery biomarkers are discussed systematically with a primary objective to evolve nanotheranostics for accomplishing EBPT.

Drug Delivery Epidemiological studies have revealed that out of 12 billion injections; improper drug deliveries cause >100 million adverse reaction, and >20 million infections every year. Hence efficient drug delivery systems are extremely important in modern medicine. Nanotechnology has enabled improvements in multi-functional drug delivery systems to improve EBPT. A descriptive overview comprising stimuli-responsive polymers, smart polymers, their biomedical applications, and major obstacles to clinical translation is now available (Kwon et al., 2012; Hansen et al., 2013). However, the basic molecular mechanism of infusion-related adverse effects of nanomedicines is yet to be established. A considerable biological variability in adverse effects with complement activation has been noticed. Hence a further research is needed to determine the exact physiological link between immunological mechanisms and genetic predisposition to hypersensitivity (Moghimi et al., 2012). Clinically-significant genetic polymorphism in immune-responsive genes is currently being explored to accelerate FDA approval and reduce the cost of healthcare system. Recently freeze-dried lettuce cells expressing vaccine biopharmaceuticals were developed to provide protection from gastric acids in the stomach but are released in the circulatory system upon digestion of the cell wall by the intestinal micro-flora. This novel approach of drug delivery provides both mucosal as well as systemic immunity against harmful toxins of bacteria, viruses, and protozoans. Similarly type-1 diabetes and hemophilia can be clinically-managed by oral delivery of auto-antigens. Pro-Insulin or Extendin-4 can be expressed in plant cells to control blood glucose levels just like exogenous Insulin administration. This novel approach confers promising strategy to control infections or inherited diseases by avoiding cumbersome purification protocols, refrigeration, and sterile conditions. Further innovations in this direction will facilitate development of biocompatible, biodegradable, environmentally-safe, and targeted drug delivery systems to accomplish EBPT (Kwon et al., 2013).

Recently hydrophilic molecules for transdermal drug delivery for skin care have been developed by estimating quantitative structure-permeability relationships (QSPR) and mechanistic models (Chen et al., 2013). However QSPR models do not provide the exact estimate of skin permeability of hydrophobic solutes. Hence further research is needed to improve skin permeability. In addition, linkers have shown potential as structural components of recombinant proteins and stable and bioactive fusion proteins. Hence naturally-occurring multi-domain proteins can be used for constructing flexible, rigid, and cleavable linkers to obtain desired PKs and controlled release of clinically-significant biomolecules *in vivo*. Although various methods used to incorporate proteins into a matrix may cause denaturation of the functional groups; the pro-drugs remain biologically–inactive before undergoing biotransformation *in-vivo* (Vig et al., 2013).

Since the pro-drug may change the biodistribution; it is important to consider its toxicity and efficacy during preclinical development. In this respect, natural and synthetic amino acids may provide better physicochemical properties. Therefore, amino acids as pro-drugs are being used for improved solubility, permeability, sustained release, i.v infusion, drug targeting, and drug stability. Particularly pulmonary drug delivery has served as an excellent route and remains the preferred route for several drugs. Therefore, dry powder inhalers, meter dose inhalers, and nebulizers have been developed to improve pulmonary drug delivery. A report summarized the rationale of pulmonary drug delivery systems (Shaikh et al., 2010). Further investigations in this direction may improve the treatment of asthma and chronic obstructive pulmonary disease (COPD) as inhalation provides direct drug targeting in the desired region. Moreover it is a needle-free treatment, avoids first pass effect, provides efficient drug response, and minimizes systemic side effects, and dose required to achieve desired therapeutic response.

NPs in PM *NPs offer distinct advantages as theranostic agents due to their small size, flexibility, increased surface to volume ratio, and surface modification with multivalent ligands to enhance molecular targeting of drugs.* Recent reports provided detailed information regarding the interaction of NPs with biological systems to facilitate their use in diagnosis, imaging, and drug delivery for nanotheranostics (Brannon-Peppas et al., 2004; Vizirianakis and Fatouros, 2012). Currently nanotheranostics has evolved to regulate genes at the transcriptional and translational level, detect cancer cells, regulate T-cell proliferation, and maintain blood glucose levels. In addition, an implant can detect blood urea levels and can restore normal levels. Another implant has been developed for artificial insemination that injects bull spermatocytes in the bovine ovary particularly during ovulation phase by detecting leutinizing hormone levels. It may be possible to treat any disease at the cellular and molecular level by detecting specific metabolic parameters by further improvising along these directions. A recent report identified nanomedicines those are currently being used in the treatment of cancer prior to FDA approval (Wieland Fussenegger, 2013). *Anticancer treatment involving polymers, liposomes, and monoclonal antibodies as well as clinical trials have been described* (Venditto and Jr Szoka, 2013). The primary focus is on the analysis of NPs containing *Camptothecin* derivatives, including two polymers and liposomal formulation. However these formulations had difficult time for FDA approval because presently-developed nanocarriers provide limited improvement in their overall performance. Irrespective of these limitations, nanotheranostics to accomplish EBPT seem quite promising.

Liposomal Drug Delivery Liposomes were first developed in early 70s to enhance drug targetability in the space occupying lesions including cysts, infarcts, tumors, and malignant cancers. Drug delivery in the tumor can be accomplished at higher concentrations as compared to normal tissue by encapsulation in the biocompatible and biodegradable liposomes. Moreover liposomal-mediated passive as well as active drug delivery can minimize the adverse effects of anticarcinogenic drugs and augments their therapeutic potential. Tumor targeting can be achieved by identifying specific receptor ligands or antibodies onto the surface of the liposome, or by developing stimulus-sensitive drug carriers such as acid or enzyme-induced drug release. In addition to tumor cells, the tumors also contain non-tumor cells such as; endothelial cells, fibroblasts, pericytes, stromal cells, mesenchymal cells, innate and adaptive immune cells which can be targeted to prevent tumor cell growth (Zhao et al., 2013). The liposomal NPs can be used to deliver anti-carcinogenic drugs to the tumor to control nonspecific uptake, interaction with blood components, and toxicity. The primary objective of liposomal encapsulation is targeting anticancer drugs to the tumor endothelial neovasculature, macrophages, and pericytes within the tumor. To target adhesion proteins including focal adhesions and adherens junction; Vinculin, polymer lipid nanoparticle (PLN) system was developed (Wang et al., 2013). The PLNs have an average size of 106 nm, positive charge, and lower encapsulation efficiency compared to poly (lacticco- glycolic) acid (PGLA) NPs, with sustained release of BSA, while PGLA NPs exhibit an initial burst release. The anti-Vinculin-conjugated PLNs could carry drug to the cytoplasm of the fibroblasts and adhered to fibronectin-fibrin complex. The unconjugated PLNs demonstrated improved gene transfection efficiency. Moreover, PLNs could be modified by using different targeting ligands for studying basic molecular mechanism of drug delivery in specific subcellular organelles including nucleus, mitochondria, Golgi body, peroxysomes, and lysosomes. Furthermore, drug transport to the brain was improved by employing targeted liposomal NPs (Lai and Fadda 2013).

Enhanced Permeability and Retention (EPR) Effect There is a significant difference between passive tumor targeting and EPR effect. Passive tumor targeting (*such as X-ray contrast agents*) has a retention period of few minutes, whereas EPR of NPs requires days to weeks and occurs due to extravasation of macromolecules or NPs through tumor neovasculature (Maeda et al., 2013). Recently methods of augmenting EPR effect for efficient delivery of drugs (*including Nitroglycerin, Angiotensin-1 Converting Enzymes (ACE) Inhibitors*) were developed to accomplish better therapeutic effect and reduced systemic toxicity. The EPR effect-based delivery of NPs was clinically-significant for tumor-targeted imaging using fluorescent or radionuclide labeling with theranostic potential. The EPR effect is extremely important for NPs and liposome delivery to cancer tissue. The EPR effect is the property by which liposomes, NPs, and macromolecular drugs accumulate in tumor tissue more specifically than normal tissues (Matsumura and Maeda., 1986; Duncan and Sat 1998; Vasey et al., 1999). EPR effect is the most popular strategy employed for targeting nanosize anticancer drugs to tumor tissues. In fact, tumor cell aggregates as small as 150- 200 μm tend to become dependent on blood for their nutritional and oxygen supply. It is now recognized that VEGF and other growth factors are primarily involved in tumor angiogenesis. *The newly formed tumor micro-vessels have no vascular smooth cell layer, and have defective endothelial cells, wide fenestrations, abnormal innervation, wider lumen, and impaired angiotensin II receptors. Tumor tissues also lack proper lymphatic drainage system which leads to abnormal molecular and fluid dynamics, especially for macromolecular drugs and*

NPs. These characteristics of EPR effect facilitate to trap and spread NPs inside the cancer tissue. In fact, the novel discovery of the EPR effect has resulted in the development of several nanomedicines, including liposome-based formulations of drugs as cancer therapeutics as described earlier. Although the use of liposomes resulted in increased accumulation of drugs in solid tumors, further improvement in therapeutic efficacy is yet to be accomplished. Imaging of the tumor localization of liposomes revealed that poor or variable performance can occur due to heterogeneous inter-subject and intra-tumoral liposome accumulation due to abnormal transport microenvironment. A major limitation of conventional anticancer chemotherapeutic agents is their lack of tumor selectivity (Greish, 2010). Moreover EPR effect can be influenced by tumor diversity, animal models, biodistribution, intracellular interaction, and release rate of cytotoxic cargo from its nanosize carrier (Greish, 2012). The EPR effect can be further enhanced by pathophysiological factors involved in the extravasation of macromolecules in solid tumors. *For example, Bradykinin, Nitric Oxide / Peroxynitrite, Prostaglandins, Vascular Permeability Factor (VEGF), Tumor Necrosis Factor and others.* Hence basic understanding of this phenomenon and its limitation are highly significant for the success of EPR-based anticancer theranostics. One of several examples is the thermal ablation with gold NPs, which can be heated up in response to near IR laser at the cancer site. This therapy works best in conjunction with chemotherapeutics or other cancer therapies (Poon and Borys., 2009). Enhanced permeability of the tumor vasculature allows macromolecules to enter the tumor interstitial space, whereas the suppressed lymphatic filtration allows their retention (Prabhakar et al., 2013). Although EPR is the basis of nanotechnology platforms to deliver drugs to tumors, progress in developing effective drugs using this approach has been hampered by heterogeneity of this effect in different tumors and limited experimental data from patients regarding its effectiveness. Kobayashi et al. (2014) recently reported that delivery of nano-sized agents is dependent on several other factors that influence the EPR effect including; *(a) regional blood flow to the tumor, (b) permeability of the tumor vasculature, (c) structural barriers imposed by perivascular tumor cells and extracellular matrix, and (d) intra-tumoral pressure.* Therapeutic NPs have advantages over low molecular weight agents with larger loading capacity, the ability to protect the payload until delivery, more specific targeting due to multi valency, and controlled/sustained drug release. However the delivery of NPs into cancer tissue is challenging because it relies only on the EPR effect that depends on the leaky nature of the tumor vasculature and the prolonged circulation of NPs, allowing slow but uneven accumulation in the tumor. Recently Stapleton et al. (2013) presented a mathematical model to describe liposome transport in solid tumors. This model is based on transport equations that describe pressure driven fluid flow across blood vessels and through the tumor and were validated by direct comparison with CT measurements of liposomes in 3 experimental models of tumor. The model was fit to liposome accumulation curves and could predict transport parameters that reflect the tumor microenvironment. Furthermore, this model attributed inter-subject heterogeneity in liposome accumulation to variations in peak interstitial fluid pressure, suggesting inter-subject and intratumoral variations of liposome drug delivery.

Pegyylation and Drug Delivery Generally *Polyethylene Glycol* (PEG) is used for the covelant conjugation of biomolecules for pharmaceutical and nanotechnological applications. Pegylation (*covalent conjugation of PEG*) provides 3 basic advantages: (*i*) *nonimmunogenicity*, (*ii*) *less entrapment of NPs in the reticuloendothelial system (RES), and* (*iii*) *slow and sustained release of drug at the target site.* It is now possible to design polymers by pegylation for theranostic applications as its protocols are now well-established. Modification of peptides and proteins can be achieved by pegylation to protect antigenic and immunogenic peptides, receptor-mediated uptake of RES, and prevent degradation by proteolytic enzymes. Various functional groups can be incorporated by pegylation to conjugate peptides and proteins. Pegylation also increases the size of the polypeptides to reduce fast renal clearance by modifying their PKs (Roberts., 1997). It is known that anticancer drug, *Paclilaxel* (PTX) has reduced water solubility and acts as a substrate for P-glycoprotein (P-gp) and cytochrome-P450. A recent study on rats demonstrated the potential of pegylated-NPs for oral *Paclitaxel* delivery (Zabaleta et al., 2012). PEG 2000 (PTX-NP2), PEG 6000 (PTX-NP6), and PEG 10,000 (PTX-NP10) were prepared for loading PTX. The intestinal permeability of PTX increased 3-7 times in the jejunum by pegylation compared to commercial product, Taxol. The PTX permeability was higher for PTX-NP2 and PTX-NP6 as compared to PTX-NP10 and maintained sustained therapeutic plasma levels for at least 48 hrs. A maximum oral bioavailability (70%) was achieved with PTX-NP2, suggesting bio-adhesive properties and inhibitory effects of pegylated NPs on P-gp and cytochrome P450. Recently drug targeting was accomplished using a single NPs platform for the clinical management of cancer and AD (Droumaguet et al., 2012). Particularly Polyisoprenoyl Gemcitabine conjugates that self-assemble as NPs showed promise for cancer thernostics (Maksimenko et al., 2013). Furthermore drug transport to the brain improved by using targeted NPs (Olivier, 2005). Several protein linkers with characteristic property, design, and functionality were developed for targeted drug delivery to accomplish EBPT (Chen et al., 2013). Further developments are being made by improving the design, functionalization, and biodegradable/biocompatible polymer-based nanocarriers (Nicolas et al., 2013). A simple procedure to synthesize multi-compartment micelles based on biocompatible poly-3-hydroxyalkanoate was developed (Babinot et al., 2013; Nicholas et al. 2013). Furthermore, clinically-significant hydrogels were developed to determine the extent of water absorption and permeation of solutes within the matrix as drug and cell carriers for constructing tissue engineering matrices (Hoffman, 2002).

Although NPs can be used for site-specific drug delivery and medical imaging, these are localized preferentially in the reticulo-endothelial system (RES) following systemic delivery. The most significant organs of the RES are lungs, liver, and spleen, where NPs undergo phagocytosis and/or endocytosis to be eliminated from the biological system within minutes. Hence amphiphilic di-blocks and multi-block copolymers- conjugated NPs were developed to prevent opsonization and recognition by macrophages (Gref, 1995). These NPs possess a hydrophilic PEG coating and a biodegradable core to encapsulate hydrophobic drugs such as Lidocaine. These NPs had significantly reduced RES accumulation, could be freeze-dried, reconstituted, and retained shelf stability. Although premature systemic clearance of NPs was reduced by modifying surfaces with pegylation; it influenced the normal performance of NPs as drug carriers (Lin et al., 2010). Hence alternative strategies including; substitute polymers, conditional removal of PEG, and surface modification to overcome limitations of PEG were introduced (Vorup-Jensen and Peer, 2010; Amoozgar and Yeo, 2012). For instance, surface modification by Polyethylene Oxide (PEO) could avoid the physiological defense depending on the particle size, extent of systemic circulation, and selectivity for target sites in the body (Stolnik et al., 1995). A further research is in progress along these directions.

Chitosans and Alignates NPs for Drug Delivery Chitosans were discovered as novel drug delivery vehicles for theranostic applications. Chitosans NPs are highly suitable drug delivery vehicles because of their biocompatibility, biodegradability, and flexibility as they can be modified and used for loading relatively unstable protein drugs, gene drugs, and anticancer drugs, via oral, nasal, i.v, and ocular routes. Alginates are bio-adhesive polymers and can be used for selective drug delivery to mucosal tissues. Wang et al. (2011) presented an excellent report on chitosan NPs, including methods of preparation, characterization, modification, *in vivo* metabolism, and clinical applications. Alginates can be synthesized from the naturally-occurring brown algae (Kelp) and can be used for trapping and/or delivery of drugs in the form of a matrix (Gombotz and Wee. 2012). Alginates are composed of linear unbranched polysaccharides having 1, 4-α-d-Manuronic acid and L-α-Glucronic acid residues which may vary in composition and sequence and are in the form of a block which can be cross-linked by the addition of divalent cations. Proteins, DNA, and cells could be incorporated into the alginate matrix while preserving their biological activity. In addition, the pore size, degradation rate, and release kinetics can be regulated by selecting suitable alginate and coating material. Gels of different morphologies were developed with alginate microbeads. Particularly, alginates were used to prepare *in situ* gelling systems for ophthalmic applications and for protecting the wounds. These properties, including nonimmunogenicity of alginates directed their application as protein delivery vectors for theranostic applications. Furthermore, *alginate/chitosan-coated nanoemulsions* were developed for oral insulin (Li et al., 2013). The alginate containing dispersion was used by adding calcium chloride and chitosan based on poly-electrolyte cross-linking, suggesting the clinical potential of alginate/chitosan nanoemulsion for an oral delivery of polypeptides and proteins. The positively charged $-NH_3^+$ groups of chitosans and negatively-charged $-COO^-$ groups of alginates are particularly suitable for developing coating materials for mucosal vaccines (Li et al., 2008). Coating onto bovine serum albumin (BSA)-loaded chitosan NPs with sodium alginate increased stability and prevented desorption of antigens in the GIT system for at least 2 hrs to meet the basic requirement of oral vaccine. Furthermore, to augment differentiation of human fetal osteoblasts, *gellan/xanthan gels* along with chitosan NPs were developed for the delivery of basic fibroblast growth factor (bFGF) and bone morphogenetic protein (BMP-7) in a dual growth factor delivery system (Dyondi et al., 2013). The sustained release of growth factors from the NPs-loaded gels facilitated improved cell proliferation and differentiation. Significantly increased alkaline phosphatase and Calcium deposition were noticed indicating that growth factors encapsulation within NPs and gels are clinically-significant for bone regeneration. The *gellan/xanthan gels* also confered antibacterial activity against pathogens involved in implant rejection. Bhoyar et al. (2012) described the detailed method and structure of gels to improve their permeability and bioavailability that can be incorporated in the novel drug delivery systems to accomplish EBPT.

Chronopharmacology in EBPT Recent advances in drug delivery methods evolved a new concept of chronophamacology which involves drug delivery in a pulsatile manner. Chronotherapy is clinically-significant where sustained release of drugs is undesirable and the drugs are extremely toxic. For instance certain anticancer drugs can cause serious adverse effects in conventional and sustained release protocols. The circadian pacemaker is localized in the suprachiasmatic nuclei and regulates biological processes including sleep-wake cycle (Bisht, 2011).

It is known that the circadian genes regulate the sleepwake cycle in order to maintain normal physiology and behavior. Hence, the circadian rhythm needs to be considered in designing the pulsatile drug delivery (PDD) of the *hormones, neuropeptides, and cytokines* that exert their physiological or pharmacological action in an oscillatory rhythm. Several FDA-approved chronopharmacological agents are now available and are being developed to provide maximum therapeutic effect with minimum adverse effects because 24 hrs rhythms are observed for the pathophysiology of chronic diseases. Hence drug delivery microsystems may facilitate accomplishing EBPT. The efficacy and toxicity of therapeutic agents would depend on the dose and time of delivery which will also be affected by PKs and PDs properties of the drug. The therapeutic effect of the pharmacological agent will be under the influence of circadian rhythm which will be influenced by biochemical, physiological, and behavioral mechanisms in the biological system. Hence a novel nanotechnology for delivering drugs in a rhythmic fashion is being developed using micropumps to minimize the chances of drug-resistance in conventional and sustained release systems. The primary objective is to determine the exact nature of the circadian rhythm, which serves as an indicator of drug release from the nano-device. Currently there is a dire need of suitable NPs or nanodevices which could be used on a routine basis for EBPT. These devices should be economical, biocompatible, biodegradable, and responsive to a rhythmic biomarker. The basic advantage of PDD nano-devices is that the release of the therapeutic agent can be controlled as and when needed. Moreover drug safety can be evaluated for personalized treatment. Recently progress has been made in the PDD systems which can treat diseases effectively; such as diabetes. Various therapeutic agents including; proteins, hormones, analgesics and other pharmacological agents are being investigated by using these nanodevices. The important issues include: *biocompatibility and toxicity of polymers, response to external stimuli, ability to accomplish required serum drug levels, shelf life, and reproducibility.*

Oral Immunotherapy (OIT) In general, the therapeutic efficacy of orally-administered drugs is reduced due to poor localization, low pH, and fast intestinal flow. Moreover orally-administered drugs are influenced by peristalsis in the GIT system which accelerates drug elimination from the biological system. Moreover the acidic environment in the stomach can easily degrade the drug. Particularly polypeptide drugs are degraded rapidly in the stomach. In addition, the drug experiences first pass effect while passing through the hepatic portal system to be metabolized by liver cytochrome P-450 isoenzymes. The drug may be *acetylated, glucronated, or sulphated* in the liver to become water soluble and eventually excreted through the renal system. Since various proteins, enzymes, peptide neurotransmitters, and hormones (*such as growth hormone and insulin*) are proteolyzed when administered orally; microneedles or micro-osmotic pumps are being developed for drug delivery in inflammatory diseases such as rheumatoid arthritis. By using microneedles and mini-osmotic pumps, a drug at minimum dose can be administered on a chronic basis. OIT seem to be well tolerated for food allergies which impact nearly 5% of US population (Kulis and Burks, 2013). To diminish the toxicity associated with oral drug delivery; novel NPs were developed for controlled drug release, improved adhesion, increased tissue penetration, and selective intestinal targeting. Currently TLR9 agonists as adjuvants in combination with OIT are being developed for targeted delivery of non-allergic herbal preparations. Several issues, such as optimal dosing, length of treatment, tolerance, and basic molecular mechanisms of protection were resolved for oral drug delivery (Chira and Desai 2012).

Particularly amino acids were used as pro-drugs to improve solubility, permeability, constant release, i.v delivery, targetability, and stability of the drugs. The oral bioavailability of drugs was improved by developing enterically-coated tablets, capsules, and liposomes. Further developments are in progress for amino acid pro-drug delivery through the GIT system. Although the role of drug transporters in the liver and kidney were investigated, there is limited information regarding the importance of influx and efflux transporters in the intestine (Wu et al., 2005). Hence drug transporters in PKs (*drug absorption and bioavailability*) gained considerable interest. Various systems including; *in-vivo* experimental models, *in situ* organ perfusion, *in vitro* tissue slices, and cell lines were developed to determine the effect of intestinal transporters on drug delivery. Recently biopharmaceutical drug disposition classification system (BDDCS) was introduced to determine the role of intestinal transporters and their enzymes on the oral drug PKs (Estudante et al., 2013). However further studies are needed in this direction.

Microfabrication for Controlled Drug Delivery Recently microdevices for controlled drug delivery were developed using integrated circuits and nanosensors for designing automatic drug delivery systems with suitable shape, size, flexibility, reservoir volume, and surface characteristics to improve EBPT. Self-folded polymeric containers were developed to encapsulate molecules, polypeptides, proteins, bacteria, fungi, and cells (Fernandes and Gracias, 2012). In addition, the oral, dermal and implantable reservoir-based drug delivery microsystems were improvised for increased drug stability and sustained release. The reservoir-based systems for targeted drug delivery could accomplish zero order kinetics, pulsatile, and/or demand dosing as compared to conventional sustained drug delivery systems. Improved version of these devices is now available for ocular applications (Zhang et al., 2012).

NPs and Endocytosis in Nanotheranostics Recently research was directed on elucidating the molecular mechanism of receptor-mediated endocytosis to determine delivery of NPs drug carriers to a specific cell *in vivo* (Peppas, 2013). In addition, strategies to improve spatiotemporal cell-signaling to enhance tissue repair were described (Xu et al., 2013). Indeed the NPs-based drug-delivery (NDD) systems improved the efficacy of drugs for theranostic applications. *As a result, the therapeutic potential of NDD systems increased with significantly reduced drug toxicity, improved bioavailability and circulation time, and controlled drug release* (Ekenseair et al., 2013). However treatment of cancer with NDD vehicle still requires improved knowledge of NPs and their PKs *in vivo*. In this respect, quantum dots (Qdots) offered potential as these have suitable surface chemistry to allow incorporation in any NDD vehicle with minimal impact on the overall characteristics and excellent optical properties for real time monitoring of drug release at the cellular and systemic level. Although clinical application of Q-dots in NDD vehicles is restricted due to potential toxicity; their core is highly suitable as organic drug carriers or inorganic contrast agents such as gold and magnetic NPs for photo-thermal therapy and magneto-transfection respectively (Probst et al., 2013). Further investigations are being made by avoiding the RES localization and by utilizing the EPR effect for tumor-specific targeting in nanotheranostics to accomplish EBPT. In addition, antibody-targeted therapy and anti-angiogenic drugs are being developed by using NPs, composed of bio-degradable as well as non-degradable polymers for personalized theranostics.

Microneedles in Nanomedicine Although microneedles were introduced as drug–delivery vehicles several years ago, their clinical significance was realized in mid-1990's with the development of nanotechnology, which developed microneedles to enhance skin permeability, drug-coated and polymer microneedles to dissolve off skin, and hallow microneedles for drug infusion into the skin (Kim et al., 2012). Currently microneedles are being used to deliver therapeutic agents, small molecules, and protein drugs. In general, hallow microneedles are used for the delivery of influenza vaccine, whereas solid microneedles are used for cosmetic applications and for ocular treatments. The successful application of microneedles depends on their proper insertion and infusion into the skin, skin recovery after removal, drug stability, safety and efficacy, storage capacity and delivery without any pain or discomfort (*such as local or systemic irritation and chances of infection*) to the patient. Further developments in microneedle nanotechnology may improve nanotheranostics for EBPT.

Nanothranostics in EBPT Recently nanotechnology improvised diagnostic and prognostic capability, and targeted drug delivery at the space occupying lesion (SOL) for personalized theranostics. Although EBPT seems impressive, the anticancer treatment compromises prognosis due to the absence of therapeutic response, drug resistance, relapse, and adverse effects of inadequate and non-targeted drug delivery. However, novel discovery of NPs has revolutionized EBPT and enabled stem cell tracking for the future development of nanotheranostics. It is now known that epigenetic changes are involved in the molecular pathogenesis of cancer. Hence basic understanding of epigenetic changes may further improve personalized nanotheranostics (Ryu et al., 2012). Recently polymeric immunomicelles were developed as nanocariers with a potential to diagnosis, targeted drug therapy, imaging, and assessing the response for the clinical management of chronic diseases. Hence multi-modality immunomicelles were developed as novel nanocarriers for personalized chemotherapy of cancer (Sawant and Jhaveri 2012); In addition to therapeutic potential, the theranostic NPs are capable of *in-vivo* non-invasive molecular imaging. Particularly optical imaging with these NPs have distinct advantages such as *sensitivity, safety, real time imaging for earlier screening, detection, treatment, and better prognosis* which will make nanotheranostics attractive to develop EBPT for achieving maximum benefit and minimum adverse effects (Mura and Couvreur, 2012).

Although cell-based therapy showed great promise, limited information regarding their exact fate *in-vivo* and precise therapeutic effect remain uncertain. Recent development of inorganic and organic NPs may facilitate tracking transplanted stem cells *in vivo* (Janowski et al., 2012). Hence nucleic acid programmable microarrays were developed using cell-free systems to generate proteins as an alternative to fluorescence-labeled approach employing nanotechnology to analyze protein function and protein-protein interaction to accomplish EBPT (Nicolini et al., 2012). For instance the limitations of fluorescence detection can be prevented by using quartz microcircuit nanogravimetry. Hence protein microarrays were developed. Similarly liposomes which selectively localize in the tumor and transport drug as well as imaging agent to accomplish theranostic capabilities for personalized treatment were developed (Petersen et al., 2012). In addition, radiolabeled liposomes may be used for evaluating their *in-vivo* performance, and in the development of liposomal drugs. Moreover multimodality fusion imaging may provide noninvasive PKs in humans. Further developments in liposomal radiolabeling and fusion imaging will facilitate EBPM. Recently theranostic NPs were utilized in chemotherapy, photodynamic and photothermal therapy, and siRNA therapy of cancer (Daka and Peer 2012). Thus instead of conventional generic treatment, patient-centered therapies are now being developed employing nanotechonolgical approaches for targeted drug delivery combined with genomics and understanding of diseases at the molecular level. To accomplish the primary objectives of EBPT; radiolabeled liposomes for imaging and siRNA for therapeutic trials were evolved. However safe, specific, and effective strategies need to be developed. Colloidal NPs can be used to examine the tissue and cell distribution profile of anticancer agents. The primary objective is to enhance the anti-tumor efficacy and reduce the systemic side effects. NPs can also be useful for the selective delivery of oligonucleotides to tumor cells. The exact knowledge about the interactions of NPs with biological system will improve their design for diagnosis, imaging, and targeted drug delivery. Certain NPs can reverse multidrug resistance (MDR) during cancer chemotherapy (Brigger et al., 2002). Hence NPs toxicity, fabrication challenges, and regulatory and ethical issues were highlighted for the progress of EBPT (Zhang et al., 2013).

Pharmaceutical Nanocarriers In general, liposomes, micelles, nonoemulsions, NPs, chitosans and alginates, gellan/xanthan gels, dendrimers, and aptamers were utilized to enhance systemic drug stability for selective localization at the SOLs with compromised vasculature. Specific targeting with increased intracellular penetration with cell-penetrating molecules and contrast properties for direct visualization *in-vivo* was achieved by stimulus-sensitive drug release employing immune-liposomes (Torchilin., 2006). Multifunctional nanocarriers can enhance the theranostic potential whereas amphiphilic copolymers can serve as micellar drug carriers (Rösler et al., 2001). Hence chemical modification of the amphiphilic copolymer building blocks-based drug delivery system were developed to enhance stability of micellar drug carriers or block copolymer containing specific ligands that allowed targeted drug delivery; or by improving micellar drug carriers by addition of auxiliary agents. The temporal control over drug release could be accomplished by improving channel kinetics of metal NPs. Furthermore, block copolymers micelles as long circulating drug nanocarriers were developed for personalized treatment (Zhang and Xu, 2012). Block copolymer micelles having polyethylene oxide can be used as hydrophilic blocks, whereas poly L-amino acid micelles can be used as hydrophobic blocks. Hydrophobic drugs include *Doxorubicin* into block copolymer micelles with prolonged systemic circulation times. The block copolymers accumulate slowly at the solid tumors and have potential in cancer theranostics similar to long-circulating liposomes. Hence basic knowledge regarding *in vivo* degradation and cellular and tissue responses which determines the compatibility of these biodegradable microspheres is extremely important to accaccomlish EBPT. PLA and PGLA microspheres carrying bone morphogenetic protein (BPM) and Leuprlin acetate and their interactions in the eye, CNS, and lymphoid tissue for vaccine development and controlled drug release were described (Shive and Anderson 1997).

Miniaturized Drug Delivery Systems It is important to have economical microdevices for transdermal and subcutaneous drug delivery. Miniaturized drug delivery systems were developed by employing osmotic principles of pumping. These devices can be simple microneedle arrays to complex systems with micropumps, micro-reservoirs, sensors, and electronic circuits for remote-controlled drug delivery (Ochoa et al., 2012). However osmotic micro-pumps do not require electrical power, provide zero order release kinetics, and can be used for wide array of applications for a prolonged period, and are not influenced by first pass effects and GIT transit time (Stevenson et al., 2012; Herrlich et al., 2012). These pumps have 3 components: *osmotic agent, solvent, and drug.* Water from the body fluids serves as a solvent and drug as an osmotic agent in a single compartment system. Two compartment system employs separate osmotic agent, and multi-compartment system utilizing solvent, drug and, osmotic agent separately. Further innovative improvements are needed for agents used during gene therapy or agents which cannot be administered orally, topically, or i.v (Meng and Hoang, 2012). These noninvasive approaches bypass physiological barriers, release appropriate dose, and ensure bioavailability of drug for the required duration to accomplish maximum efficacy. Recently micro-electromechanical systems (MEMS) were developed for radiolabeling, nanomedicine delivery for cancer treatment, and sustained ocular drug delivery (Li et al., 2012a)

Further improvements of MEMS actuators, valves, and other microstructures for on-demand dosing may provide better performance. A regulated valve was developed for intra-thecal delivery of insulin and other drugs using MEMS (Li et al. 2012b). In addition to bolus and continuous flow delivery systems, a piezoelectronically-controlled silicon valve, equipped with pressure sensors was developed for controlled drug release from a mechanically-pressurized reservoir. These microdevices have clinical significance in neuronal hearing loss associated with equilibrium disorders and tinnitus, which may be recovered by employing regenerative therapeutic approaches for targeted and sustained drug delivery (Pararas et al., 2012). These micro-devices promise to repair and regenerate hearing and CNS disorders of aging patients for which there is currently no better treatment option.

Recent Studies with Q-Dot NPs In order to determine the PKs and therapeutic potential of bone marrow-derived mononuclear stem cells (MNCs) in experimental model of acute ischemic stroke (AIS), the researchers labeled these cells with 3nm and 5nm Cd/Se quantum dots (Q-Dots) NPs (Brenneman et al., 2012). Digital fluorescence imaging and confocal microscopic analyses provided evidence that MNCs exhibit preferential chemotaxis in the peri-infarct region and are exponentially-eliminated as a function of time, suggesting a therapeutic window of MNCs-mediated neuronal recovery. Subsequently the researchers provided a detailed description of cell-based therapy in AIS and discovered that MNCs provide neuroprotection in oxygen and glucose-deprived cultured cortical neurons (*in vitro model of AIS*) by modulating microglia and elucidated the basic molecular mechanism of MNCs-mediated neuroprotection (Yang et al., 2012; Mishra et al., 2011). Treatment of MNCs in AIS rats increased brain regional interleukin-10 (IL-10), which led us to propose that cerebral cortex neurons are protected through MNCs-mediated paracrine release of an anti-inflammatory cytokine, IL-10 by binding to its specific receptor. Furthermore IL-10 provides anti-inflammatory action by activating upstream PI-3 kinase and downstream STAT3-mediated signaling (Sharma et al., 2010). The researchers discovered for the first time IL-10 receptors on the murine cortical cultured neurons. These findings were further confirmed by examining the effect of trans-catheter injection of MNCs on the viability and cytokine release of MNCs (Khoury et al., 2010). The researchers established that MNCs are highly primitive and can readily release anti-inflammatory cytokines such as IL-10 and other trophic factors to provide therapeutic effect in AIS and other neurodegenerative diseases (Sharma et al., 2011). Several other molecular mechanism(s) of MNCs-mediated neuroprotection remain unexplored. *In-vivo* molecular imaging with [18]FdG and ^{18}F-DOPA as PET imaging biomarkers, strongly supported the therapeutic role of metallothioneins (MTs) in stem cells as potent antioxidant zinc-binding proteins in progressive neurodegenerative diseases (Sharma and Ebadi, 2012). Hence MTs induction in stem cells can enhance their therapeutic potential in chronic neurodegenerative diseases (Sharma and Ebadi, 2011a). Based on these novel findings, the researchers proposed to investigate the pharmacological properties of NPs employing   MTs   and   Charnoly   Body   (CB)   as   universal   biomarkers   of neuroprotection/neurodegeneration (Sharma and Ebadi, 2011b). Further studies in this direction will not only promote nanotheranostics but also provide further insight regarding the safety and toxicity of NPs to accomplish EBPT.

α-Synuclein Index (SI) as a Biomarker for Drug Discovery The researchers discovered SI as an early and sensitive biomarker of progressive neurodegenerative α-synucleinopathies (Sharma, 2013); MTs inhibit α-synucleinopathies by inhibiting CB formation and by acting as free radical scavengers and as anti-inflammatory agents. Hence, in addition to CB; MTs and α-synuclein index may be used as novel biomarkers of drug discovery to accomplish EBPT.

Charnoly Body as Universal Biomarker of EBPT The author discovered that Charnoly Body (CB) is a pre-apoptotic biomarker of compromised mitochondrial bioenergetics (Sharma and Ebadi 2014). Oxidative and nitrative stress induces free radical overproduction to cause mitochondrial degeneration and form pleomorphic, compact multi-lamellar, electron-dense membrane stacks (*named as Charnoly Body: CB*). The CB formation occurs due to nutritional stress and/or exposure to environmental neurotoxins (*kainic acid, domoic acid, and acromelic acid)*, or toxic NPs in the most vulnerable cells such as developing hippocampal or cerebellar Purkinje neurons due to mitochondrial degeneration. Usually CB is phagocytosed by lysosomal activation characterized by chronolophagy (*to describe degenerated mitochondrial autophagy*). Depending on the extent of acute or chronic exposure to toxic NPs; free radical-mediated mitochondrial degeneration results in lysosomal-sensitive or lysosomal-resistant CB formation. Lysososomal-sensitive CB can be readily subjected to charnolophagy, resulting in neuroprotection during acute phase as a basic molecular mechanism of energy-driven intracellular detoxification; whereas lysosomal-resistant CB may inhibit charnolophagy during chronic phase, resulting in the formation of intraneuronal inclusions and apoptosis due to the release of toxic substances (cytochrome C, Iron, Casase-3, apoptosis inducing factor, and Ca^{2+}) from the degenerating mitochondria due to CB sequestration and BCl_2 down-regulation, and 18KD translocator protein (TSPO) delocalization, resulting in progressive neurodegenerative diseases and cardiovascular diseases. CB formation compromizes epigenetic modifications in health and disease because DNA methylation and histone acetylation requires the presence of S-adenosyl methionine, which is synthesized in the mitochondria and requires ATP and methyl transferase. Furthermore intra-mitochondrial synthesis of various steroid hormones is also down-regulated as a result of free radical-mediated CB formation. These molecular events facilitate further neurodegeneration. Hence novel drugs may be developed to prevent TSPO delocalization and early epigenetic modifications due to free radical overproduction and increased synthesis of mitochondrial DNA oxidation product, 8-OH, 2dG.

Accumulation of CBs at the junction of axon hillock may block proximo-distal flow of enzymes, neurotransmitters, growth factors, and mitochondria, resulting in blockade of axoplasmic transport to induce cognitive impairments. Nutritional rehabilitation with omega-3 and polyunsaturated fatty acids (PUFA), protein-rich diet, physiological zinc, and MTs prevent CB formation.

In general non-specific induction of CB formation occurs in the hyper-proliferating cells with conventional cancer treatment. Depending on the extent of acute or chronic exposure of toxic drugs or NPs; free radical-mediated mitochondrial degeneration results in lysosomal-sensitive or resistant CB formation. Lysosomal-sensitive CB can be easily subjected to charnolophagy, resulting in cellular recovery due to intracellular sanitation; whereas lysosomal-resistant CB inhibits charnolophagy, resulting in the formation of intra-neuronal inclusions and apoptosis due to mitochondrial degeneration, causing progressive neurodegenerative diseases and cardiovascular diseases. Nonspecific induction of CB formation may cause alopecia, myelosuppression (*anemia, neutropenia, and thrombocytopenia*), GIT disturbance, neurodegeneration, testicular dysgenesis, amenorrhea, craniofacial abnormalities in fetal alcohol syndrome victims, atherosclerotic plaque rupture, and infertility in MDR malignancies. Hence drugs may be developed to target cancer stem cell specific CB formation to inhibit charnolophagy for the prevention and/or treatment of malignancies, whereas specific drugs inhibiting CB formation and augmenting charnolophagy will be beneficial for the treatment of neurodegenerative and cardiovascular diseases involving charnolopathy at the subcellular, molecular, genetic, and epigenetic levels. Eventually CB and charnolophagy-targeted agonists and antagonists will have minimum or no adverse effects. Furthermore, the author proposed primarily 3 types of NPs, which could be developed for CB targeting including: (a) inert or neutral; without any influence on CB formation; (b) toxic; augmenting CB formation, and (c) protective; ROS scavengers-loaded NPs having therapeutic potential in neurodegenerative and cardiovascular diseases by either preventing or inhibiting CB formation. Hence CB formation or its elimination at the subcellular level may be used as a universal biomarker of novel drug discovery in addition to structural and functional characterization of NPs and/or drugs for EBPT applications (Sharma, 2014; Sharma et al., 2013; Sharma and Ebadi, 2014; Sharma et al., 2014; Sharma et al., 2013; Sharma and Ebadi, 2014, Sharma 2015).

SiRNA-Mediated Gene Silencing with Fusion Proteins in PM Winkler (2011) described the use of fusion proteins for target therapy using siRNA which can be accomplished if the basic issues of pharmaceutical development are addressed such as; specific Arginine-rich peptides for siRNA loading capacity, stability, with reduced toxicity and immunogenicity. In addition to liposomal and polymeric NPs; fusion proteins may be used for targeted delivery and release of the siRNA after cellular uptake. This fusion consists of a protein binder and an oligonucleotide including polymers and dendrimers respectively. Recently FDA approved 20 antibodies for therapy. Hence researchers are now using antibody derivatives as the targeting component of fusion proteins for siRNA delivery. To accomplish EBPT, individual gene targets can be used with the same delivery agent without purification (Watkins et al., 2010). Protamine-fusion protein was first used for specific siRNA delivery (Chen et al., 1995; Caravella and Lugovskoy, 2010). The heavy chain Fab fragment of an HIV-1 envelope antibody was fused to a truncated Protamine for complexation of nucleic acids and a plasmid encoding the bacterial toxin ETA was transported into HIV-infected cells. A protein consisting of a single-chain antibody specific for the tumor surface protein ErbB2 and a truncated protamine fusion protein was used to deliver luciferase plasmid into antigen-positive cells for siRNA complexation (Li et al., 2001; Song et al., 2005). This fusion protein can transport siRNA to the tumor tissue *in vitro* and in an animal xenografts, resulting in down-regulation of the targeted mRNA, suppressing immune activation and inflammatory processes. In other experiment, a 65 aa double-stranded RNA binding domain was fused to TAT protein for binding and enhancing cellular uptake of siRNA (Peer et al., 2007).

Gene targets were knocked down after treating mice intra-nasally. High target down-regulation and low toxicity were reported without any significant selectivity. Furthermore, conjugates of TAT peptides with poly-amido-amine (PAMAM) dendrimers were synthesized to enhance oligonucleotide uptake, however this approach was unable to increase uptake of siRNA and gene-silencing (Wen et al., 2007), whereas packaging siRNAs in polylysine prevented Toll-like receptor activation. Similar effects were possible for the other fusion proteins (Kumar et al., 2008).

It is known that the tripeptide Arg-Gly-Asp (RGD) binds to αvβ3 integrin, which is expressed on endothelial cells during tumor angiogenesis. Tethering the RGD peptide increased binding to integrin-positive cells, and intracellular accumulation of imaging agents (Eguchi et al., 2009). There was no enhancement of the RGD-targeted dendrimer in cell-culture model due to enhanced membrane permeation mediated by the cationic surface groups. However, tissue penetration was increased by the RGD conjugation in a 3D cell-culture model and a larger portion of the siRNA was delivered to the tumor (Waite et al., 2009). Hence dendrimers may be developed for targeted delivery if specific uptake and gene-silencing are determined and cytotoxicity issues are resolved. For both polymeric as well as for dendrimeric carriers, the distinction between fusion proteins and NPs was diffuse, as aggregation to multimolecular structures was noticed (Kang et al., 2005). Packaging siRNAs in poly-lysine prevented Toll-like receptor activation, and similar effects were possible for the fusion proteins (Shukla et al., 2005) Recently protamine-derived peptides or oligo-arginines were used due to the ease of their preparation and availability. Complexation strategies such as dendrimeric structures may improve loading capacity, but may also increase the particle size. In addition, unspecific cellular uptake and toxic effects may arise when using charged complexing agents. Hence optimal size and structure have to be elucidated for safe and effective theranostics. In addition, it is important to select carefully the siRNA structure and sequence. Usually partially 2α-O-modified oligonucleotides and LNAs (*locked nucleic acids*) are used in siRNA technology, however optimization of antisense oligonucleotides is crucial for the success of nucleic acid-based therapeutics (Kunath et al., 2003; Sioud et al., 2010);. Hence comprehensive knowledge of chemical modifications pertinent to efficiency, target selectivity, and endosomal escape is required.

CB As Universal Biomarker in Nanothranostics. The researchers reported that CB is a universal biomarker of cell injury (Sharma and Ebadi, 2014). Free radicals-induced genetic and epigenetic changes may induce CB formation. Nutritional stress, environmental toxins, toxic NPs, chronic diseases, microbial (bacteria, virus, fungus, etc.) infections, drug addiction and aging augment CB formation due to down-regulation of nuclear DNA, mitochondrial DNA, and microRNA, which participate in cell injury and apoptosis involved in progressive neurodegenerative diseases, cardiovascular diseases, and cancer. Nutritional rehabilitation, physiological zinc, and MTs prevent CB formation by acting as free radical scavengers and eliminate CBs by an active process called "charnolophagy". During acute phase, charnolophagy occurs to prevent further release of toxic substances such as cytochrome C, Iron sulfur proteins, Bax, BID, and apoptosis inducing factor (AIF) from the degenerating mitochondria to provide cytoprotection as an efficient molecular mechanism of intracellular detoxification, whereas during chronic phase, lysosomal-resistant CB formation occurs, which participates in the accumulation of precipitated proteins as intracellular inclusions, involved in progressive neurodegenerative and cardiovascular diseases. Hence miRNA and CB formation may be used as biomarkers for theranostic applications. Furthermore CB-specific antagonists and charnolophagy agonists may be developed to provide neuro-protection and cardio-protection and vice versa for the eradication of MDR malignancies, before developing specific structures and nucleotide sequences for thernostic applications. For cancer chemotherapy, NPs may be designed with distinct tumor characteristics for both cell-surface antigen and the siRNA-mediated target gene silencing (Vester and Wengel, 2004).

MicroRNA in EBPT There is a significant correlation between EBPT and miRNAs. Recent advances in molecular biology emphasized the clinical significance of microRNA in neurodegenerative diseases, cardiovascular diseases, and cancer. MicroRNAs are single-stranded 19-24 nucleotides non-coding segments, involved in the transcriptional regulation of genes, and have key regulatory role in various cell processes including mRNA and protein expression. MicroRNAs have been implicated in disease progression and regression; hence can be used as sensitive biomarkers for EBPT. In addition, polymorphisms in miRNA encoding, their targets, and factors involved in maturation can be used as novel PGx biomarkers in cancer (Leachman et al., 2010). Dysregulated miRNAs expression is involved in MDR malignancies. Hence miRNAs can be used as molecular targets to evaluate drug response in personalized treatment. PGx investigations highlighted genes that contribute to individual patient's drug sensitivity, resistance, and toxicity. It was also designated the cause of inter-individual variation in the expression and function of genes, including the role of microRNA, DNA methylation, copy number variations, and SNPs (Shukla et al., 2010). *It is now well established that miRNAs regulate apoptosis, cell cycle, differentiation, cytoskeletal organization at the post-transcriptional level by either down-regulating the target genes by binding at the coding region, or by inhibiting the translation at the 3'- untranslational region. In addition, miRNAs in the body fluids can be used for the diagnosis, prognosis, clinical outcome, and response to treatment in various clinical conditions* (Avci and Baran, 2013). Particularly miRNAs have a crucial role in cancer etiology and in the post-transcriptional regulation of genes involved in neurodegeneration via CB formation. Hence miRNA-mimics and miRNA silencing molecules may be developed to modulate miRNA expression in tumors as theranostic agents (Dreussi et al., 2012); In fact aging model of *C alegans* indicated that 73 out of 139 miRNAs have sequence homology to human miRNAs (Fabbri, 2013; Ibáñez-Ventoso and Driscoll, 2009). MiRNAs control neuronal cell fate during development and alter gene expression of the non-coding RNA during progressive neurodegenerative disorders and can be detected in the peripheral mononuclear cells (Ibáñez-Ventoso and Driscoll, 2009; Klinge, 2009; Maes et al. 2010). Several disorders of aging in female population after menopause can be attributed to functional decline in Estrogen. Furthermore, abnormal microRNA expression has been associated with *Estrogen-Responsive Breast Cancer* and the target genes involved in the aging process (Lie et al., 2014).

Epigenetic Changes and microRNA Recent evidence supports that epigenetic changes are involved in chromatin remodeling and can contribute to fetal metabolic programming by methylation of DNA at the cytosine residues and acetylation of histones. These epigenetic changes can be modulated by miRNAs to influence gene expression during undernutrition, environmental neurotoxicity, or fetal Alcohol exposure. Maternal undernutrition during conception may also increase the risk of developing insulin resistance during adulthood (Sookoian et al., 2013). In singleton fetuses, prenatal undernutrition resulted in reduced expression of PIK3CB, PRKCZ, and pPRKCZ (Thr410) genes in skeletal muscle. In PIUN singletons, there was increased expression of IRS1, PDPK1, and SLC2A4 genes. In twins, PCUN caused increased expression of IRS1, AKT2, PDK1 and PRKZ, PRKCZ, while PIUN also induced increased expression of IRS1 and PRKCZ and SLC2A4 SLC2A4 genes in fetal muscle. *There were specific changes in the expression of 22 microRNAs in skeletal muscle, providing evidence that maternal undernutrition during conception induces changes in the* *microRNAs, which may alter the insulin-signaling in the skeletal muscle suggesting association between prenatal undernutrition and insulin resistance in adult life. In addition, stem cell pluripotency and differentiation are governed by methylation at cytosine residues and modulated by histone acetylation-deacetylation.* Hence nutritional and environmental stress (including toxins and microbial infections) may induce deleterious changes in the developing fetus. Furthermore, miRNA can influence the epigenetic changes leading to future risk of metabolic syndromes, fatty liver, insulin resistance (**Tomasetti et al., 2014**), and even Zika Viral-induced microcephaly due to neuronal CB formation in the developing brain. The author proposed primarily two types of tissue-specific CBs depending on the nature of mitochondria. (i) Monoamine oxidase-A and monoamine oxidase-B specific CB which can be localized in the hippocampus and striatal regions respectively to cause AD, PD, MDDs, and several other neurodegenerative α-syncuelinopathies beyond the scope of this chapter.

Regulation of Mitochondrial Function by miRNAs It is known that the maintenance of cellular energy and homeostasis depends on the normal function of mitochondria which plays a pivotal role in the apoptotic pathway and their dysfunction is associated with chronic diseases. The role of miRNAs in the regulation of the mitochondrial bioenergetics, and in modulating metabolic pathways in tumor suppression and theranostic application was summarized (Chan et al., 2009). Reprogramming of the energy metabolism was proposed as an emerging feature of cancer diagnosis and prognosis. MicroRNAs localization in the mitochondria emerged as key regulators of metabolism. MicroRNAs can modulate mitochondrial proteins encoded by nuclear genes. The miRNAs regulate signaling pathways in mitochondria, and may be deregulated in various diseases including cancer. Hence modulation of miRNAs levels may provide novel theranostic strategies for the treatment of mitochondria-related diseases. Recently pulmonary arterial endothelial cells were used as representative cell types and the Iron-sulfur cluster assembly proteins (ISCU1/2) as targets for down-regulation by hypoxia-induced miRNA 210 (miR-210). ISCU1/2 induced assembly of Iron-sulfur clusters (*involved in electron transport and redox reactions*). By upregulating miR-210 and down-regulating ISCU1/2; the structural integrity of Iron sulfur clusters was impaired. Downregulation of ISCU1/2 during hypoxia was associated with induction of MiR-210, which decreased the activity of Iron-sulfur proteins involved in regulating mitochondrial metabolism, including ubiquinone-NADH–oxido-reductase (complex-1) and acotinase, resulting in the down-regulation of oxidative phosphorylation and hence bioenergetics and other functions, suggesting clinically-significant association of miRNA, Iron-sulfur cluster proteins, hypoxia, and mitochondrial functions in cellular metabolism and adaptation to stress. Further investigations in this direction are needed to improve various clinically-significant aspects of nanotheranostics as discussed in this chapter. Moreover, the elucidation of the role of miRNAs in the regulation of mitochondrial bioenergetics will elucidate yet undiscovered molecular mechanisms involved in the progression and regression of CB in cancer and other chronic diseases. Eventually, this knowledge will promote the development of noninvasive and innovative nanotheranostics with minimum or no adverse effects. In addition, future development of membrane penetrating peptides may prove beneficial for targeted drug delivery in specific cellular organelle; including peroxysomes, golgi body, mitochondria, nucleus, and lysosomes and other intraceullar organallae to ultimately accomplish successful EBPT of chronic illnessess.

CONCLUSION

Nanotechnology provides better, safe, effective, and economical personalized theranostic options for cancer and other drug-resistant chronic diseases including AD, PD, chronic drug addiction, and MDDs, where conventional medical treatment has limited prospectus. Hence future development in innovative NPs, nanomaterials, and nanodevices for targeted drug delivery utilizing chronopharmacological approaches may provide better theranostics and reduce the cost of time-consuming, cumbersome, and potentially painful, and futile therapeutic options with serious adverse effects. PM can design time-and cost-effective theranostic protocols for each patient while taking into consideration genetic predisposition and individual variability to accomplish best treatment options with minimum or no adverse effects. For instance, treatment with patient-specific stem cells is a promising effort in this direction. Recently, micellar NPs for the topical and transdermal drug delivery of pharmaceuticals and personal care products were developed (Lee et al. 2010). Particularly, specific CB and/or chronolophagy agonists and antagonists may be developed for the effective treatment of neurodegenerative diseases, cardiovascular diseases, and cancer. In addition to possible therapeutic strategies with siRNA; the miRNAs are involved in post-transcriptional control and may be de-regulated in chronic diseases and aging (Wang, 2009). Recently lactosyl *Gramicidine*-based lipid NPs (Lac-GLN) for targeted delivery of anti-mir-155 to hepatocellular carcinoma were developed (Zhang et al., 2013). Further studies to explore the exact pathophysiological significance of dysregulated miRNAs in compromised mitochondrial bioenergetics causing CB formation in chronic illnesses will expand our nanotheranostics capability (Hamburg et al., 2010). Eventually molecularly well-defined and genetically-sculptured practice of EBPT developing novel NPs and nano-drug delivery devices/systems will confer painless treatment without any adverse effects, which will improve the quality of our life. Hence the future of nanotheranostics to accomplish EBPT seems quite promising.

REFERENCES

Ahmed, N., Fessi, H. & Elaissari, A. (2012). Theranostic applications of nanoparticles in cancer. *Drug Discov. Today*, *17*, 928-34.

Amoozgar, Z. & Yeo, Y. (2012). Recent advances in stealth coating of nanoparticle drug delivery systems. *Wiley Interdiscip Rev. Nanomed. Nanobiotechnol*, *4*, 219-233.

Avci, C. B. & Baran, Y. (2013). Use of microRNA in PM. M. Yousef and Allmer J (eds) miRNomics: MicroRNAs biology and Computational Analysis. *Methods in Mol Biol*, *1107*, 243-56. Springer Verlag Heidelberg Vol 1107.

Babinot, J., Renard, E. & Droumaguet, B. L. (2013). Facile Synthesis of Multicompartment Micelles Based on Biocompatible Poly(3-hydroxyalkanoate). *Macromol Rapid Commun*, *34*, 362-368.

Bhoyar, N., Giri, T. K., Tripathi, D. K., Alexander, A. & Ajazuddin. (2012). Recent Advances in Novel Drug Delivery System Through Gels: Review. *J. Pharm. & Allied Health Sci.*, *2*, 21-39.

Bisht, R. (2011). Chronomodulated drug delivery system: A comprehensive review on the recent advances in a new sub-discipline of 'chronopharmaceutics'. *Asian J. Pharm.*, *5*, 1-8.

Brannon-Peppas, L. & Blanchette, J. O. (2004). Nanoparticle and targeted systems for cancer therapy. *Adv. Drug. Deliv. Rev*, *56*, 1649-1659.

Brenneman, M., Sharma, S., Harting, M., et al. (2010). Autologous bone marrow mononuclear cells enhance recovery after acute ischemic stroke in young and middle-aged rats. *J. Cerebral Blood Flow & Metabolism*, *30*, 140-149.

Brigger, I., Dubernet, C. & Couvreur, P. Nanoparticles in cancer therapy and diagnosis. *Adv. Drug Deliv. Rev.*, 2002, *54*, 631-51.

Caravella, J. & Lugovskoy, A. Design of next-generation protein therapeutics. *Curr. Opin. Chem. Biol.*, 2010, 14, 520-28.

Chabenne, A., Moon, C., Ojo, C., Khogali, A., Nepal, B. & Sharma, S. (2014). Biomarkers in Fetal Alcohol Syndrome (Recent Update) *Biomarkers & Genomic. Med.*, *6*, 12-22.

Chan, S. Y., Zhang, Y. Y., Hemann, C., Mahoney, C. E., Zweier, J. L. & Loscalzo, J. (2009). MicroRNA-210 controls mitochondrial metabolism during hypoxia by repressing the Iron-sulfur cluster assembly proteins ISCU1/2. *Cell Metab.*, *10*, 273-84.

Chen, L., Han, L. & Lian, G. (2013). Recent advances in predicting skin permeabilityof hydrophilic solutes. *Adv. Drug Deliv. Rev.*, *65*, 295-05.

Chen, N. T., Cheng, S. H. & Souris, J. S. (2013). Theranostic applications of mesoporous silica nanoparticles and their organic/inorganic hybrids. *J. Mater. Chem. B*, *1*, 3128-35.

Chen, S. Y., Zani, C., Khouri, Y. & Marasco, W. A. (1995). Design of a genetic immunotoxin to eliminate toxin immunogenicity. *Gene Ther*, *2*, 116–123.

Chen, X., Zaro, J. L. & Shen, W. C. (2013). Fusion protein linkers: Property, design and functionality. *Adv. Drug Deliv. Rev*, *65*, 1357-1369.

Chirra, H. D. & Desai, T. A. (2012). Emerging microtechnologies for the development of oral drug delivery devices. *Adv. Drug Deliv. Rev.*, *64*, 1569-1578.

Cho, I. K., Moran, S. P., Paudyal, R., et al., (2014). Longitudinal Monitoring of Stem Cell Grafts *In vivo* Using Magnetic Resonance Imaging with Inducible Maga as a Genetic Reporter. *Theranostics*, *4*, 972-89.

Clairambault, J. (2009). Modelling Physiological and Pharmacological Control on Cell Proliferation to Optimise Cancer Treatments. *Mathematical Modelling of Natural Phenomena*, *4*, 12-67.

Daka, A. & Peer, D. (2012). RNAi-based nanomedicines for targeted personalized therapy, *Adv. Drug Deliv. Rev.*, *64*, 1508-1521.

Deng, H., Zhong, Y., Du, M., et al. (2014). Theranostic Self-Assembly Structure of Gold Nanoparticles for NIR Photothermal Therapy and XRay Computed Tomography Imaging. *Theranostics*, *4*, 904-918.

Draz, M. S., Fang, B. A., Zhang, P., et al. (2014). Nanoparticle-Mediated Systemic Delivery of siRNA for Treatment of Cancers and Viral Infections. *Theranostics*, *4*, 872-92.

Dreussi, E., Biason, P., Toffoli, G. & Cecchin, E. (2012). miRNA pharmacogenomics: the new frontier for PM in cancer. *Pharmacogenomics*, *13*, 1635-1650.

Droumaguet, B. L., Nicolas, J., Brambilla, D., et al. (2012). Versatile and efficient targeting using a single nanoparticulate platform: application to cancer and Alzheimer's disease. *ACS Nano*, *6*, 5866-5879.

Duncan, R. & Sat, Y. N. (1998). "Tumour targeting by enhanced permeability and retention (EPR) effect". *Ann. Oncol, 9* (Suppl.2), 39.

Dyondi, D., Webster, T. J. & Banerjee, R. (2013). A nanoparticulate injectable hydrogel as a tissue engineering scaffold for multiple growth factor delivery for bone regeneration. *Int. J. Nanomed., 8,* 47-59.

Eguchi, A., Meade, B. R., Chang, Y. C., et al. (2009). Efficient siRNA delivery into primary cells by a peptide transduction domain-dsRNA binding domain fusion protein. *Nat. Biotechnol., 27,* 567-71.

Ekenseair, A. K., Kasper, F. K. & Mikos, A. G. (2013). Perspectives on the interface of drug delivery and tissue engineering. *Adv. Drug Deliv. Rev., 65,* 89-92.

Estudante, M., Morais, J. G., Soveral, G. & Benet, L. Z. (2013). Intestinal drug transporters: An overview. *Adv. Drug Deliv. Rev., 65,* 1340-1356.

Etheridge, M. L., Campbell, S. A., Erdman, A. G., Haynes, C. L., Wolf, S. M. & McCullough, J. (2013). The big picture on nanomedicine: the state of investigational and approved nanomedicine products, Nanomedicine: *Nanotech, Biol & Med, 9,* 1-14.

Fabbri, M. (2013). MicroRNAs and cancer: towards a PM. *Curr Mol Med, 3,* 751-756.

Fan, C. H., Lin, W. H., Ting, C. Y., et al. (2014). Contrast-Enhanced Ultrasound Imaging for the Detection of Focused Ultrasound-Induced Blood-Brain Barrier Opening. *Theranostics,* 2014, *4,* 1014-25.

Fernandes, R. & Gracias, D. H. (2012). Self-folding polymeric containers for encapsulation and delivery of drugs., *Adv. Drug Deliv. Rev., 64,* 1579-1589.

Gajewicz, A., Rasulev, B., Dinadayalane, T. C., et al. (2012). Advancing risk assessment of engineered nanomaterials: Application of computational approaches. *Adv. Drug Deliv. Rev., 64,* 1663-93.

Gombotz, W. R. & Wee, S. F. (2012). Protein release from alginate matrices. *Adv. Drug Deliv. Rev., 64,* 194-205.

Gref, R., Domb, A., Quellec, P., et al. (1995). The controlled intravenous delivery of drugs using PEG-coated sterically stabilized nanospheres. *Adv Drug Deliv Rev, 16,* 215-33.

Greish, K. (2010). Enhanced permeability and retention (EPR) effect for anticancer nanomedicine drug targeting. *Methods Mol. Biol., 624,* 25-37.

Gremse, F., Theek, B., Kunjachan, S., et al. (2014). Absorption Reconstruction Improves Biodistribution Assessment of Fluorescent Nanoprobes Using Hybrid Fluorescence-mediated Tomography. *Theranostics, 4,* 960-971.

Griesh, K. (2012). Enhanced permeability and retention effect for selective targeting of anticancer nanomedicine: are we there yet? *Drug Discov. Today Technol., 9,* 161-166.

Hamburg, M. A. & Collins, F. C. (2010). The Path to PM. *New Eng. J. Med., 363,* 301-304.

Hansen, S., Claus-Michael Lehr, C. M. & Schaefer, U. F. (2013). Modeling the human skin barrier - Towards a better understanding of dermal absorption. *Adv. Drug Deliv. Rev., 65,* 149-51.

Hayashi, K., Nakamura, M., Miki, H., et al. (2014). Magnetically Responsive Smart Nanoparticles for Cancer Treatment with a Combination of Magnetic Hyperthermia and Remote-Control Drug Release. *Theranostics, 4,* 834-844.

Herrlich, S., Spieth, S., Messner, S. & Zengerle, S. R. (2012). Osmotic micropumps for drug delivery. *Adv. Drug Deliv. Rev., 64,* 1617-1627.

Ho, D., Sun, X. & Sun, S. (2011). Monodisperse magnetic nanoparticles for theranostic applications. *Acc. Chem. Res., 44,* 875-882.

Hoffman, A. S. (2002). Hydrogels for biomedical applications. *Adv Drug Deliv. Rev.*, *54*, 3-12.

Hondroulis, E., Zhang, R., Zhang, C., et al. (2014). Immuno Nanoparticles Integrated Electrical Control of Targeted Cancer Cell Development Using Whole Cell Bioelectronic Device. *Theranostics*, *4*, 919-930.

Ibáñez-Ventoso, C. & Driscoll, M. (2009). MicroRNAs in C. elegans Aging: Molecular Insurance for Robustness? *Curr. Genomics*, *10*, 144-153.

Janowski, M., Bulte, J. W. & Walczak, P. (2012). Personalized nanomedicine advancements for stem cell tracking. *Adv. Drug Deliv. Rev.*, *64*, 1488-507.

Jayasena, B. & Subbiah, S. (2011). "A novel mechanical cleavage method for synthesizing few-layer graphenes". *Nanoscale Res. Lett.*, *6* (1), 9501.

Jian, J., Liu, C., Gong, Y., et al., (2014). India Ink Incorporated Multifunctional Phase-transition Nanodroplets for Photoacoustic/Ultrasound Dual modality Imaging and Photoacoustic Effect Based Tumor Therapy. *Theranostics*, *4*, 1026-1038.

Jing, L., Liang, X., Li, X., et al. (2014). Mn-porphyrin Conjugated Au Nanoshells Encapsulating Doxorubicin for Potential Magnetic Resonance Imaging and Light Triggered Synergistic Therapy of Cancer. *Theranostics*, *4*, 858-871.

Kang, H., Delong, R., Fisher, M. H. & Juliano, R. L. (2005). TAT-conjugated PAMAM dendrimers as delivery agents for antisense and siRNA oligonucleotides. *Pharm. Res*, *22*, 2099-2006.

Khoury, R. E. l., Misra, V., Sharma, S., et al. (2010). The effect of Trans-Catheter Injections on Viability and Cytokine Release of Mononuclear Cells. *Am. J. Neurorad.*, *31*, 1488-1492.

Kim, T. H., Lee, S. & Chen, X. (2013). Nanotheranostics for PM. *Expert Rev. Mol. Diagn.*, *13*, 257-269.

Kim, Y. C., Park, J. H. & Prausnitz, M. R. (2012). Microneedles for drug and vaccine delivery. *Adv. Drug Deliv. Rev.*, *64*, 1547-1568.

Klinge, C. M. (2009). Estrogen Regulation of MicroRNA Expression. *Curr Genomics*, *10*, 169-183.

Kobayashi, H., Watanabe, R. R. & Choyke, P. L. (2014). Improving Conventional Enhanced Permeability and Retention (EPR) Effects; What Is the Appropriate Target? *Theranostics*, *4*, 81-89.

Kulis, M. & Burks, W. A. (2013). Oral immunotherapy for food allergy: Clinical and preclinical studies. *Adv. Drug Deliv. Rev.*, *65*, 774-781.

Kumar, P., Ban, H. S., Kim, S. S., et al. (2008). T cell-specific siRNA delivery suppresses HIV-1 infection in humanized mice. *Cell*, *134*, 577-586.

Kunath, K., Merdan, T., Hegener, O., Haberlein, H. & Kissel, T. (2003). Integrin targeting using RGD-PEI conjugates for *in vitro* gene transfer. *J. Gene Med.*, *5*, 588-599.

Kwon, G. S. & Kataoka, K. (2012). Block copolymer micelles as longcirculating drug vehicles. *Adv. Drug Deliv.*, *64*, 237-245.

Kwon, K. C., Nityanandam, R., Stewart, J. & Daniell, H. (2013). Oral delivery of bioencapsulated exendin-4 expressed in chloroplasts lowers blood glucose level in mice and stimulates insulin secretion in beta-TC6 cells. *Plant Biotechnol. J.*, *11*, 77-86.

Lai, F., Fadda, A. M. & Sinico, C. (2013). Liposomes for brain delivery. *Expert opinion on Drug Deliv.*, *10*, 1003-1022.

Leachman, S. A., Hickerson, R. P., Schwartz, M. E., et al. (2010). First-in-human mutation-targeted siRNA Phase Ib trial of an inherited skin disorder. *Mol. Ther.*, *18*, 442-446.

Lee, R. W., Shenoy, D. B. & Sheel, R. (2010). Micellar Nanoparticles: Applications for Topical and Passive *Transdermal Drug Delivery*. Chapter 2: p 37-58. Handbook of Non-Invasive Drug Delivery Systems. (Non-Invasive and Minimally-Invasive Drug Delivery Systems for Pharmaceutical and Personal Care Products) A volume in Personal Care & Cosmetic Technology.

Li, G. H., Yang, P. P., Gao, S. S. & Zu, Y. Q. Synthesis and micellar behavior of poly (acrylic acid-b-styrene) block copolymers. *Coll Polymer Sci*, 2012a, *290*, 1825-31.

Li, T., Evans, A. T., Chiravuri, S., Gianchandani, R. Y. & Gianchandani, Y. B. (2012). Compact, power-efficient architectures using microvalves and microsensors, for intrathecal, insulin, and other drug delivery systems. *Adv. Drug Deliv. Rev.*, *64*, 1639-1649.

Li, X., Qi, J., Xie, Y., et al. (2013). Nanoemulsions coated with alginate/ chitosan as oral insulin delivery systems: preparation, characterization, and hypoglycemic effect in rats. *Int. J. Nanomed.*, *8*, 23-32.

Li, X., Stuckert, P., Bosch, I., Marks, J. D. & Marasco, W. A. (2001). Single-chain antibody-mediated gene delivery into erbb2-positive human breast cancer cells. *Cancer Gene Ther.*, *8*, 555-565.

Li, X. Y., Kong, X. Y., Shi, S., et al. (2008). Preparation of alginate coated chitosan microparticles for vaccine delivery. *BMC Biotech.*, *8*, 89-100.

Lie, S., Morrison, J. L., Williams-Wyss, O., et al. (2014). Periconceptional undernutrition programs changes in insulin-signaling molecules and microRNAs in skeletal muscle in singleton and twin fetal sheep. *Biol. Reprod.*, *9*, 90-95.

Lin, W. J., Juang, L. W., Wang, C. L., Chen, Y. C., Lin, C. C. & Chang, K. L. (2010). Pegylated Polyester Polymeric Micelles as a Nano-carrier: Synthesis, Characterization, Degradation, and Biodistribution. *J. Expt. & Clin. Med.*, *2*, 4-10.

Liu, S. (2013). Epigenetics advancing personalized nanomedicine in cancer therapy. *Adv. Drug Deliv. Rev.*, *64*, 1532-1543.

Liu, Z. & Li, Z. (2014). Molecular Imaging in Tracking Tumor-Specific Cytotoxic T Lymphocytes (CTLs). *Theranostics*, *4*, 990-1001.

Maeda, H., Nakamura, H. & Fang, J. (2013). The EPR effect for macromolecular drug delivery to solid tumors: Improvement of tumor uptake, lowering of systemic toxicity, and distinct tumor imaging *in vivo*. *Adv. Drug. Deliv. Rev.*, *65*, 1375-1385.

Maes, O. C., Chertkow, H. M., Wang, E. & Schipper, H. M. (2010). MicroRNA: Implications for Alzheimer's disease and other human CNS disorders. *Curr. Genomics*, *10*, 154-168.

Maksimenko, A., Mougin, J., Mura, S., et al. (2013). Polyisoprenoyl gemcitabine conjugates self-assemble as nanoparticles, useful for cancer therapy. *Cancer Lett.*, *334*, 346-353.

Matsumura, Y. & Maeda, H. (1986). "A new concept for macromolecular therapeutics in cancer chemotherapy: mechanism of tumoritropic accumulation of proteins and the antitumor agent smancs". *Cancer Res*, *46*, 6387-6392.

Meng, E. & Hoang, T. (2012). MEMS-enabled implantable drug infusion pumps for laboratory animal research, preclinical, and clinical applications. *Adv. Drug Deliv. Rev.*, *64*, 1628-1638.

Mertens, M. E., Frese, J., Bölü kbas, D. A., et al., (2014). FMN-Coated Fluorescent USPIO for Cell Labeling and Non-Invasive MR Imaging in Tissue Engineering. *Theranostics*, *4*, 1002-1013.

Misra, V., Yang, B., Sharma, S. & Savitz, S. (2011). Cell Based Therapy for Stroke. In Therapy for Neurological injury. Ed Charles S Cox Jr. Chapter 7, pp. 143-162. Humana Press. Springer Science.

Moghimi, S. M., Wibroe, P. P., Helvig, S. Y., Farhangrazi, S. Z. & Hunter, A. C. (2012). Genomic perspectives in inter-individual adverse responses following nanomedicine administration: The way forward. *Adv. Drug Deliv. Rev.*, *64*, 1385-1393.

Mura, S. & Couvreur, P. (2012). Nanotheranostics for PM. *Adv. Drug Deliv. Rev.*, *64*, 1394-1416.

Nanotechnology Information Center: Properties, Applications, Research, and Safety Guidelines". *American Elements*. (Retrieved 13 May 2011).

Nicholas, A. & Peppas, N. A. (2012). An introduction to the most cited papers in the history of Advanced Drug Delivery Reviews (1987–2012). *Adv. Drug Deliv. Rev.*, *48*, 139-1357.

Nicolas, J., Mura, S., Brambilla, D., Mackiewicz, N. & Couvreur, P. (2013). Design, functionalization strategies and biomedical applications of targeted biodegradable/ biocompatible polymer-based nanocarriers for drug delivery. *Chem. Soc. Rev.*, *42*, 1147-1235.

Nicolini, C., Bragazzi, N. & Pechkova, E. (2012). Nanoproteomics enabling personalized nanomedicine. *Adv. Drug Deliv. Rev.*, *64*, 1522-1531.

Ochoa, M., Mousoulis, C. & Ziaie, B. (2012). Polymeric microdevices for transdermal and subcutaneous drug delivery. *Adv. Drug Deliv. Rev.*, *64*, 1603-1616.

Ohdo, S., Koyanagi, S. & Matsunga, N. (2010). Chronopharmacological strategies: Intra- and inter-individual variability of molecular clock. *Adv. Drug Deliv. Rev.*, *62*, 885-897.

Olivier, J. C. (2005). Drug Transport to Brain with Targeted Nanoparticles. *NeuroRx*, *2*, 108–119.

Pararas, E. L., Borkholder, D. A. & Borenstein, J. T. (2012). Microsystems technologies for drug delivery to the inner ear. *Adv. Drug Deliv. Rev.*, *64*, 1650-1660.

Peer, D., Zhu, P., Carman, C. V., Lieberman, J. & Shimaoka, M. (2007). Selective gene silencing in activated leukocytes by targeting siRNAs to the integrin lymphocyte function-associated antigen-1. *Proc. Natl Acad Sci. USA*, *104*, 4095-4100.

Peppas, N. A. (2013). Historical perspective on advanced drug delivery: How engineering design and mathematical modeling helped the field mature. *Adv. Drug Deliv. Rev.*, *65*, 5-9.

Petersen, A. L., Hansen, A. E., Gabizon, A. & Andresen, T. L. (2012). Liposome imaging agents in PM. *Adv. Drug Deliv. Rev.*, *64*, 1417-1435.

Poon, R. T. & Borys, N. (2009). "Lyso-thermosensitive liposomal Doxorubicin: a novel approach to enhance efficacy of thermal ablation of liver cancer". *Expert Opin Pharmacother.*, *10*, 333-343.

Prabhakar, U., Maeda, H., Jain, R. K., et al. (2013). Challenges and key considerations of the enhanced permeability and retention effect for nanomedicine drug delivery in oncology. *Cancer Res*, *73*, 2412-2417.

Probst, C. E, Zrazhevsky, P., Bagalkot, V. & Gao, X. (2013). Quantum dots as a platform for nanoparticle drug delivery vehicle design. *Adv. Drug Deliv. Rev.*, *65*, 703-719.

Roberts, M. J., Bentley, M. D. & Harris, J. M. (1997). Chemistry for peptide and protein PEGylation. *Adv. Drug Deliv. Rev.*, *28*, 25-42.

Rösler, A. A., Vandermeulen, G. W. M. & Klok, H. A. (2001). Advanced drug delivery devices via self-assembly of amphiphilic block copolymers. *Adv. Drug Deliv. Rev*, *53*, 95-108.

Ryu, J. H., Koo, H., Sun, I. C., et al., (2012). Tumor-targeting multi-functional nanoparticles for theragnosis: new paradigm for cancer therapy. *Adv. Drug Deliv. Rev.*, *64*, 1447-1458.

Sanvicens, N. & Marco, M. P. Multifunctional nanoparticles-Properties and prospectus for their use in human medicine. P. 425, Elsevier Publishers 2008.

Sawant, R. R., Jhaveri, A. M. & Torchilin, V. P. (2012). Immunomicelles for advancing personalized therapy. *Adv. Drug Deliv. Rev.*, *64*, 436-446.

Shaikh, S., Nazim, S., Khan, T., Shaikh, A., Zameeruddin, M. & Quazi, A. Recent Advances in Pulmonary Drug Delivery System: A Review. *Int J Appl Pharm*, 2010, *2*, 27-31.

Sharma, S. & Ebadi, M. (2012). *In-Vivo* Molecular Imaging in Parkinson's Disease. In Parkinson's Disease, CRC Press, Eds M. Ebadi and R. Pfieffer. Chapter 58, pp. 787-802, CRC Press Boca Rotan, Florida USA.

Sharma, S., Bing, Y., Brenneman, M., et al., (2010). Bone Marrow Mononuclear Cells Protect Neurons and Modulate Microglia in Cell Culture Models of Ischemic Stroke. *J. Neurosci. Res.*, *88*, 2869-2876.

Sharma, S. & Ebadi, M. (2014). Charnoly body as Universal Biomarker of Cell Injury. *Biomarkers & Genomic Med*, *6*, 89-98.

Sharma, S. & Ebadi, M. (2011). Metallothioneins as early and sensitive biomarkers of redox signaling in neurodegenerative disorders. Inst. Integ. *Omics Appl. Biotech.*, *2*, 98-106.

Sharma, S. & Ebadi, M. (2014). Significance of Metallothioneins in Aging Brain. *Neurochem. Int.*, *65*, 40-48.

Sharma, S. & Ebadi, M. (2011). Therapeutic potential of metallothioneins as anti-inflammatory agents in polysubstance abuse. *Inst. Integ. Omics Appl. Biotech. J.*, *2*, 50-61.

Sharma, S., Moon, C. S., Khogali, A., et al., (2013). Biomarkers of Parkinson's Disease (Recent Update). *Neurochem. Int.*, *63*, 201-229.

Sharma, S., Nepal, B., Moon, C. S., et al., (2014). Psychology of craving. *Open. Jr. of Med. Psych.*, *3*, 120-125.

Sharma, S., Rais, A., Sandhu, R., Nel, W. & Ebadi, M. (2013). Clinical significance of metallothioneins in cell therapy and nanomedicine. *Int. J. Nanomed.*, *8*, 1477-1488.

Sharma, S., Yang, B., Xi, X., Grotta, J., Aronowski, J. & Savitz, S. (2011). IL-10 Directly Protects Cortical Neurons by Activating PI-3 Kinase and STAT-3 Pathways. *Brain Res.*, *1373*, 189-194.

Sharma, S. (2014). Molecular Pharmacology of Environmental Neurotoxins. In Kainic Acid: Neurotoxic Properties, Biological Sources, and Clinical Applications. p301, Chapter 85. Nova Science Publishers. New York.

Sharma, S. (2013). Charnoly Body as a Sensitive Biomarker in Nanomedicine. International Translational Nanomedicine Conference, Boston, MASS, July 25-27, 2013.

Sharma, S. (2014). Nanotheronostics in Evidence-Based PM *Current Drug Targets*, *15*, 10 3

Shive, M. S. & Anderson, J. M. (1997). Biodegradation and biocompatibility of PLA and PLGA microspheres. *Adv. Drug Deliv. Rev.*, *28*, 5-24.

Shukla, R., Thomas, T. P., Peters, J., Kotlyar, A., Myc, A. & Baker, J. R. (2005). Tumor angiogenic vasculature targeting with pamam dendrimer–RGD conjugates. *Chem Commun, 46*, 5739-5741.

Shukla, S., Sumaria, C. S. & Pradeepkumar, P. I. (2010). Exploring chemical modifications for siRNA therapeutics: A structural and functional outlook. *Chem. Med. Chem., 5*, 328-349.

Sioud, M. (2010). Recent advances in small interfering RNA sensing by the immune system. *Nat Biotechnol, 27*, 236-242.

Song, E., Zhu, P., Lee, S. K., et al. (2005). Antibody mediated *in vivo* delivery of small interfering RNAs via cell-surface receptors. *Nat. Biotechnol, 23*, 709-717.

Sookoian, S., Gianotti, T. F., Burgueño, A. L. & Pirola, C. J. (2013). Fetal metabolic programming and epigenetic modifications: a systems biology approach. *Pediat. Res., 73*, 531-542.

Stapleton, S., Milosevic, M., Allen, C., et al., (2013). A Mathematical Model of the Enhanced Permeability and Retention Effect for Liposome Transport in Solid Tumors. *PLos One, 8*, E81157.

Stevenson, C. L., Santini, Jr. J. T. & Langer, R. (2012). Reservoir-based drug delivery systems utilizing microtechnology. *Adv. Drug Deliv. Rev., 64*, 1590-1602.

Stolnik, L, Illum, L, Davis, S. S., (1995). Long circulating microparticulate drug carriers. *Adv. Drug Deliv. Rev., 16*, 195-214.

Sulek, K., Han, T. L., Villas-Boas, S. G., et al. (2014). Hair Metabolomics: Identification of Fetal Compromise Provides Proof of Concept for Biomarker Discovery. *Theranostics, 4*, 953-959.

Sun, Y., Kim. H. S., Park, J., et al. (2014). MRI of Breast Tumor Initiating Cells Using the Extra Domain-B of Fibronectin Targeting Nanoparticles. *Theranostics, 4*, 845-857.

Swami, A., Shi, J., Gadde, S., et al. (2012). Nanoparticles for targeted and temporally-controlled drug delivery. Chapter 2, S. Svenson and R.K. Prud;home (eds) Multifunctional Nanoparticles for Drug Delivery Applications: Imaging, Targetting, and Delivery. *Nanostructure Science and Technology*, 9-29. Springer Verlag Publishers.

Tomasetti, M., Neuzil, J. & Dong, L. (2014). MicroRNAs as regulators of mitochondrial function: role in cancer suppression. *Biochim. Biophys. Acta., 1840*, 1441-1453.

Torchilin, V. P. (2006). Multifunctional Nanocarriers. *Adv. Drug Deliv. Rev., 58*, 1532-1555.

Turker, N. S., Heidari, P., Kucherlapati, R., Kucherlapati, M. & Mahmood, U. (2014). An EGFR Targeted PET Imaging Probe for the Detection of Colonic Adenocarcinomas in the Setting of Colitis. *Theranostics, 4*, 893-903.

Vasey, P. A., Kaye, S. B., Morrison, R., et al. (1999). "Phase I clinical and pharmacokinetic study of PK1[N-(2-hydroxypropyl)methacrylamide copolymer Doxorubicin]: first member of a new class of chemotherapeutic agents-drug-polymer conjugates. Cancer Research Campaign Phase I/II Committee". *Clin. Cancer Res., 5*, 83-94.

Venditto, V. J. Jr. & Szoka, F. C. (2013). Cancer Nanomedicines: So many papers and so few drugs. *Adv. Drug Deliv, Rev., 65*, 80-88.

Vester, B. & Wengel, J. (2004). LNA (locked nucleic acid): high-affinity targeting of complementary RNA and DNA. *Biochem, 43*, 13233-13241.

Vig, B. S., Huttunen, K. M., Laine, K. & Rautio, J. (2013). Amino acids as promoieties in prodrug design and development. *Adv. Drug. Deliv. Rev., 65*, 1375-1385.

Vizirianakis, I. S. & Fatouros, D. G. (2012). Personalized nanomedicine: paving the way to the practical clinical utility of genomics and nanotechnology advancements. *Adv. Drug Deliv. Rev.*, *64*, 1359-1362.

Vorup-Jensen, T. & Peer, D. (2012). Nanotoxicity and the importance of being earnest. *Adv. Drug Deliv. Rev.*, *64*, 1661-1662.

Waite, C. L. & Roth, C. M. (2009). Pamam-RGD conjugates enhance siRNA delivery through a multicellular spheroid model of malignant glioma. *Bioconjug. Chem.*, *20*, 1908-2016.

Wang, E. (2009). MicroRNA Regulation and its Biological Significance in PM and Aging. *Curr. Genomics*, *10*, 143.

Wang, J., Örnek-Ballanco, C., Xu, J., Yang, W. & Yu, X. (2013). Preparation and characterization of vinculin-targeted polymer–lipid nanoparticle as intracellular delivery vehicle. *Int. J. Nanomed.*, *8*, 39-46.

Wang, J. J., Zeng, Z. W., Xiao, R. Z., et al. (2011). Recent advances of chitosan nanoparticles as drug carriers. *Int. J. Nanomed*, *6*, 765-774.

Watkins, J., Marsh, A., Taylor, P. C. & Singer, D. R. (2010). PM: The impact on chemistry. *Ther. Deliv.*, *1*, 651-665.

Wen, W. H., Liu, J. Y., Qin, W. J., et al. (2007). Targeted inhibition of hbv gene expression by single-chain antibody mediated small interfering RNA delivery. *Hepatol*, *46*, 84-94.

Wieland, M. & Fussenegger, M. (2013). Reprogrammed cell delivery for PM. *Adv. Drug Deliv. Rev.*, *64*, 1477-1487.

Winkler, J. (2011). Nanomedicines based on recombinant fusion proteins for targeting therapeutic siRNA oligonucleotide. *Ther. Deliv.*, *2*, 891-905.

Wu, C. Y. & Benet, L. Z. (2005). Predicting drug disposition via application of BCS: transport/absorption/ elimination interplay and development of a biopharmaceutics drug disposition classification system. *Pharm. Res.*, *22*, 11-23.

Xu, S., Olenyuk, B. Z., Okamoto, C. T. & Hamm-Alvarez, S. F. (2013). Targeting receptor-mediated endocytotic pathways with nanoparticles: Rationale and advances. *Adv. Drug. Deliv. Rev.*, *65*, 121-138.

Yang, B., Strong, R., Sharma, S., et al. (2011). Therapeutic Time Window and Dose-Response of Autologous Bone Marrow Mononuclear Cells for Ischemic Stroke. *J. Neurosci. Res.*, *89*, 833-839.

Zabaleta, V., Ponchel, G., Salman, H., Agüeros, M., Vauthier, C. & Irache, J. M. Oral administration of paclitaxel with pegylated poly(anhydride) nanoparticles: permeability and pharmacokinetic.

Zeng, Z., Parekh, P., Li, Z., Shi, Z. Z., Tung, C. H. & Zu, Y. (2014). Specific and Sensitive Tumor Imaging Using Biostable Oligonucleotide Aptamer Probes. *Theranostics*, *4*, 945-952.

Zhang, L. Y., Mena, J., Sun, J., et al. (2012). "Electrospray of multifunctional microparticles for image-guided drug delivery", Proc. SPIE 8233, Reporters, Markers, Dyes, Nanoparticles, and Molecular Probes for Biomedical Applications IV, 823303 (February 9, 2012).

Zhang, M., Zhou, X., Wang, B., et al. (2013). Lactosylated gramicidin-based lipid nanoparticles (Lac-GLN) for targeted delivery of anti-miR-155 to hepatocellular carcinoma. *J. Control Release*, *168*, 251-261.

Zhang, X. Q., Xu, X., Bertrand, N., Pridgen, E., Swami, A. & Farokhzad, O. C. (2012). Interactions of nanomaterials and biological systems: Implications to personalized nanomedicine. *Adv. Drug Deliv. Rev.*, *64*, 1363-84.

Zhang, Y., Chan, H. F. & Leong, K. W. (2013). Advanced materials and processing for drug delivery: The past and the future. *Adv. Drug Deliv. Rev.*, *65*(1), 104-120.

Zhao, G. & Rodriguez, B. L. (2013). Molecular targeting of liposomal nanoparticlesto tumor microenvIronment. *Int. J. Nanomed.*, *8*, 61-71.

Zhu, J., Huang, H., Dong, S., Ge, L. & Zhang, Y. (2014). Progress in Aptamer-Mediated Drug Delivery Vehicles for Cancer Targeting and Its Implications in Addressing Chemotherapeutic Challenges. *Theranostics*, *4*, 931-944.

BIOMARKERS IN PERSONALIZED THERANOSTICS OF NEURODEGENERATIVE DISEASES

Chapter 8

BIOMARKERS IN PERSONALIZED THERANOSTICS OF FETAL ALCOHOL SYNDROME

ABSTRACT

Ethanol consumption during pregnancy is a serious problem and is increasing globally among young women. *Development of biomarkers of fetal Alcohol syndrome (FAS) that can identify children at risk for adverse neurobehavioral consequences could lead to interventions earlier in life. Moreover animal models of fetal Alcohol spectrum disorders (FASD) in biomarker discovery can help in this most challenging area.* The FASD biomarkers include classical biomarkers (indirect) of Alcohol-induced pathology (mean corpuscular volume, γ-glutamyl transferase, aspartate aminotransferase, alanine aminotransferase, acetaldehyde-derived conjugates, and derivatives of non-oxidative Ethanol metabolism (fatty acid ethyl esters, ethyl glucuronide, ethyl sulphate, and phosphadityl Ethanol). Since Ethanol and acetaldehyde can be measured few hours after Ethanol intake in blood, urine, and sweat, these can be used to detect recent Ethanol exposure. Magnetic resonance spectroscopic biomarkers including; N-Acetyl Aspartate, indicator of brain regional neuronal density; Choline, a precursor of the neurotransmitter, Acetyl Choline, implicated in learning and memory and in the synthesis of Glycerophocholine, involved in membrane synthesis; and Glutamate and Creatine are reduced in FAS. Glutamate is a precursor for the synthesis of inhibitory neurotransmitter, GABA; and Creatine, for the high energy phosphates. Furthermore, reduced BDNF, Somatostatin, Complexin, Taurine, Glutathione, Myoinositol, Leptin and increased IGF and NMDA receptor excitotoxicity can be estimated in FAS. Imapired Methionine-Homocysteine cycle may also cause deleterious effect on protein, DNA methylation, and Histone acetylation in FAS victims. *In addition to meconium* fatty acid ethyl esters, *MRI, PET and SPECT imaging* facilitate earlier theranostic intervention for less Alcohol-related disabilities which cannot be confirmed in the absence of maternal drinking history. In addition, brain volume, isocortical volume, thickness, and surface area are reduced following prenatal exposure to Ethanol. Hence *novel discovery of biomarkers like Charnoly Body (CB) is needed to define cognitive impairments, and individual behavioral, physical, and genetic factors which could lead to having children with FASD for their successful EBPT. (**Note:** Ethanol and Alcohol have been written synonymously in this chapter)*

Keywords: fetal alcohol syndrome, biomarkers, Charnolybody, early diagnosis, prognosis

INTRODUCTION

Alcohol and several other drugs are now frequently abused alone or in combination in the entire world (Martin, 2008). Ethanol is a teratogen whose consumption among women of childbearing age is increasing gradually. Landgraf et al. (2013) recently described that fetal Alcohol syndrome (FAS) belongs to the spectrum of fetal Alcohol spectrum disorders (FASD) that affects 0.02-0.8% of all annual births with increased number of undetected cases. FAS has severe life-determining consequences for the affected individual and his family members because it can cause early morbidity and mortality. Since FAS as well as fetal Alcohol effect (FAE) represent the most preventable causes of mental retardation and birth defects, identification of Alcohol abuse early during pregnancy is exceedingly important to avoid deleterious consequences on the fetal brain development. Hence, extensive work is needed to incorporate the knowledge on fetal Alcohol effects among women of the childbearing age. Moreover, awareness and training among health care professionals may play a pivotal role in the early diagnosis of FASD.

A detailed description about animal models of FAS, Alcohol related birth defects, and Alcohol related neurodevelopmental disorders is available in a source book written by Cudd (2008). In addition, Johnston and Bronski (1991) wrote an excellent review on animal models of craniofacial abnormalities in FAS victims. In their earlier studies, Onley et al. (2002) discovered that a single episode of Ethanol intoxication can trigger apoptotic neurodegeneration in the developing rat or mouse brain and proposed that the NMDA antagonist and GABA mimetic properties of Ethanol are responsible for its apoptogenic effect. Other drugs that block NMDA glutamate receptors or mimic GABA at $GABA_A$ receptors, also trigger apoptotic neurodegeneration in the developing brain. Although the underlying mechanism remains uncertain, these novel findings explain the molecular basis of reduced brain mass and neurobehavioral abnormalities in human FAS. In addition to Ethanol, several other agents have NMDA antagonist or GABA-mimetic properties, such as drugs that may be abused by pregnant mothers [Phencyclidine (Angel Dust), Ketamine (Special K), Nitrous Oxide (Laughing Gas), Barbiturates, Benzodiazepines], and medicines used in obstetric and pediatric neurology (Anticonvulsants), and anesthesiology (general anesthetics are either NMDA antagonists or GABA-mimetics).

The primary limitation of animal models in FAS research is that the window of vulnerability coincides with the developmental period of synaptogenesis, also known as the brain growth-spurt period, which in rodents is a postnatal event, but in humans extends from the sixth month of gestation to several years after birth. Hence extrapolation and translation of animal data to human FAS could be misleading. Moreover the lack of a convincing molecular biomarker has hindered FASD research and treatment. Thus the primary objective of biomarker research is to objectively evaluate, evidence-based, clinically relevant, easily applicable, early diagnostic picture of FAS. Recently following diagnostic criteria for FAS were recommended: at least one deficit of growth, 3 defined facial characteristics, and one structural or functional abnormality of the CNS must be present during clinical evaluation of FAS victim. However confirmation of intrauterine Alcohol exposure is not considered as a prerequisite for the FAS diagnosis. This guideline constitutes an unbiased evidence-based approach for the FAS diagnosis which includes a pocket guide for a quick overview during routine clinical practice.

The FAS represents the most severe form of disorders, including characteristic craniofacial abnormalities, stunted growth, and behavioral impairments, caused by complex gene-environment interactions in addition to Ethanol. FASD and FAS can lead to physical, cognitive, and behavioral disabilities, whose early diagnosis is important for primary prevention with total abstinence during pregnancy and secondary prevention in newborns to reduce risk of deleterious consequences in later life. Recently significant efforts have been made to understand the underlying molecular mechanisms of FAS by identifying molecular diagnostic biomarkers in neonatal meconium and by performing 3D MRI. However, further investigations are needed to implement this knowledge on fetal effects of Ethanol, and multidisciplinary approach to increase awareness among women about the deleterious consequences of consuming even small amounts of Ethanol during pregnancy (Memo et al., 2013).

As a leading cause of intellectual impairments, FAS has significant social and public health impact as it is associated with a broad range of neurobehavioral deficits (Pulsifer, 1996). Clinical identification of FASD group is difficult because they do not exhibit all the physical features of FAS, and the physiological biomarkers for gestational Alcohol exposure have limitations. Hence determination of a profile based on the neurobehavioral effects of prenatal Alcohol exposure would allow more accurate identification of FAS. The development of such a profile is aimed at identifying those who are affected by prenatal Alcohol exposure, and not simply those who have been exposed to Alcohol prenatally (Vagnarelli et al., 2011). Hence determination of a profile based on the neurobehavioral effects of increased prenatal Alcohol exposure would allow more accurate identification of affected victims (Mattson and Riley, 2011).

The exact molecular mechanism underlying fetal developmental abnormalities caused by maternal Ethanol consumption remain uncertain. Unfortunately, the diagnosis of FAS and FAE is made after birth, when the damage has become irreversible and permanent. Laboratory diagnosis can help prevent this damage and make a valuable contribution in assessing prenatal Alcohol abuse. Especially the clinical utility of blood/breath Alcohol, γ-Glutamyl transferase (γ-GT), mean corpuscular volume (MCV), HAA, and carbohydrate-deficient transferrin (CDT) in pregnancy, is highly significant. Although none of these biomarkers as such has adequate sensitivity and specificity; the diagnostic accuracy is enhanced when these are estimated in combination (Cook, 2003).

This chapter highlights recent literature on biomarkers as maternal risk factors for FASD and emphasizes that this risk is multidimensional including; factors related to quantity, frequency, and timing of Alcohol abuse, maternal age, number of pregnancies, frequency of child birth, body size, body mass index (BMI), nutritional status, socioeconomic status, metabolism, religion, spirituality, depression, drug abuse, and social relationships. A systematic brief description of various biomarkers which can be used as a basic guideline for the evaluation and clinical management of FAS during early stages is highlighted in this chapter.

Although the first trimester is considered as the most vulnerable period, it is now realized that intrauterine exposure to Ethanol may cause fetal damage throughout entire gestational period. Falk et al. (2006, 2008) reported that individually, Alcohol, tobacco, and illicit drugs (Cocaine or Amphetamine) are harmful to the developing fetus during pregnancy. However determining the harm resulting from multiple drug abuse during pregnancy is a most challenging task. Moreover, unpredictable interactive (*additive or synergistic*) effects of the drugs abused simultaneously during pregnancy may have long-term deleterious consequences on the child's health and development. It has been noticed that intrauterine Ethanol-exposed adolescents are highly prone to develop drug dependence later in their life and Ethanol neurotoxicity is enhanced by Nicotine in these individuals. Moreover, interaction of Alcohol and Cocaine is more harmful than the use of each drug individually because of the formation of the highly toxic metabolite, Cocoethylene (McCance et al. 1995; Pennings et al. 2002). Hence FAS must be a diagnosis of exclusion and must be differentiated from conditions caused by other embryotoxic agents such as environmental neurotoxins (Kainic acid, Domoic acid, Acromelic acid), malnutrition, microbial infection, and genetic syndromes that share similar morphological features. By performing microPET imaging with ^{18}F-DOPA and ^{18}FdG on Cocaine and Meth-Amphetamine (METH)-intoxicated C57BL/6J mice, the researchers discovered that these drugs cause reduction in the striatal dopaminergic neurotransmission. The striatal ^{18}F-DOPA and the myocardial ^{18}FdG uptakes were further reduced when Cocaine and METH were administered along with Ethanol, suggesting that Alcohol accentuates Cocaine and METH neurotoxicity and may be considered as the gateway to multiple drug abuse (Sharma and Ebadi, 2008). Moreover, various other neurotransmitters and their receptors may be impaired in FAS; for example dopaminergic, cholinergic, GABA-ergic, glutamatergic, and serotonergic systems are all significantly impacted in FAS. Hence Alcohol consumption should be absolutely prevented at any stage of pregnancy, as it may seriously influence the brain regional synaptic neurotransmission.

Ideal Biomarker of FAS An ideal biomarker for detecting Alcohol abuse among pregnant women should have the following characteristics: the capacity to detect low-to-moderate levels of drinking over a prolonged period, a high probability of detecting drinking during pregnancy (*sensitivity*); and a low rate of false-positive results (*specificity*). In addition, biomarker should be easily obtainable from a biological sample by a noninvasive and clinically acceptable procedure; with little or no sample preparation steps, and simple economical analytical procedure(s) of its estimation, to provide rapid results. Unfortunately, none of the presently available FAS biomarkers sufficiently satisfies more than one or two of these criteria.

Clinical Consequences of Intrauterine Alcohol Usually still birth, preeclampsia, abortion, and fatality have been noticed depending on the concentration and frequency of maternal Alcohol consumption during pregnancy. In addition to FAS; *Trout syndrome, sudden infant death syndrome (SIDS), and autism may occur as illustrated in* Figure 8. Trout syndrome is characterized by impairment in the brain regional serotonergic neurotransmission due to point mutation in the serotonin transporter causing facial grimace, head, neck, and facial twitches and ticks, which remain persistent until adolescent life. In some individuals these symptoms may remain persistent even after the age of 20.

Classification of FAS Biomarkers FAS biomarkers can be broadly classified as *in-vitro and in-vivo* biomarkers and can be further divided as *(i) clinical biomarkers, (ii) molecular biomarkers, (iii) omics biomarkers, (iv) imaging biomarkers, (v) meconium biomarkers (vi) cord blood biomarkers, (vii) placental biomarkers, (viii) plasma biomarkers, (ix) and urinary biomarkers.* There are primarily 8 major types of FAS biomarkers including (i) clinical biomarkers (ii) molecular biomarkers (iii) omics biomarkers (iv) imaging *biomarkers (v) meconium biomarkers (vi) cord blood biomarkers, (vi) anatomical biomarkers, and (viii) neurobehavioral biomarkers as illustrated in* Figure 9.

Clinical Consequences of FAS

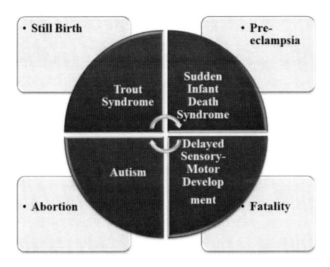

Figure 8. *Clinical consequences of intrauterine Alcohol*. This diagram illustrates clinical consequences of intrauterine Alcohol exposure to a developing fetus. Alcohol induces deleterious effects on the developing fetus and the severity of fetal damage depends on the strength and frequency of Alcohol consumption during pregnancy. In general sill birth, preeclampsia, abortion, and fatality have been noticed. Fetal Alcohol can also induce fetal Alcohol syndrome (FAS), Trout syndrome, sudden infant death syndrome (SIDS), and autism as illustrated in this figure.

Significant FAS Biomarkers

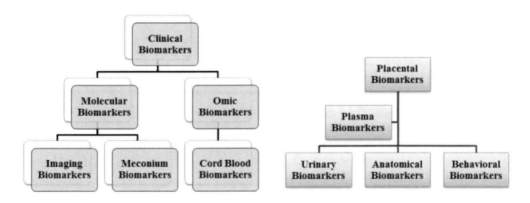

Figure 9. Biomarkers *of FAS* In general biomarkers of FAS can be divided into two major categories including (i) in-vitro biomarkers and (ii) *in-vivo* biomarkers. FAS biomarkers can be divided into following eight major types including: (i). Clinical biomarkers (ii) Molecular biomarkers (iii) Omics biomarkers (iv) Imaging biomarkers (v) Meconium biomarkers (vi) cord blood biomarkers (vi) Anatomical biomarkers, and (viii) Neurobehavioral biomarkers.

Temporal Window of FAS Biomarkers Usually <1drink/day is considered low, 2 drinks/day moderate, and >14 drinks/week are considered severe. According to the U.S.

National Institute of Alcohol Abuse and Alcoholism, about 70% of American adults drink at low-risk levels or do not drink at all. (35% of Americans do not consume Alcohol.) About 28% of American adults drink at levels that put them at risk for Alcohol dependence and Alcohol-related problems. According to New York Times report, a person is affected by the amount of Alcohol consumed, not the type. Beer and wine are not "safer" than hard liquor; they simply contain less Alcohol per ounce. By definition"one drink" as 12 ounces of beer, 8 - 9 ounces of malt liquor, 5 ounces of wine, or 1.5 ounces (a jigger or shot) of 80-proof liquor. Therefore, 12 ounces of beer is equivalent to 5 ounces of wine, or a 1.5 ounce short of hard liquor. Moderate drinking, particularly red wine, may decrease the risk of heart disease. However, even moderate drinking should be avoided in certain circumstances, such as before driving a vehicle, during pregnancy, when taking medications that may interact with Alcohol, or if a medical condition that may be worsened by drinking. Moderate drinking is defined as: no more than two drinks a day for men and one drink a day for women. Low-risk drinking is defined as: No more than 4 drinks a day, or 14 drinks per week, for men. No more than 3 drinks per day, or 7 drinks per week, for women (both men and women over age 65 should not drink more than this amount). At-risk (heavy) drinking is defined as: >14 drinks per week, or four drinks in a day, for men. More than seven drinks per week, or three drinks a day, for women. People who consume Alcohol are considered: at low risk for Alcohol-related problems if they drink within low-risk limits; at increased risk if they drink more than either the single-day limits or the weekly limits; at highest risk if they drink more than both the single-day limits and the weekly limits. Certain people are at much higher risk for the harmful effects of Alcohol, such as older subjects with high blood pressure or those taking medications for arthritis or pain. [For detailed description please refer to Single et al. (2000)].

The estimation and quantitation of biomarkers for the differential diagnosis of FAS has a critical temporal window. For example, within hrs of birth; breath, blood, and urine Alcohol levels can be estimated to assess the severity of maternal Alcohol abuse even at low doses. Moderate Alcohol consumption can be detected by estimating urinary Ethyl Glucronide (EThG) within first 5 days of delivery, *whereas % carbohydrate deficient transferrin (CDT) and Phosphatidyl Ethanolamine (PEThE) can be detected within <3 weeks. γ-Glutamyl transferase (GGT) and mean corpuscular volume (MCV) can be detected within < 3 weeks; and hair analysis of FAEE, EtG, and PEth can be performed within <3 months in the hair, plasma, and meconium samples as illustrated in* Figure 10. Ideally weeks and months are the target areas for the development of better biomarkers of FAS. *Furthermore, several in-vitro biochemical biomarkers of FAS including (i) mean corpuscular volume, MCV (ii) Alanine transferase (iii) fatty acid ethyl esters (FAEE), γ-Glutamyl transferase (GGT), Acetaldehyde–derived conjugates, Ethyl glucronide, Ethyl sulphate, Aspartate amino transferase, derivatives of nonoxidative Ethanol metabolism, derivatives of nonoxidative Ethanol metabolism, phosphatidyl-ethanolamine may facilitate early FAS diagnosis and/or treatment.* Particularly, *direct maternal biomarkers including γ-Glutamyl transferase (GGT), Aspartate amino transferase (AST), Alanine amino transfrase, MCV, carbohydrate deficient transferrin (CDT), and the ratio of 5-HTOL/5-HIAA have been estimated in FAS as illustrated in* Figure 11.

Temporal Sequence of FAS Biomarker Detection

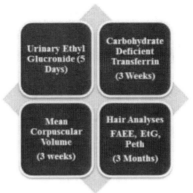

Figure 10. *Temporal window of biomarkers detectability*: Different fetal Alcohol syndrome (FAS) biomarkers can be detected within hrs, days, weeks and months depending on the amount of Alcohol consumed during pregnancy. Soon after delivery within hrs, breath Alcohol, blood Alcohol, and urine Alcohol can be detected at even low doses of Alcohol; Moderate Alcohol consumption may be detected by estimating % carbohydrate-deficient transferrin (CDT) and phosphatidyl Ethanolamine (PEth). Higher concentration of Alcohol may have deleterious consequences. Urinary Ethanol and ethylene glucronide can be estimated within weeks, whereas mean corpuscular volume (MCV), gamma glutamyl transferase (GGT), meconium FAEE, and hair analysis of FAEE, Ethylene glucronide, and phosphatidyl Ethanolamine can be detected within months in the FAS victims as illustrated in this diagram.

In-Vitro Biochemical FAS Biomarkers

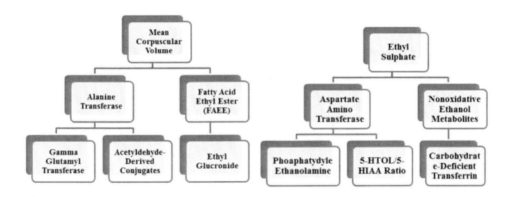

Figure 11. *In-vitro biomarkers of FAS*: In general *in vitro* FAS biomarkers can be divided into following catagories: (i) Mean corpuscular volume (ii) Alanine transferase (iii) Fatty acid ethyl esters (FAEE), Gamma glutamyl transferase (GGT), Acetaldehyde–derived conjugates, ethyl glucornide, ethyl sulphate, Aspartate amino transferase, Derivatives of nonoxidative Ethanol metabolism, Aspartate amino transferase, derivatives of nonoxidative Ethanol metabolism, phosphatidyl Ethanolamine. These *in-vitro* biomarkers can be analyzed to facilitate early FAS and its prevention and/or treatment.

Trait Biomarkers vs State Biomarkers of FAS In general, FAS biomarkers can be divided in two broad categories: *(i) trait biomarkers and (ii) state biomarkers.* Trait biomarkers include platelet Adenyl cyclase activity and increased β-Endorphins responsiveness. State biomarkers are of two types: (i) indirect and (ii) direct. The indirect and direct biomarkers can be subdivided into spot or short-term abuse and chronic long term abuse respectively. For spot or short-term use, Ethanol in blood, breath, and urine, EtG in urine and blood, FAEE in serum, PEtH in blood, EtS and EtP in urine and blood, TICS or β-Carboline in urine or blood, can be estimated. For chronic long-term Alcohol abuse, FAEE in hair and meconium, EtG in hair and meconium, Cocoethylene in hair, Acetaldehyde adducts of proteins in erythrocytes and hair, and β-Carboline in hair samples can be estimated. *The direct biomarkers can be sub-divided into spot or short-term (5-HTOL/5HIAA) and can be detected in urine. Particularly, for chronic or long term use, GGT in urine, ALT and AST in serum, MCV in blood, CDT in urine, Sialic acid and its index of serum Apolipoproteins, β-Hexosaminidase in the serum, Methanol in blood, and Dolicohol in blood and urine, can be estimated as illustrated in* Figure 12.

Clinical Biomarkers of FAS Clinical biomarkers can be sub-divided as: *(i) anatomical biomarkers, (ii) developmental biomarkers, (iii) neurological biomarkers, (iv) delayed motor learning, (v) and impaired hand writing as illustrated* in Figure 13. In general, *anatomical biomarkers include, (i) facial abnormalities (ii) micrognathia (iii) small size lips, (iv) reduced frontal lobe development, (v) and reduced eye blinking. However, these anatomical biomaekrs are highly specific to FAS.*

Direct Biomarkers of FAS

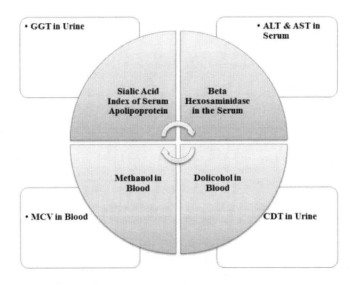

Figure 12. *Direct Maternal Biomarkers of FAS:* Direct maternal biomarkers include gamma glutamyl transferase (GGT), Aspartate amino transferase (AST), Alanine amino transfrase, Mean corpuscular volume, and carbohydrate deficient transferrin (CDT). In addition, the ratio of 5-HTOL/5-HIAA is also significantly increased in FAS as illustrated in this diagram.

Clinical Biomarkers of FAS

(a)   (b)

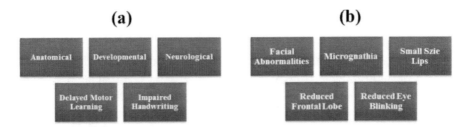

Figure 13. *Classification of FAS Biomarkers*: In general FAS biomarkers may be divided in two broad categories (i) Trait biomarkers and (ii) state biomarkers as presented in this diagram. Trait biomarkers include platelet adenyl cyclase activity and increased β-endorphins responsiveness. State biomarkers are of two types including indirect biomarkers and direct biomarkers. The indirect and direct biomarkers can be subdivided into spot or short-term use and chronic long term use respectively. For spot or short-term use, the researchers can estimate Ethanol in blood breath, and urine, EtG in urine and blood, FAEE in serum, PEtH in blood, EtS and EtP in urine and blood, TICS or β-carboline in urine or blood. For chronic long-term use, the researchers can estimate FAEE in hair and meconium, EtG in hair and meconium, cocoethylene in hair, acetaldehyde adducts of proteins in erythrocytes, in hair, and β-carboline in hair. Direct biomarkers can be sub-divided into spot or short-term use (5-HTOL/5HIAA) in urine. For chronic or long term use GGT in urine, ALT and AST in serum, MCV in blood, CDT in urine, sialic acid in serum, sialic acid index of serum apolipoproteins, β-hexosaminidase in the serum, and Methanol in blood, dolicohol in blood and urine.

Morphological Biomarkers of FAS It is known that not all women who consume Alcohol during pregnancy have children with FASD; as genetic factors, nutritional status, and basal metabolic index (BMI) can also play a significant role in Ethanol teratogenesis. However FASD comprises severe cognitive and structural birth defects including *short stature, small head, cleft lip/palate, small jaw, wide-set eyes, dental abnormalities, and digit abnormalities*. Interestingly, mutations in an inwardly rectifying potassium channel, Kir2.1, cause a similar birth defects as noticed in FASD. In other words, FASD phenocopies the traits conveyed by Kir2.1 mutations. Recently Bates, (2013) reported that Alcohol targets Kir2.1 to cause the birth defects associated with FASD. Clinical, genetic, biochemical, electrophysiological, and molecular evidence has also identified Kir2.1 as a molecular target for FASD development and therapeutic treatment. Furthermore, Downing et al. (2012) examined gene expression in embryos and placentae from C57BL/6J (B6) and DBA/2J (D2) mice following prenatal Alcohol exposure. B6 fetuses were susceptible to morphological malformations while D2 were relatively resistant. Affymetrix Mouse Genome 430 v2 microarray analysis exhibited altered expression of genes, involved in methylation, chromatin remodeling, protein synthesis, and mRNA splicing. Few genes were differentially expressed between Maltose-exposed tissues and tissues that did not receive Ethanol during intrauterine life. Gene classes up-or down-regulated in B6 were primarily involved in mRNA splicing, transcription, and translation. Several other genes were identified with altered expression, including specific for B6, a strain susceptible to Ethanol teratogenesis. Lack of strain-specific effects in D2, suggested that there are few gene expression changes that induce resistance.

Increasing body of evidence from neuroimaging studies on individuals with FASD has supported functional links between prenatal Alcohol exposure and neuromorphological deficits. Yang et al. (2012) collected the structural MRI data from 69 children and adolescents with FASD and 58 nonexposed controls from 3 sites using free surfer to detect cortical thickness changes across the entire brain in FASD and their associations with facial dysmorphology. Subjects with FASD exhibited thicker cortices than controls in frontal, temporal, and parietal regions. Analyses revealed differences in left inferior frontal cortex. In addition, increased inferior frontal thickness was correlated with reduced palpebral fissure length. Consistent with previous reports, findings of this study are supportive of regional increases in cortical thickness serving as a biomarker for impaired brain development in FASD. The associations between thickness and dysmorphic measures suggested that the severity of brain anomalies may be reflected by that of the face. Ocular defects have been reported in about 90% of children with FAS, including microphthalmia, loss of neurons in the retinal ganglion cell (RGC) layer, optic nerve hypoplasia, and dysmyelination. Estimations of the numbers of neurons in the ganglion cell layer and dorsolateral geniculate nucleus (dLGN), and a detailed analysis of RGC morphology were carried out in transgenic mice exposed to Ethanol during the early postnatal life. Dursun et al. (2011) performed a study in male and female transgenic mice expressing yellow fluorescent protein (YFP) under the control of Thy-1 (thymus cell antigen 1) regulator on a C57 background. In the Alcohol exposure group, out of 13 morphological parameters examined in RGCs, soma was significantly reduced and dendritic tortuosity increased. A decrease in total dendritic field area and an increase in the mean branch angle were also observed. Interestingly, RGC dendritic elongation and a decrease in the spine density were observed in the IC group, as compared to Ethanol-exposed and control subjects. There were no significant effects of Alcohol exposure on total retinal area, suggesting that early postnatal Ethanol exposure affects development of the visual system, reducing the numbers of neurons in the ganglion cell layer and in the dLGN, and altering RGCs' morphology. VandeVoort et al. (2011) performed an *in vitro* study on rhesus monkey ESC lines (ORMES-6 and ORMES-7) which were treated with different concentrations of Ethanol, Estradiol, or Acetaldehyde with or without Estradiol for 4 weeks. Although control ESCs remained unchanged, abnormal morphology in the Ethanol and Acetaldehyde groups was observed before two weeks of treatment. Immunofluorescence staining biomarkers (TRA-1-81 and alkaline phosphatase) indicated a loss of ESC pluripotency in the 1.0% Ethanol group. ORMES-7 was more sensitive to the deleterious effects of Ethanol than ORMES-6. Estradiol increased sensitivity to Ethanol in the ORMES-6 and ORMES-7 cell line. The morphological changes and labeling for pluripotency, proliferation, and apoptosis demonstrated how Ethanol influences the development of cells in culture and their differentiation suggesting that the effects of Ethanol may be mediated through metabolic pathways regulating Acetaldehyde formation, however the molecular mechanism of accentuation by Estradiol in some cases is yet to be determined. Furthermore, Ethanol exposure on gestational day (GD) seven, in the mice has been shown to result in ventromedian forebrain deficits along with facial anomalies of FAS. Morphological changes in the forebrains of Ethanol-exposed embryos included cerebral hemispheres that were too close in proximity or rostrally united, enlarged foramina of Monro or united lateral ventricles, and hippocampal and ventromedian forebrain deficiency. In GD 12.5 control and Ethanol-exposed embryos, *in situ* hybridization employing probes for Nkx2.1 or Fzd8 to distinguish the preoptic area and medial ganglionic eminences (MGEs) from the lateral ganglionic eminences, confirming the selective loss of ventromedian tissues. Immunohistochemical labeling of oligodendrocyte progenitors with Olig2, a transcription factor necessary for their specification, and of GABA showed Ethanol-induced reductions. Furthermore, Godin et al. (2011) investigated delayed consequences of ventromedian forebrain loss, MGE-derived somatostatin-expressing interneurons in the sub-pallial region of GD 17 fetal mice. *Somatostatin-expressing interneurons were dysmorphic in the Ethanol-exposed fetuses. Morphological biomarkers including facial abnormalities, micrognathia, small lip size, reduced frontal lobe development, and reduced eye blinking, observed in FAS are illustrated* in Figure 14.

Neurological Biomarkers of FAS *In general, typical neurological biomarkers of FAS include mental retardation, reduced memory retention, slow learning, abnormal behavior, reduced intelligence, and aggressive behavior as illustrated in* Figure 15. *In-vivo* neuroimaging studies have focused primarily on Alzheimer's disease (AD), pediatric brain cancer, and FAS, in addition to mapping the normal brain. Such efforts necessitate coordination of image data collection protocols, ontology development, computational requirements, data archiving, and sharing. Multicenter neuroimaging trials, consortia, and collaborations enabled the acquisition of large-scale datasets that can be used to predict clinical outcomes as well as guide in selecting treatment options for FAS (Van Horn and Toga., 2009). The symptoms of FAS include neurological and immunological dysfunctions that are linked to cell reduction. Neural stem cells (NSC) and hematopoietic stem cells (HSC) may be targets for the cytotoxic effects of Ethanol. Furthermore, protein kinase C (PKC) signal transduction systems may be involved in Ethanol-induced cell death. Hao et al. (2003) exposed CD34+ human fetal liver HSC and CD133+/nestin+ human NSC to 0.1-10 mM Ethanol. Classic and novel PKC isozyme protein expressions in the membrane fraction of cells were differentially affected by EtOH. Concentrations of EtOH capable of inducing NSC, but not HSC death also changed apoptosis-associated PKC isozyme expression in NSC, but not in HSC. Thus, PKC expression may mediate the susceptibility of NSC to Ethanol-induced cytotoxicity via signal transduction pathways. The toxic effect of Ethanol on NSC may lead to decreased neural cell number in FAS indicating that the susceptibility of NSC is not simply due to their being stem cells. This also indirectly explains the relative lack of hematopoietic problems associated with FAS.

Morphological Biomarkers of FAS

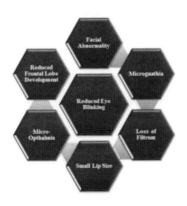

Figure 14. *Clinical biomarkers of FAS*: Clinical biomarkers can be divided into following catagories: (i) Anatomical biomarkers (ii) Developmental biomarkers (iii) Behavioral biomarkers (iv) Neurological biomarkers, and (v) impaired handwriting as illustrated in this diagram.

Typical Neurological Biomarkers of FAS

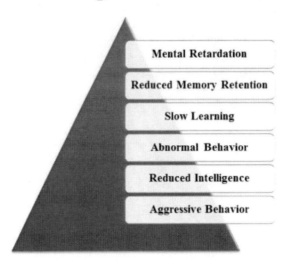

Figure 15. *Neurological biomarkers of FAS*: In general neurological biomarkers of FAS are mental retardation, reduced memory retention, slow learning, abnormal behavior, and reduced intelligence and aggressive behavior as illustrated in this diagram.

Molecular Biomarkers of FAS The molecular pathogenesis of FAS has not been well elucidated. In a previous study, Lee et al. (1997) performed mRNA differential display analyses to identify potential biomarkers for FAS. Out of ~1,080 mRNA transcripts in mouse embryos, the levels of three mRNAs were altered. Two of these mRNAs (one novel and one encoding HSP-47) were also modulated by another teratogen, 3-Methylcholanthrene. The third mRNA, encoding α-Tropomyosin, was specifically up-regulated by Ethanol. The level of α-Tropomyosin protein (31 kDa), a brain specific isoform was elevated in the Ethanol-exposed embryos. Several well-known medications, such as Aspirin, Cimetidine, and Ranitidine, interact with Alcohol metabolism leading to a higher level of blood Alcohol concentration (BAC) (*Baraona et al. 1994; Fraser 1998; Gentry et al. 1999*). Given that BAC is a reliable predictor of the severity of Alcohol-mediated brain injury in preclinical studies, any drug that interferes with Alcohol metabolism and results in an increase in BAC may be a cofactor in increasing Alcohol-mediated damage (Bonthius and West 1988, 1990). In another example, Johnson et al. (1991) showed that cigarette smoking reduces peak BAC in humans, and preclinical studies supported these findings (Gilbertson and Barron 2005; Parnell et al. 2006). Although decreasing BAC in the presence of Nicotine may suggest a smaller deleterious effect from Alcohol to experience "high" from Alcohol or to drink to the point of inebriation, this decrease in BAC may promote additional Alcohol abuse, which may lead to an accumulation of Acetaldehyde, a toxic metabolite of Alcohol that exerts further damage to the developing fetus. Ismail et al. (2010) reviewed the teratogenic effects of Alcohol, strategies for detecting maternal Alcohol consumption, identification of fetal biomarkers, and prevention measures for FAS. Furthermore, Roehsig et al. (2010) developed a method for the determination of eight FAEEs as potential biomarkers (Ethyl laurate, Ethyl myristate, Ethyl palmitate, Ethyl palmitoleate, Ethyl stearate, Ethyl oleate, Ethyl linoleate and Ethyl arachidonate) in meconium samples using GC-MS. FAEEs could be detected in Alcohol-exposed newborns and in some non-exposed newborns, yet the concentrations were lower than those measured in exposed cases. Previous studies in C57BL/6J and C57BL/6N mice provide evidence that Alcohol-induced pathogenesis follows early changes in gene expression within specific molecular pathways in the developing embryo. Dutta et al. (2008) used a murine model to screen amniotic fluid for biomarkers to discriminate between FAS-positive and FAS-negative pregnancies. B6J and B6N litters were treated with Alcohol (exposed) or saline (control) on day 8 of gestation. Amniotic fluid was subjected to Trypsin digestion for the analysis by matrix-assisted laser desorption-time of flight mass spectrometry. Multidimensional protein identification system detected reduced peaks to α-Fetoprotein (AFP). Traves et al. (2007) estimated serum biomarkers to determine the structural integrity of the intestine in response to exposure to Ethanol in utero which reduced apoA-IV levels in serum at birth, regardless of body weight, suggesting that circulating apoA-IV could be used as a clinical biomarker of FAS. In addition Barr et al. (2005) reported that rodents that are prenatally exposed to Ethanol exhibit a wide range of cognitive deficits, including impairments in memory, attention, and executive function. To determine a molecular substrate for cognitive dysfunction in adulthood, these investigators measured presynaptic proteins complexin I and II in a rat model of FAS. Prenatal exposure to Ethanol did not alter presynaptic proteins in the hippocampus or Synaptophysin in the prefrontal cortex. However, rats prenatally exposed to Ethanol displayed significantly reduced Complexin I and II in the prefrontal cortex compared to control animals, indicating a selective loss of complexin in the frontal cortex. These proteins are important for activity-dependent neurotransmission and mediate synaptic plasticity and cognition. In an earlier study Lee et al. (1997) determined the molecular mechanisms underlying Alcohol-induced ocular anomalies in Xenopus embryos which were exposed to various concentrations of Alcohol, and the subsequent effects on eye development and biomarker gene expression. In addition, Peng et al., (2004) investigated the role of reactive oxygen species (ROS) and reactive nitrogen species (RNS) in FAS-associated ocular injury, by using two antioxidant enzymes, Catalase and Peroxiredoxin 5, which were over-expressed in the blastomeres of the two-cell stage Xenopus embryos. Exposure of Xenopus embryos to Alcohol caused marked ocular anomalies, including microphthalmia, incomplete closure of the choroid fissure, and malformation of the retina. Alcohol reduced the expression of several eye biomarker genes, of which TBX5, VAX2, and Pax6 were highly vulnerable. Overexpression of Catalase and of cytosolic and mitochondrial Peroxiredoxin 5 restored the expression of these biomarkers and decreased the frequency of ocular malformation. These enzymes also reduced Alcohol-induced ROS production, but only Peroxiredoxin 5 inhibited RNS formation suggesting that both oxidative and nitrative stresses contribute to Alcohol-induced fetal ocular injury.

Meconium Biomarkers of FAS *The biomarkers of FAS that can be detected from the meconium include: fatty acid ethyl ester, (ii) ethyl glucronate, (iii) phosphatidyl Ethanolamine (iv) and ethyl sulphate.* Their estimation can provide a reliable measure of Alcohol consumption during pregnancy as these are quite stable and can be estimated even after 2-3 months of delivery as presented in Figure 16. Thon et al. (2013) reported that in addition to self-reports and questionnaires, biomarkers are of relevance in the diagnosis and therapy for Alcohol abuse disorders. Traditional biomarkers such as γ-Glutamyl transpeptidase (GGT) or mean corpuscular volume (MCV) are indirect and are subject to the influence of age, gender, and non-Alcohol related diseases, whereas Ethyl glucuronide (EtG), Ethyl sulphate (EtS) and Phosphatidyl-ethanol (PEth) are direct metabolites of Ethanol that are positive only after Ethanol intake; hence represent useful diagnostic tools for identifying

Alcohol abuse more accurately than traditional biomarkers. Each of these biomarkers remains positive in serum and urine for a considerable length of time after the cessation of Ethanol intake. Their application include routine clinical use, emergency room settings, proof of abstinence in Alcohol rehabilitation programs, driving under the influence, workplace testing, assessment of Alcohol intake in the context of liver transplantation and FAS. Due to these unique properties, these biomarkers open up new avenues for prevention, interdisciplinary collaboration, diagnosis, and therapy for Alcohol-related disorders. Natekar et al. (2012) studied all cases where both chronic Cocaine and Alcohol consumption, and determined values of hair Cocaine, Benzoylegconine (BE), CE, and FAEEs as biomarker of chronic Alcohol consumption. Cocaine and BE concentrations were associated with increased FAEE. Positive hair CE results had high specificity for chronic excessive Alcohol consumption among Cocaine users. Thus with no established safe level of Alcohol in pregnancy, identification of CE in hair of pregnant women who use Cocaine can serve as a biomarker for FASD.

Since pregnant women tend to underreport Alcohol drinking by questionnaires, a number of biomarkers have been proposed and evaluated for their capability to highlight gestational drinking behavior. These include classical biomarkers of Alcohol-induced pathology (MCV), GGT, AST and ALT, Acetaldehyde-derived conjugates, and derivatives of non-oxidative Ethanol metabolism (FAEEs, EtG, EtS, and PEth). Since Ethanol itself and Acetaldehyde can be measured few hours after Ethanol intake in blood, urine and sweat; they are only useful to detect recent Ethanol exposure. Joya et al. (2012) reviewed analytical procedures for the determination of these biomarkers during pregnancy and related prenatal Ethanol exposure. In addition, these investigators presented toxicological applications of their procedures. Increasing evidence indicates that neurons and glia are direct targets of Alcohol, but may also be vulnerable to molecules produced in peripheral systems as a result of Alcohol exposure. Diagnostics and therapies can take advantage of these processes and biomarkers, and these may be applicable to CNS pathology in FASD (Kane et al., 2012). In addition, Vagnarelli et al. (2011) performed a study to evaluate the experience, knowledge and confidence of Italian and Spanish neonatologists and pediatricians with respect to the diagnosis of FAS and FASD, and to evaluate awareness of maternal drinking patterns during pregnancy. Neonatologists and pediatricians rated confidence in the ability to diagnosis FAS and FASD as low, with over 50% responders felt the need for more knowledge regarding FAS and FASD identification in newborn and children. However they did not feel confident about accurately diagnosing FAS and FASD. Arose et al. (2011) prospectively identified heavily drinking pregnant women who consumed on average 4 or more drinks of Ethanol per day (≥ 48 g/day) and assessed growth in 69 of their offspring and an unexposed control group of 83 children, measuring serum IGF-I, IGF-II, IGF-binding protein 3 (IGFBP-3) and leptin. Exposure to Ethanol during pregnancy increased IGF-I and IGF-II and decreased leptin during early childhood suggesting that this hormone should be explored as a potential biomarker for prenatal Alcohol exposure. It has been also shown that Alcohol alters DNA methylation patterns and inhibits neural stem cell differentiation (Zou et al., 2011) whereas Emodin prevents Ethanol-induced developmental anomalies in cultured mouse fetus which requires further study (Yon et al., 2013).

Meconium Biomarkers of FAS

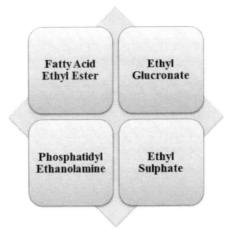

Figure 16. *Meconium Biomarkers of FAS*: This diagram illustrates various biomarkers of FAS which can be detected from the meconium. These include fatty acid ethyl ester, (ii) ethyl glucronate, (iii) phosphatidyl Ethanolamine (iv) ethyl sulphate.

Van Horn and Toga, (2009) reported that multicenter neuroimaging trials, consortia, and collaborations enable the acquisition of large-scale, purpose-driven datasets that can be used to model and predict clinical outcomes as well as guide clinicians in selecting treatment options for neurological disease. Furthermore, Cook (2003) reported that the classic biomarkers of Alcohol exposure, including blood/breath Alcohol, γ-glutamyl transferase (γ-GT), mean corpuscular volume (MCV), hemoglobin-associated acetaldehyde (HAA) and carbohydrate deficient transferrin (CDT), are valuable biomarkers for the early and accurate diagnosis of FAS. However confirmation of PAE is required as a diagnostic criterion for the children adversely affected by PAE who do not manifest the physical features associated with FAS. Bakhireva et al. (2013) performed a study to evaluate the feasibility and cost of PAE screening by measuring phosphatidyl-ethanol (PEth) in dried blood spot (DBS) cards. Specimens were sent for PEth analysis by liquid chromatography-tandem mass spectrometry. PAE screening by PEth in DBS was simpler and cost-effective and majority of infants had enough blood after the routine heel prick to fill an additional card. Joya et al. (2012) reviewed procedures for the determination of biomarkers during pregnancy and related prenatal exposure. They reported that fetal Alcohol disorders are preventable, but self-reported Alcohol consumption could be misleading and impede effective treatment. This study evaluated the relationship between blood PEth and Alcohol abuse in a sample of reproductive age women. The relationship between total Alcohol consumption and PEth was stronger in women with recent heavy drinking days. The relationship between drinking and PEth varied considerably between individuals, and sensitivity for a certain amount of drinking was low at a highly specific cutoff concentration. Hence PEth is a highly sensitive biomarker of moderate and heavy Alcohol consumption and may complement the use of self-report Alcohol screens when additional objective biomarkers of Alcohol abuse are needed. However, choosing a highly valid cutoff concentration for PEth to differentiate various levels of Alcohol consumption may not be feasible (Stewart et al., 2010).

Cord Blood Biomarkers of FAS

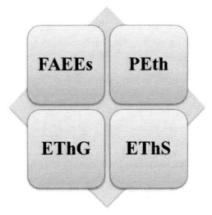

Figure 17. *Cord Blood Biomarkers of FAS*: This diagram illustrates various biomarkers of FAS which can be estimated from the cord blood. These include Fatty acid ethyl esters, phosphatidyl Ethanolamine, ethyl glucronate, and ethyl sulphate.

Cord Blood Biomarkers of FAS Accurate confirmation of PAE is required as a diagnostic criterion for the majority of children adversely affected by PAE who do not manifest the physical features associated with FAS. *Cord blood biomarkers of FAS can be detected and estimated. These include FAEEs, PEth, EThG, and EThS as presented* in Figure 17.

Omic Biomarkers of FAS Although several molecular and genetic biomarkers have been discovered, none of them is really selective. *Omics biomarkers of the FAS can be divided into (a) proteomic biomarkers (b) metabolomic biomarkers (c) lipidomic biomarkers (d) glycomic biomarkers and (e) genomic biomarkers as illustrated* in Figure 18.

Omic Biomarkers of FAS

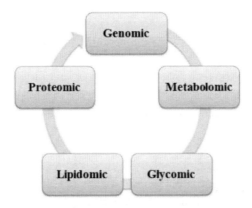

Figure 18. *Omic Biomarkers* A flow diagram illustrating various omic biomarkers including Proteomic biomarkers, (ii) metabolomics biomarkers (iii) Lipidomic biomarkers (iv) Glycomic biomarkers, and Genomic biomarkers.

In addition, urinary ethyl sulfate can be estimated to determine the severity of FAS.

Imaging Biomarkers of FAS *Imaging biomarkers of FAS include CT biomarkers, PET imaging biomarkers, (iii) MRI imaging and MR spectroscopy, and (iv) ultrasound imaging* as illustrated in Figure 19. Histological studies in animals characterized developmental cerebral cortical abnormalities that result from prenatal Ethanol exposure. Additionally, MRI identified abnormalities associated with fetal Ethanol exposure in the cerebral cortices of children and adolescents. Leigland et al. (2013) performed postmortem MRI experiments on rodents, during time periods relative to late human gestation through adulthood, to characterize anomalies associated with FASD throughout development. By determining how histologically identified abnormalities are manifested in MRI measurements specifically during the critical early time points, neuroimaging-based biomarkers of FASD can be identified at much earlier ages in humans, thus reducing the impact of these disorders. Cerebral cortical volume, thickness, and surface area were characterized by MRI in Long-Evans rat pups born from dams that were Ethanol-treated, maltose/dextrin-treated, or untreated throughout gestation at 6 developmental time points (1-60 days). Brain volume, isocortical volume, isocortical thickness, and isocortical surface area were reduced following prenatal exposure to Ethanol. Significant differences were observed throughout the range of time points studied. Additionally, regional patterns in cortical thickness differences suggested primary sensory areas that were particularly vulnerable to gestational Ethanol exposure. In earlier studies, Ikonomidou et al. (2000) reported that Ethanol treatment on postnatal day seven (P7) causes brain cell death and could be used as a model of late gestational Alcohol exposure. Adult mice that received P7 Ethanol had reduced total brain volume with multiple brain regions being reduced in both males and females. Immunohistochemistry indicated reduced frontal cortical parvalbumin immunoreactive (PV + IR) interneurons and Cux1+IR layer II pyramidal neurons. Biomarkers of adult hippocampal neurogenesis differed between sexes, with only Ethanol treated males showing increased Doublecortin and Ki67 expression in the dentate gyrus, with increased neurogenesis. However, Coleman et al. (2012) reported increased adult neurogenesis in males, but not in females, which is consistent with differential adaptive responses to P7 Ethanol toxicity between the sexes suggesting that one day of Ethanol exposure, e.g., P7, causes persistent adult brain dysmorphology.

In-Vivo Imaging Biomarkers of FAS

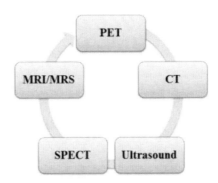

Figure 19. *Imaging Biomarkers of FAS*: This flow diagram illustrates imaging biomarkers of FAS which include CT biomarkers, PET imaging biomarkers, (iii) MRI imaging and MR spectroscopy, and (iv) Ultrasound imaging.

MRI and MRS as Theranostic Biomarkers of FAS In addition to MRI, high-resolution magnetic resonance spectroscopy (MRS) has provided a lead in our basic understanding of brain regional neurochemicals that are altered as a result of deleterious consequences of FAS in the developing brain. MRS biomarkers of FAS including N-Acetyl Aspartate, which is indicator of brain regional neuronal density; Choline, which is a precursor of the neurotransmitter, Acetyl Choline implicated in learning memory; and in the synthesis of Glycerophocholine involved in membrane synthesis; Glutamate, which is significantly reduced in FAS. Glutamate is a precursor for the synthesis of GABA, an inhibitory neurotransmitter, and Creatine is required for the high energy phosphate synthesis are reduced. Reduced Taurine, Glutathione, Myoinositol, and NMDA receptor excitotoxicity have also been discovered in the FAS. Moreover, Methionine-Homocysteine cycle may impact protein, DNA, and Histone methylation during FAS. Several other neurochemicals may be altered in FAS and can be estimated by magic angle spinning high resolution MRS analysis (*beyond the scope of this chapter*). *In addition, urinary analysis of ethyl sulphate can be made to further confirm FAS diagnosis.*

Domoate Neurotoxicity and its Relevance to FAS Ingestion of Domoic acid (DA)-contaminated seafood results in a severe neurotoxic disease known as amnesic shellfish poisoning (ASP). Clinical signs of ASP include seizures and neuronal damage from activation of iontropic glutamate receptors. Qiu et al. (2006) evaluated the contribution and temporal involvement of NMDA, non-NMDA and metabotropic-type Glutamate receptors (GluRs) in DOM-induced neuronal death using rat primary mixed cortical cultures. Co-application of antagonists for AMPA/kainite (NDQX) and NMDA-type GluRs (D-AP5) but not for metabotropic GluRs reduced DOM toxicity induced by either of three EC_{50} dose/duration paradigms. Maximal protection offered by D-AP-5 and NBQX either extended or not to the 30 to 60 min period after DOM exposure respectively. Antagonists were infective if applied with a 2-h delay, indicating the presence of a critical time window for neuronal protection after DOM exposure. Neuronal swelling was seen as early as 10 min post-DOM, which was linked to depolarization and release of endogenous Glutamate. The finding that NMDAR-mediated depolarization triggers release of endogenous Glutamate supports that DOM toxicity is regulated by iGluRs. In addition Lefebre et al. (2009) examined the transcriptome of whole brains from zebra fish receiving intracoelomic (IC) injection of DOM at both symptomatic and asymptomatic doses. A majority of zebra fish exhibited clinical signs of neuroexcitotoxicity within 5-20 min of IC injection. Microarray analysis yielded 306 differentially expressed genes represented by signal transduction, ion transport, and transcription factor function categories suggestive of neuronal apoptosis following induction of protective adaptive pathways. In addition, potential molecular biomarkers of neuropathic injury, including the zebrafish homologs of human NDRG4, were identified and were relevant to exposure below that causes neurobehavioral injury. Similar to Ethanol, DOM intoxication contributed to reproductive failure in Calforia sea lions (Goldstein et al., 2009). Furthermore, application of DOM to hippocampal slices produced a chemical form of long-term potentiation (LTP) of CA-1 field synaptic potentials that could not be blocked by NMDA antagonist MK-801 but could be blocked by Calcium-Calmodulin dependent protein kinase-II (CAMKII) (p-Thr286) or cAMP-dependent protein kinase (PKA) inhibitor H-89. Furthermore, DOM-potentiated slices exhibited decreased autophosphorylated CAMK-II (P-Thr286), the effect that is also dependent on the activity of CaMKII and PKA. In addition increased phosphorylation of α-Amino-3-Hydroxy-5-Methyl-4-Isozazole Propionic acid

(AMPA) receptor subunit GluR1 (p-Ser831) was observed in DOM-potentiated slices. Thus impaired regulation of CaMKII and GluR1 phosphorylation occurred after DOM application. However, Tetanus-induced LTP as well as increased phosphorylation of CaMKII (p-Thr286) were reduced in DOM-potentiated slices. Compared with brief exposure, slices recovering from prolonged exposure did not show potentiation or altered levels of CaMKII (p-Ther 286) or GluR (-Ser831). However, decreased phosphorylation of GluR1 and Ser845 was seen. The impairment of Tetanus LTP and misregulation of CaMKII and GluR1 phosphorylation may partially explain DOM neurotoxicity and underlie the molecular basis of memory deficit (Qiu et al., 2009). Furthermore, local microinjections of DOM into the hippocampus of rats produced degeneration of CA-1 and CA3 pyramidal neurons and dentate gyrus granule cells (Sutherland et al., 1990; Dakshinamurti et al., 1991, Sharma and Dakshinamurti, 1992; Dakshinamurti. et al., 1993). DOM-treated rats exhibited anterograde amnesia for spatial information in the Morris water Maze task. DOM microinjection in the hippocampal CA-3 region caused generalized bilateral electrical seizure discharge activity. Local hippocampal administration of GABA resulted in neuronal recovery from DOM-induced seizures. Other GABA inhibitors such as Picrotoxin and Pentylene Tetrazole also induce seizure activity in rats by inhibiting GABA ergic neurotransmission (Sharma and Ebadi 1993; Sharma et al., 1994). Intrauterine exposure to DOM caused selective loss of neurons in the hippocampal CA3 and dentate gyrus regions as noticed in patients with AD (Dakshinamurti et al., 1993). Recently Pérez-Gómez and Tasker (2013) reported evidence of cell proliferation and increased neurogenesis in rat hippocampal slice cultures (OHSC) after a transient excitotoxic injury to the hippocampal CA1 region induced by low concentrations of DOM. A study investigated the key intracellular pathways responsible for DOM-induced neurogenesis in OHSC including the effects of transient excitotoxicity on the expression of BDNF, a regulator of progenitor cell mitosis. However chronic intrauterine Ethanol exposure caused significant reduction in the serum BDNF levels. In addition, recent studies revealed that Somatostatin (SST) diminishes presynaptic Glutamate release by activating SST type-2 receptors (SST2R). SST exerts an anticonvulsant action in some experimental models of seizures. Kozhemyakin et al. (2013) studied the basic molecular mechanism of action of SST on excitatory synaptic transmission at the Schaffer collateral-CA1 synapses and the ability of SST to treat SE in rats using patch-clamp electrophysiology and video-EEG monitoring of seizures. SST reduced action potential-dependent EPSCs (sEPSCs) at Schaffer collateral-CA1 synapses at concentrations up to 1μM; higher concentrations had no effect or increased the sEPSC frequency. SST also prevented paired-pulse facilitation of evoked EPSCs and did not alter action-potential-independent miniature EPSCs (mEPSCs). The effect of SST on EPSCs was inhibited by the SST2R antagonist Cyanamid-154806 and was mimicked by the SST2R agonists, Octreotide and Lanreotide. Both SST and Octreotide reduced the firing rate of CA1 pyramidal neurons. Intracerebroventricular administration of SST, either attenuated Pilocarpine-induced SE or delayed first grade 5 seizure by 11min. Similarly, Octreotide or Lanreotide prevented or attenuated SE in >65% of animals. Compared to the Pilocarpine, Octreotide was highly potent in attenuating hippocampal stimulation-induced SE within 60 min of SE onset, suggesting that SST, through the activation of SST2Rs, diminishes presynaptic glutamate release and attenuates SE. In addition chronic supplementation of Taurine to mice ameliorated the age-dependent decline in memory acquisition and retention. Concomitant with the amelioration in cognitive function, Taurine caused alterations in the GABA-ergic and Somatonergic neurotransmission. These changes included increased GABA and Glutamate, increased expression of GAD and Somatostatin, decreased hippocampal β-2/3 subunits of the GABA$_A$ receptor expression, an increase in the number of Somatostatin-positive neurons, and amplitude and duration of population spikes from CA1 in response to Schaefer collateral stimulation and enhanced paired pulse facilitation in the hippocampus. These alterations of the inhibitory system oppose those naturally induced by aging, suggesting a protective role of Taurine. In addition, Shen et al. (2013) discovered that Taurine affects gene expression of various subunits of the GABA$_A$ receptors and GAD. Hence further studies to examine the effects of Taurine on gene expression will increase our understanding of age-related Taurine-mediated neurochemical changes in the GABA-ergic system that is impaired in FAS and will be important in elucidating the age-related decline in cognitive functions of FAS. Furthermore, FAS children suffer from ocular abnormalities including micro-opthalmia and reduced eye blinking which is currently assigned to impaired somatostanergic neurotransmission. Both CA1 pyramidal and SOM interneurons share a common cellular mechanism that leads to the learning-induced increased intrinsic excitability (McKay et al., 2013). Dong et al. (2013) determined the effects of Ginsenosides Rb1(GSRb1) on learning and memory and expression of Somatostatin (SS) in the hippocampus and frontal cortex in rat model of sleep deprivation (SD). GSRb1 enhanced the expression of Somatostatin in SD rats and subsequently improved their learning and memory abilities. Grigoriev et al. (2012) studied the effect of Somatostatin on presynaptic NMDA receptors and postsynaptic GABA, NMDA, and AMPA receptors in the rat brain. Somatostatin inhibited NMDA-induced $^{45}Ca^{2+}$ uptake into synaptosomes isolated from rat brain cortex, potentiated AMPA receptors, and inhibited hippocampal NMDA receptors; it also potentiated or inhibited GABA receptor currents suggesting that Somatostatin modulates the function of ionotropic Glutamate and GABA receptors and is involved in cognitive and neurodegenerative processes in the mammalian brain. Hence SOM may have neuromodulatory role in FAS which needs to be established further.

Hogberg et al. (2011) evaluated DOM-induced toxicity in immature and mature primary cultures of neurons and glial cells from rat cerebellum by measuring mRNA expression of selected genes. These investigators also assessed if the induced toxicity is mediated through activation of the AMPA/KA and/or the NMDA receptor. The expression of neuronal biomarkers was affected after DOM exposure in both immature and mature culture. However the mature culture seemed to be more sensitive to the treatment, as the effects were observed at lower concentrations and at earlier time points than the immature cultures. The DOM effects were completely prevented by the antagonist of AMPA/KA receptor (NBQX), while the antagonists of the NMDA receptor (AVP) partly blocked the DOM-induced effects. The DOM-induced effect was partly prevented by the neurotransmitter, GABA. DOM-exposure also affected the mRNA levels of the aBQX, AVP, and GABA. Although Ethanol neurotoxicity could be attenuated by NMDA receptor antagonist, MK-801; the doses required for neuroprotection were very high or even toxic.

Differential Toxicity of Ethanol Recent studies indicated that Ethanol specifically causes deleterious effect on the hippocampal progenitor cells as compared to hematopoietic stem cells. This could be due to early development of the hippocampus during intrauterine life as compared to hematopoietic stem cells or may be due to genetic and or intrinsic vulnerability of hippocampal progenitor cells, or due to the early development of NMDA receptors in this highly vulnerable region implicated in learning, intelligence, memory and behavior, those are impaired in the FAS victims. A further study is needed to establish the exact neurochemical role of Somatostatin, Synaptophysin, and BNDF in the hippocampal region of the FAS victims which will further improve our knowledge on the basic molecular mechanisms of memory consolidation in normal and FAS victims and possible strategies for its prevention and treatment.

Fetal Alcohol Syndrome and Depression It has been shown that women who drink heavily and who borne children with FASD are likely to have heavy drinking in their families of origin and procreation and also in their peer groups (May et al. 2009). Moreover depression is the most common complaint among mothers of children with FASD (Flynn and Chermack 2008; Rubio et al. 2013; Henderson et al., 2013). Mothers of FASD children in some countries use other drugs in addition to Alcohol. Smoking and drinking among mothers of FASD children may also affect the mood. The researchers recommended tryptophan-rich diet to alleviate symptoms of depression as it occurs due to brain regional depletion of Serotonin (Faisal et al., 2013). As such 5-HT cannot pass through the blood brain barrier. However its precursor, tryptophan can easily pass through the blood brain barrier, which in the presence of Pyridoxine (Vitamin-B_6) facilitates the synthesis of brain regional 5-HT by decarboxylation of 5-Hydroxy Tryptophan. Hence diet rich in Tryptophan and Vitamin B_6 may alleviate various symptoms of depression particularly in pregnant women consuming Alcohol. Very few studies are as yet available in this direction.

Neuroprotective and Therapeutic Strategies of FAS Recently the researchers have recommended some neuroprotective and therapeutic strategies for the clinical management of FAS. *These include Thiamine, Vitamin B_6, Folate, Choline, Octanol, MK-801, and Antioxidants such as Zinc, Glutathione and Vitamin C, Vitamin D, and Vitamin E*, which may alleviate neurobehavioral symptoms of FAS by acting as free radical scavengers. In adults, chronic abuse of Alcohol may cause *Vernicke's syndrome characterized by confabulations; however Thiamine (Vitamin B_1) can ameliorates these symptoms*. (*A detailed description of the neuroprotective and therapeutic strategies of FAS is beyond the scope of this chapter*). The researchers discovered Charnoly Body (CB) formation in the developing undernourished rat cerebellar Purkinje neurons due to degeneration of mitochondria (Sharma et al. 20013 a,c). Charnoly bodies are electron-dense multi-lamellar (usually penta or hepta-lamellar) structures that are formed in the developing Purkinje cell dendrites as a consequence of free radical generation due to undernutrition during intrauterine and early postnatal life. Simultaneously low molecular weight, Cysteine-rich, metal binding (Zn^{2+}) proteins, Metallothioneins (MTs) are induced during Ethanol intoxication and in the developing undernourished brain to provide neuroprotection by acting as free radical scavengers and by inhibiting CB formation (Sharma et al., 2013a, Sharma et al., 2013b). Hence CB formation may be considered as an early biomarker of FASD. CB formation is a reversible transitory stage between apoptosis and neurodegeneration and can be prevented by nutritional rehabilitation. Keen et al. (2010) suggested that moderate deficiencies of a single nutrients, such as Zn can act as a permissive factor for FASD and that adequate nutritional status or through exogenous supplementation may provide protection from the deleterious effects of FAS. Furthermore, these investigators proposed multiple mechanisms that underlie the teratogenicity of Ethanol. MTs may provide neuroprotection in genetically-engineered mice models of other neurodegenerative disorders including PD, AD, and aging (Ebadi et al., 2005; Sharma and Ebadi, 2014). However detailed studies regarding their exact role in FAS remains unknown. Further studies in this direction may help in the discovery of innovative biomarkers to provide better opportunities for the early differential diagnosis of FASD, their prevention, and/or successful EBPT.

MICROCEPHALY IN DEVELOPING BRAIN

The author proposed that fetal Alcohol expsure, Zinc deficiency, heavy metal ions (Lead, Mercury) environmental toxins, and/or Zika viral infection alone or in combination induce CB formation in the neuronal cells in utero to causes microcephaly in the developing human brain. CB was discovered in the developing undernourished rat cerebellar Purkinje neurons (Sharma and Ebadi, 2014) and in the intrauterine Domoic acid-exposed mice hippocampal and hypothalamic neurons (Sharma, 2014). The incidence of CB is increased with the severity of nutritional and environmental neurotoxic insult. Recently the researchers reported CB as a universal biomarker of cell injury and as a novel diagnostic biomarker in nanomedicine and chronic drug addiction (Sharma et al, 2013; Sharma, 2015). CB is also observed in the cellular and animal models of fetal Alcohol syndrome, PD, AD, vascular dementia, chronic drug addiction, and intrauterine exposure to environmental neurotoxins including, KA, Domoic acid, Acromelic acid, PCBs and lead (Sharma et al., 2014, Jagtap et al., 2015). At the ultrastructural level, CB appears as a pleomorphic, electron-dense multi-lamellar, quasi-crystalline, stack of degenerated mitochondrial membranes causing progressive neurodegeneration in the highly vulnerable neurons of the developing brain and may be induced by Zika virus infection during intrauterine life from the infected parents. CB is a pre-apoptotic biomarker of compromised mitochondrial bioenergetics which is formed in the most vulnerable cell in response to nutritional stress, environmental toxins, and/or drug of abuse as described above due to free radical overproduction and mitochondrial genome down-regulation. Accumulation of CB at the junction of axon hillock impairs axoplasmic flow in the synaptic terminals causes cognitive impairment, early morbidity, and mortality in chronic malnutrition and drug addiction (Sharma et al.,, 2015; Chabenne et al., 2015). Early event in CB formation including: $\Delta\Psi$ collapse, down-regulation of mitochondrial ubiquinone-NADH-oxidoreductase, and 8-OH-2dG can be detected as CB rudiments to evaluate clinical symptoms of acute drug addiction as epigenetic modulators of DNA methylation and histone acetylation as a consequence of fetal Alcohol exposure and/or Zika virus infection. During chronic phase, CB can be detected at the ultrastructure level. Antioxidants such as MTs, inhibit CB formation as free radical scavengers by regulating zinc-mediated transcriptional activation of genes involved in growth, proliferation, differentiation, and development as the researchers established in gene-manipulated human dopaminergic (SK-N-SH and SHY5Y) cells and in mouse models of neurodegeneration and multiple drug abuse. Hence novel drugs may be developed to prevent Zika virus-induced CB formation or enhance charnolophagy as an efficient molecular mechanism of intracellular detoxification during acute phase and novel CB antagonists may be developed to avert microcephaly by employing CB as an early, sensitive and specific biomarker to detect, prevent and effectively treat Zika Virus infection-induced or other forms of microcephaly.

Zika virus is a mosquito-transmitted infection related to dengue, yellow fever and West Nile virus. Currently, it remains unknown how Zika virus infection causes microcephaly which was first detected in Pernambuco (Brazil) in May 2015. By November 2015, Zika virus infection was declared as a health emergency in Brazil and currently there is no vaccine available against its infection. The C.D.C. advised pregnant women to avoid going to regions where Zika virus is being transmitted. Travelers were advised to prevent mosquito bites by staying in screened or air-conditioned rooms or sleep inside the mosquito nets, apply insect repellent and wear long pants, long sleeves, shoes, and hats. No specific antiviral medication has been recommended for people infected with the Zika virus. The symptoms usually require rest, nourishment and other supportive care. The newborns should be tested for infection with the Zika virus, if their mothers have visited in any country experiencing an outbreak and if the mothers' own tests are positive. Zika virus infection may be associated with visual and auditory defects, even if the child does not suffer microcephaly. The new guidance applies only to infants of mothers who report symptoms of Zika virus infection — a rash, joint pain, red eyes, or fever — while living abroad in an affected country or within two weeks of travel to these places.

About 62 locations mostly in the Caribbean, Central America and South America have been affected by Zika virus infection. The children exposed to Zika virus infection may become burden to society rest of their life. It is now proposed that Zika virus-induced CB formation in the developing brain may enhance free radical overproduction due to mitochondrial oxidative and nitrative stress to cause lipid peroxidation which induce structural and functional breakdown of polyunsaturated fatty acids in the highly vulnerable developing plasma membranes and enhances further neurodegeneration. Hence novel drugs may be developed to inhibit CB formation during acute phase and augment charnolophagy during chronic phase of Zika virus infection as a basic molecular mechanism of intracellular detoxification for the normal growth and development of embryonic brain and avert the deleterious consequences of Zika virus infection as described earlier. Zika virus-infected pregnant mother may be treated by providing nutritional rehabilitation and antioxidant-rich well-nourished Alcohol-free diet to prevent CB formation implicated in microcephaly in the developing brain. CB sequestration during chronic untreated phase may induce further neurodegeneration by releasing Cytochrome C, Caspases and apoptosis-inducing factors from the degenerating mitochondrial membranes due to peroxynitrite ($ONOO^-$) ion stress. ROS-mediated lipid peroxidation of mitochondrial membranes causes down-regulation of microRNA, involved in the transcriptional regulation of ubiquinone-NADH –Oxidoreductase (Complex-1), which is the rate limiting enzyme complex involved in electron transport chain during ATP synthesis. Furthermore, mitochondrial membrane transorter (TSPO: 18KDa protein) involved in cholesterol transport impairs steroid hormones synthesis including dihydroepindiaterone, testosterone, estrogen, and progesterone involved in not only mitochondrial membrane stabilization, but also lysosomal membranes in the cell. CB formation is also accompanied with down-regulation of outer mitochondrial membrane enzymes, monoamine oxidase-A and monoamine oxidase-B involved in the regulation of 5-HTergic and NEergic, and DA-ergic neurotransmission in the brain as described in author's recent book "Monoamine Oxidase Inhibitors "Clinical Pharmacology, Benefits, and Potential Health Risks" published by Nova Science Publishers, New York, U.S.A. Moreover, it is well known that Ethanol enhances mitochondrial monoamine oxidases to facilitate depletion of brain regional 5-HTergic and DA-ergic neurotransmission. Hence proper nutrition, sanitary conditions, and abstinence from drugs of abuse (*particularly Nicotine, Ethanol*) can prevent and/or minimize Zika virus-induced CB formation to have children with normally-developed brain. The most important strategy should be to maintain environmental protection by eradicating the mosquito growth particularly in the Caribbean and tropical regions globally, in addition to nutrition and healthy life style avoiding drugs of abuse such as Ethanol and tobacco during pregnancy. Some women should get blood tests, and all should get ultrasound scans.

It is now known that mosquitoes of the Aedes species, which can breed in a small pools of water and usually bite during the day, disseminate Zika infection. Although the yellow fever mosquito, Aedes aegypti spread most Zika cases, mosquito is common in the US only in Florida, along the Gulf Coast, and in Hawaii – although it has been found in Washington, D.C., in hot weather. The Asian Aedes albopictus, is also known to transmit the virus, but it is uncertain how efficiently. Although the virus is spread by mosquitoes, there has been one report of possible spread through blood transfusion and one of possible spread through sex. The virus has been detected in the semen. Although it was discovered in the Zika forest in Uganda in 1947 and in Africa and Asia, it did not spread in the Western Hemisphere until last May, when an outbreak occurred in Brazil. Some may have immune defenses against the virus, so it is spreading rapidly. The WHO warned that the Zika virus is spreading in the Americas and that as many as 4 million people could be infected by the end of this year. CDC advised pregnant women against travel to ~30 countries, mostly in the Caribbean and Latin America, where the outbreak is increasing.

Microcephaly is rare, and may have several other causes including: infection of the fetus with rubella (German measles), cytomegalovirus or toxoplasmosis (cat-litter disease); poisoning of the fetus by Alcohol, Mercury or radiation; or severe maternal malnutrition and diabetes. It is also caused by several gene mutations, including Down syndrome, in addition to Zika virus infection. It has circulated in the same regions as dengue and chikungunya, and compared to those two painful infections – nicknamed "break-bone fever" and "bending-up fever" – Zika was usually mild. The virus might have reached Asia from Africa at least 50 years ago. However, the exact cause still remains unknown. In 2013, French Polynesia doctors confirmed 42 cases of *Guillain-Barrê syndrome*, which can cause paralysis. The CDC guidelines are complex—and may change. In general, pregnant women who have visited any area with Zika transmission should consult a doctor. Those who have had symptoms of infection like fever, rash, joint pain and bloodshot eyes during their trip or within two weeks of returning should have a blood test for the virus. Even women with no symptoms may have been infected—80% of those who get the virus do not feel ill — and there is no evidence that babies are hurt only when the mother is apparently ill. Tests for the virus itself only work in the first week or so after infection. Tests for antibodies can be done later, but they may yield false positives if the woman has had dengue, yellow fever or even a yellow fever vaccine. Pregnant women who have been to affected regions–whether they have symptoms or not, and whether they have negative or positive blood tests–should eventually have an ultrasound scan to see if their fetuses are developing microcephaly or calcification of the skull. Unfortunately, an ultrasound cannot detect microcephaly before the end of the second trimester. Some women also should have amniocentesis to test the fluid around the fetus for Zika virus. But amniocentesis involves piercing the amniotic sac with a long needle through the abdomen; it is slightly risky for the fetus and is not recommended before 15 weeks of gestation. Several pharmaceutical companies are working on rapid tests for the detection of Zika virus infection. The C.D.C. also distributes test kits and training materials to state health departments during outbreaks. The Pan American Health Organization believes that the virus will spread locally in every country in the Americas except Canada and Chile. In ~15% of cases, a small head is just a small head, and there is no effect on the infant. But in the remainder of cases, the infant's brain may not have developed properly during pregnancy or may have stopped growing in the first years of life. These children may experience developmental delays, intellectual deficits or hearing loss in addition to genetic abnormalities. Microcephaly can also be triggered by infections of the fetus, including German measles (also known as rubella), toxoplasmosis (a disease caused by a parasite, often in cat feces) and cytomegalovirus. Microcephaly may also result if a pregnant woman consumes Alcohol, zinc deficient, is severely malnourished, or has diabetes. If the defect occurs in a child's first years, it may be a result of a brain injury during labor. There is no treatment for microcephaly. "There is no way to fix the problem, just therapies to deal with the downstream consequences. Simultaneous infection with other viruses, may be contributing to the rise; hence Zika virus may not be the main cause, although currently evidence suggests that it is. It remains unknown how common microcephaly has become in Brazil's outbreak. About 3 million babies are born in Brazil each year. About 150 cases of microcephaly are reported, and it has reported ~4,000 cases.

The researchers discovered that dopamine metabolites, DOPAC and HVA are neurotoxic and induce apoptosis in cultured dopaminergic neuron by augmenting free radical-induced mitochondrial degeneration and eventually augmenting CB formation implicated in apoptosis and progressive neurodegeneration. MTs are low molecular weight (6-7kDa) cysteine-rich, zinc-binding antioxidant proteins that provide neuroprotection by storing, buffering, and donating zinc ions. MTs provide coenzyme Q_{10} and zinc-mediated transcriptional activation of genes involved in growth, proliferation, and differentiation, which is inhibited during fetal alcohnol exposure and/or microbial infection. In neurodegenerative disease, MTs inhibit CB formation by serving as free radical scavengers. The most promising diagnostic biomarker is the analysis of α-synuclein in the CSF samples. However, α-synuclein concentrations may be modulated by several other disease-modifying agents (Sharma and Ebadi, 2003; Sharma et al., 2013b; Sharma and Ebadi, 2013; Arain et al., 2013).

Charnoly Body-Mediated Microcephaly

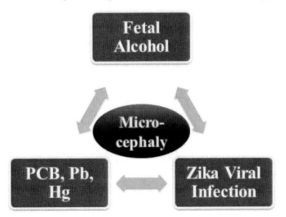

Figure 20. *Charnoly Body-Mediated Microcephaly* A pictorial diagram representing risk factors involved in Charnoly body-mediated microcephaly. Various risk factors including (i) fetal Alcohol, environmental neurotoxins (poly-chlorobiphynyls: PCBs, lead: Pb, and mercury, Hg), and Zika viral infection alone or in combination can induce Charnoly Body (CB) formation in the developing neuronal cells in utero to cause apoptosis, and eventually microcephaly in the new born child. Early environmental protection, personal hygiene, well-nourished diet, and antioxidants can prevent microcephaly.

It is proposed that *in-vitro* estimation of α-Synuclein index (SI) and ex-vivo detection of CB formation may further facilitate confirming diagnosis of Zika virus infection at early stages of disease onset and implementing proper therapeutic interventions. Attention is now turning to stratification of Zika virus infection into certain at-risk groups defined by genotype. The application of multimodality biomarker screening to these populations may be more beneficial. Since CB formation as a pre-apoptotic hallmark of compromised mitochondrial bioenergetics is now well-established; it can be used as an early diagnostic biomarker of Zika virus-induced or other risk factor-induced microcephaly and novel drug discovery during early phase to enhance charnolophagy during chronic phase and facilitate early clinical management of Zika Virus infection and its deleterious effects in the developing brain due to microcephaly. Peripheral platelets and lymphocytes of Zika virus infected mothers may facilitate detecting CB formation. Recent studies emphasized the involvement of CB in the genetic predisposition to neurodegenerative disorders and cancer (Li et al., 2014), in Aβ deposition (Zhang et al, 2015), and the therapeutic potential of MTs as potent antioxidants, anti-apoptotic, and anti-inflammatory factors to prevent CB sequestration which will further facilitate developing new diagnostic as well as therapeutic strategies for personalized treatment of Zika virus-induced microcephaly as well as numerous other neurodegenerative disorders of unknown etiopathogenesis (Yamamoto et al., 2015). Furthermore, discovery of novel CB-targeted biomarkers may provide better personalized treatment and association between fetal Alcohol exposure and/or Zika Virus-induced microcephaly and neurodegeneration in the developing brain as proposed in this chapter. *Various risk factors including (i) fetal Alcohol, environmental neurotoxins (poly-chlorobiphynyls: PCBs, lead: Pb, and mercury, Hg), and Zika viral infection alone or in combination can induce CB formation in the developing neuronal cells in utero to cause apoptosis, and eventually microcephaly in the new born child. Early environmental protection, personal hygiene, well-nourished diet, and antioxidants, in addition to personalized intrauterine diagnosis during first trimester of pregnancy could prevent microcephaly as illustrated in Figure 20.*

CONCLUSION

Alcohol consumption during any phase of pregnancy is deleterious. Alcohol induces most significant deleterious effects during first trimester (gastrulation period) of pregnancy, which may be further complicated with intrauterine exposure to environmental toxins and/or microbial infections including different viral infections. Differential diagnosis of FAS is still a challenge. Hippocampal Somatostatin and BDNF are reduced in FAS. Particuarly hippocampal neuronal progenitor cells are highly susceptible to Ethanol. It is proposed that Zika virus infection in utero compromises mitochondrial bioenergetics to enhance free radical overproduction and lipid peroxidation. These deleterious events induce CB formation in the highly vulnerable developing neurons and induce apoptosis to cause early neurodegeneration and microcephaly. Early therapeutic interventions to inhibit CB formation by nutritional rehabilitation, physiological zinc supplementation, antioxidants, and healthy life-style choices (including personal and environmental hygiene) may go a long way in the prevention and/or treatment of microcephaly induced due to intrauterine Alcohol abuse, toxins, and/or microbial infections.

REFERENCES

Aros, S., Mills, J. L., Iñiguez, G., Avila, A., Conley, M. R., Troendle, J., Cox, C. & Cassorla, F. (2011). Effects of prenatal Ethanol exposure on postnatal growth and the insulin-like growth factor axis. *Horm Res Paediatr.*, *75*, 166-173.

Bakhireva, L. N., Savich, R. D., Raisch, D. W., Cano, S., Annett, R. D., Leeman, L., Garg, M., Goff, C. & Savage, D. D. (2013). The feasibility and cost of neonatal screening for prenatal Alcohol exposure by measuring phosphatidylEthanol in dried blood spots. *Alcohol Clin Exp Res.*, *37*, 1008-1015.

Baraona, E., Gentry, R. T. & Lieber, C. S. (1994). Bioavailability of Alcohol: role of gastric metabolism and its interaction with other drugs. *Digestive Disorders*, *12*, 351–367.

Barr, A. M., Hofmann, C. E., Phillips, A. G., Weinberg, J. & Honer, W. G. (2005). Prenatal Ethanol exposure in rats decreases levels of complexin proteins in the frontal cortex. *Alcohol Clin Exp Res.*, *29*, 1915-1920.

Bates, E. A. (2013). A potential molecular target for morphological defects of fetal Alcohol syndrome: Kir2.1. *Curr Opin Genet Dev.*, *23*, 324-329.

Bonthius, D. J. & West, J. R. (1988). Blood Alcohol concentration and microencephaly: A dose-response study in the neonatal rat. *Teratology*, *37*, 223–231.

Bonthius, D. J. & West, J. R. (1990). Alcohol-induced neuronal loss in developing rats: increased brain damage with binge exposure. *Alcoholism: Clinical And Experimental Research*, *14*, 107–118.

Buske, C. & Gerlai, R. (2011). Early embryonic Ethanol exposure impairs shoaling and the dopaminergic and serotoninergic systems in adult zebrafish. *Neurotoxicol Teratol.*, *33*, 698-707.

Chabenne, A., Moon, C., Ojo, C., Khogali, A., Nepal, B. & Sharma, S. (2015). Biomarkers in Fetal Alcohol Syndrome (Recent Update) *Biomarkers and Genomic Medicine*, *6*, 12-22.

Coleman, L. G., Jr. Oguz, I., Lee, J., Styner, M. & Crews, F. T. (2012). Postnatal day 7 Ethanol treatment causes persistent reductions in adult mouse brain volume and cortical neurons with sex specific effects on neurogenesis. *Alcohol.*, *46*, 603-612.

Cook, J. D. (2003). Biochemical markers of Alcohol use in pregnant women. *Clin Biochem.*, *36*, 9-19.

Cudd, T. A. (2008). Animal models for studying fetal Alcohol syndrome, Alcohol related birth defects, and Alcohol related neurodevelopmental disorders. Source Book for *Models for Biomedical Research*. Ed. P.M. Conn, Humana Press. P 603.

Dakshinamurti, K., Sharma, S. K. & Geiger, J. D. (2003). Neuroprotective actions of pyridoxine. *Biochim Biophys Acta.*, *1647*, 225-229.

Dakshinamurti, K., Sharma, S. K. & Sundaram, M. (1991). Domoic acid induced seizure activity in rats. *Neurosci Lett.*, *127*, 193-197.

Dakshinamurti, K., Sharma, S. K., Sundaram, M. & Watanabe, T. (1993). Hippocampal changes in developing postnatal mice following intrauterine exposure to domoic acid. *J Neurosci.*, *13*, 4486-4495.

Dong, J., Wang, J., Fang, J., Feng, R., Yuan, Z., Lu, K., Jin, Y. & Zeng, L. (2013). [Effects of ginsenosides Rb1 on learning and memory and expression of somatostatin in sleep deprivation rats]. *Zhejiang Da Xue Xue Bao Yi Xue Ban.*, *42*, 197-204.

Downing, C., Flink, S., Florez-McClure, M. L., Johnson, T. E., Tabakoff, B. & Kechris, K. J. (2012). Gene expression changes in C57BL/6J and DBA/2J mice following prenatal Alcohol exposure. *Alcohol Clin Exp Res.*, *36*, 1519-1529.

Downing, C., Flink, S., Florez-McClure, M. L., Johnson, T. E., Tabakoff, B. & Kechris, K. J. (2012). Gene expression changes in C57BL/6J and DBA/2J mice following prenatal Alcohol exposure. *Alcohol Clin Exp Res.*, *36*, 1519-1529.

Dursun, I., Jakubowska-Doğru, E., van der List, D., Liets, L. C., Coombs, J. L. & Berman, R. F. (2011). Effects of early postnatal exposure to Ethanol on retinal ganglion cell morphology and numbers of neurons in the dorsolateral geniculate in mice. *Alcohol Clin Exp Res.*, *35*, 2063-2074.

Dutta, S., Turner, D., Singh, R., Ruest, L. B., Pierce, W. M. Jr. & Knudsen, T. B. (2008). Fetal Alcohol syndrome (FAS) in C57BL/6 mice detected through proteomics screening of the amniotic fluid. *Birth Defects Res A Clin Mol Teratol.*, *82*, 177-186.

Ebadi, M., Brown-Borg, H., Garrett, S., Singh, B., Shavali, S. & Sharma, S. (2005). Metallothionein-Mediated Neuroprotection in genetically-Engineered Mice Models of Parkinson's Disease and Aging. *Molecular Brain Res.*, *134*, 67-75.

Faisal, S., Patel, A., Mattison, C., Bose, S., Krishnamohan, R., Sweeney, E., Sandhu, S., Nel, W., Rais, A., Sandhu, R., Ngu, N. & Sharma, S. (2013). Effect of diet on, serotonergic neurotransmission in depression. *Neurochemistry International.*, *62*, 324-329.

Falk, D., Yi, H. Y. & Hiller-Sturmhöfel, S. (2006). An epidemiologic analysis of co-occurring Alcohol and tobacco use and disorders: Findings from the National Epidemiologic Survey on Alcohol and Related Conditions. *Alcohol Research & Health*, *29*, 162–171.

Falk, D., Yi, H. Y. & Hiller-Sturmhöfel, S. (2008). An epidemiologic analysis of co-occurring Alcohol and drug use and disorders: Findings from the National Epidemiologic Survey on Alcohol and Related Conditions (NESARC). *Alcohol Research & Health*, *31*, 100–110.

Farooq, M. U., Bhatt, A. & Patel, M. (2009). Neurotoxic and cardiotoxic effects of Cocaine and Ethanol. *Journal of Medical Toxicology*, *5*, 134–138.

Flynn, H. A. & Chermack, S. T. (2008). Prenatal Alcohol use: the role of lifetime problems with Alcohol, drugs, depression, and violence. *J. Stud. Alcohol Drugs.*, *69*, 500-509

Fraser, A. G. (1998). Is there an interaction between H2-antagonists and Alcohol? *Drug Metabolism and Drug Interactions*, *14*, 123–145.

Gentry, R. T., Baraona, E., Amir, I., et al. (199). Mechanism of the aspirin-induced rise in blood Alcohol levels. *Life Science*, *65*, 2505–2512.

Gilbertson, R. J. & Barron, S. (2005). Neonatal Ethanol and Nicotine exposure causes locomotor activity changes in preweaning animals. *Pharmacology, Biochemistry, and Behavior*, *81*, 54–64.

Godin, E. A., Dehart, D. B., Parnell, S. E., O'Leary-Moore, S. K. & Sulik, K. K. (2011). Ventromedian forebrain dysgenesis follows early prenatal Ethanol exposure in mice. *Neurotoxicol Teratol.*, *33*, 231-239.

Godin, E. A., O'Leary-Moore, S. K., Khan, A. A., Parnell, S. E., Ament, J. J., Dehart, D. B., Johnson, B. W., Allan Johnson, G., Styner. M. A. & Sulik, K. K. (2010). Magnetic resonance microscopy defines Ethanol-induced brain abnormalities in prenatal mice: effects of acute insult on gestational day 7. *Alcohol Clin. Exp. Res.*, *34*, 98-111.

Goldstein, T., Zabka, Y. S., Ddelong, R. L., Wheeler, E. A., Yiltalo, G., Bargu, S., Silver, M., Leighfield, T., Van Dolah, F., Langlois, G., Sidor, I., Dunn, J. L. & Gulland, F. M. (2009). The role of domoic acid in abortion and premature parturition of Calfornia sea lions (Zalophus Californicus) on San Miguel island, California. *Journal of Wildlife Diseases.*, *45*, 91-108.

Grigoriev, V. V., Petrova, L. N., Gabrelian, A. V., Zamoyski, V. L., Serkova, T. P. & Bachurin, S. O. (2012). Effect of somatostatin on presynaptic and postsynaptic glutamate receptors and postsynaptic GABA receptors in the neurons of rat brain. *Bull. Exp. Biol. Med.*, *154*, 10-12.

Hao, H. N., Parker, G. C., Zhao, J., Barami, K. & Lyman, W. D. (2003). Differential responses of human neural and hematopoietic stem cells to Ethanol exposure. *J. Hematother. Stem Cell Res.*, *12*, 389-399.

Henderson, K. M., Clark, C. J., Lewis, T. T., Aggarwal, N. T., Beck, T., Guo, H., Lunos, S., Brearley, A., Mendes de Leon, C. F., Evans, D. A. & Everson-Rose, S. A. (2013). Psychosocial distress and stroke risk in older adults. *Stroke.*, *44*, 367-372.

Hoyme, H. E., May, P. A., Kalberg, W. O., et al. (2005). A practical clinical approach to diagnosis of fetal Alcohol spectrum disorders: Clarification of the 1996 Institute of Medicine Criteria. *Pediatrics*, *115*, 39–47.

Ikonomidou, C., Bittigau, P., Ishimaru, M. J., et al. (2000). Ethanol-induced apoptotic neurodegeneration and fetal Alcohol syndrome. *Science*, *287*, 1056–1060.

Ismail, S., Buckley, S., Budacki, R., Jabbar, A. & Gallicano, G. I. (2010). Screening, diagnosing and prevention of fetal Alcohol syndrome: is this syndrome treatable? *Dev Neurosci.*, *32*, 91-100.

Jagtap, A., Gawande, S. & Sharma, S. (2015). Biomarkers in Vascular Dementia (A Recent Update) *Biomarkers and Genomic Medicine*, *7*, 43-56.

Johnston, M. C. & Bronsky, P. T. (1991). Animal models for human craniofacial malformations. *J Craniofac Genet Dev Biol.*, *11*, 277-291.

Joya, X., Friguls, B., Ortigosa, S., Papaseit, E., Martínez, S. E., Manich, A., Garcia-Algar, O., Pacifici, R., Vall, O. & Pichini, S. (2012). Determination of maternal-fetal biomarkers of prenatal exposure to Ethanol: a review. *J Pharm Biomed Anal.*, *69*, 209-222.

Kane, C. J., Smith, S. M., Miranda, R. C. & Kable, J. (2012). Proceedings of the 2010 annual meeting of the Fetal Alcohol Spectrum Disorders Study Group. *Alcohol.*, *46*, 107-114.

Keen, C. L., Uriu-Adams, J. Y., Skalny, A., Grabeklis, A., Grabeklis, S., Green, K., Yevtushok, L., Wertelecki, W. W. & Chambers, C. D. (2010). The plausibility of maternal nutritional status being a contributing factor to the risk for fetal Alcohol spectrum disorders: the potential influence of zinc status as an example. *Biofactors.*, *36*, 125-135.

Kozhemyakin, M., Rajasekaran, K., Todorovic, M. S., Kowalski, S. L., Balint, C. & Kapur, J. (2013). Somatostatin type-2 receptor activation inhibits glutamate release and prevents status epilepticus. *Neurobiol Dis.*, *54*, 94-104.

Landgraf, M. N., Nothacker, M. & Heinen, F. (2013). Diagnosis of fetal Alcohol syndrome (FAS): German guideline version 2013. *Eur J Paediatr Neurol.*, *17*, 437-446.

Lee, I. J., Soh, Y. & Song, B. J. (1997). Molecular characterization of fetal Alcohol syndrome using mRNA differential display. *Biochem Biophys Res Commun.*, *240*, 309-313.

Lefebre, K. A., Tilton, S. C., Bammier, T. K. & Bever, R. P. (2009). Srinouanprachan S, Stapleton PL, Farin FM, Gallagher EP. Gene expression profiles in zebrafish brain after acute exposure to domoic acid at symptomatic and asymptomatic doses. *Toxiclological Sciences.*, 65-77.

Leigland, L. A., Ford, M. M., Lerch, J. P. & Kroenke, C. D. (2013). The influence of fetal Ethanol exposure on subsequent development of the cerebral cortex as revealed by magnetic resonance imaging. *Alcohol Clin. Exp. Res.*, *37*, 924-932.

Li, Z., Lin, Q., Ma, Q., Lu, C. & Tzeng, C. M. (2014). Genetic predisposition to Parkinson's disease and cancer. *Curr Cancer Drug Targets.*, *14*(3), 310-321.

Mao, H., Diehl, A. M. & Li, Y. X. (2009). Sonic hedgehog ligand partners with caveolin-1 for intracellular transport. *Lab Invest.*, *89*, 290-300.

Marrs, J. A., Clendenon, S. G., Ratcliffe, D. R., Fielding, S. M., Liu, Q. & Bosron, W. F. (2010). Zebrafish fetal Alcohol syndrome model: effects of Ethanol are rescued by retinoic acid supplement. *Alcohol.*, *44*, 707-715.

Mattson, S. N. & Riley, E. P. (2011). The quest for a neurobehavioral profile of heavy prenatal Alcohol exposure. *Alcohol Res Health.*, *34*, 51-55.

May, P. A., Gossage, J. P., Kalberg, W. O., et al. (2009). Prevalence and epidemiologic characteristics of FASD from various research methods with an emphasis on recent in-school studies. *Developmental Disabilities Research Reviews*, *15*, 176–192.

McKay, B. M., Oh, M. M. & Disterhoft, J. F. (2013). Learning increases intrinsic excitability of hippocampal interneurons. *J Neurosci.*, *33*, 5499-5506.

Memo, L., Gnoato, E., Caminiti, S., Pichini, S. & Tarani, L. (2013). Fetal Alcohol spectrum disorders and fetal Alcohol syndrome: the state of the art and new diagnostic tools. *Early Hum Dev.*, *89*, S40-S43.

Molina, J. C., Spear, N. E., Spear, L. P., Mennella, J. A. & Lewis, M. J. (2007). The International society for developmental psychobiology 39th annual meeting symposium: Alcohol and development: beyond fetal Alcohol syndrome. *Dev Psychobiol.*, *49*, 227-242

Natekar, A., Motok, I., Walasek, P., Rao, C., Clare-Fasullo, G. & Koren, G. (2012). Cocaethylene as a biomarker to predict heavy Alcohol exposure among Cocaine users. *J Popul Ther Clin Pharmacol.*, *19*, e466-472.

Nunez, C. C., Roussotte, F. & Sowell, E. R. (2011). Focus on: structural and functional brain abnormalities in fetal Alcohol spectrum disorders. *Alcohol Res Health.*, *34*, 121-31.

Olney, J. W., Wozniak, D. F., Farber, N. B., Jevtovic-Todorovic, V., Bittigau, P. & Ikonomidou, C. (2002). The enigma of fetal Alcohol neurotoxicity. *Ann Med.*, *34*, 109-119.

Parnell, S. E., Dehart, D. B., Willis T. A., et al. (2006). Maternal oral intake mouse model for fetal Alcohol spectrum disorders: Ocular defects as a measure of effect. *Alcoholism: Clinical and Experimental Research*, *30*, 1791–1798.

Parnell, S. E., O'Leary-Moore, S. K., Godin E. A., et al. (2009). Magnetic resonance microscopy defines Ethanol-induced brain abnormalities in prenatal mice: Effects of acute insult on gestational day 8. *Alcoholism: Clinical and Experimental Research*, *33*, 1001–1011.

Peng, Y., Yang, P. H., Guo, Y., Ng, S. S., Liu, J., Fung, P. C., Tay, D., Ge, J., He, M. L., Kung, H. F. & Lin, M. C. (2004). Catalase and peroxiredoxin 5 protect Xenopus embryos against Alcohol-induced ocular anomalies. *Invest Ophthalmol Vis Sci.*, *45*, 23-29.

Pérez-Gómez, A. & Tasker, R. A. (2013). Transient domoic acid excitotoxicity increases BDNF expression and activates both MEK- and PKA-dependent neurogenesis in organotypic hippocampal slices. *BMC Neurosci.*, *14*, 72.

Pulsifer, M. B. (1996). The neuropsychology of mental retardation. *J Int Neuropsychol Soc.*, *2*, 159-176.

Qiu, S., Jebelli, A. K., Ashe, J. H. & Curras-Collazo, M. C. (2009). Domoic acid induces long-lasting enhancement if CA-1 field responses and impairs tetanus-induced long-term potentiation in rat hippocampal slices. *Toxicological Sciences*, *111*, 140-150.

Qiu, S., PaK, C. W. & Curras-Collazo, M. C. (2006). Sequential involvement of distinct glutamate receptors in Domoic acid-induced neurotoxicity in rat mixed cortical cultures: Effect of multiple dose/Duration Paradigm, chronological age, and repeated exposure. *Toxicological Sciences.*, *89*, 243-256.

Roehsig, M., de Paula, D. M., Moura, S., Diniz, E. M. & Yonamine, M. (2010). Determination of eight fatty acid ethyl esters in meconium samples by headspace solid-phase microextraction and gas chromatography-mass spectrometry. *J Sep Sci.*, *33*, 2115-2122.

Rubio, J. M., Olfson, M., Villegas, L., Pérez-Fuentes, G., Wang, S. & Blanco, C. (2013). Quality of life following remission of mental disorders: findings from the National Epidemiologic Survey on Alcohol and Related Conditions. *J. Clin. Psychiatry.*, *74*, 445-450.

Sharma, S., Gawande, S., Jagtap, A., Abeulela, R. & Salman, Z. Fetal Alcohol Syndrome; Prevention, Diagnosis, & Treatment. In Alcohol Abuse: Prevalence, Risk Factors. Nova Science Publishers, New York, U.S.A. 2015.

Sharma, S., Moon, C. S., Khogali, A., Haidous, A., Chabenne, A., Ojo, C., Jelebinkov, M., Kurdi, Y. & Ebadi, M. (2013). Biomarkers in Parkinson's disease (recent update). *Neurochem. Int.*, *63*, 201-229.

Sharma, S., Rais, A., Sandhu, R., Nel, W. & Ebadi, M. (2013). Clinical significance of metallothioneins in cell therapy and nanomedicine. *Int J Nanomedicine.*, *8*, 1477-1488.

Sharma, S. K., Bolster, B. & Dakshinamurti, K. (1994). Picrotoxin and pentylene tetrazole induced seizure activity in pyridoxine-deficient rats. *J. Neurol. Sci.*, *121*, 1-9.

Sharma, S. & Ebadi, M. (2008). SPECT Neuroimaging in Translational Research of CNS Disorders. *Neurochem. Internat.*, *52*, 352-362.

Sharma, S. & Ebadi, M. (2014). Significance of Metallothioneins in Aging Brain. *Neurochemistry International.*, *65*, 40-48.

Sharma, S. (2014). Molecular Pharmacology of Environmental Neurotoxins. In Kainic Acid: Neurotoxic Properties, Biological Sources, and Clinical Applications. Nova Science Publishers. New York. P1-47.

Sharma, S. (2014). Nanotheranostics in Evidence Based Personalized Medicine. *Current Drug Targets.*, *15*, 915-930.

Sharma, S. & Ebadi, M. (2013). Antioxidant Targeting in Neurodegenerative Disorders. Ed. I. Laher, Springer Verlag. Germany. Chapter 85, p. 1-30.

Sharma, S. & Ebadi, M. (2014). Charnoly body as a Universal Biomarker of Cell Injury. *Biomarkers and Genomic Medicine*, *6*, 89-98.

Sharma, S., Moon, C. S., Khogali, A., Haidous, A., Chabenne, A., Ojo, C., Jelebinkov, M., Kurdi, Y. & Ebadi, M. (2013). Biomarkers of Parkinson's Disease (Recent Update). *Neurochemistry International.*, *63*, 201-229.

Sharma, S. K. & Dakshinamurti, K. (1992). Seizure activity in pyridoxine-deficient adult rats. *Epilepsia.*, *33*, 235-47.

Sharma, S. K. & Dakshinamurti, K. (1993). Suppression of domoic acid induced seizures by 8-(OH)-DPAT. *J Neural Transm Gen Sect.*, *93*, 87-98.

Sharma, S. K. & Ebadi, M. (2003). Metallothionein attenuates 3-morpholinosydnonimine (SIN-1)-induced oxidative stress in dopaminergic neurons. *Antioxid Redox Signal.*, *5*, 251–264.

Shen, C. H., Lempert, E., Butt, I., Neuwirth, L. S., Yan, X. & El, Idrissi, A. (2013). Changes in gene expression at inhibitory synapses in response to taurine treatment. *Adv Exp Med Biol.*, *775*, 187-194.

Single, E., Ashley, M. J., Bondy, Rankin, S. J. & Rehm, J., (2000). Evidence Regarding the Level of Alcohol Consumption Considered to be Low-Risk for Men and Women. *Australian Commonwealth Department of Health and Aged Care Final Report.*, Vol 6, pp. 1-76.

Sowell, E. R., Johnson, A., Kan, E., Lu, L. H., Van Horn, J. D., Toga, A. W., O'Connor, M. J. & Bookheimer, S. Y. (2008). Mapping white matter integrity and neurobehavioral correlates in children with fetal Alcohol spectrum disorders. *J. Neurosci.*, *28*, 1313-1319.

Stewart, S. H., Law, T. L., Randall, P. K. & Newman, R. (2010). PhosphatidylEthanol and Alcohol consumption in reproductive age women. Alcohol *Clin Exp Res.*, *34*, 488-492.

Sutherland, R. J., Hoesing, J. M. & Whishaw, I. Q. (1990). Domoic acid, an environmental toxin, produces hippocampal damage and severe memory impairment. *Neuroscience Letters.*, *120*, 221–223.

Thon, N., Weinmann, W., Yegles, M., Preuss, U. & Wurst, F. M. (2013). [Direct Metabolites of Ethanol as Biological Markers of Alcohol Use: Basic Aspects and Applications.] *Fortschr Neurol Psychiatr.*, *81*(9), 493-502.

Través, C., Coll, O., Cararach, V., Gual, A., de Tejada, B. M. & López-Tejero, M. D. (2007). Clinical approach to intestinal maturation in neonates prenatally exposed to Alcohol. *Alcohol Alcohol.*, *42*, 407-412.

Ullah, I., Ullah, N., Naseer, M. I., Lee, H. Y. & Kim, M. O. (2012). Neuroprotection with metformin and thymoquinone against Ethanol-induced apoptotic neurodegeneration in prenatal rat cortical neurons. *BMC Neurosci.*, *19*, 13, 11.

Vagnarelli, F., Palmi, I., García-Algar, O., Falcon, M., Memo, L., Tarani, L., Spoletini, R., Pacifici, R., Mortali, C., Pierantozzi, A. & Pichini, S. (2011). A survey of Italian and Spanish neonatologists and paediatricians regarding awareness of the diagnosis of FAS and FASD and maternal Ethanol use during pregnancy. *BMC Pediatr.*, *11*, 51.

Van Horn, J. D. & Toga, A. W. (2009). Multisite neuroimaging trials. *Curr Opin Neurol.*, *22*, 370-378.

VandeVoort, C. A., Hill, D. L., Chaffin, C. L. & Conley, A. J. (2011). Ethanol, acetaldehyde, and estradiol affect growth and differentiation of rhesus monkey embryonic stem cells. Alcohol *Clin Exp Res.*, *35*, 1534-1540.

Vaurio, L., Crocker, N. & Mattson, S. N. (2010). Fetal Alcohol spectrum disorders. In: Davis, A.S., ed. The Handbook of Pediatric Neuropsychology. New York: Springer Publishing Company, pp. 877–886.

Yamamoto, T., Uchiyama, T., Higuchi, Y., Asahina, M., Hirano, S., Yamanaka, Y., et al. (2015). Subthalamic Nucleus Deep Brain Stimulation Modulate Catecholamine Levels with Significant Relations to Clinical Outcome after Surgery in Patients with Parkinson's Disease. *PLoS ONE*, *10*(9).

Yang, Y., Phillips, O. R., Kan, E., Sulik, K. K., Mattson, S. N., Riley, E. P., Jones, K. L., Adnams, C. M., May, P. A., O'Connor, M. J., Narr, K. L. & Sowell, E. R. (2012). Callosal thickness reductions relate to facial dysmorphology in fetal Alcohol spectrum disorders. *Alcohol Clin Exp Res.*, *36*, 798-806.

Yang, Y., Roussotte, F., Kan, E., Sulik, K. K., Mattson, S. N., Riley, E. P., Jones, K. L., Adnams, C. M., May, P. A., O'Connor, M. J., Narr, K. L. & Sowell, E. R. (2012). Abnormal cortical thickness alterations in fetal Alcohol spectrum disorders and their relationships with facial dysmorphology. *Cereb Cortex.*, *22*, 1170-1179.

Yon, J. M., Lin, C., Oh, K. W., Baek, H. S., Lee, B. J., Yun, Y. W. & Nam, S. Y. (2013). Emodin prevents Ethanol-induced developmental anomalies in cultured mouse fetus through multiple activities. *Birth Defects Res B Dev Reprod Toxicol.*, *98*, 268-275.

Zhang, S., Lei, C., Liu, P., Zhang, M., Tao, W., Liu, H. & Liu, M. (2015). Association between variant amyloid deposits and motor deficits in FAD-associated presenilin-1 mutations: A systematic review. *Neuroscience & Biobehavioral Reviews*, *56*, 180–192.

Zhou, F. C., Balaraman, Y., Teng, M., Liu, Y., Singh, R. P. & Nephew, K. P. (2011). Alcohol alters DNA methylation patterns and inhibits neural stem cell differentiation. *Alcohol Clin. Exp. Res.*, *35*, 735-746.

Chapter 9

BIOMARKERS IN PERSONALIZED THERANOSTICS OF PARKINSON'S DISEASE

ABSTRACT

Early diagnosis of PD poses a significantly challenge, because typical clinical symptoms including body tremor, muscular rigidity, and postural irregularity appear very late when >60-80% nigrostriatal dopaminergic neurons are already destroyed. Although PET neuroimaging with ^{18}F-DOPA can provide quantitative estimate of loss of nigrostriatal neurons, and ^{18}FdG neuroimaging can provide information regarding brain regional mitochondrial bioenergetics, these noninvasibe *in-vivo* imaging modalities alone or in combination with other imaging modalities are still very costly and not easily accessible to the general public. Hence there is quest for the novel discovery of peripheral biomarker(s) which could be used for the successful EBPT of PD. In this chapter various basic and clinical presymptomatic and symptomatic biomarkers are described to differentially diagnose and treat PD patient. It is envisaged that these biomarkers may find their universal acceptance as specific biomarkers for the early personalized treatment of PD. Although some of the biomarkers such as hyposmia, hypogustia, depression, can be diagnosed early during disease progression, these are nonspecific and donot provide the exact estimate of disease progression/regression. (For more details please refer to author's recent publication: Sharma, S., Moon, C.S., Khogali, A., Haidous, A., Chabenne, A., Ojo, C., Jelebinkov, M., Kurdi, Y., Ebadi, M., 2013. Biomarkers of Parkinson's Disease (Recent Update). *Neurochemistry International. 63, 201-229*).

Keywords: nigrostriatal, dopaminerifc neurons, ^{18}F-DOPA, ^{18}FdG, peripheral biomarker

INTRODUCTION

Parkinson's disease (PD) is the second most common neurodegenerative disease affecting mostly the aging population over sixty. Although neuronal loss may occur early, cardinal symptoms, including tremors, muscle rigidity, drooping body posture, drooling, walking difficulty, and autonomic symptoms appear late when >60-65% nigrostriatal dopaminergic neurons are already destroyed. Neuroprotective therapy starting at such an 'advanced stage' may prove futile to halt the neurodegenerative process. Novel discovery of early, sensitive, specific, and economical biomarkers may facilitate early, non-invasive, and effective individualized treatment of PD. In this chapter various biomarkers, which can be used effectively for the personalized treatment of PD are described in brief.

Definition of A Biomarker A biomarker is a characteristic that can be measured and evaluated as an indicator of normal biological and pathogenic processes or pharmacologic responses to a therapeutic intervention. Biomarkers are used in: (a) confirmation of diagnosis (b) epidemiological screening, (c) predictive testing, (d) monitoring disease progression, (e) drug development, (f) evaluating response to treatment, and (g) elaborating brain–behavior.

Rationale of Biomarkers Research As describe above, >60% of the NS dopaminergic neurons are already destroyed before a neurologist can establish the diagnosis of idiopathic PD. Neuroprotective therapy at this 'advanced stage' may prove referectory to halt the degenerative process. Hence, identification of patients at risk at earlier stages is essential to accomplish therapeutic success. Early diagnosis of neurodegenerative disorders such as PD, AD, and MDD is extremely important to slowdown the progression of disease at initial stage. Novel diagnostic biomarkers for the early clinical management of PD are α-synuclein index, Charnoly body, and metallothioneins (MTs).

Definitions of a Biomarker Depending on the type of information provided, biomarkers can be classified as clinical, neuroimaging, biochemical, genetic or proteomic biomarkers. Biomarkers serve a wide variety of purposes, including confirmation of diagnosis, epidemiological screening, predictive testing, monitoring disease progression following diagnosis, drug development, response to treatment, and learning brain behavior. Modern therapeutic strategies for PD focus primarily on reducing the severity of symptoms using dopaminergic medications. However this approach has limited therapeutic potential for the clinical management of PD. Hence there is a dire need of specific and sensitive biomarkers discovery for PD to improve drug development related to the disease.

Classification of PD Biomarkers

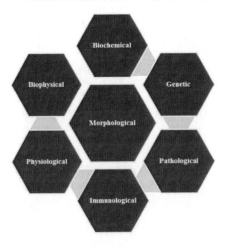

Figure 21. *Classification of PD Biomarkers* A diagrammatic representation of various PD biomarkers. In general, PD biomarkers can be divided into 7 major disciplines including: (i) Biochemical (ii) Biophysical, (iii) Genetic (iv) Pathological, (v) Immunological, (vi) Physiological, and (vii) Morphological.

Gerlich et al. (2012) suggested that the biomarker should be: linked to fundamental features of PD neuropathology and mechanisms underlying neurodegeneration in PD; correlated to disease progression as assessed by clinical rating scales; able to monitor the exact disease status; pre-clinically validated; confirmed by at least two independent investigators and results published in peer-reviewed journals; most important, inexpensive, non-invasive, simple to use, and technically validated. Reliable biomarkers can be used for early diagnosis, tracking disease progression, and development of effective treatments of PD. Presently there are no reliable biomarkers to detect early neurodegeneration in PD and monitor effects of drug candidates on the disease process. Some biomarker candidates seem promising, such as neuromelanin antibodies, pathological forms of α-Synuclein, DJ-1, gene expression pattern, metabolomics, and protein profiling. Parkinson's Progression Markers Initiative (PPMI) has been founded to tackle problems associated with the development of promising biomarkers that can be used for early diagnosis and evaluating disease progression.

The Michael J. Fox Foundation has initiated the step to identify clinical, imaging, and biological markers of PD. Initially the emphasis is being geared to fluid biomarkers including α-Synuclein, DJ-1, amyloid β, and tau in the CSF and Urate in the blood. This study is expected to enroll 400 newly diagnosed patients who are not yet on medication and who have evidence of dopamine transporter (DAT) loss on imaging with SPECT and 200 healthy age-matched controls. The acquired data and biological specimens, stored in a central repository will be available to the research community. The PPMI will provide a valuable resource to augment further academic and industry-initiated studies and innovations, and promising biomarker candidates. Eventually, well-defined biomarkers that are consistent in many labs will be established.

Biomarker Classification In general various biomarkers of PD can be divided into two major catagories; (i) premotor (preclinical); (ii) motor (clinical). These biomarkers can be further subdivided into two categories: (i) *in-vitro*; (ii) *in- vivo*. Based on the currently available information, PD biomarkers can be divided as (a) clinical (b) biochemical (c) biophysical (d) physiological (e) genetic (f) morphological (g) immunological, and (h) pathological categories as illustrated in Figure 21.

Biomarkers in PD Sharma et al. (2013) reported that PD is the second most common neurodegenerative disorder mostly affecting the aging population over sixty. Cardinal symptoms including, tremors, muscle rigidity, drooping posture, drooling, walking difficulty, and autonomic symptoms appear when a significant number of nigrostriatal dopaminergic neurons are already destroyed. Hence the researchers need early, sensitive, specific, and economical peripheral and/or central biomarker(s) for the differential diagnosis, prognosis, and treatment of PD. These can be classified as clinical, biochemical, genetic, proteomic, and neuroimaging biomarkers. Novel discoveries of genetic as well as nongenetic biomarkers may be utilized for the personalized treatment of PD during preclinical (premotor) and clinical (motor) stages. Premotor biomarkers including; hyper-echogenicity of substantia nigra, olfactory and autonomic dysfunction, depression, hyposmia, deafness, REM sleep disorder, and impulsive behavior may be noticed during preclinical stage. Neuroimaging biomarkers (PET, SPECT, MRI), and neuropsychological deficits can facilitate differential diagnosis. Single-cell profiling of dopaminergic neurons has identified pyridoxal kinase and lysosomal ATPase as biomarker genes for PD prognosis. Promising biomarkers include: fluid biomarkers, neuromelanin antibodies, pathological forms of α-Syn, DJ-1, amyloid β and tau in the CSF, patterns of gene expression, metabolomics, urate, as well as protein profiling in the blood and CSF samples. In addition, reduced brain regional N-acetyl-aspartate is a biomarker for the *in vivo* assessment of neuronal loss using magnetic resonance spectroscopy and T_2 relaxation time with MRI. To confirm PD diagnosis, the PET biomarkers include [^{18}F]-DOPA for estimating dopaminergic neurotransmission, [^{18}F]dG for mitochondrial bioenergetics, [^{18}F]BMS for mitochondrial complex-1, [^{11}C](R)-PK11195 for microglial activation, SPECT imaging with ^{123}IFlupane and βCIT for dopamine transporter (DAT), and urinary Salsolinol and 8-Hydroxy, 2-Deoxyguanosine for neuronal loss.

This chapter has described the merits and limitations of recently discovered biomarkers and proposed Coenzyme Q_{10}, mitochondrial Ubiquinone-NADH oxidoreductase, Melatonin, α-Synuclein index, Charnoly body, and MTs as novel biomarkers to confirm PD diagnosis for early and effective personalized treatment of PD. Pre-symptomatic clinical biomarkers, such as hypogustia and hyposmia are non-specific to early diagnose PD.

Lewy bodies PD is the second most common age-related neurodegenerative disorder with movement disorder and is characterized clinically by Parkinsonism and pathologically by selective loss of DAergic neurons in the substantia nigra, characterized by bradykinesia, postural instability, resting tremor, and rigidity. The neuropathological hallmark of PD is the existence of proteinaceous inclusions of α-Synuclein, known as Lewy bodies and Lewy neurites, in some of the remaining dopaminergic neurons. Overexpression of the wild type or mutant α-Synuclein affects the generation of new neurons in the hippocampal dentate gyrus in experimental models of PD. Point mutations in α-Synuclein, Parkin, and Ubiquitin was detected in sporadic PD population with or without Lewy body pathogenesis. Juvenile Parkinson's disease was noticed among juvenile Japanese with Parkin gene mutation; however Lewy body was absent in these patients, indicating that Lewy body may not be used as an exclusive theranostic biomarker of PD.

Depression in PD The incidence of depression is 40% among PD patients. Hippocampal dysfunction with reduced neurogenesis plays a significant role in the pathogenesis of depression, a non-motor symptom in PD. However, personalized antidepressant treatment in PD is still lacking. A study explored if impaired hippocampal neurogenesis in the A53T transgenic animal model of PD may be restored by oral administration of the selective serotonin reuptake inhibitor (SSRI), Fluoxetine. The expression of transgenic mutant A53T synuclein in developing dentate gyrus neurons and early expression of the transgene linked to a severely impaired neurogenesis was investigated. Fluoxetine increased neurogenesis in the hippocampus three fold in treated A53T mice compared to controls. The pro-neurogenic effect of chronic Fluoxetine was related to an increased proliferation of neural precursor cells in the DG, and to a lesser extent by induction of differentiation into mature neurons. Fluoxetine induced brain and glial cell-derived neurotrophic factor indicated potential of SSRI-dependent mechanisms to stimulate hippocampal neurogenesis in experimental models of α-Synuclein and may lead to improved neuropsychiatric symptoms of PD (Kohl et al., 2012).

Genetic Biomarkers It is now well-established that genetic mutations (duplications, triplications or missense mutations) in the α-Synuclein gene can lead to PD, but even in these patients, age-dependent physiological changes or environmental exposures appear to be involved in disease progression. In addition, autosomal dominant missense mutations in the gene for leucine-rich repeat kinase 2 (LRRK2/PARK8) have been recognized as a cause of PD. G2019S, the disease-causing mutant of LRRK2, has significant effects on the kinase activity of LRRK2:

1. Wild-type LRRK2 activity was inhibited by Manganese.
2. G2019S mutation abrogated this inhibition.

Based on these findings, it was reported that LRRK2 may be a sensor of cytoplasmic Manganese levels and that the G2019S mutant has lost this function. Hence dysregulation of neuronal Manganese homeostasis can play a crucial role in the etiology of PD. Furthermore, mutations in five genes [α-Synuclein (SNCA), Parkin, PTEN-induced kinase 1 (PINK1), DJ-1, Leucine-rich repeat kinase 2 (LRRK2)] account for 2-3% of all cases with parkinsonism, are clinically indistinguishable from idiopathic PD. The functional role of PINK1 and LRRK2 as kinases is now well-established, whereas mutations in the ATP13A2 gene have been linked to Kufor-Rakeb syndrome. ATP13A2 encodes lysosomal ATPase and exhibits increased expression of PARK9 in the brains of sporadic cases, suggesting a potential role in the idiopathic PD.

CSF Biomarkers of PD Three CSF biomarkers; total-tau (T-tau), phospho-tau (P-tau) and the 42 amino acid form of β-amyloid (Amyloid-β-42) have recently been discovered. These biomarkers have high sensitivity to differentiate early and incipient AD from normal aging, depression, Alcohol dementia, and PD, but lower specificity against other dementias, such as frontotemporal dementia and Lewy body dementia. If CSF biomarkers are used together with the information from the clinical examination, laboratory tests, and brain-imaging with SPECT and MRI, they may have a significant role in the clinical evaluation of MCI cases.

Recently, the impact of the transcription factor Sim1 in the differentiation of mDA and rostral serotonergic (5-HT) neurons *in vivo* has been explored using Sim1-/- mouse embryos and newborn pups, and *in vitro* by gain- and loss-of-function approaches. A selective reduction in the number of dorsal raphe nucleus (DRN) serotonergic (5-HT) neurons was noticed in Sim1-/- newborn mice. In contrast, serotonergic (5-HT) neurons of the raphe nuclei as well as dopaminergic neurons were not affected. In addition, the analysis of the underlying molecular mechanism revealed that tryptophan hydroxylase 2 (Tph2) and the transcription factor Pet1 are regulated by Sim1. Transcription factor Lhx8 and the modulator of 5-HT(1A)-mediated neurotransmitter release, Rgs4, exhibited increased expression in ventral hindbrain, compared to midbrain and are target genes of Sim1. These results demonstrated a selective transcription factor dependence of the serotonergic (5-HT) cell groups, and introduced Sim1 as a regulator of DRN acting upstream of Pet1 and Tph2. Moreover, Sim1 may act to modulate serotonin release via regulating RGS4 suggesting that subpopulations of neurotransmitter phenotype use distinct transcription factors to control the expression of shared properties.

A recent review has assessed the efforts in developing CSF biomarkers for AD and the status of CSF biomarker in schizophrenia, depression, PD and MS (Flood et al., 2011). Abnormally phosphorylated forms of the microtubule-associated protein, tau was found in the brains of AD patients. Tau could be detected in CSF, two assays based on well-defined monoclonal tau antibodies were developed to study these proteins in CSF. One assay detected normal and abnormal forms of tau (CSF-tau); the other was specific for phosphorylated tau (CSF-PHFtau). More than 88% of AD patients had a CSF-PHF tau value higher than the controls. This study demonstrated that elevated tau/PHF tau levels are noticed in CSF of AD patients. However, a considerable overlap existed with other forms of dementia, including

VAD and FLD. Hence CSF-tau and CSF-PHF tau may be useful biochemical markers to discriminate AD from normal aging, PD, and depressive pseudodementia.

General In Vitro Biomarkers of PD These biomarkers can be detected from CSF, blood, serum, plasma, and urine samples; by estimating DJ-1 concentration in the CSF, neuromelanin antibody, platelet complex-1 activity, urinary 8-OH-2dG, reduced CSF Glutathione-SH, α-Synuculein, Parkin, Ubiquitin, brain-derived neuronal factor (BDNF), Cytokines, Monoamines, Tetrahydroisoquinolines (TIQs: Salsolinol), plasma Homocysteine, Osteopontin, and Monoamine oxidase-B (MAOB).

The neurobehavioral biomarkers in PD are primarily, depression, hyposmia, hearing loss, micrographia, impaired handwriting, agraphia, loss of urinary bladder control, and impaired circadian rhythm which may appear early during PD progression as presented in Figure 22. The various clinical biomarkers of PD can be characterized by several clinical biomarkers, which may facilitate in the diagnosis of this devastating disease. The most important clinical biomarkers include: body tremor, falling, postural irregularities, drooling, bradykinesia, visiospatial and color discrimination, reduction in sympathetic skin response, walking difficulty, nocturia, incontinence, imcompitence, impaired circadian rhythm, anosmia, hypogustia, SMI deficit, Cardiac Sympathetic innervation, deafness, and muscle rigidity as illustrated in Figure 23. The early diagnosis of PD can be accomplished by performing the analyses of *in-vivo* imaging biomarkers. Clinically most significant *in-vivo* biomarkers of PD include: (i) PET biomarkers (^{18}F-DOPA), SPECT biomarkers (^{123}I-Iofupan, ^{123}I-CTI), sleep EEG, somnograhy, MRI, muscle action potential, ultrasonography (to determine striatal Iron levels) as illustrated in Figure 24. The most important *in vitro* PD biomarkers can be estimated from blood, CSF, and urine are (i) CSF α-Synuclein, CSF Glutathione, Parkin, BDNF, Ubiquitin, TIQ, Salsolinol, plasma homocysteine, monoamines, CSF ostopontin, CSF DJ-1, platelet complex-1 activity, neuromelanin antibody, urinary 8-hydroxy 2 deoxy guanosine, and cytokines as Figure 25 illustrates.

Neurobehavioral Biomarkers of PD

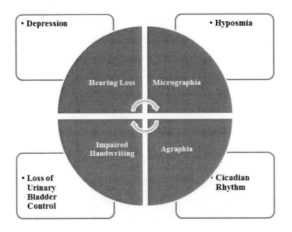

Figure 22. *Neurobehavioral Biomarkers in PD* The neurobehavioral biomarkers in PD are primarily, depression, hyposmia, hearing loss, micrographia, impaired handwriting, agraphia, loss of urinary bladder control, and impaired circadian rhythm which may appear early during PD progression.

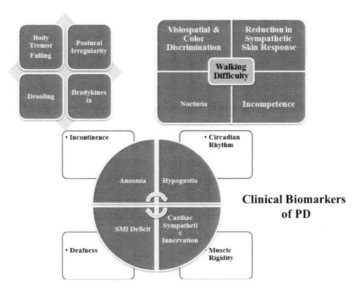

Figure 23. *Clinical Biomarkers of PD* Pictorial diagrams to illustrate various clinical biomarkers of PD. PD can be characterized by several clinical biomarkers, which may facilitate in the diagnosis of this devastating disease. The most important clinical biomarkers include: body tremor, falling, postural irregularities, drooling, bradykinesia, visiospatial and color discrimination, reduction in sympathetic skin response, walking difficulty, nocturia, incotinence, imcompitence, impaired circadian rhythm, anosmia, hypogustia, SMI deficit, cardiac sympathetic innervation, deafness, and muscle rigidity.

In-Vivo Biomarkers in PD

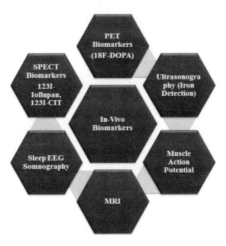

Figure 24. *In-Vivo Biomarkers of PD* A diagram illustrating biomarkers which can be used for the early diagnosis of PD by performing the analyses of *in-vivo* imaging biomarkers. Clinically most significant *in-vivo* biomarkers of PD include: (i) PET biomarkers ([18]Fd-DOPA), SPECT biomarkers (^{123}I-Iofupan, ^{123}I-CTI), sleep EEG, somnograhy, MRI, muscle action potential, ultrasonography (to determine striatal Iron levels).

In-Vitro Biomarkers of PD
(Blood, CSF, Saliva, Urine)

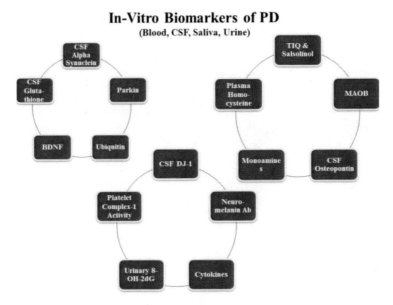

Figure 25. *In-Vitro Biomarkers of PD* Pictorial diagrams illustrating various *in-vitro* biomarkers of PD. The most important invitro PD biomarkers which can be estimated from blood, CSF, and urine are (i) CSF alpha synuclein, CSF Glutathione, Parkin, BDNF, Ubiquitin, TIQ, Salsolinol, plasma homocysteine, monoamines, SCF ostopontin, CSF DJ-1, platelet complex-1 activity, neuromelanin antibody, urinary 8-hydroxy 2 deoxy guanosine, and cytokines.

Omic Biomarkers in PD

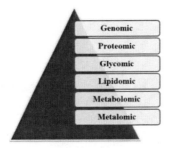

Figure 26. *Omic Biomarkers of PD* In general, omic biomarkers of PD can be characterized as: (a) genomic, (b) proteomic, (c) glycomic, (d) lipidomic, (e) metabolomics, (f) metalomic, which can be estimated from Fluid samples (blood, serum, plasma, CSF, saliva, and urine samples of a PD patient. There are primarily three major metabolites including: proteins, RNA, and DNA. The metabolomics biomarkers include: lipid, sugars, toxins etc. The determination of various proteins and their analyses is performed in proteomics, and genomic analyses include: DNA sequencing, next generation sequencing to detect single nucleotide polymorphism (SNPs), and microarray analyses.. Metalomic analyses of biological fluids (serum, plsmaa, CSF, urine) samples and brain biopsy samples can be performed by treating with 0.4N perchloric acid to exctract metal ions. The samples are homogenized and centrifuged to collect the supernatants, which are used to analyze metal ions, employing' atomic absorption spectrophotometer which can detect metal ions in part per billion. The main limitation of atomic absorption spectrometer is that the researchers require several electrical lamps as standards to quantitatively estimated the concentrations of each metal ion. Which is costly, time consuming, and cumbersome. Each time the electrical lamp is changed the settings and alignments are altered, which can pose a problem in the detection of accurate concentration in the biological samples. Inductively-coupled plasma mass spectrophotometer (ICP-MS) provides an accurate estimate of 34 metal ions in a biological samle of 10 ul within 20 min. Moreover this metod does not require any specialized training to prepare the sample. The ICP-MS estimation is matrix independent and does not require any extraction protocols. The argon plasma torch burns at 5000-7000°C. The sample at this extremely high temperature is dehydrated, atomized, and ionized within a fraction of a second for the detection of its ionization potential. The position of the ionization spectra identifies the metal ion and its peak estimates the concentration, which is estimated by compter analyses employing user-friendly computer software. The striatal Iron levels are 2.5 times high in the patients suffering from PD as compared to normal aging subjects of the same age.

In general, omic biomarkers of PD can be characterized as: (a) genomic, (b) proteomic, (c) glycomic, (d) lipidomic, (e) metabolomics, (f) metalomic, which can be estimated from fluid samples (blood, serum, plasma, CSF, saliva, and urine samples of a PD patient as illustrated in Figure 26. There are primarily three major metabolites including: proteins, RNA, and DNA. The metabolomics biomarkers include: lipid, sugars, toxins, etc. The determination of various proteins and their analyses is performed in proteomics, and genomic analyses include: DNA sequencing, next generation sequencing to detect single nucleotide polymorphism (SNPs), and microarray analyses. Metalomic analyses of biological fluids (serum, plasma, CSF, urine) samples and brain biopsy samples can be performed by treating with 0.4N perchloric acid to exctract metal ions. The samples are homogenized and centrifuged to collect the supernatants, which are used to analyze metal ions, employing' atomic absorption spectrophotometer which can detect metal ions in parts per billion. The main limitation of atomic absorption spectrometer is that the researchers require several electrical lamps as standards to quantitatively estimate the concentrations of each metal ion. Which is costly, time consuming, and cumbersome. Each time the electrical lamp is changed the settings and alignments are altered, which can pose a problem in the detection of accurate concentration in the biological samples. Inductively-coupled plasma mass spectrophotometer (ICP-MS) provides an accurate estimate of 34 metal ions in a biological sample of 10 ul within 20 min. Moreover this method does not require any specialized training to prepare the sample. The ICP-MS estimation is matrix independent and does not require any extraction protocols. The argon plasma torch burns at 5000-7000°C. The sample at this extremely high temperature is dehydrated, atomized, and ionized within a fraction of a second for the detection of its ionization potential. The position of the ionization spectra identifies the metal ion and its peak estimates the concentration, which is estimated by computer analyses employing user-friendly computer software. The striatal Iron levels are 2.5 times high in the patients suffering from PD as compared to normal aging subjects or the same age. The lipidomic biomarkers of PD can be analyzed by lipidomics analyses including: lipid isolation, lipid analyses, pathway analyses of lipids, to eventually determine the precise lipid-protein interactions. Usually gas chromatography is employed to conduct lipidomic analyses as illustrated in Figure 27. The pathological biomarkers of PD can be divided into five major parts. These are α-Synuclein index (which is a ratio of nitrative α-Synulclein vs native α Synuclein), Charnoly body formation, Lewy body formation, striatal Iron accumulation to assess the loss of nigrostriatal DA-ergic neurons as shown in Figure 28. The neuroprotective biomarkers of PD can be various antioxidants including: Glutathione, Melatonin, Coenzyme Q10, Metallothionein, Ubiquinone NADH oxidoreductase (a rate limiting enzyme complex-1 for the oxidative phosphorylation in electron transport chain, and neuromelanin, which can be estimated to determine the severity of PD progression. In general, the nigrostriatal concentration of these neuroprotective antioxidant biomarkers is significantly reduced in PD patients as shown in Figure 29. A patient suffering from PD is trapped in a vicious circle of (a) depression (b) sleep disorders. Usually REM sleep is significantly impaired in PD patients and they suffer from a triad accompanied with depression, sleep disturbance, and nocturia as illustrated in Figure 30.

Lipidomic Biomarkers in PD

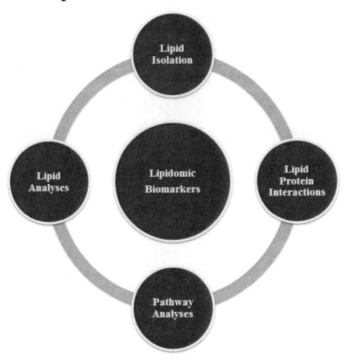

Figure 27. *Lipidomic Biomarkers of PD* A diagram illustrating lipidomic biomarkers of PD those are analyzed by lipidomics analyses including: lipid isolation, lipid analyses, pathway analyses of lipids, to eventually determine the precise lipid-protein interactions. Usually gas chromatography is employed to conduct lipidomic analyses.

Pathological Biomarkers in PD

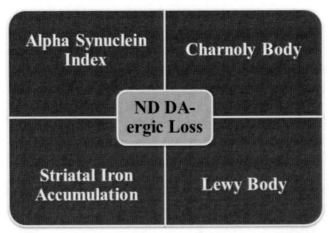

Figure 28. *Pathological Biomarkers of PD* A diagram illustrating pathological biomarkers of PD which can be divided into five major parts. These are alpha Synuclein index (which is a ratio of nitrative alpha synulclein vs native alpha synuclein), Charnoly body formation, Lewy body formation, striatal Iron accumulation to assess the loss of nigrostriatal DA-ergic neurons.

Neuroprotective Biomarkers in PD

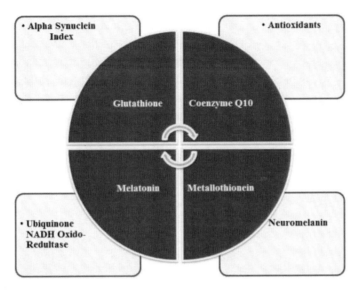

Figure 29. *Neuroprotective Biomarkers of PD* The neuroprotective biomarkers of PD can be alpha synuclein indexand various antioxidants including: Glutathione, melatonin, coenzyme Q10, metallothionein, ubiquinone NADH oxidoreductase (a rate limiting enzyme complex-1 for the Oxidative phosphorylation in electron transport chain, and neuromelanin, which can be estimated to determine the severity of PD progression. In general, the nigrostriatal concentration of these neuroprotective antioxidant biomarkers is significantly reduced in PD patients.

PD Triad

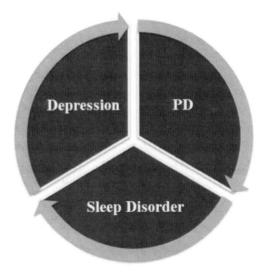

Figure 30. *PD Vicious Circle* A patient suffering from PD is trapped in a vicious circle of (a) depression (b) sleep disorders. Usually REM sleep is significantly impaired in PD patients and they suffer from nocturia.

PET Biomarkers ^{18}F-DOPA and [18]FdG have been used extensively as sensitive noninvasive and early diagnostic PET biomarkers of progressive neurodegenerative disorders such as PD, AD, and drug addiction. ^{18}F-DOPA and [18]FdG were recently utilized as sensitive and early biomarkers of microPET imaging of genetically-engineered α-Synuclein, MTs, and MTs over-expressing wv/wv mice. The primary objective of this study was to establish that MTs are neuroprotective agents as anti-inflammatory, antiapoptotic, and antioxidant proteins in PD and other neurodegenerative disorders such as AD, MDD, and drug addiction. Since wv/wv mice exhibit progressive loss of striatal dopaminergic neurons, whereas MTs transgenic (MT_{trans}) mice live long; the researchers proposed to transplant mesenchymal fetal stem cells derived from MT_{trans} embryos in wv/wv mice striatal regions and evaluate their therapeutic potential by performing [18]F- DOPA microPET neuroimaging. Progressive reduction in ^{18}F-DOPA occurs as a consequence of oxidative and nitrative stress in wv/wv mice. Since brain regional MTs and CoQ_{10} were significantly reduced in wv/wv mice, a sensitive colorimetric enzyme- linked immunosorbant assay (ELISA) was developed for the estimation of brain regional MTs and HPLC-UV method for the estimation of CoQ_{10} from genetically-engineered rare biological samples of α-Synuclein-Metallothioneins triple gene knock out (α-SynMTtko) mice. Crossbreeding of wv/wv mice with MT_{trans} mice developed a progeny of MTs over-expressing wv/wv with significantly improved striatal [18]FdG as well as ^{18}F-DOPA in MTs-over-expressing (wv/wv-MTs) mice, authenticating the hypothesis that MTs provide CoQ_{10}-mediated neuroprotection by rejuvenating the down-regulated mitochondrial (ubiquinone-NADH-oxidoreductase) complex-1, a rate limiting enzyme complex involved in oxidative phosphorylation and ATP synthesis for maintaining the mitochondrial bioenergetics and prevent CB formation (Sharma and Ebadi 2005; Sharma et al., 2006; Sharma and Ebadi, 2008; Sharma and Ebadi, 2013a). The researchers discovered that Cocaine and METH induce significant reduction in the striatal [18]Fd-DOPA uptake in C57BL6J mice. The uptake of [18]Fd-DOPA was further reduced when Ethanol was co-administered simultaneously with Cocaine and METH-abused mice, suggesting that Ethanol augments Cocaine and METH neurotoxicity (Sharma and Ebadi, 2008). The distribution kinetics of ^{18}F-DOPA was significantly impaired in wv/wv mice (Sharma and Ebadi 2005). A progressive reduction in the striatal ^{18}F-DOPA was observed in wv/wv mice as function of aging (Sharma et al., 2006).

In-Vivo Molecular Imaging Biomarkers The underlying pathological mechanisms leading to tremor, coexistent dementia and depression in PD and the role of imaging as a biomarker for testing neuroprotective agents have been considered. Measuring hippocampal volume with MRI has provided clinically important information about several neuropsychiatric disorders. Smaller hippocampal volumes have been reported in: epilepsy, AD, dementia, mild cognitive impairment, the aged, traumatic brain injury, cardiac arrest, PD, HD, Cushing's disease, herpes simplex encephalitis, Turner's syndrome, Down's syndrome, survivors of low birth weight, schizophrenia, major depression, posttraumatic stress disorder, chronic Alcoholism, personality disorder, obsessive-compulsive disorder, and antisocial personality disorders, whereas, significantly larger hippocampal volumes have been correlated with autism and children with fragile X syndrome. Preservation of hippocampal volume has been reported in: congenital hyperplasia, children with fetal Alcohol syndrome, anorexia nervosa, attention-deficit hyperactivity disorder (ADHD), bipolar disorder, and panic disorder. Standard univariate analysis of neuroimaging data revealed neuroanatomical and functional differences between healthy individuals and patients suffering from a wide range of neurological and psychiatric disorders. Furthermore, Support-Vector-Machine (SVM), an alternative form of analysis, allows categorization of an individual's previously unseen data into a predefined group using a classification algorithm, developed on a training data set. SVM has been successfully applied in the diagnosis, treatment and prognosis of progressive neurodegenerative disorders including, PD, AD, MDD, schizophrenia, and drug addiction, using both structural and functional neuroimaging data. Recent advances in tracer kinetic modeling, MRI to PET co-registration, radiochemistry techniques, instrumentation and image processing have paved the way for increased emphasis on functional imaging studies of neuropsychiatric disorders of the elderly including PD. Several radiotracers are now employed as biomarkers of dopamine storage capacity, vesicular monoamine, and dopamine transporter availability. In addition, Transcranial Sonography and Molecular Imaging have been employed to differentially diagnose PD. Midbrain/nigral structural abnormalities can be demonstrated *in-vivo* with both Transcranial sonography (TCS) and diffusion tensor MRI (DTI). Transcranial ultrasound has shown susceptibility factors for PD related to Iron overload in the substantia nigra. In addition, PET and SPECT ligands can be employed to demonstrate dysfunction in the dopaminergic neurotransmission.

Omics Biomarkers Omic biomarkers of PD can be sub-divided into lipidomic, metabolomics, neuroproteomic, and genomic biomarkers as described below:

(a) *Lipidomics* The advent of soft ionization procedures such as electrospray ionization (ESI) and atmospheric pressure chemical ionization (APCI) made it possible for the studies of various lipid structures in the brain, including phospholipids, ceramides, sphingomyelin, cerebrosides and cholesterol. Lipid analyses delineated metabolic defects in disease conditions including mental retardation, PD, schizophrenia, AD, depression, brain development, and ischemic stroke. Additionally, proteomic strategies for characterizing lipid-metabolizing proteins in the CSF have been described. These proteins may be potential therapeutic targets since they transport lipids required for neuronal growth or convert lipids into molecules that control brain physiology. Hence, combining lipidomics and proteomics will enhance the existing knowledge of disease pathology and increase the chances of discovering specific biomarkers and biochemical mechanisms of neurological diseases including PD to accomplish EBPT.

(b) *Metabolomics* CNS disorders are linked to disturbances in metabolic pathways related to neurotransmitter systems (Dopamine, Serotonin, GABA, and Glutamate); fatty acids such as Arachidonic acid cascade; oxidative stress, and mitochondrial function. Recently, metabolomics and its promise for biomarker discovery was emphasized for early diagnosis of schizophrenia, major depressive disorder (MDD), bipolar disorder (BD), amyotrophic lateral sclerosis (ALS), and PD. Metabolomics promises to improve current, single metabolites-based clinical assessments by identifying biomarkers that embody global biochemical changes in disease, predict prognosis, or side effects of medication.

(c) *Neuroproteomics* Common features of neurodegenerative diseases comprise failure of the ubiquitin proteasome system and increased levels of metal ions in the brain. Parkin is a ligase involved in ubiquitin-proteasome pathway and mutations in the parkin gene are the most common cause of recessive familial PD. Iron and Zinc are involved in several metabolic processes and are related to modulation of neuroproteomics of PD.

(d) *Genomics* Gene expression changes in neuropsychiatric and neurodegenerative disorders, and gene responses to therapeutic drugs, may provide new and efficient ways to identify CNS targets for drug discovery. Gene-based candidates for PD include: ubiquitin-proteosome system; Scavengers of reactive oxygen species (ROS); Brain-derived neurotrophic factor (BDNF), TrkB receptor, Early growth response-1, Nurr-1, Signaling through protein kinase C and RAS pathways. The genomic biomarkers may also facilitate in the EBPT of PD alone and/or in combination with other omic biomarkers described above.

Premotor/Preclinical Biomarkers A long preclinical or asymptomatic period may occur in PD, which prevents early PD diagnosis. Marked degeneration of the substantia nigra and loss of striatal dopamine occur before clinical symptoms become obvious. Nonmotor signs (*depression or sensory changes*) often precede motor signs after several years. More economical alternative to costly and highly inaccessible biomarkers (eg *PET detection of striatal dopamine reduction*). Recent cohort study sought to determine the relationship between the risk factors hyperechogenicity of the substantia nigra (SN+) and/or positive family history of PD (faPD+) and putative premotor markers of PD (Liepelt-Scarfone et al., 2011). SN+ exhibiting the highest association with premotor biomarkers suggested that SN+ might be a reliable biomarker of neurodegeneration in PD.

Pre-symptomatic Biomarkers As a chronic progressive disease, PD has a pre-symptomatic period during which the pathological process has begun, but motor signs required for the clinical diagnosis are absent. Recently proposed staging systems of PD have suggested that degeneration may occur initially in areas outside the substantia nigra, suggesting that non-motor manifestations may be used as biomarkers of pre-symptomatic PD.

Sex Hormones Clinical and experimental evidence have supported a role of steroid-dopamine interactions in the pathophysiology of schizophrenia, depression, and PD. Animal studies demonstrated effects of Estrogens, Progesterone, and Androgens on various biomarkers of dopaminergic neurotransmission. Hence specific steroidal receptor agonists and selective Estrogen receptor modulators (SERMs) could find applications as adjunct treatments in neurological disorders including PD.

Systemic Biomarkers Molecular Pathology biomarkers of PD include: α-Synuclein index, Lewy body formation, nigrostriatal dopaminergic loss, and striatal Iron accumulation

Systemic Biomarkers (Serotonin as a Biomarker) A few studies suggested that damage to brain serotonergic neurons might play a significant role in certain characteristics of PD, including depression. PET studies determined that SERT binding levels in PD were lower than those in controls in all examined brain areas, with the changes statistically significant in orbitofrontal cortex, caudate, putamen, and midbrain. Tritiated Imipramine binding in platelets was used to evaluate Serotonin activity in depression in previous studies. However Imipramine binding in platelets proved ineffective diagnostic tool for depression and PD.

Advanced End Glycation Products (AGE) It is known that proteins or lipids that become glycated after exposure to sugars, which promotes the deposition of proteins due to the protease resistant crosslinking between the peptides and proteins. The age-related neurodegenerative disorders are accompanied with abnormal accumulation or aggregation of proteins: Amyloid β, tau, α-Synuclein, Prions: glycated and the extent of glycation is correlated with α-Synuclein (α-Syn) [Small soluble protein across presynaptic terminals in the CNS, involved in the regulation of DAergic neurotransmission] is upregulated in a discrete population of presynaptic terminals of the brain during a period of acquisition-related synaptic rearrangement, which triggers the abnormal deposition and accumulation of the modified proteins.

MicroRNA Analysis in PD MicroRNAs are highly crucial for the normal development / survival of dopaminergic and other neurons in the CNS. α-Synuclein mRNA remains under negative control of at least 2 microRNAs (miR-7 and miR-153). Regulation of candidate genes by specific microRNA species, profiling approaches are revealing variations in the abundance of certain microRNAs relevant to PD. It was reported that miR-133b is deficient in the PD midbrain and miR-34b/34c is decreased in affected brain regions in PD and Lewy body disease.

α-Synuclein Induced Microglial Activation in PD α-Synuclein incites microglial activation via toll-like receptors (TLRs) activation, which causes increased expression of TLRs. TLRs mediate down stream pathways to induce increased expression of proinflammatory cytokines. Morphological changes were consistent with enhanced inflammation within 24 hrs. α-Synuclein was the first gene to be linked to PD and forms a principal constituent of Lewy bodies *"Lewy bodies: abnormal aggregates of protein that develop inside nerve cells in PD. Overexpression of α-synuclein triggers Lewy body formation, which disrupt vital recycling processes in neurons due to accumulation in the presynaptic terminals to cause.* hypertrophy in these terminals. PD patients exhibit α-Synuclein Positive staining in Lewy bodies. Hence, pathologicaly, PD can be characterized by loss of midbrain dopamine neurons, presence of large proteinaceous α-Synuclein-positive intracellular inclusions, oxidatively modified molecules, and activated microglia. In addition, α-Synuclein directly activates microglia inciting the production of pro-inflammatory molecules and alters the expression of Toll-like receptors (TLRs). TLR expression changes occur in PD which may influence the theranostic response

Neuroinflammatory Biomarkers in PD Generally, PD is a slow progressive neurodegenerative disease. Mutations in α-Synuclein lead to autosomal-dominant, early-onset PD in some families, and α-Synuclein is found in Lewy bodies of all PD patients Pro-inflammatory cytokine NFkβ is significantly increased, whereas mitochondrial ubquinone-NADH oxidoreductase (complex-1) is significantly down-regulated in PD, which may impair striatal mitochondrial bioenergetics to induce progressive DA-ergic neurodegeneration due to CB formation.

Cytokines as Biomarkers in PD Cytokines are immunological messengers which facilitate both intra- and inter-system communication. Cytokines are the key players in the neuroinflammatory cascades associated with the neurodegenerative process in PD. Cytokines are induced in depression and other cognitive (memory impairment, dementia) and affective disturbances (anxiety); hence are associated with high co-morbidity, with neurodegenerative diseases like PD, AD, MDD, schizophrenia, and chronic drug addiction.

Brain-Derived Neurotrophic Factor (BNDF) BDNF is the *most* widely distributed neurotrophin in the CNS and serves important roles in synaptic plasticity and neuronal survival. BDNF production and secretion is significantly influenced in neurodegenerative diseases and mood disorders: depression, eating disorders, and schizophrenia. BDNF has been implicated in the induction of long-term synaptic potentiation (LTP) to enhance and consolidate learning and memory processes. BDNF is now considered a key molecules modulating brain plasticity. Hence it can be used as a sensitive biomarker of impaired memory and general cognitive function in PD, AD, and aging. In addition, gonadal steroids are involved in the regulation of several CNS processes, including: mood, affective and cognitive functions during reproductive aging. Recent studies have reported altered levels of BDNF in the circulation (serum or plasma) of patients with major depression, bipolar disorder, AD, HD, and PD. Correlations between serum BDNF levels and affective, cognitive and motor symptoms have also been reported.

Multimodality Biomarkers Multimodality biomarkers are be explored for the future diagnosis of PD, which incorporate combination of clinical, laboratory, imaging, and genetic data. Genetics, imaging, and CSF analyses indicates "α-Synuclein aggregation & disturbances of other candidate proteins are associated with dementia in PD" Miscellaneous biomarkers of PD including α-Synuclein Index, Charnoly Body (CB) formation, Lewy body formation, increased striatal Iron, reduced Ferritin, and reduced Pyridoxal kinase activity.

α-Synuclein Index as Biomarker of PD The author discovered α-Synuclein Index (ratio of nitrated α-synuclein: native α-synuclein) as a sensitive diagnostic biomarker for the early clinical management of PD (Sharma et al., 2003). Selegiline, a monoamine oxidase-B inhibitor provides neuroprotection in the cultured dopaminergic neurons via MTs induction by acting as an anti-apoptotic, anti-inflammatory, and as an antioxidant protein. MTs inhibit CB formation by acting as free radical scavengers and by activating Zinc-mediated transcriptional regulation of genes involved in growth, proliferation, differentiation, and development (Sharma and Ebadi, 2014). Hence, MTs can be used as early and effective redox-sensitive theranostic biomarkers for the clinical management of PD and drug addiction.

MTs Inhibit Charnoly Body (CBs) Formation MTs provide neuroprotection by inhibiting nitration of α-Synuclein involved in neurodegenerative α-Synucleinopathies. Hence α-Synuclein index and MTs may be utilized for the clinical diagnosis and prognosis of PD.

Charnoly Bodies (CBs) The author discovered CB formation in developing undernourished rat Purkinje neurons as pleomorphic, multilamellar, aggregated electron-dense membrane stacks of degenerated mitochondria due to enhanced lipid peroxidation and oxidative stress. CB can be used as a diagnostic biomarker which is induced as a harmful consequence of oxidative and nitrative stress in the CNS due to degeneration of mitochondrial membranes due to ROS-mediated structural and functional breakdown of polyunsaturated fatty acids in the plasma membranes. Charnoly Body's formation is augmented in nutritional stress or in response to environmental neurotoxic insult, where as MTs inhibit CBs formation and neurodegenerative α-Synucleinopathies by inhibiting α-Synuclein index and by acting as free radical scavengers to provide mitochondrial neuroprotection.

Calcium Binding Proteins, TRPCs TRPCs were down-regulated in human cultured dopaminergic neurons when exposed to 1-methyl, 4-phenyl, pyridinium. Hence can be considered as potential early and sensitive biomarkers for the *in-vitro* assessment of the Lewy body pathogenesis and PD (Bolimuntha et al., 2005).

NAP (Davunetide) in PD NAP is 8 amino acid peptide that provide neuroprotection from activity-dependent neuroprotective protein (ADNP) a molecule that is essential for CNS formation. It is involved in increasing memory scores in patients from amnestic mild cognitive impairment and enhances functional behaviors in schizophrenia patients.

Lithium and PD Lithium has neuroprotective properties and serves as an inhibitor of glycogen synthase kinase 3 (GSK3). Lithium has been reported as a mediator of Ethanol neurotoxicity. It has been utilized in the treatment of acute brain injuries, chronic neurodegenerative diseases, and ALS. Lithium is known to ameliorate Ethanol-induced neuroapoptosis.

Ethanol and PD Ethanol is a teratogen and involved in fetal Alcohol spectrum disorders (FASD) as it causes apoptosis in the developing brain & behavioral deficits, leading to Wernicke-Korsakoff syndrome and neurodegeneration

Complexins Complexins is a cytoplasmic neuronal protein which binds to the SNARE protein complex (*SNAREpin*) with a high affinity. It controls fast synchronous neurotransmitter release. Genetic elimination of Complexins causes reduction in neurotransmitter release, schizophrenia, HD, depression, bipolar disorder, PD, AD, traumatic brain injury, Wernicke's encephalopathy, and fetal Alcohol syndrome. In addition, concentration of plasma copper, Ceruloplasmin (CRP), non-ceruloplasmin-bound Cu (NCBC), and MTs = biomarkers for neurodegenerative diseases. Increased levels of Cu have been noticed in the plasma of AD, PD, and vascular dementia (VD) patients.

C-Reactive Protein and other Proteins in PD CRP is elevated in response to the inflammatory component of the diseases. The levels of MTs was proportional to VD. Cu/CRP and Cu/MTs ratios are both indicative of disease progression for AD patients. Genetic transfer of MTs may serve as potential treatment modalities for neurodegenerative disorders, including PD, AD, and ALS. Transplantation of genetically modified cells into the brain represents a promising strategy for the delivery and expression of specific neurotrophic factors, neurotransmitter-synthesizing enzymes, and cellular regulatory proteins for intervention in neurodegenerative diseases.

Pharmacological Biomarkers- Folate and Vit B_{12} The pharmacological biomarkers, Folate and Vit B12 are essential for methylation of Homocysteine to Methionine in the brain. Increased plasma Homocysteine levels are associated with CVAs and a compromised blood-brain barrier. Problem with transmethylation pathway abnormal S-Adenosylmethionine (SAM) is associated with neurodegenerative diseases including PD. Patients with disorders in this pathway may be prone to irreversible neurological symptoms including PD.

Neuroprotective Biomarkers in PD The author proposed possible neuroprotective biomarkers of PD including: Melatonin, Antioxidants, Glutathione, α Synuclein index. CoQ_{10} has antioxidant properties and enhances the mitochondrial complex I activity (*which is defective in PD*). Future studies are needed to establish this correlation.

Nonmotor Biomarkers in PD It is now realized that non motor symptoms increase with progression of PD. A significant number of people with PD reported that they experienced problems with olfaction, taste, nocturia, depression and constipation prior to diagnosis which may help to serve as potential biomarker(s) of PD.

Sleep Disturbance in PD Abnormal idiopathic REM sleep behavior is present in 50% of patients with PD. Abnormal sleep is characterized by loss of atonia, resulting in motor activity during dreams related to NMS biomarkers. Excessive daytime sleepiness is common in PD and has been associated with PD-related dementia. Epworth sleepiness scale scores were higher in PD patients without dementia and PD patients with dementia than controls. Scores > 10 was observed in PD patients with dementia excessive daytime sleepiness observed in PD patients with dementia. No data is yet available on Melatonin secretion in these patients. The Epworth Sleepiness Scale (ESS) is a scale intended to measure daytime sleepiness that is measured by use of a very short questionnaire. This can be helpful in diagnosing sleep disorders. The questionnaire asks the subject to rate his or her probability of falling asleep on a scale of increasing probability from 0 to 3 for 8 different situations that most people engage in during their daily lives, though not necessarily every day. The scores for the eight questions are added together to obtain a single number. A number in the 0–9 range is considered to be normal while a number in the 10–24 range indicates that expert medical advice should be sought.

Hyposmia in PD In association with other cognitive problems, hyposmia is a non motor sign of PD, the interrelation is still under investigation. Morley et al. (2011) established that there was a correlation between olfactory dysfunction and neuropsychiatric manifestations. Worse olfaction was associated with poorer memory- suggesting that olfactory dysfunction could be a possible biomarker for PD.

Depression in PD About 50% of patients with PD are affected patients. The underlying mechanism of depression in PD is complex and involves biological, psychosocial, and therapeutic factors.

Biological factors Degeneration of mesencephalic dopaminergic neurons (mDA) is associated with PD. Defects in the Serotonergic system are related to depression, 5-HT system is markedly affected in the parkinsonian brain. Low 5-HT combined with altered network activity within the basal ganglia are involved in depression in PD. Tryptophan-rich diets may alleviate symptoms of depression. These findings include evidence that depression is a side effect of deep brain stimulation (DBS) of the subthalamic nucleus (STN), a treatment option in advanced PD.

Depression (Other factors) Depressed PD patients have less suicidal ideations, but suffer more anxiety. Some PD patients may have past history of depression. Particularly, female gender, and patients with greater left brain involvement were more prone to depression.

Electrophysiological Biomarkers in PD The excitability threshold to transcranial stimulation (TCS) was found to be lower in patients with PD as compared to ALS patients. Hence this could be a significant biomarker for PD. Transcranial magnetic stimulation (TMS) is a noninvasive method to cause depolarization or hyperpolarization in the neurons of the brain. TMS uses electromagnetic induction to induce weak electric currents using a rapidly changing magnetic field; this can cause activity in specific or general parts of the brain with minimal discomfort, allowing the functioning and interconnections of the brain to be studied.

CONCLUSION

PD is the most prevalent neurodegenerative disorder. The nigrostriatal DAergic neuronal losses as a consequence of incrased α-Synuclein index, CB formation, and Lewy body pathogenesis are the hallmarks of PD, and are reflected as motor impairments, muscle rigidity, and body tremors, secondary to destruction of about 65% of dopaminergic neurons. Hence there is a quest for the novel discovery of specific biomarkers, which could be used on a routine basis for the successful EBPT of PD. Althoug clinical biomarkers discussed in this chapter can aid in early detection, thse are nonspecific, hence there is a dire need for multimodality PD biomarkers for the prompt management of this devastating clinical condition.

REFERENCES

Bollimuntha, S., Singh, B., Shavali, S., Sharma, S. & Ebadi, M. (2005). TRPC-1-Mediated Inhibition of MPP$^+$ Toxicity in Human SH-S-Y5Y Neuroblastoma Cells. *J. Biol. Chem.*, *280*, 2132-2140.

Flood, D. G., Marek, G. J. & Williams, M. (2011). Developing predictive CSF biomarkers— A challenge critical to success in Alzheimer's disease and neuropsychiatric translational medicine. *Biochemical Pharmacology*, *81*, 1422–1434.

Gerlach, M., Hendrich, A., Hueber, R., Jost, W., Winkler, J., Woitalla, D. & Riederer, P. (2008). The early detection of Parkinson's disease: unmet needs. *Neurodegener Dis.*, *5*, 137–139.

Gerlach, M., Maetzler, W., Broich, K., Hampel, H., Rems, L., Reum, T., Riederer, P., Stöffler, A., Streffer, J. & Berg, D. (2012). Biomarker candidates of neurodegeneration in Parkinson's disease for the evaluation of disease-modifying therapeutics. *J. Neural. Transm.*, *119*, 39–52.

Kohl, Z., Winner, B., Ubhi, K., Rockenstein, E., Mante, M., Münch, M., Barlow, C., Carter, T., Masliah, E. & Winkler, J. (2012). Fluoxetine rescues impaired hippocampal neurogenesis in a transgenic A53T synuclein mouse model. *Eur. J. Neurosci.*, *35*, 10-19.

Liepelt-Scarfone, I., Behnke, S., Godau, J., Schweitzer, K. J., Wolf, B., Gaenslen, A. & Berg, D. (2011). Relation of risk factors and putative premotor markers for Parkinson's disease. *J. Neural Transm. (Vienna).*, *118*(4), 579-585.

Morley, J. F., Weintraub, D., Mamikonyan, E., Moberg, P. J., Siderowf, A. D. & Duda, J. E. (2011). Olfactory dysfunction is associated with neuropsychiatric manifestations in Parkinson's disease. *Mov. Disord.*, *26*, 2051-2057.

Sharma, S. & Ebadi, M. (2005). Distribution Kinetics of ^{18}F-DOPA in Weaver Mutant Mice. *Molecular Brain Research*, *139*, 23-30.

Sharma, S., Krause, G. & Ebadi, M. (2008). Basic Requirements of Quality Control of PET Radiopharmaceuticals. *Proceedings of the International Atomic Energy Agency*, Bangkok, Thailand, Nov 10-14, 2007.

Sharma, S. & Ebadi, M. (2008). Therapeutic Potential of Metallothioneins in Parkinson's Disease. In New Research on Parkinson's Disease. Eds: Timothy F. Hahn & Julian Werner, Nova Science Publishers, New York, pp. 1-28.

Sharma, S. & Ebadi, M. (2008). SPECT Neuroimaging in Translational Research of CNS Disorders. *Neurochem. Internat.*, *52*, 352-362.

Sharma, S. & Ebadi, M. (2013). *In-Vivo* Molecular Imaging in Parkinson's Disease. In Parkinson's Disease. Eds. RF. Pfeiffer, ZK Wszolek, M. Ebadi. IInd Edition, Chapter 58, CRC Press Taylor & Francis Group. Boca Rotan, FL, USA. pp. 787-802

Sharma, S. & Ebadi, M. (2013). Antioxidant Targeting in Neurodegenerative Disorders. Ed. I. Laher, Springer Verlag. Germany. Chapter 85, p. 1-30.

Sharma, S., Moon, C. S., Khogali, A., Haidous, A., Chabenne, A., Ojo, C., Jelebinkov, M., Kurdi, Y. & Ebadi, M. (2013) Biomarkers of Parkinson's Disease (Recent Update). *Neurochem. Internat.*, *63*, 201-229.

Sharma, S., Rais, A., Sandhu, R., Nel, W. & Ebadi, M. (2013). Clinical significance of metallothioneins in cell therapy and nanomedicine. *International Journal of Nanomedicine.*, *8*, 1477–1488.

Sharma, S., Refaey, H. El. & Ebadi, M. (2006). Complex-1 activity and ^{18}F-DOPA uptake in genetically engineered mouse model of Parkinson's disease and the neuroprotective role of coenzyme Q_{10}. *Brain Res. Bull.*, *70*, 22-32

Sharma, S., Carlson, E. & Ebadi, M. (2003). The Neuroprotective Actions of Selegiline in Inhibiting 1-Methyl, 4-Phenyl, Pyridinium Ion (MPP$^+$)-Induced Apoptosis in Dopaminergic Neurons. *J. Neurocytology*, *32*, 329-343.

Sharma, S., Kheradpezhou, M., Shavali, S., EI Refaey, H., Eken, J., Hagen, C. & Ebadi, M. 2004. Neuroprotective Actions of Coenzyme Q_{10} in Parkinson's Disease. *Methods in Enzymology.*, *382*, 488-509.

Chapter 10

BIOMARKERS IN PERSONALIZED THERANOSTICS OF ALZHEIMER'S DISEASE (RECENT UPDATE)

ABSTRACT

Alzheimer disease (AD) is an age-related neurodegenerative disorder, characterized by loss of memory and cognitive function. It is the most common cause of dementia in elderly and is a global health concern as the population of people aged 85 and older, is growing alarmingly. Although pharmacotherapy for the treatment of AD has improved, lot of work remains to treat this devastating disease. AD pathology begins even before the onset of clinical symptoms. Because therapies could be more effective if implemented early in the disease progression, it is highly prudent to discover reliable biomarkers, to detect its exact pathophysiology during early pre-symptomatic stage. Biomarker(s) with high sensitivity and specificity would facilitate AD diagnosis at early stages. Currently, CSF amyloid β 1-42, total tau, and phosphorylated tau181 are used as AD biomarkers. This chapter describes conventional and potential *in-vitro* and *in-vivo* AD biomarkers. Particularly, *in-vitro* transcriptomic, proteomic, lipidomic, and metabolomic; body fluid biomarkers (C-reactive proteins, Homocysteine, α-Sunuclein Index, and Dehydroepiandrosterone sulphate) from blood, serum, plasma, CSF, and saliva; and neuronal, platelets, and lymphocyte microRNA, mtDNA, and Charnoly Body (CB) may be detected. *In-vivo* physiological and neurobehavioral biomarkers are evaluated by analyzing computerized EEG, event-related potentials, circadian rhythm, and multimodality fusion imaging including: CT, MRI, SPECT, and PET. More specifically, PET imaging biomarkers representing reduced fronto-temporal ^{18}FdG uptake, increased ^{11}C or ^{18}F-PIB uptake, ^{11}C-PBR28 to measure 18 kDa translocator protein (TSPO), a biomarker for inflammation; and 3-D MRI (ventriculomegaly)/MRS are performed for early and effective clinical management of AD, with an ultimate quest to accomplish EBPT.

Keywords: disease specific biomarkers, Charnolybody, α-synuclein index, metallothioneins, brain derived nerve growth factor, Alzheimer's disease, differential diagnosis

INTRODUCTION

Although AD has been studied for >100 years, the exact cause(s) and pathogenic mechanism(s) are yet to be established. Despite increasing global prevalence, the precise pathogenesis and diagnosis of neurodegenerative dementias remain controversial, and basic understanding of the disease and the molecular mechanism of cholinergic neuronal loss in AD remain unknown. AD is the most common cause of dementia among the elderly that involves complex neurodegeneration. Although AD starts 20-30 years before first clinical symptoms become evident, it is difficult to diagnose accurately in its early stages. As AD is a slowly progressing disease, the evaluation of effects of candidate drugs requires extensive clinical as well as long-term treatment trials. Moreover, the efficient disease-modifying treatment and ideal diagnostic methods for AD are currently unavailable. The updated guidelines recognize three distinct stages of AD: (a) preclinical AD, (b) MCI due to AD, and (c) AD with dementia. Specific biomarkers which could accurately distinguish these three stages are yet to be discovered for the successful personalized treatment of AD. Obviously, there is a dire need for novel biomarkers and pre-clinical models to accomplish early indication of treatment response. Treatment of AD is hampered by the lack of easily accessible biomarkers that could detect disease and predict disease risks accurately. Although fluid biomarkers of AD provide indications of disease stage, they are unreliable predictors of disease progression or treatment response, as most of them are measured in CSF, which limits their routine clinical applicability.

The neuropathologic process underlying AD begins several years, before the onset of memory impairment. In general, AD is characterized by the presence of Aβ plaques in the cerebral cortex, which result from the action of the enzymes β-secretase and γ-secretase on Amyloid Precursor Protein (APP). The pathological hallmarks of AD include: (a) accumulation of Aβ, (b) activation of astrocytes and microglia, and (c) impaired cholinergic neurotransmission. Epidemiological and laboratory studies also support vascular injury and inflammation, as pathological events in AD. Early-onset familial AD is an autosomal dominant disorder caused by mutations in the APP, presenilin-1 (PSEN1), or presenilin 2 gene.

Most clinical chemistry tests rely on old technology, and are neither sensitive nor specific. Usually, multiple cellular processes including regulation of Aβ peptide, tau, inflammation, and cell death are associated with AD. The brain regional Aβ deposition is one of the most important hallmarks of AD. Although tau pathology is correlated with neuronal loss, how its accumulation triggers neurotoxic events remains uncertain. AD is characterized by proteolytic cleavage of tau protein, which initiates neuronal demise. Recent advances in neuroimaging suggest that it is possible to detect Alzheimer-associated neuropathological changes well before the onset of dementia; however the increasing prevalence of AD is becoming one of the most significant health and economic challenges in the entire world. In fact, AD shares several characteristics of abnormal brain aging. It is the most common cause of dementia involving progressive deterioration of neuronal networks, accounting for 60-80% of the reported cases. Although the exact pathophysiological mechanism of AD is yet to be established, it is reported that apart from Aβ and tau protein; a number of other factors including cardiovascular risk factors, inflammation, and lipid metabolism may also play a crucial role in the etiopathogenesis of AD (Fiolaki et al., 2014).

There is now a serious effort for the novel discovery of reliable biomarkers for AD that could be used on a routine basis to assist in the differential diagnosis, inform disease progression, and monitor therapeutic response. Recently Desican et al (2013) developed *in-vivo* biomarkers for the clinical evaluation of AD and discussed how assessment strategies might incorporate neuroimaging biomarkers to inform patients, families, and clinicians when memory impairment prompts a search for diagnosis and management options. Although the understanding of dementia in the old subjects has advanced, more research is needed among diversified racial, ethnic, and socioeconomic groups, and biomarkers discovery in neuroimaging, modifiable risk factors, and therapy.

The most common clinical syndromes of old age are alzheimer's dementia, vascular dementia, and mixed dementia with diversified etiologies. Recently, epidemiology, prevalence, clinical presentation, neuropathology, imaging features, risk factors, and treatment options of AD in the old population were described (gardner et al., 2013). it is realized that single neuropathological entities such as Alzheimer's dementia and Lewy body pathology appear to have lesser relevance to cognitive decline, while mixed pathology with AD, vascular disease (cortical microinfarcts), and hippocampal sclerosis have more relevance. It is proposed that risk factors for dementia include a low level of education, poor mid-life general health, reduced physical activity, depression, and delirium, whereas Apolipoprotein e (apo-e) genotype, hypertension, hyperlipidemia, and elevated peripheral inflammatory biomarkers appear to have less relevance. Hence therapeutic strategies require further investigations; Nevertheless the oldest old may be more prone to adverse effects compared with younger patients and targeted therapies may be less efficacious since single pathologies are less frequent in AD.

Usually AD develops for an unknown period and may remain undiagnosed for several years before clinical manifestation of cognitive impairments become evident. Current AD treatments offer only a symptomatic relief, because it is diagnosed when the pathology is already advanced, whereas treatments may be most effective in the early phases of pathology. Hence, the identification of sensitive and specific biomarker(s) is crucial to accomplish novel drug discovery, early differential diagnosis, and effective clinical management of AD.

This chapter presents systematically current knowledge about various *in-vitro* and *in-vivo* biomarkers including (i) CSF, serum, and PET imaging biomarkers, (ii) broadly classified omics *(lipidomics, proteomics, genomics, transcriptomics, and metabolomics)* biomarkers, (iii) and miscellaneous biomarkers including proinflammatory C-*reactive proteins*, α-*Synuclein index, and Charnoly Body* (CB) in neurons, lymphocytes, platelets, and the cells from the buccal mucosa. More specifically, the author has discussed *in-vitro* biomarkers of body fluids including; CSF, serum, and blood platelets, and *in-vivo* multimodality CT, MRI/MRS, SPECT, and PET fusion imaging, for the early diagnosis and clinical management of AD with minimum and/or no adverse effects. Furthermore, he has highlighted the importance of conventional, putative, and potential biomarkers and provided recent knowledge for basic medical scientists as well as for clinical doctors, interested in the early diagnosis, prognosis and effective treatment of AD. Although AD and Lewy body diseases (LBD) including; PD, PD with dementia (PDD), and dementia with Lewy bodies (DLB), are common causes of geriatric cognitive impairments; AD and LBD are often found in the same patients at autopsy; therefore, biomarkers that can detect the presence of both pathologies in living subjects are needed.

Recently Aβ, soluble Aβ precursor protein, and autoantibodies have emerged as potential biomarkers for the diagnosis and treatment of AD. The author has discussed the clinical significance and limitations of these emerging AD biomarkers with a primary objective to highlight the efforts of the blood-based biomarker interest group, an international group of experts in the field of in-vivo molecular imaging biomarkers, omics biomarkers, neurobehavioral biomarkers and physiological biomarkers. It is envisaged that this chapter will enlighten basic guidelines for beginners and refreshment for those who are experts in the field of AD biomarker development.

Hippocampal Dysfunction in AD It is known that animal models and AD patients exhibit reorganization in hippocampal and cortical neuro-circuitry which is triggered by an early imbalance between excitation and inhibition, leading to altered neuronal activity. Although precise molecular mechanisms underlying these changes remains unknown, either soluble or fibrillar forms of Aß are implicated to network alterations in AD. However, Aβ over-production in animal models is not directly linked to over-excitation. It is hypothesized that early changes in the excitation-inhibition balance within the hippocampus produces only slight changes in the hippocampal activity in the beginning (Goutagny and Krantic, 2013). A basic concept was introduced, according to which the subtle changes in θ and γ EEG rhythms might occur during the early stages of AD and could be used as a predictor for the disease. It is proposed that Aβ could be a promising target for disease-modifying therapeutic strategies like passive immunotherapy with anti-Aβ monoclonal antibodies (mAbs) in AD (Moreth et al., 2013).

Neurochemical biomarkers in CSF include alterations of Aβ that facilitate the diagnosis of AD. Hence the levels of Aβ in CSF and plasma could play an important role in the early clinical management of AD. These strategies have significant impact on the outcome of such studies, since the biomarkers can be used to monitor the activity of anti-Aβ mAbs. In this context, the clinical trials of Solanezumab were primarily based on the Aβ levels in CSF and plasma, whereas those of Bapineuzumab were based on cognitive performance; however, there is limited information about the basic molecular mechanisms altering the levels of these biomarkers, and no biomarker has yet been proven successful predictor for AD therapy. The Aβ biomarkers allow for the determination of free and bound anti-Aβ mAb to monitor the concentration of bioactive drugs and provide directions to the molecular mechanism of action.

Diagnostic Challenge in AD Although diagnostic tools for AD involve neuropsychological testing and neuroimaging techniques, the identification of reliable, early and non-invasive biomarkers remains a major challenge. While definitive diagnosis requires a pathological evaluation at autopsy, neurodegenerative changes are believed to begin several years before the clinical presentation of cognitive deficit. Therefore, there is a dire need for reliable biomarkers to aid in the early detection of disease to implement preventative strategies. Recently new biomarkers and novel criteria for the diagnosis of AD and guidelines for physicians were proposed (Kapoor, 2013; Howe, 2013). Since the characteristics of different pathological processes in AD brain and how these relate to each other remains uncertain; this motivated further exploration using binding studies in postmortem brains with molecular imaging tracers to facilitate the development of specific biomarkers to accurately determine basic molecular mechanism of disease progression. In general, attempts to develop AD therapies have been unsuccessful because there is no means to target an effective therapeutic window. Although CNS biomarkers are promising, these are impractical for high-throughput population-based screening. Therefore, a peripheral, blood-based biomarker which would improve early diagnosis, enable pre-symptomatic detection, and facilitate targeting of disease-modifying treatments is suggested (Rembach et al., 2013).

The plasma, platelets, and cellular fractions, are now being explored as peripheral biomarkers for AD. Some of these biomarkers for clinical application have been highlighted. Generally, AD can be histopathologically characterized by the presence of three biomarkers: *(a) senile plaques (rich in Aβ peptide), (b) neuronal fibrillary tangles (rich in phosphorylated tau protein), and (c) synaptic loss.* However, definitive biomarkers for this devastating disease are still awaited. Despite detailed understanding of the molecular mechanism involved in its pathogenesis, and millions of dollars of investment in drug discovery and clinical trials, no single drug has yet been approved for its effective treatment since the advent of cholinesterase inhibitors and Memantine. The use of currently approved drugs in Phase II and III clinical trials was recently reviewed (Léger and Massoud, 2013). Driven by the increasing knowledge from Phase III failures and improvements in early detection of biomarkers, there is evidence to support that AD cure is around the corner.

A rare form of AD, caused by autosomal-dominant mutations, affects carriers with 100% certainty and at a younger age. Studying families with these mutations allows investigation of the temporal sequence of biomarker changes in AD. A study determined whether the pupil flash response (PFR), previously reported to be altered in sporadic AD, is different in pre-symptomatic mutation carriers (Frost et al., 2013). Researchers collected pupil response data from cognitively normal participants in the Dominantly Inherited Alzheimer's Network (DIAN) Study during 2010-2011. Participants were from a single family harboring an Aβ precursor protein genetic mutation (APPGlu693Gln). Six carriers and six non-carriers were available for pupil testing. Pupil response parameter comparison between mutation carriers and non-carriers exhibited 75% recovery time which was longer in mutation carriers and percentage recovery 3.5 seconds after stimulus was less in mutation carriers, indicating that PFR changes occur pre-symptomatically in autosomal dominant AD mutation carriers, supporting further investigation of PFR for early detection of AD.

Risk Factor Genes as Biomarkers in AD Although Apo-E ε4 is the robust risk gene, recently 10 novel genes that increase the risk of developing AD have been identified by applying genome-wide association studies. These genes encode for proteins that are involved in the metabolism of cholesterol, activation of the immune system, and synaptic cell membrane processes. Based on the identification of these risk genes, new hypotheses on the pathological mechanisms for AD have been proposed. However, these hypotheses partly replace and partly supplement the previous Aβ pathway hypothesis. Several new risk genes in AD have been identified. The researchers summarized the genetic factors related to AD, based on findings in Alzgene, a database of genetic association studies in AD, a literature search in PubMed, and their own experience in dementia research (Rongve et al., 2013). Mutations of the genes APP, PSEN1 and PSEN2 cause half of all cases of the onset autosomal dominant form of AD, or how much of the development of the disease in an individual that is explained by genetics, is between 60- 80% in the late onset form of AD. The new risk genes point to the discovery of potential for new biomarkers for specific disease processes and to potential new targets for future disease modifying therapies.

Biomarkers Detectability and Accuracy Biomarkers are often measured with error due to imperfect lab conditions or variability within subjects. Using an internal reliability sample of the biomarker, a parametric bias-correction approach was developed for estimating diagnostic measures including sensitivity, specificity, and the Youden index with its optimal cut-point, positive and negative predictive values, and positive and negative diagnostic likelihood ratios when the biomarker was subjected to measurement error (White and Xie, 2013). These investigators derived the asymptotic properties of the likelihood-based estimators and demonstrated that they are consistent and normally distributed and proposed confidence intervals and confidence bands for the receiver operating characteristic (ROC) curves. This approach eliminated the bias due to measurement error. They also derived the asymptotic bias of naïve estimates and discussed conditions in which naïve estimates of the diagnostic measures are biased toward estimates when the biomarker is ineffective or are biased, and recommended collecting an internal reliability sample during the biomarker discovery phase to evaluate the performance of biomarkers with proper adjustment for error. Hence ROC analysis is currently used to find the optimal combination of biomarkers. Two new biomarker combination methods that make use of the covariate information were proposed (Liu and Zhou, 2013). The first method is to maximize the area under the covariate-adjusted ROC curve (AAUC). To overcome the limitations of the AAUC measure, these investigators proposed the area under covariate-standardized ROC curve (SAUC) as an extension of the covariate-specific ROC curve. With simulation studies, the optimal AAUC and SAUC methods were compared with the optimal AUC method that ignores the covariates. The biomarker combination methods were illustrated by an example from AD research. The results indicated that the optimal AAUC combination performs well. Based on these findings the investigators confirmed that the optimal SAUC method is flexible, and allows the results to be generalized to different populations. The proposed optimal AAUC and SAUC approaches address the covariate adjustment problem in estimating the optimal biomarker combination. Hence the optimal SAUC method is preferred, because the biomarker combination rule can be easily evaluated for different populations.

There is now interest in the development of methods to validate novel biomarkers for AD diagnosis. Previously, a proteomic panel of CSF biomarker candidates that differentiated AD and non-AD CSF with accuracy >90% was discovered. Information about these CSF proteins can be used to develop multiple reaction monitoring (MRM) based analytical assays, which provide excellent opportunities to quantify changes in protein expression in biological samples, as well as, validation among multiple labs. Furthermore, MRM assay demonstrates reproducibility for CSF biomarkers in AD (Choi et al., 2013).

MRM quantification results of Aβ1-40, Aβ1-42, Retinol-binding protein, and Cystatin C, correlated very well with those from ELISA. The analysis showed that 12 out of 16 selected targets exhibit similar trend in protein expression as reported in the literature. The AD biomarkers can be grossly divided as (a) *in-vitro biomarkers derived* from the serum, saliva, and urinary samples of AD patients, (b) and *in-vivo biomarkers*, derived from multimodality fusion imaging of CT, MRI, PET, SPECT, computerized EEG, and ultrasound. The ex-vivo biomarkers can be derived from the biopsy samples of the animal models of AD and rarely from the biopsy brain sample of an AD patient. Various pathological biomarkers can be derived from the brain autopsy samples of an AD patient to accomplish EBPT of AD as illustrated in Figure 31. This chapter describes various *in-vitro biomarkers*, *in-vivo* biomarkers, pathological biomarkers, and miscellaneous biomarkers including Charnoly Body (CB) and α-Synuclein index (SI), discovered originally by our group for the differential diagnosis, prognosis, and personalized treatment of AD.

AD BIOMARKERS IN EBPM

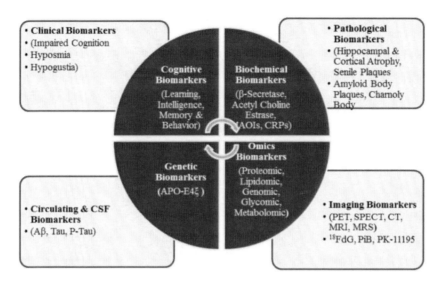

Figure 31. *AD Biomarkers in EBPM* In general AD biomarkers can be clssified as (i) clinical biomarkers, (ii) cicrulating biomarkers, (iii) pathological biomarkers, and (iv) imaging biomarkers. Cognitive biomarkers can be evaluated based on learning, intelligence, memory, and behavior, where as biochemical biomarkers including: β-secretase, acetyl choline esterase, MAOIs, and CRPs can be estimated from the CSF and serum samples of AD patients. Genetic biomarkers particularly APO-E4€ and omics biomarkers: proteomic, lipidomic, genomic, glycomic, and metabolomics biomarkers can further facilitate accomplishing EBPT of AD.

There are primarily two major types of AD biomarkers including: *in-vitro* biomarkers and (ii) *in-vivo* biomarkers. The invitro biomarkers can be further sub-divided into biochemical and urinary biomarkers, and *in-vivo* biomarkers can be sub-divided into molecular biomarkers and ex-vivo biomarkers as described in the text and illustrated in Figure 32. The bodily fluid AD biomarkers include: CSF biomarkers, serum lipid triglycerides, and cholesterol, pro-inflammatory cytokines, CRP, BDNF, and blood platelets as biomarkers which may facilitate early diagnosis of AD as Figure 33 illustrates. Various omic biomarkers of AD include: proteomic biomarkers, genomic biomarkers, glycomic biomarkers, lipidomic biomarkers, and metabolomics biomarkers, in addition to microRNA which can be employed to accomplish PM as shown in Figure 34. Various *in-vivo* biomarkers which can be employed for the personalized treatment of AD are: PET imaging biomarkers including: reduced brain regional [18]FdG uptake and increased ^{18}F-PiB uptake, AD biomarkers for personalized treatment, multiple diagnostic biomarkers, MRI morphological biomarkers, fronto-temporal atrophy, ventriculomegaly, and demyelination, MRS biomarkers: reduced NAA, PCr/Cr Ratio, Reduced choline and glutamate as shown in Figure 35. Various physiological/behavioral biomarkers, electrophysiological biomarkers, circadian biomarkers, epidemiological biomarkers, neuropsychological biomarkers, and biomarkers used for personalized treatment for the early personalized diagnosis and treatment of AD as shown in Figure 36. Various pathological biomarkers including: APOE polymorphism, neuropathological biomarkers, and biomarkers in VaD and AD. Amyloid beta, and CRP biomarkers to differentiate AD vs VaD and biomarkers in BPD and AD as presented in Figure 37. Misclaneous AD biomarkers of

AD include mitochondrial biomarkers 8-OH, 2dG and Charnoly body; (ii) PUFA as a biomarker to assess brain regional myelination. α-synuclein as a biomarker (α-synuclein index), CB as a biomarkers, Domoic acid as an AD probe, hormones as AD biomarkers: GH, estrogen, and progesterone as Figure 38 illustrates.

In-Vitro and In-Vivo AD Biomarkers

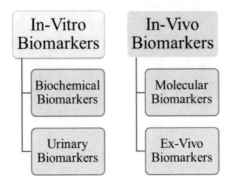

Figure 32. *In-Vitro and In-Vivo AD Biomarkers* A systematic diagram illustrating primarily two major types of AD biomarkers including: *in-vitro* biomarkers and (ii) *in-vivo* biomarkers. The *in-vitro* biomarkers can be further sub-divided into biochemical and urinary biomarkers, and *in-vivo* biomarkers can be sub-divided into molecular biomarkers and ex-vivo biomarkers as described in the text.

Bodily Fluid AD Biomarkers

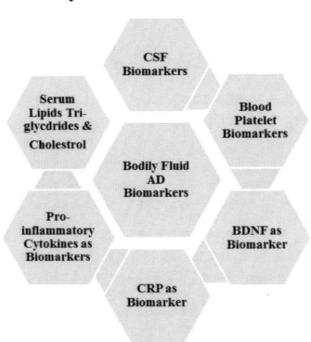

Figure 33. *Bodily Fluid AD Biomarkers* A diagram illustrating bodily fluid AD biomarkers including: CSF biomarkers, serum lipid triglycerides, and cholesterol, pro-inflammatory cytokines, CRP, BDNF, and blood platelets as biomarkers which may facilitate early diagnosis of AD.

Omic AD Biomarkers

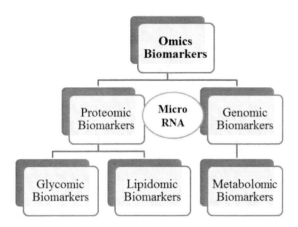

Figure 34. *Omic Biomarkers of AD* A schematic diagram illustrating various omic biomarkers of AD. The omice biomarkers of AD include: proteomic biomarkers, genomic biomarkers, glycomic biomarkers, lipidomic biomarkers, and metabolomics biomarkers, in addition to microRNA which can be employed to accomplish PM.

In-Vivo Imaging AD Biomarkers

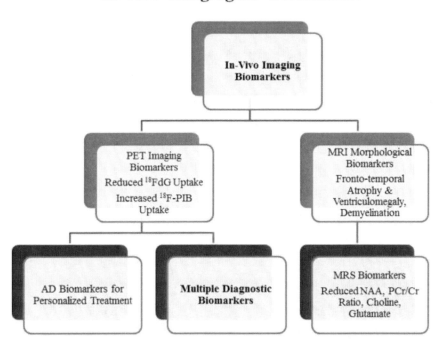

Figure 35. *In-Vivo Imaging Biomarkers of AD* A pictorial representation of various *in-vivo* biomarkers which can be employed for the personalized treatment of AD are: PET imaging biomarkers including: reduced brain regional ^{18}FdG uptake and increased ^{18}F-PiB uptake, AD biomarkers for personalized treatment, multiple diagnostic biomarkers, MRI morphological biomarkers, fronto-temporal atrophy, ventriculomegaly, and demyelination, MRS biomarkers: reduced NAA, PCr/Cr Ratio, Reduced choline and glutamate.

Physiological and Behavioral AD Biomarkers

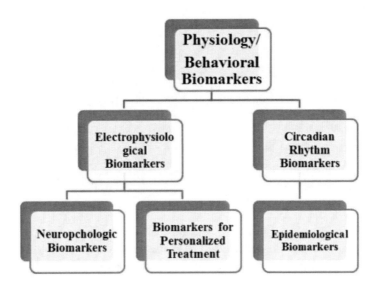

Figure 36. *Physiological/Behavioral Biomarkers of AD* A diagram illustrating various physiological/behavioral biomarkers, electrophysiological biomarkers, circadian biomarkers, epidemiological biomarkers, neuropsychological biomarkers, and biomarkers used for personalized treatment for the early personalized diagnosis and treatment of AD.

Pathological AD Biomarkers

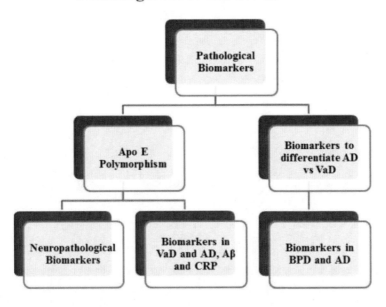

Figure 37. *Pathological Biomarkers of AD* A pictorial diagram illustrating various pathological biomarkers including: APOE polymorphism, neuropathological biomarkers, and biomarkers in VaD and AD. Amylod beta, and CRP biomarkers to differentiate AD vs VaD and biomarkers in BPD and AD.

Miscellaneous AD Biomarkers

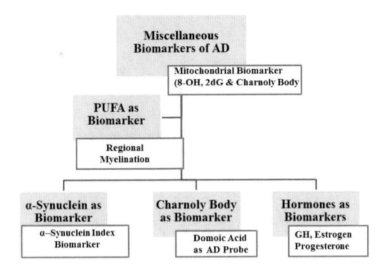

Figure 38. *Misclaneous AD Biomarkers* A systematic diagram illustrating misclaneous AD biomarkers. Mitochondrial biomarkers 8-OH, 2dG and Charnoly body; (ii) PUFA as a biomarker to assess brain regional myelination α-synuclein as a biomarker (α-synuclein index), CB as biomarkers, Domoic acid as an AD probe, hormones as AD biomarkers: GH, estrogen, and progesterone.

Potential therapeutic biomarkers of AD including: Glutathione, N-acetyl cysteine, PUFA, B-Vitamins, Vitamin D, Melatonin, Curcumin, Flavinoids, antioxidants, Coenzyme Q10, and micronutrients, Zinc and Magnesium which can be supplemented in the diet of AD patient for better clinical prognosis and outcome personzed treatment of AD as illustrated in Figure 39. The general over view of biomarkers for personalized treatment of AD. These biomarkers can be classified into 8 main headings: (a) clinical biomarkers (b) circulating and CSF biomarkers, (c) imaging biomarkers, (d) pathological biomarkers, (e) cognitive biomarkers, (f) genetic biomarkers, (g) biochemical biomarkers, and (h) omic biomarkers. All these biomarkers have their own merits and limitations. No specific biomarker can precisely confirm AD diagnosis. Hence these are analyzed in combination to authenticate the early diagnosis for the personalized treatment of AD. Generally clinical biomarkers include: cognitive impairments, hyposmia, and hypogustia; circulating and CSF biomarkers include: amylod-β, Tau, and phosphorylated tau, and imaging biomarkers include: CT/SPECT/PET/MRI. MRS analyses. Three most common PET biomarkers are ^{18}FdG, ^{18}F-PiB and ^{11}C-PK-11195 to assess brain regional glucose metabolism, amyloid-β burden, and microglial inflammation respectively. Pathological biomarkers include hippocampal and corical atrophy, senile plaques, amyloid body plaques, and Charnoly Body (CB) aggregates. Cortical, hippocampal, and callosal atrophy can also be determined by performing MRI *in vivo*. Cognitive biomarkers include: impairments in learning, intelligence, memory, and behavior. Biochemical biomarkers, which can facilitate AD diagnosis include: β-secretase, Amyloid Precursor Protein, acetyl choline esterase, MAOIs, and C-reactive proteins. One of the most important genetic biomarker is apolipoprotein E4ζ. The omics biomarkers include: genomic, proteomic, metabolomics, glycomic, lipidomic, and metalomic analyses. These biomarkers in combination can provide an accurate diagnosis for the personalized treatment of AD.

Potential Therapeutic AD Biomarkers

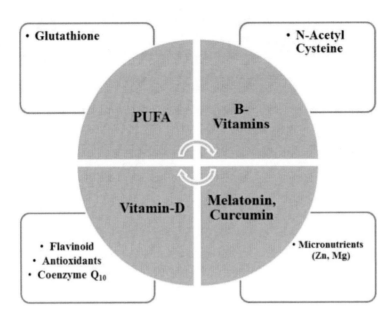

Figure 39. *Potential Therapeutic Biomarkers of AD* A pictorial diagram illustrating potential therapeutic biomarkers of AD including: Glutathione, N-acetyl cysteine, PUFA, B-Vitamins, Vitamin D, Melatonin, Curcumin, Flavinoids, antioxidants, Coenzyme Q10, and micronutrients, Zinc and Magnesium which can be supplemented in the diet of AD patient for better clinical prognosis and outcome for the personalized treatment of AD.

IN-VITRO MOLECULAR BIOMARKERS IN AD

Several *in-vitro* biomarkers have been developed for an early and differential diagnosis of AD, with limited success. CSF Aβ1-42, total tau (T-tau) and phosphorylated tau181 (P-tau) are finding increasing utility as biomarkers of AD. In general, a combined approach of analyzing *in-vivo* as well as *in-vitro* biomarkers has facilitated accurate diagnosis of AD. Although the pharmacotherapy for the treatment of AD has improved, a lot of work is needed to eventually treat this devastating disorder. In general, *in-vitro* biomarkers can be derived from the blood, CSF, saliva, and urinary samples of AD patients. Various bodily fluid biomarkers can facilitate confirming AD diagnosis. In addition, *in-vivo* biomarkers can be divided as molecular biomarkers and ex-vivo biomarkers by taking biopsy samples from animal models and autopsy samples from AD patients. The effect of 12-15LO on tau levels and metabolism and the mechanism involved by using genetic and pharmacologic approaches were investigated (Inoue et al., 2013). While no significant differences were observed in the levels of tau for both groups, compared with controls; Tg2576 mice overexpressing 12-15LO revealed increased phosphorylated tau at two specific epitopes, Ser 202/Thr 205 and Ser 396. *In vitro* and *in vivo* studies showed that 12-15LO modulates tau metabolism via the cdk5 kinase pathway. Associated with these changes were biochemical markers of synaptic pathology. Moreover, 12-15LO-dependent alteration of tau metabolism was independent from an effect on Aβ. These findings provided a novel pathway by which 12-15LO modulates endogenous tau metabolism making this protein a pharmacologic target for the effective treatment of AD and related tauopathies.

CSF Biomarkers in AD Recently several biomarkers of dementia were validated based on the neuropathological processes occurring in the brain. However the lack of pathologically validated biomarkers and their high variability; the combinations of these biomarkers may represent a more precise analytical and diagnostic tool in the complex plethora of degenerative dementia. CSF biomarkers are generally used for the diagnosis of dementia (Sancesario and Bernardini, 2015). Opposite changes in the level of amyloid-β_{1-42} versus total tau and phosphorylated-tau_{181} in the CSF reflect the specific pathology of AD in the brain. These biomarkers can differentiate AD from controls and from the major types of dementia, and can evaluate the disease progression from MCI to AD. In the absence of specific biomarkers reflecting the pathologies of the other forms of dementia, such as Lewy Body disease, frontotemporal degeneration, Creutzfeldt-Jakob disease, the evaluation of biomarkers of AD pathology is used to exclude rather than to confirm AD. Other biomarkers do not adequately relate to the underlying pathology. In addition, Progranulin (PGRN) was proposed as a selective biomarker of frontotemporal dementia with mutations in the PGRN gene; the 14-3-3 protein is a highly sensitive and specific biomarker for Creutzfeldt-Jacob disease, but has to be used carefully in differentiating rapid progressive dementia; and α-Synuclein is a candidate biomarker of the diversified neurodegenerative α-synucleinopathies.

OMICS BIOMARKERS IN AD

Various types of omics biomarkers are being explored for the development of novel disease specific biomarker of AD. The omic biomarkers can be broadly classified as proteomic biomarkers, genomic biomarkers, metabolomics biomarkers, lipidomic biomarkers, and glycomic biomarkers. The analysis of these biomarkers requires bioinformatics approach and extensive computer analysis for feature selection. In addition recently microRNAs have been detected in the plasma and CSF samples of AD patients. The omics biomarkers can be broadly classified as proteomic, genomic, metabolomis, lipidomic, and glycomic.

Genomic Instability in AD It is reported that maintenance of metabolic systems relating to accurate DNA replication and repair is critical for lifelong human health (Lee et al., 2015). Should this homeostatic balance become impaired, genomic instability emerges, compromising the structural and functional integrity of the genome, which may result in impaired gene expression and human disease. Both genomic instability and micronutrient imbalance have been implicated in diseases associated with accelerated aging which potentially leads to an increased risk for the future development of clinically-defined neurodegenerative disorders. Cognitive decline leading to the clinical diagnosis of MCI predicts an increased risk in later life of developing AD. Although knowledge on the impact of dietary factors in relation to MCI and AD risk is improving, it is still inadequate. Particularly the role of nutrient combinations (i.e., *nutriomes*) has not been thoroughly investigated. Currently, there is a dire need for preventative strategies as well as the reproducible diagnostic biomarkers that will allow identification of those individuals with increased risk for neurodegenerative diseases. Growing evidence suggests cells originating from different somatic tissues derived from individuals that have been clinically diagnosed with neurodegenerative disorders, exhibit increased frequencies of DNA damage compared to tissues of cognitively healthy individuals which could be due to malnutrition. This report discussed current evidence and lacunae in the present knowledge relating to genome instability biomarkers and blood micronutrient profiles from MCI and AD patients that may contribute to the increased risk of these diseases.

Micro RNA as Biomarkers of AD MicroRNAs (miRNAs) are class of small noncoding molecules that play an important role in the regulation of gene expression at the post-transcriptional level. Due to their ability to modulate different genes, these are highly suitable to function as key regulators during immune cell differentiation, and their dysfunction can contribute to pathological conditions associated with neuro-inflammation. MiRNAs belong to the class of regulatory RNA molecules of ~22 nt length and regulate ~60% of all genes through post-transcriptional gene silencing (RNAi). They have potential as useful biomarkers for clinical applications because of their stability and ease of detection in many tissues, especially blood. Circulating profiles of miRNAs discriminate different tumor types, indicate staging and progression of the disease and as prognostic biomarkers. Recently their role in neurodegenerative diseases, both as diagnostic biomarkers as well as elucidating basic disease etiology was highlighted. Expression levels of miRNAs have potential as diagnostic biomarkers as they circulate and their tissue specific profiles can be identified in plasma, CSF, and urine. Recent developments in sequencing technology provide unique opportunities to develop biomarker discovery from the profile of a miRNA in body fluids specific to neurodegenerative diseases. Recently a circulating 7-miRNA signature (hsa-let-7d-5p, hsa-let-7g-5p, hsa-miR-15b-5p, hsa-miR-142-3p, hsa-miR-191-5p, hsa-miR-301a-3p and hsa-miR-545-3p) in plasma was reported, which could distinguish AD patients from normal controls (NC) with >95% accuracy (Kumar et al., 2013). There was a >2 fold difference for all miRNAs between the AD and NC samples. Pathway analysis, taking into account enriched target mRNAs for these miRNAs was also carried out, suggesting that the disturbance of multiple enzymatic pathways including lipid metabolism could play a significant role in AD etiology.

The application of miRNA sequencing in biomarker identification from biological fluids and its translation into clinical practice was recenty highlighted (Cheng et al., 2013). A novel miRNA-based signature for detecting AD from blood samples by applying NGS to miRNAs from blood samples of 48 AD patients and 22 unaffected controls, yielding a total of 140 mature miRNAs with significantly changed expression levels was presented (Leidinger et al., 2013). Of these, 82 had higher and 58 had lower abundance in AD patient samples. These investigators selected 12 miRNAs for an RT-qPCR analysis on a larger cohort of 202 samples, comprising not only AD patients and healthy controls but also patients with other CNS illnesses. These included MCI, which represents a transitional period before the development of AD, multiple sclerosis, PD, MDD, bipolar disorder, and schizophrenia. Target enrichment analysis of the selected 12 miRNAs indicated their involvement in CNS development, neuron projection development, and morphogenesis. Using this 12-miRNA signature, these researchers differentiated between AD and controls with an accuracy of 93%, a specificity of 95%, and a sensitivity of 92%. The differentiation of AD from other neurological diseases was possible with accuracies between 74% to 78%. The differentiation of the other CNS disorders from controls yielded even higher accuracies indicating that deregulated miRNAs in blood might be used as biomarkers in the diagnosis of AD or other neurodegenerative diseases.

A recent study confirmed that miRNA may be potential biomarkers of AD (Bekris et al., 2013). These investigators demonstrated that miRNAs in human brain or biofluids are differentially expressed according to disease status, tissue type, neuritic plaque score, or Braak stage. Post-mortem brain (PMB) miRNA were profiled using microarrays and validated using qRT-PCR. Five qRT-PCR-validated miRNAs were measured in a sample of PMB, CSF and plasma from the same subjects. Plasma miR-15a was associated with plaque score in the sample, suggesting that miRNA in human biofluids may offer utility as biomarkers of AD. Indeed, the circulating miRNAs is opening a new era in systemic and tissue-specific biomarker research, highlighting new inter-cellular and inter-organ communication mechanisms (Oliveiri et al., 2013). Circulating miRNAs might be active messengers eliciting a systemic response as well as non-specific "by-products" of cell activity and even of cell death; in either case they have the potential to be clinically significant biomarkers for numerous pathophysiological processes, including inflammatory responses and inflammation-related diseased conditions. The current evidence indicates that miRNAs can exert two opposite roles, i.e., activating as well as inhibiting inflammatory pathways. The inhibitory action relates to the need for activating anti-inflammatory mechanisms to inhibit pro-inflammatory signals, like the NF-κB pathway and to prevent cell and tissue destruction. Thus miRNA-based anti-inflammatory mechanisms may acquire a crucial role during aging, where a chronic, low-level pro-inflammatory status is sustained by the cell senescence secretome and by activation of immune cells as a function of time. This process entails age-related changes, especially in extremely old age, in those circulating miRNAs that are capable of modulating the inflammatory status (inflamma-miRs). A number of such circulating miRNAs seem to be promising biomarkers for the age-related diseases that share a common chronic, low-level pro-inflammatory status, such as cardiovascular disease (CVD), type 2 diabetes mellitus (T2DM), AD, rheumatoid arthritis (RA), and cancers.

Recent studies addressed the role of miRNAs in the differentiation of progenitor cells into microglia and in the activation process, clarifying the origin of adult microglia and the contribution of the CNS environment to microglial phenotype, in health and disease. Altered expression of miRNAs was associated with AD, MS, and ischemic injury, suggesting their significance as disease–specific biomarkers and new therapeutic targets. Advances in miRNA-mediated regulation of microglial development and activation were summerized (Guedes et al., 2013). These investigators discussed the role of specific miRNAs in the maintenance and switching of microglial activation states and their potential both as biomarkers of inflammation as well as new therapeutic targets for the modulation of microglial behavior in the CNS. A further study is needed to elucidate the exact pathophysiological significance of miRNAs as biomarkers of AD and other neurodegenerative disorders (Zhou and Xu, 2015).

Long Noncoding RNA as a Biomarker in AD It remains unknown if long noncoding RNAs (lncRNAs) may play a role in AD pathogenesis (Sood et al., 2015). The investigators identified AD-associated lncRNAs by reannotation of microarray data based on postmortem tissue samples of AD patients and matched elderly controls and found 24 upregulated and 84 downregulated lncRNAs in AD patients compared with controls. The most downregulated lncRNAs in AD were highly expressed in the brain but not in other tissues. Gene set enrichment analysis identified a downregulated lncRNA n341006 in association with protein ubiquitination pathway, and upregulated lncRNA n336934 linked to cholesterol homeostasis. Interestingly, lncRNA expression signatures could predict tissue types with equal accuracy as protein-coding genes, but the number of lncRNAs required for optimal prediction was less than protein-coding genes. This study provided a resource for AD-associated lncRNAs for the development of lncRNA biomarkers and the identification of functional lncRNAs involved in AD pathogenesis.

Transcriptomics in AD Diagnosis In a recent study, transcriptomic approach was applied to build the first multi-tissue RNA expression signature by gene-chip profiling from sedentary subjects who reached 65 years of age in normal health (Kim et al., 2013). A total of 150 probe-sets from an accurate classifier of young versus older muscle tissue and RNA classifier performed in independent cohorts of human muscle, skin and brain tissue, represented a biomarker for biological age. By employing the Uppsala Longitudinal Study of Adult Men birth-cohort, these investigators demonstrated that the RNA classifier is insensitive to confounding lifestyle biomarkers, while greater gene score at age 70 years was associated with better renal function at age 82 years and longevity. The gene score was 'up-regulated' in healthy hippocampus with age, and when applied to blood RNA profiles from two independent age-matched dementia case-control data sets the healthy controls had greater gene scores than those with cognitive impairment. Alone, or when combined with previously described prototype AD RNA 'disease signature', the healthy aging RNA classifier was diagnostic for AD. These authors identified a novel and multi-tissue RNA signature of healthy aging that can act as a diagnostic biomarker of health, using a peripheral blood sample. This RNA signature had potential to assist biomarker research aimed at finding treatments for and/or management of AD and other aging-related conditions.

Proteomic Biomarkers in AD The researchers need biomarkers for pre-symptomatic diagnosis, treatment, and monitoring of AD. CSF is selected because its proteome reflects the composition of the brain. Ideal biomarkers have low inter-individual variability among control subjects to minimize overlaps between clinical groups. Proteins, studied as potential biomarkers, play important roles in numerous physiological activities and diseases. Moreover genetic variation may modulate corresponding protein levels and point to the role of these variants in AD pathophysiology. Effects of individual SNPs have been analyzed for the plasma protein levels using GWAS data and proteomic data with 132 quality-controlled analytes from 521 caucasian participants. Linear regression analysis detected 112 significant associations between 27 analytes and 112 SNPs. 107 out of these 112 associations were tested in the Indiana Memory and Aging Study (IMAS) cohort for replication and 50 associations were replicated and uncorrected in the same direction of effect as those in the ADNI. Novel associations including that of rs7517126 with plasma complement factor H-related protein 1 (CFHR1) level accounted for 40% of total variation of the protein level (Oh et al., 2013). An association of rs6677604 with the same protein was noticed. Although these two SNPs were not in the strong linkage disequilibrium, 61% of total variation of CFHR1 was accounted for by rs6677604 without additional variation by rs7517126, when both SNPs were tested together. 78 other SNP-protein associations in the ADNI sample exceeded genome-wide significance, confirming gene-protein associations for IL-6 receptor, chemokine CC-4, angiotensin-converting enzyme (ACE), and angiotensinogen, although the direction of effect was reversed in some cases. This study was among the first analyses of gene-protein product relationships integrating proteomics and targeted genes extracted from a GWAS array.

A Sensitive Biosensor for the Detection of Aβ Recently, a carbon nanotube (CNT) film-based nanobiosensor with a metal semiconductor field effect transistor (MESFET) was developed. A gold top gate was deposited on the middle of the CNT channel and probe antibodies were immobilized on the gold top gate with an antibody-binding protein, protein G or Escherichia coli outer membrane (OM) with autodisplayed Z-domains of protein A. These CNT-MESFET biosensors exhibit a higher sensitivity than the CNT-FET biosensor with probe antibodies immobilized using a chemical linker, since the antibody-binding proteins control the orientation of immobilized antibodies. In addition, nonspecific binding is inhibited by E. coli OM. Using the CNT-MESFET biosensors with E. coli OM containing Z domain, these investigators detected Aβ in human serum at 1pg/mL without labeling, which was lower than the limit of detection using ELISA, suggesting that CNT-MESFET biosensors might be clinically useful for early diagnosis of AD. Recently a process of multi-affinity fractionation (MAF) and quantitative label-free liquid chromatography tandem mass spectrometry (LC-MS/MS) for CSF biomarker was developed by (i) identifying sources of technical variability, (ii) assessing subject variance and residual technical variability for CSF proteins, and (iii) testing its ability to segregate samples on the basis of biomarker characteristics (Perrin et al., 2013). These investigators used 14 aliquots of pooled CSF and 2 aliquots from 6 cognitively normal individuals, enriched for low-abundance proteins by MAF, digested proteolytically, randomized again, and analyzed by nano-LC-MS. Among 11,433 aligned charge groups, 1360 relatively abundant ones were annotated by MS2, yielding 823 unique peptides. Analyses, including Pearson correlations of LC-MS ion chromatograms, performed for all sample comparisons, identified several sources of technical variability: i) incomplete MAF and Keratins; ii) globally-or segmentally-decreased ion current in isolated LC-MS analyses; and iii) oxidized Methionine-containing peptides. Exclusion of these sources yielded 609 peptides representing 81 proteins most of which showed low coefficients of variation whether they were quantified from the mean of all or only the two most-abundant peptides. Clustering, using 24 proteins selected for high subject variance, yielded perfect segregation of pooled and individual samples, indicating that LC-MS/MS can measure scores of CSF proteins with low variability and can segregate samples according to desired criteria. Thus, this technique has a potential for biomarker discovery in AD.

Lipidomic Biomarkers in AD. Lipids serve diversified functions in cellular homeostasis including; membrane organization, for membrane function and protein/protein or protein/lipid interaction, energy storage, and in signal transduction. Lipidomics is defined as "the full characterization of lipid molecular species and their biological roles with respect to expression of proteins involved in lipid metabolism and function, including gene regulation" (Naudí et al., 2015). Human brain contains a large amount of lipids and diversity of lipid molecular species. Perturbations in lipid homeostasis may result in abnormal cellular function. Recent advances in lipidomics enabled to view AD pathogenesis, and revealed that lipid aberrations are implicated in the disease progression. These researchers suggested that, the study of brain lipidomics can help to unravel the diversity, and to disclose the specificity of these lipid traits, and its alterations in neural (neurons and glial) cells, groups of neural cells, brain, and fluids such as CSF and plasma; thus helping to discover potential biomarkers of human brain aging and AD. They discussed the lipid composition of the adult human brain, considered a brief approach to lipid definition, classification, and tools for the analysis that emerged with lipidomics, and turn to the lipid profiles in human brain and how lipids affect CNS function. Finally, they focused on the current status of lipidomics in human brain aging and AD, and highlighted that neurolipidomics will enhance our knowledge regarding physiological and pathological functions of brain cells and will elucidate the concept of selective neuronal vulnerability. Furthermore, the lipid alternations, which affect amyloid plaque and neurofibrillary tangles formation and accumulation, as well as to neuronal and synaptic dysfunction in cells and animal models were highlighted (Xiang et al., 2015). Hence lipid abnormalities observed in the human CSF, plasma, and serum in association with AD could serve as potential biomarkers to differentially diagnose and monitor the disease in future.

Metabolomic Biomarkers in AD Metabolomics is gaining momentum in the investigation of neurological pathologies such as AD, PD, and ALS. The magnitude of emotional, physical, and financial burden related to these three devastating pathologies can be deduced considering that ~20 million people worldwide suffer from these three pathologies. The recent applications of metabolomics were overviewed to investigate the neurodegenerative diseases (Ibáñez et al., 2015). Novel metabolomics strategies are now being developed to map perturbations in biochemical pathways linked to neurodegeneration. These pathologies can begin years or even decades before the onset of clinical symptoms, and thus, metabolomics is being used to discover preclinical biomarkers of these neurological diseases. Metabolomics is a powerful technique for discovering novel biomarkers and biochemical pathways to improve EBPT. The main advantage of metabolomics is that it enables assessment of global metabolic profiles of biofluids and discovery of new biomarkers distinguishing disease status, with the possibility of enhancing clinical diagnosis. Identifying multiple novel biomarkers for neurological diseases enhanced with recent advances in metabolomics that are more accurate than conventional procedures. CSF, which is known to be a rich source of small-molecule biomarkers for neurological and neurodegenerative diseases, and is in close contact with diseased areas in neurological disorders, could be used for AD diagnosis. It is expected that metabolomics will drive CSF analysis, improve the development of AD treatment, and will result in greater benefits to public health.

Recently, the use of ultra-high performance liquid chromatography-time-of-flight mass spectrometry (UHPLC-TOF MS) was introduced to analyze CSF samples from patients with different AD stages (Ibenez et al., 2013). To obtain wide metabolome coverage, two different chromatographic separation modes, namely reversed phase (RP) and hydrophilic interaction chromatography (HILIC), were used. The two methods, RP/UHPLC-MS and HILIC/UHPLC-MS, were applied to analyze CSF samples from 75 patients related to AD progression. Significant differences in CSF samples from subjects with different cognitive status related to AD progression were detected, obtaining potential biomarkers together with a classification model by means of a multivariate analysis. The proposed model predicted the development of AD biomarkers with an accuracy of 98.7% and specificity and sensitivity >95%. Although the majority of AD clinical trials have focused on anti-Aβ treatments, other therapeutic approaches may be necessary. The ability to monitor changes in cellular networks that include both Aβ and non-Aβ pathways is essential to increase our understanding of the etiopathogenesis of AD and subsequent development of cognitive symptoms and dementia. Metabolomics is a powerful tool that detects metabolites that reflect changes downstream of genomic, transcriptomic, and proteomic fluctuations, and represents an accurate biochemical profile of the organism in health and disease (Trushina and Mielke, 2013). Hence this approach could identify biomarkers for early AD diagnosis, discover novel therapeutic targets, and monitor therapeutic response and disease progression. Moreover, given the considerable parallel between mouse and human metabolism, the use of metabolomics provides translation of animal research into human studies for drug development. Different aspects of CSF metabolomics and their significance in the post-genomic era, emphasizing the importance of small-molecule metabolites in this emerging field were highlighted (Zhang et al., 2013).

A metabolomic analysis of serum and saliva obtained from patients with dementias, including AD, frontotemporal lobe dementia (FTLD), and Lewy body disease (LBD), as well as from age-matched healthy controls was performed (Tsuruoka et al., 2013). By performing CE-TOFMS, these investigators discovered that 6 metabolites in serum *(β-alanine, creatinine, hydroxyproline, glutamine, iso-citrate, and cytidine)* and 2 in saliva *(arginine and tyrosine)* are significantly different between dementias and controls. By multivariate analysis confirmed serum as a more efficient biological fluid for diagnosis compared to saliva; additionally, 45 metabolites were identified as candidate biomarkers that could discriminate at least one pair of diagnostic groups from the healthy control group. These metabolites provided a unique opportunity for diagnosing dementia-type by multiphase screening. Moreover, diagnostic-type-dependent differences are observed in various TCA cycle compounds detected in serum, indicating that glucose metabolic pathways may be altered in neurodegenerative dementia patients. This pilot study revealed changes in metabolomic profiles between various dementias. Moreover impaired cerebral glucose metabolism, a pathophysiological feature, may be a critical biomarker to evaluate the pathogenesis of AD.

GENETIC BIOMARKERS IN AD

Mutations in known AD genes account for 1% to 3% of patients, and almost all are dominantly inherited. Recessive inheritance of complex phenotypes can be linked to long (>1-megabase [Mb]) runs of homozygosity (ROHs) detectable by SNP arrays. A study was performed to evaluate the association between ROHs and AD in an African American population known to have a risk for AD up to 3X higher than white individuals (Ghani et al., 2015). This was the first study of African American data set previously genotyped on different genome-wide SNP arrays. Global and locus-based ROH measurements were analyzed using raw or imputed genotype data from 2 case-control subsets grouped based on SNP array: AD Genetics Consortium data set *(871 cases and 1620 control individuals)* and Chicago Health and Aging Project-Indianapolis Ibadan Dementia Study data set (279 cases and 1367 control individuals). These investigators examined the entire data set using imputed genotypes from 1917 cases and 3858 control individuals. The ROHs >1 Mb, 2 Mb, or 3 Mb were investigated separately for global burden evaluation, consensus regions, and gene-based analyses. The African American cohort had a low degree of inbreeding. In the AD Genetics Consortium data set, a higher proportion of cases with ROHs >2 Mb or >3 Mb was detected. In the Chicago Health and Aging Project-Indianapolis Ibadan Dementia Study data set, a significant 202-kilobase consensus region on Chr15q24 and a cluster of 13 significant genes on Chr3p21.31 was identified. A total of 43 of 49 nominally significant genes common for both data sets also mapped to Chr3p21.31. Analyses of imputed SNP data confirmed the association of AD with global ROH and a gene-cluster on Chr3p21.31. In addition, association between AD and CLDN17, encoding a protein from the Claudin family members was suggested as AD biomarkers. This was the first study of increased burden of ROHs among patients with AD from an outbred African American population, which could reflect either the cumulative effect of multiple ROHs to AD or the contribution of specific loci harboring recessive mutations and risk haplotypes in a subset of patients. Hence sequencing is essential to uncover AD variants in a specific ethenic group.

Single Nucleotide Polymorphism (SNP) in AD It is well established that SNPs contribute most of the genetic variation to the human genome. SNPs associate with many complex and common diseases like AD. Hence discovering SNP biomarkers at different loci can improve early diagnosis and treatment of these diseases. Bayesian network (BN) provides a framework for representing interactions between genes or SNPs. A different BN structure learning algorithms was applied in WGS data for detecting the causal AD SNPs and gene-SNP interactions (Sherif et al., 2015). These researchers focused on polymorphisms in the top 10 genes associated with AD, identified by GWA studies. New SNP biomarkers associated with AD were rs7530069, rs113464261, rs114506298, rs73504429, rs7929589, rs76306710, and rs668134. These findings demonstrated the effectiveness of using BN as biomarkers for identifying AD causal SNPs and supported that the SNP set detected by Markov blanket based methods had a significant association with AD, achieves better performance than both naïve Bayes, and tree augmented naïve Bayes. Minimal augmented Markov blanket reached accuracy of 66.13% and sensitivity of 88.87% versus 61.58% and 59.43% in naïve Bayes.

Apolipoprotein E ε4 Polymorphism in AD It is now known that the ApoE gene has three common alleles (ε 2, ε 3, and ε 4) and is linked to health outcomes and longevity. The ε2 allele has neuroprotective effects, whereas the ε 4 allele is a risk factor for cardiovascular disease and AD. However, the relationships of Apo-E with mortality and physical function remains uncertain. Individuals who carry the Apo-E ε4 polymorphism have an increased risk of late-onset AD. However, because possession of the ε4 allele confers an increased risk for the diagnosis of dementia, it was problematic in older individuals to dissociate the influence of ε4 on cognitive capacity as distinct from its influence on clinical diagnosis. A statistical approach that attempts to influence diagnostic group members (AD, MCI, healthy control) from the influence of Apo-E ε4 genetic status on cognitive functioning was applied (Foster et al., 2013). The phenotype hypothesis predicted that ε4-positive individuals will show cognitive deficits independent of the development of AD, whereas the prodromal/preclinical AD hypothesis proposed that the effect of Apo-E status on cognitive performance is a function of the increased risk of dementia in individuals with the ε4 allele. These hypotheses were evaluated in the Australian Imaging, Biomarkers and Lifestyle cohort to determine whether ε4 status and age-related neuropsychological performance could be explained by recruiting people with MCI into the healthy control group. As interactions between the ε4 allele and age have been reported in cognitive functioning within healthy elderly populations, it was determined whether the inclusion of MCI individuals may drive this relationship. Neuropsychological tests were administered to 764 healthy control subjects, 131 individuals with MCI, and 168 individuals with AD. The effect of the ε4 allele on cognitive performance was assessed using a statistical mediation analysis and supplemented with Bayesian methods to address limitations associated with Fisherian/Neyman-Pearsonian significance. These findings supported the prodromal/preclinical AD hypothesis.

The Social EnvIronment and Biomarkers of Aging Study (SEBAS) were used to examine the relationship between Apo-E polymorphisms and physical and pulmonary function in

1,000 Taiwanese adults aged 53 years and older (Vasunilashorn et al., 2013). Measures of physical function included self-reported difficulties with respect to activities of daily living (ADLs) and other physical functions and performance-based measures of grip strength (kg), walking speed (m/s) over a distance of 3 m, and chair stand speed (stand/s). Peak expiratory flow rate was also measured as an indicator of pulmonary function. There were no significant relationships between Apo-E carrier status and the measures of pulmonary function suggesting that the Apo-E gene may not be a risk factor for functional decline in AD.

SNP in Inflammatory Genes and AD It is realized that SNP in genes encoding immunological mediators can affect the biological activity of molecules by regulating transcription, translation, or secretion, modulating the genetic risk of inflammatory damage in AD. Polymorphisms in 10 inflammatory genes were compared to genotype distribution across outpatients with late-onset AD and noncognitively impaired subjects, and controlling for ancestry heritage and ApoE genotype. Almost 40% lower chance of AD was noticed among homozygotes of the IL10-1082A allele (rs1800896). Dichotomization to ApoE and mean ancestry levels did not affect protection, except among those with greater European or minor African heritage. The IL-10 locus seemed to affect the onset of AD in the genetic ancestry of Brazilian older adults. Age and the Apo-E ε4 allele are risk factors for AD, but whether female sex is also a risk factor remains controversial. A study estimated the effects of ApoE ε4 and sex on age-specific morphometric and clinical decline in late-onset sporadic AD (Holland et al., 2013). By using linear mixed-effects models, these investigators examined the effect of age, ApoE ε4, and sex on longitudinal brain atrophy and clinical decline among cognitively-healthy older individuals and individuals with MCI and AD. They also evaluated the relationship between these effects and CSF biomarkers of AD pathology. ApoE ε4 significantly accelerated rates of decline in women as compared to men. Although the magnitude of the sex effect on rates of decline was as large as those of ε4, their relationship to CSF biomarkers was weaker, suggesting that in addition to ApoE ε4 status, diagnostic and therapeutic strategies should be considered to evaluate the effect of female sex on the AD pathogenesis.

It was reported that the importance of biomarker research for psychiatric disorders is delayed by symptom-related diagnostic categories that are only distantly associated with biological mechanisms (Bagdy and Juhasz, 2013). In neuropsychiatric disorders that have high heritability (schizophrenia, autism, and AD), genomic research provided significant GWAS results. In contrast, in moderately heritable psychiatric disorders (anxiety disorders, unipolar major depression), the development of symptoms, in addition to risk genes, was primarily dependent on specific environmental risk factors. Thus, controlling for heterogeneity, and not simply increasing the number of subjects, was crucial for significant psychiatric GWAS findings that warrant the collection of detailed data and information about relevant environmental exposures. Thus gene-gene interactions and intermediate phenotypes or psychiatric and somatic co-morbidities, by identifying similar cases within a diagnostic category, could further increase the weak effects of individual genes that limit their usefulness as biomarkers. Hence methods that are suitable to identify biologically homogeneous subgroups within a given psychiatric disorder are necessary to enhance biomarker research.

Epigenetic Biomarkers in AD Within putative biomarkers, peripheral BDNF levels correlated significantly with cognitive decline in AD, although conflicting results were reported. Sirtuin 1 (Sirt1) serum levels are lower in AD patients and Presenilin 1 (Psen1) is expressed by blood cells (Carboni et al., 2015). In addition, DNA methylation is altered in AD patients, suggesting that epigenetic mechanisms play a significant role in AD pathophysiology. A study investigated promoter methylation levels of potential biomarkers in AD patients and controls. Peripheral blood DNA methylation levels were analyzed by methylation-specific primer real-time PCR. BDNF promoter methylation did not differ between AD patients and controls. Sirt1 promoter revealed minimal levels of methylation which did not display significant differences between groups. Similarly, no significant difference was noticed between AD patients and controls in Psen1 methylation, showing a large variability among subjects. Although peripheral BDNF expression was associated with differential promoter methylation in psychiatric and neurological disorders, these results suggested different mechanisms in AD. The finding that the control of Sirt1 protein levels in blood was not exerted through the repression of mRNA expression by promoter hypermethylation was in agreement with previous data. In contrast, other studies reported that Psen1 methylation may be increased or decreased in AD patients. Hence further studies are needed to confirm that peripheral levels of the potential AD biomarker proteins BDNF, Sirt1, and Psen1 are not regulated by different promoter methylation.

Detection of Biomarkers by ELISA It is reported that, in addition to research and drug development, neurochemical biomarkers have a central role in the diagnosis and clinical management of AD (Andreasson et al., 2015). The ELISA is commonly used for the measurement of low-abundance biomarkers. However, it may be associated with systematic and random errors. This urges the need for more rigorous control of assay, regardless of its use in a research setting, in routine clinical practice, or drug development. The aim of a method validation is to present evidence that a method fulfills all the requirements for its intended application. Although much was published on which parameters to investigate in a method validation, limited information is available on how to perform the corresponding experiments. To remedy this, SOPs with step-by-step instructions for validation parameters were included together with a validation report template, which allows better presentation of the results.

Type-2 Diabetes and Biomarkers of Neurodegeneration Recently, it was investigated whether type 2 diabetes mellitus (T2DM) influences neurodegeneration in a manner similar to AD, by augmenting Aβ or tau (Moran et al., 2015). These investigators studied the associations of T2DM with cortical thickness, brain Aβ load, and CSF Aβ and tau in AD patients. All (n = 816) received MRI, and a subsample underwent brain amyloid imaging (n = 102) and CSF Aβ and tau measurements (n = 415). There were 124 patients with T2DM (mean age 75.5 years) and 692 without T2DM (mean age 74.1 years). After adjusting for age, sex, intracranial volume, APO ε4 status, and cognitive diagnosis, T2DM was associated with lower bilateral frontal and parietal cortical thickness (mL). T2DM was associated with increased CSF total tau and phosphorylated tau, but was not associated with ^{11}C-PiB SUV ratio in any brain region or with CSF Aβ$_{42}$ levels. The association between T2DM and cortical thickness was attenuated by 15% by the inclusion of phosphorylated tau, suggesting that T2DM may promote neurodegeneration independent of AD dementia, and its effect may be driven by tau phosphorylation. Hence the mechanism(s) through which T2DM may promote tau phosphorylation requires further investigations.

Selective Tau Ligands As Biomarker(s) in AD It is well-established that abnormally aggregated tau protein is central to the pathophysiology of AD, frontotemporal dementia, progressive supranuclear palsy, corticobasal degeneration, and chronic traumatic encephalopathy. The post-mortem cortical density of hyperphosphorylated tau tangles correlated with pre-morbid cognitive dysfunction and neuronal loss (Dani et al., 2015). Selective PET ligands including $[^{18}F]$ THK5117, $[^{18}F]$ THK5351, $[^{18}F]$ AV1451 (T807) and $[^{11}C]$ PBB3 provided *in vivo* imaging information about the timing and distribution of tau in the early phases of neurodegeneration. Hence these could be used as potential biomarkers for both confirming diagnosis and tracking disease progression. These investigators discussed the challenges posed in developing selective tau ligands as biomarkers, their state of development and the recent information about AD diagnosis, prognosis, and treatment.

Brain Targeted SurR9-C84A Nanocarriers in AD The chronic systemic administration of d-Galactose in C57BL/6J mice demonstrated a relatively high oxidative stress, amyloid-β expression, and neuronal cell death. Enhanced pyknotic nuclei and caspase-3, and reduced neuronal integrity biomarkers further confirmed the aforesaid insults. However, concomitant treatment with the recombinant protein (SurR9-C84A) and the anti-transferrin receptor antibody conjugated SurR9-C84A (SurR9+TFN) nanocarriers showed improvement in neuronal health. The FDA-approved, biodegradable poly (lactic-co-glycolic acid) (PLGA) nanocarriers enhanced the biological half-life and the efficacy of the treatments. These nanocarriers lowered the Aβ expression, enhanced the neuronal integrity biomarkers and maintained the basal levels of endogenous survivin that is essential for attenuating the caspase activation and apoptosis. Hence the brain targeted SurR9-C84A nanocarriers alleviate the d-Galactose induced neuronal insults and has potential for future brain targeted nanomedicine applications.

Amyloid-β As a Fluid Biomarker in AD In general, AD biomarkers are used to assess the risk or presence of the disease, diagnose AD in an early stage, and provide objective and reliable estimates of disease progression. Various biomarkers that can be detected from the blood, serum, plasma, and/or CSF samples of a patient suspected to have MCI or AD can be categorized as fluid biomarkers. As mentioned earlier, plasma and serum samples are relatively easier to obtain compared to CSF; moreover it does not require specialized training as compared to CSF tapping. In addition, blood platelets can be used for the detection of Aβ-1-42 and C-reactive protein (CRP). These two biomarkers are elevated among AD patients and can be detected in the CSF; however routine and easy sample accessibility is a limitation. Aβ is a specific and sensitive biomarker, which can accurately pre-diagnose AD. When Aβ peptide is released by proteolytic cleavage of APP, some solubilized forms are detected in CSF and plasma, which makes these peptides promising candidate as biomarkers. The Aβ demonstrates >80% sensitivity and specificity, in distinguishing AD from dementia and will provide a future for diagnosis and eventually treatment of AD (Bateman et al., 2006; Jorge et al., 2010). Aβ is composed of a family of peptides produced by proteolytic cleavage of the type I transmembrane spanning glycoprotein, APP. Within Senile plaques, Aβ protein species exists in residue 40 or 42, but Aβ-42 form is crucial in the pathogenesis of AD (Hansson et al., 2010).

Although Aβ42 makes up <10% of total Aβ, it aggregates at much faster rates than Aβ40 (Harald et al., 2010). Aβ42 is the initial and major component of senile plaques. While the most accepted hypothesis for mechanisms of Aβ-mediated "neurotoxicity" is structural damage to the synapse, various other mechanisms such as; oxidative stress, altered calcium homeostasis, induction of apoptosis, structural damage, chronic inflammation, and neuronal formation of amyloid have been proposed (Deborah et al., 2008). Furthermore, Aβ42/Aβ40 ratio is considered as a promising biomarker for AD. As Aβ42 failed to be a reliable biomarker in plasma, attention was drawn for alternative biomarkers (Rival et al., 2009). Enzymatic digestions, including β- and γ- secretase, cleave APP into various types of Aβ protein. Most β-secretase activity originates from an integral membrane aspartyle protease encoded by the β-site APP-cleaving enzyme 1 gene (BACE1). A sensitive and specific BACE1 assay was developed to assess CSF BACE1 activity in AD. Increased BACE1 expression and enzymatic activity were detected in subjects with AD. Hence elevated BACE 1 activity may contribute to the amyloidogenic process in AD and could be a potential candidate biomarker to monitor amyloidogenic APP' metabolism in the CNS (Zetterberg, et al., 2008).

Soluble Aβ precursor protein (sAPP) as a Biomarker in AD APP is an integral membrane protein whose *proteolysis* generates *β-amyloid* ranging from 39- to 42- amino acid peptide. Although biological function of APP remains unknown, it is predicted that APP may play a role during *neuroregeneration*, and regulation of neural activity, connectivity, *plasticity*, and memory. Recent researches showed that sAPP present in CSF may serve as a potential biomarker of AD. The researchers tested performance of sAPP α and β (Seubert et al., 1992). Significant increase in sAPP α and sAPP β were noticed in patients with AD, compared to normal subjects. However, the CSF level of α-sAPP and β-sAPP generated contradictory result. Although many researches reported that the CSF level of α sAPP increases in AD patients, some reported no significant change. Therefore more studies are needed to confirm the validity of sAPP as a biomarker for AD.

Recently three candidate CSF biomarkers that reflect AD pathology were identified: Aβ, total tau protein (t-tau), and phosphorylated tau protein at AD-specific epitopes (p-tau). These biomarkers are useful in confirming the AD diagnosis and have predictive value when patients are in the MCI stage. However, their predictive value in cognitively-skillful subjects remains uncertain. A review of the studies published between 1993 and 2011, summarized the role of CSF biomarkers for AD in healthy elderly (Randall et al., 2013).

Abnormalities in the CSF profiles of patients with DLB using a combination of decreased Aβ-42 and increased tau levels were evaluated. With clinical deterioration, the abnormalities in the CSF profile became more pronounced, indicating that DLB can be distinguished from PD, in spite of both being synucleinopathies. However the pathophysiology of increased tau and decreased Aβ levels in these conditions has to be elucidated further, since both proteins are involved in the pathogenesis of AD, but no clear explanation is proposed for DLB yet. Frequently used diagnostic biomarkers are Aβ-42, tau, and phospho-tau, which are measured in CSF, and allow a reasonable, but not full, distinction of AD patients and controls. Besides Aβ-42, additional proteolytic cleavage products of the Aβ protein precursor (AβPP) have been investigated as potential biomarkers including α-secretase cleaved soluble AβPP ectodomain (sAβPPα). Some studies found a reduction of sAβPPα, whereas others reported an increase in the CSF of AD patients. The divergent findings may result from the detection of sAβPPα with antibodies, such as 6E10, which do not exclusively detect sAβPPα, but also the alternative β-secretase cleavage product sAβPPβ'. Hence the sAβPPα-specific antibody 14D6 was used to develop an ELISA which detects sAβPPα in cell culture supernatants, in human CSF, and in serum (Taverna et al., 2013). This assay was used to analyze sAβPPα levels in CSF and serum of AD patients and controls. The assay detected a mild, but significant increase in sAβPPα in the CSF of AD patients compared to non-demented controls, while a mild reduction was observed in serum. Thus the 14D6 antibody assay in CSF allowed a better distinction of AD patients from controls compared to the 6E10 antibody assay. In addition, the levels of Aβ and p-tau, are associated with the risk of progression from normal cognition to onset of clinical symptoms during preclinical AD.

It was examined whether cognitive reserve (CR) modifies this association (Soldan et al., 2013). CSF was obtained from 239 participants (mean age, 57.2 years) who were followed for up to 17 years with clinical and cognitive assessments. A composite score based on the National Adult Reading Test, vocabulary, and years of education was used as an index of CR. The increased risk of progression from normal cognition to symptom onset was associated with lower CR, lower Aβ, and higher p-tau. There was no interaction between CR and Aβ, suggesting that the protective effects of higher CR are equivalent across the range of amyloid levels. However, both tau and p-tau interact with CR, indicating that CR is more protective at lower levels of tau and p-tau. Furthermore, the dynamics of CSF tau and Aβ biomarkers in AD patients from prodromal pre-symptomatic to severe stages of dementia have not been clearly defined. To clarify this issue, the CSF tau and Aβ biomarker data from 142 of the ADNI study subjects [18 AD, 74 mild cognitive impairment (MCI), and 50 cognitively normal subjects (CN)] were analyzed (Toledo et al., 2013). These studies were conducted for up to 48 months for the analyses of CSF $Aβ_{1-42}$, phosphorylated tau (p-tau_{181}), and total tau (t-tau). The analysis revealed that for $Aβ_{1-42}$ and p-tau_{181} biomarkers there were subjects with stable CSF biomarkers and subjects who showed a decrease ($Aβ_{1-42}$, 9.2 pg/ml/year) or increase (p-tau_{181}, 5.1 pg/ml/year) of these values. Low baseline $Aβ_{1-42}$ values were associated with increases in p-tau_{181}. High baseline p-tau_{181} values were not associated with changes in $Aβ_{1-42}$ levels. When the subjects with normal baseline biomarkers and stable concentrations during follow-up were excluded, the time to reach abnormal CSF levels and the mean AD values was shortened, suggesting that there is a distinct population of ADNI with abnormal changes in CSF p-tau_{181} and $Aβ_{1-42}$ levels, and these results supported that $Aβ_{1-42}$ changes precede p-tau_{181} changes. Furthermore, these investigators reported the assessment of α-Synuclein (α-Syn) in CSF and its association with CSF tau (t-tau), phosphorylated tau_{181} (p-tau_{181}), and amyloid $beta_{1-42}$ ($Aβ_{1-42}$) in subjects of ADNI (n = 389). A significant correlation was observed between α-Syn and t-tau in controls, as well as in patients with AD and MCI. However, the correlation was unspecific to subjects in the ADNI cohort, as it was also seen in PD patients and controls enrolled in the Parkinson's Progression Markers Initiative (PPMI; n = 102). A bimodal distribution of CSF α-Syn was observed in the ADNI cohort, with high levels of α-Syn in the subjects with abnormally increased t-tau values. Although a correlation was noted between α-Syn and p-tau_{181}, there was a mismatch (α-Syn-p-tau_{181}-Mis), i.e., higher p-tau_{181} levels accompanied by lower α-Syn levels in ADNI patients. Based on these findings it was hypothesized that α-Syn-p-tau_{181}-Mis is a CSF signature of LBD pathology and that their estimations improves the diagnostic sensitivity/specificity of CSF biomarkers and better predicts cognitive impairments in AD patients. The diagnostic guidelines of AD include neuroimaging and CSF biomarkers, to increase the certainty whether a patient has an ongoing AD neuropathology or not. *Hence the CSF biomarkers; total tau (T-tau), hyperphosphorylated tau (P-tau) and amyloid-β (Aβ-42) reflect the core pathologic features of AD, which reflect neuronal loss, intracellular neurofibrillary tangles, and extracellular senile plaques.* These biomarkers may facilitate early disease detection. Rosén et al (2013) summarized the CSF biomarker data available from each of the stages based on results derived from blood and CSF biomarker analyses.

The core AD CSF biomarkers had high diagnostic accuracy both for AD with dementia and to predict incipient AD (*MCI due to AD*). Longitudinal studies on healthy elderly and cross-sectional studies on patients with dominantly inherited AD mutations also found biomarker changes in cognitively skillful at-risk individuals. Hence this will be significant if disease-modifying treatment becomes available, given that it will probably be most effective early in the disease. Since measurements vary between studies and laboratories, standardization of analytical as well as pre-analytical procedures is essential. Apart from having diagnostic roles, biomarkers may also be utilized for prognosis, disease progression, development of new therapeutic strategies, monitoring prognosis and for increasing the knowledge about pathologic processes coupled to the disease. Although several candidate biomarkers were detected in CSF, these were harder to find in the blood. Recent analyses on blood samples, derived from AD patients, presented encouraging results which need to be verified in independent studies. Moreover the overlapping clinical features of AD and DLB make differentiation difficult in the clinical setting (Luo et al., 2013).

CSF Visinin-Like Protein-1 as a Biomarker in AD It is now realized that evaluating the CSF biomarkers in AD and DLB patients could facilitate clinical diagnosis. In this context, CSF Visinin-like protein-1 (VILIP-1), a calcium-mediated neuronal injury biomarker, was proposed as a novel biomarker for AD (Braunewell, 2012). The aim of this study was to investigate the diagnostic utility of CSF VILIP-1 and VILIP-1/$A\beta_{1-42}$ ratio to distinguish AD from DLB. Levels of CSF VILIP-1, t-tau, p-tau$_{181P}$, $A\beta_{1-42}$, and α-synuclein were measured in 61 AD patients, 32 DLB patients, and 40 normal controls using ELISA. The CSF VILIP-1 level significantly increased in AD patients compared with both normal controls and DLB patients. The CSF VILIP-1 and VILIP-1/$A\beta_{1-42}$ levels had sufficient diagnostic accuracy to allow the detection and differential diagnosis of AD. Additionally, CSF VILIP-1 levels were positively correlated with t-tau and p-tau$_{181P}$ within each group and with α-Synuclein in the AD and control groups suggesting that CSF VILIP-1 could be a useful diagnostic biomarker for AD, differentiating it from DLB.

BDNF and Proinflammatory Biomarkers in AD The circulating biomarker BNDF, is significantly reduced in the CSF as well as serum samples of AD patients, whereas pro-inflammatory cytokines TNFα, NFkβ, and IL-1β may be increased; however the results are ambiguous and currently no definite consensus has reached to authenticate the diagnosis based on the analysis of pro-inflammatory cytokines. As CSF IL-10 is increased during the disease progression, it may be considered as a biomarker of progressive neurodegeneration in AD. Similarly lipid profile exhibits fluctuations in the CSF and serum samples of AD patients. In general, serum cholesterol is linked to AD progression. However, increased serum or CSF cholesterol levels could not be considered the most accurate and reliable biomarker of AD. Furthermore, BDNF Val66Met polymorphism is implicated in AD-related cognitive impairment. The relationship between BDNF Val66Met and Aβ on cognitive decline, hippocampal atrophy, and Aβ accumulation over 36 months in 165 healthy adults enrolled in the *Australian Imaging, Biomarkers and Lifestyle* study (Lim et al., 2012; Lim et al. 2013).

Healthy adults with high Aβ, Met carriers showed moderate-to-large declines in episodic memory, executive function, and language, and increased hippocampal atrophy over 36 months, compared with Val/Val homozygotes. BDNF Val66Met was not related to rates of change in cognition or hippocampal volume in healthy adults with low Aβ. BDNF Val66Met did not relate to the amount of Aβ or to the rate of Aβ accumulation in either *group* indicating that high Aβ levels coupled with Met carriage may be useful prognostic biomarkers of cognitive decline and hippocampal degeneration in the preclinical stage of AD. In a study, the potential of BDNF, complement factor H (CFH), TNFα, IL-10, and Hsp90 as serum biomarkers were investigated in a cohort of the AD Turkish population because these biomarkers are associated with AD (Gezen-Ak et al., 2013). Three groups of patients, early-onset AD (EOAD; age of onset < 65; n = 22), late-onset AD (LOAD; age of onset > 65; n = 54), and MCI (n = 30), were compared with age-matched healthy controls using ELISA. The serum BDNF levels decreased and TNFα levels increased in the EOAD and LOAD groups compared to the age-matched healthy controls. There was a correlation between serum TNFα and IL-10 levels in the LOAD and healthy control groups. Serum CFH levels in the LOAD and MCI patients were decreased compared with controls. Serum Hsp90 levels in the EOAD, LOAD, and MCI patients were decreased compared with controls. The protein misfolding, the inflammatory response, and decreased neurotrophic factor synthesis were related to AD type brain pathology, and suggested that these alterations can be detected from serum samples. Hence for accurate early diagnosis of AD, it is important to determine alterations in multiple biomarkers in large-scale population studies. A number of studies have suggested blood measures of inflammatory proteins as putative biomarkers.

Recently, 27 cytokines and related proteins in 350 subjects with AD, subjects with MCI and elderly normal controls were estimated where longitudinal change in cognition and baseline neuroimaging measures of atrophy were made (Leung et al., 2013). Five inflammatory proteins associated with evidence of atrophy on MRI data in whole brain, ventricular and entorhinal cortex measures were identified. Six analytes showed significant changes in patients with fast cognitive decline compared to those with intermediate and slow decline. Particularly IL-10 was associated with brain atrophy in AD as evidenced by neuroimaging and with both clinical and imaging evidence of severity of disease and might therefore have potential as a biomarker of disease progression.

CRP as a Biomarker in AD The exact functional relationship between plasma CRP and AD remains unknown. Recent studies reported that CRP participates in the systemic response to inflammation (Yarchoan et al., 2013). These investigators measured plasma CRP in 203 AD, 58 MCI and 117 normal aging subjects and administered Mini-Mental State Examinations (MMSE) during a 3-year follow-up period to investigate CRP's relationship with diagnosis and progression of cognitive decline. Subjects adjusted for age, sex, and education, subjects with AD had significantly lower levels of plasma CRP than subjects with MCI and normal aging. However, there was no significant association between plasma CRP at baseline and subsequent cognitive decline as assessed by longitudinal changes in MMSE score supporting reduced levels of plasma CRP in AD and its potential utility as a biomarker for the diagnosis of AD. Furthermore, It is known that Disintegrin and Metallopeptidase 10 (ADAM10) are significantly reduced in AD patients compared with healthy subjects. A study evaluated whether platelet ADAM10 correlates with the clock drawing test (CDT) scores, which is a measure of visuospatial ability and executive function in AD patients. This study was performed on 30 elderly patients with probable AD and 25 healthy controls, matched by age, gender, and educational status (Manzine et al., 2013). Platelet proteins were analyzed by SDS-PAGE and ADAM10 was identified by immunoblotting. The Spearman's correlation coefficient between ADAM10 and CDT was obtained for each group. The area under the curve (AUC) was used to compare the ROC curves. The CDT scores and platelet ADAM10 expression were significantly different between patients with AD and controls. In AD patients, there was a positive correlation between ADAM10 expression and CDT scores. The combination of ADAM10 and CDT was better to confirm the AD diagnosis than the AUCs of

ADAM10 and CDT, suggesting association of ADAM10 and cognitive test as a reliable biomarker of AD.

Butyrylcholinesterase (BuChE) Activity Modulates Inflammatory Cytokines in AD Butyrylcholinesterase (BuChE) activity is associated with activated astrocytes in AD brain. The BuChE-K variant exhibits 30%-60% reduced ACh hydrolyzing capacity. It was investigated if genetic heterogeneity in BuChE affects CSF biomarkers of inflammation and cholinoceptive glial function (Darreh-Shori et al., 2013). AD patients were BCHE-K-genotyped. Proteomic and enzymatic analyses were performed on CSF and/or plasma. BuChE genotype was linked with CSF levels of GFAP, S100B, IL-1β, and TNF-α. BCHE-K noncarriers displayed 100%-150% higher GFAP and 64%-110% higher S100B than BCHE-K carriers, who had 40%-80% higher IL-1β and 21%-27% higher TNF-α compared with noncarriers. A high level of CSF BuChE correlated with higher CSF levels of astroglial markers and several factors of the innate complement system, but lower levels of pro-inflammatory cytokines. These patients also displayed beneficial clinical findings, such as high cerebral glucose utilization, low β-amyloid load, and less severe progression of clinical symptoms. *In vitro* analysis on human astrocytes confirmed the involvement of a regulated BuChE status in the astroglial responses to TNF-α and ACh. Histochemical analysis in a rat model of nerve injury-induced neuro-inflammation, and showed assembly of astroglia in proximity of BuChE-immunolabeled sites suggesting that BuChE enzymatic activity plays an important role in regulating inflammation and activity of cholinoceptive glial cells. The dissociation between astroglial biomarkers and inflammatory cytokines indicated that a proper activation and maintenance of astroglial function is a beneficial response, rather than a disease-driving mechanism. Further studies are needed to explore the therapeutic potential of manipulating BuChE activity and astroglial functional status in AD.

CHF5074 As a Novel Anti-Inflammatory Microglial Modulator in AD As neuro-inflammation is an early event in the pathogenesis of AD, selective anti-inflammatory drugs could lead to preventive measures. A study evaluated the safety, tolerability, PKs, and pharmacodynamics of CHF5074, a new microglial modulator, in a 12-week, double-blind, placebo-controlled, parallel groups study involving 96 MCI patients (Ross et al., 2013). Subjects were allocated into three successive study cohorts to receive titrated doses of CHF5074 (200, 400 or 600 mg/day) or placebo. Vital signs, cardiac safety, neuropsychological performance and clinical lab parameters were assessed. Plasma samples were collected for measuring drug concentrations, CD40 ligand (sCD40L) and TNF-α. At the end of treatment, CSF samples were collected after the last dose to measure drug levels, β-amyloid1-42 (Aβ42), tau, phospho-tau181, sCD40L, and TNF-α. Ten patients did not complete the study: one in the placebo group (consent withdrawn), two in the 200-mg/day treatment group (consent withdrawn and unable to comply) and seven in the 400-mg/day treatment group (five AEs, one consent withdrawn and one unable to comply). The frequent adverse events were diarrhea, dizziness and back pain. CHF5074 total body clearance depended on the gender, age and glomerular filtration rate. CHF5074 CSF concentrations increased in a dose-dependent manner. At the end of treatment, mean sCD40L and TNF-α in CSF were inversely related to the CHF5074 dose. Plasma levels of sCD40L in the 600-mg/day group were lower than those measured in the placebo group. No significant differences between treatment groups were found in neuropsychological tests but a positive dose-response relationship was found on executive function in ApoE-4 carriers, suggesting that CHF5074 is well tolerated in MCI patients after a 12-week treatment up to 600 mg/day and affects CNS biomarkers of neuro-inflammation.

Platelet Biomarkers in AD Although CSF measures of tau and amyloid proteins are now accepted as diagnostic tools to aid the clinical diagnosis of AD, CSF is not routinely obtained in most clinical settings. Hence there is a need to discover peripheral biomarkers that may enable detection of AD-specific proteins in blood or blood derivatives. Platelets contain proteins found in neuronal cell lines, including tau protein. Since tau protein is a characteristic of AD-neuropathology, a biochemical analysis of tau at the microtubule-binding and C-terminal region, as well as two tau phosphorylation sites (Ser202/Thr205 and Thr181) in 25 AD and 26 was conducted in control subjects using platelets (Mukaetova-Ladinska et al., 2013). Platelet tau protein estimates did not discriminate between AD and control individuals. However, subjects with MMSE 24-27 had elevated C-terminal tau protein compared to those with MMSE >27, whereas older AD subjects (>80 years) showed higher t-tau protein in comparison to younger AD (<80 years) and controls (<80 years) confirming that platelet tau protein can be estimated, and requires further study as these biomarkers may be useful in indicating early stages of cognitive impairment in AD. Platelets may be of particular interest because they express APP and impaired processing in AD.

New biomarkers, derived from neuroimaging and CSF analyses, have helped to identify anatomical and biochemical biomarkers of VaD and AD. Nevertheless, there is a significant difference between the two entities. While it is clear that VaD is a heterogeneous entity, AD is considered to be a single disorder. Nobody attempts to use Cerebral Autosomal Dominant Arteriopathy with Sub-cortical Infarcts and Leukoencephalopathy (CADASIL) as a template to develop treatment for sporadic VaD. On the other hand, early-onset AD is used to develop therapy for sporadic AD. The problems relating to this false concept and its consequences were discussed recently (Korczyn, 2013). In addition, Sultana et al. (2013) discovered elevated levels of oxidative stress biomarkers in the mitochondria isolated from lymphocytes of subjects with MCI compared to cognitively healthy individuals. An increase in mitochondrial oxidative stress in MCI was associated with MMSE score, Vitamin E, and β-Carotene content. A proteomic analysis revealed that alteration in the Thioredoxin-dependent peroxide reductase, Myosin light polypeptide 6, and ATP synthase subunit β, might be important in the pathogenesis of AD. Hence increased understanding of oxidative stress and protein alterations in peripheral tissues might help in developing biomarkers to combat this devastating disorder.

Biomarkers in Disease-Modifying Drug Development Recently, efforts were directed to develop "disease-modifying drugs" for AD which include drugs to reduce Aβ production, prevent Aβ aggregation, promote Aβ clearance, target tau phosphorylation and assembly, and other novel approaches (Caraci et al., 2013). Active and passive immunotherapy is also a strategy to enhance Aβ clearance. Unfortunately several candidate disease-modifying drugs have failed in phase III clinical trials conducted in mild to moderate AD patients. A study validated an assay for amyloid-precursor protein (sAPP)-α and -β in platelets of AD and MCI patients, compared to healthy young and old controls (Plagg et al., 2015). Platelet extracts (25 μg) were incubated with or without recombinant BACE1 (β-secretase, 8U) at 37°C and low pH and the levels of sAPP-α and sAPP-β were measured by ELISAs. sAPP-α levels were not different between AD, MCI and control subjects. However, sAPP-β levels in MCI and AD were elevated. When recombinant BACE1 was added, no changes were noticed in sAPP-α levels, but the sAPP-β levels were increased. The sAPP-β processing was specific and selective after 2.5 hours at 37°C, and was mediated by exogenous BACE1, because it was blocked by a BACE1 inhibitor and BACE1 enzyme levels were enhanced in AD patients suggesting that quantitative analysis of platelet sAPP-β by ELISA may be a novel diagnostic biomarker for MCI and AD.

A relation between Aβ accumulation and Neprilysin (NEP), an Aβ degrading enzyme, was proposed but studies of NEP and the levels of the pathological hallmarks of AD, Aβ and tau, in CSF are limited. The enzyme activity of NEP in serum and CSF was measured, using a sandwich ELISA and a fluorescence resonance energy transfer (FRET) assay, respectively, in patients with AD, frontotemporal dementia (FTD), Creutzfeldt-Jakob disease (CJD), and depression (Sorensen et al., 2013). Results were correlated with the levels of CSF AD biomarkers Aβ-42, p-tau, and t-tau. In serum, no differences in NEP-like activity or concentration were noticed between the groups and there were no correlations between NEP and AD biomarkers. In CSF, no influence of age or gender on NEP levels or enzyme activity was observed. However, NEP concentration was lower and the specific activity was higher in FTD compared to AD. Aβ-42 levels in CSF did not correlate with NEP concentration in the AD, CJD, or depression groups, but NEP-like activity and Aβ-42 levels correlated in the FTD group. In AD and depression, the NEP-like activity in CSF correlated with levels of p-tau, and, in the AD group, it also was correlated with t-tau levels suggesting that the relation between the specific activity of NEP and t-tau and p-tau is a characteristic trait of AD. Thus the correlation between NEP and Aβ-42 in FTD needs further investigation (Ishii, 2013).

TECHNICAL AND CLINICAL ISSUES IN BIOMARKER ESTIMATIONS

Biomarker Estimations from CSF Aliquots A study determined whether CSF biomarker concentrations are affected by aliquot storage volume and whether addition of detergent-containing buffer mitigates any observed effects (Toombs et al., 2013). AD and control CSF was distributed into polypropylene tubes in aliquots of different volumes (50-1500 μL). Aβ1-42, t-tau and p-tau were measured with and without addition of 0.05% Tween-20. The concentrations of Aβ1-42 increased two-fold with aliquot storage. A volume increase of 10 μL caused an Aβ1-42 increase of 0.95pg/mL in controls, and 0.60 pg/mL in AD samples. Following addition of Tween-20, the positive relationship between Aβ1-42 and aliquot volume disappeared. T-tau and P-tau remained unaffected indicating that CSF aliquot storage volume has a significant impact on the concentration of Aβ1-42. Hence the introduction of a detergent buffer at the initial stage of aliquot preparation may be a solution to this problem.

Diagnostic Accuracy of CSF Vs MRI Biomarkers in AD A study compared the early utility of AD biomarkers in the CSF with brain MRI to ascertain the diagnostic accuracy of both techniques used in combination (Monge Argilés et al., 2014). Thirty patients with MCI were examined using 1.5 Tesla brain MRI and AD biomarker analysis in CSF. MRI studies were evaluated according to the Korfs visual scale. CSF biomarkers were analyzed using INNOTEST reagents for $A\beta_{1-42}$, total-tau and phospho-tau_{181p}. By 2 years, 15 of the original 30 patients (50%) developed AD (according to NINCDS-ADRA criteria). Although the predictive utility of AD biomarkers in CSF was greater than that of MRI; using both techniques together yielded a sensitivity and a negative predictive value of 100%. Normal results on both complementary tests ruled out progression to AD within 2 years. These results demonstrated higher diagnostic accuracy of biomarkers in CSF than that of MRI biomarkers. However combined use of both techniques was highly accurate for either early diagnosis or exclusion of AD in patients with MCI.

Infuence of Hypertension (HTN) on CSF Biomarkers in AD It is known that in HTN, cerebral hemodynamic is changed, and the threshold for BP at which perfusion is safely maintained is higher. This shift may increase the brain's vulnerability to lower BP in subjects with vascular disease. A study investigated whether reduction in mean arterial pressure (MAP) was related to changes in CSF biomarkers of AD in cognitively healthy elderly with and without HTN (Glodzik et al., 2014). The relationships among MAP, memory decline, and hippocampal atrophy were also examined. A total of 77 subjects were assessed twice, 2 ± 0.5 years apart. At both time points, all subjects underwent medical and neuropsychological evaluations, lumbar punctures, and MRI examinations. Hyper- and normotensive subjects did not differ in their CSF biomarkers, hippocampal volumes (HipVs), or memory scores at baseline. In the entire group the increase in tau phosphorylated at Threonine 181 (p-tau$_{181}$) was associated with a decline in verbal episodic memory and HipV reduction. However, longitudinal decrease in MAP was related to memory decline and an increase in p-tau$_{181}$ only in subjects with HTN suggesting that the hypertensive group may be sensitive to BP reductions.

Mitochondrial DNA as Biomarker in AD It is important to identify a novel biomarker that precedes clinical symptoms of AD. By using qPCR, mitochondrial DNA (mtDNA) in CSF from study participants, selected from a cohort of 282 subjects, that were classified, according to their concentrations of Aβ1-42, t-tau, and p-tau, and by the presence or absence of dementia, in: asymptomatic subjects at risk of AD, symptomatic patients diagnosed with sporadic AD, pre-symptomatic subjects having PSEN1 mutations and patients diagnosed with fronto-temporal lobe degeneration (FTLD) (Podlesniy et al., 2013). Equivalent studies were performed in a separate validation cohort of sporadic AD and FTLD patients. In addition, mtDNA copy number in cultured cortical neurons from mutant Amyloid Precursor Protein/Presenilin1 (APP/PS1) transgenic mice was measured. *Asymptomatic patients at risk of AD, and symptomatic AD patients, but not FTLD patients, exhibited a significant decrease in mtDNA in the CSF.* In addition, pre-symptomatic subjects carrying pathogenic PSEN1 gene mutations showed low mtDNA in CSF before the appearance of AD related biomarkers in CSF. Moreover, mtDNA in CSF classified with high sensitivity and specificity AD patients against either controls or patients with FTLD. Furthermore, cultured cortical neurons from APP/PS1 transgenic mice had less mtDNA, before the appearance of altered synaptic biomarkers. Thus low levels of mtDNA in CSF may be a novel biomarker for the early detection of preclinical AD. These findings supported the hypothesis that mtDNA depletion is a pathophysiological factor of neurodegeneration in AD. In addition platelets have been widely proposed as biomarkers in studies of mitochondrial function and aging-related and neurodegenerative diseases. Defects in mitochondrial function are found not only in the substantia nigra of PD patients but also in their platelets. Similarly, it is evident in the platelet mitochondria of AD patients. The researchers discovered that genetically-engineered mouse models of PD and mitochondrial genome knock out (Rh$_{mgko}$) cultured human dopaminergic (SK-N-SH) neurons possess significantly reduced ubiquinone-NADH oxidoreductase (Complex-1), CoQs, and are highly susceptible to neurotoxins, including 1-Methyl, 4-Phenyl, 1,2,3,6 Tetrahydropydine (MPTP), 6-Hydoxydopamine, and Rotenone (Sharma et al., 2006). Downregulation of mtDNA in cultured human SK-N-SH and SH-S-Y5Y neurons augmented

CB formation and apoptosis as confirmed by multiple fluorochrome Comet assay (Sharma et al., 2004). Furthermore, mitochondrial aerobic metabolism function and protein expression in platelets of MS patients and controls, mitochondrial aconitase, superoxide dismutases 1 and 2 (SOD1 and SOD2), and respiratory complex enzyme activities in platelets of MS patients and control subjects were studied (Iñarrea et al., 2014). Lipid peroxidation, SOD1, and cytochrome c expressions were investigated. Mitochondrial aconitase activity was higher in MS patients than in controls. A significant increase in all respiratory complex activities in MS patients was observed. Mitochondrial lipid peroxidation was higher in MS patients. Significant changes in cytochrome c and mitochondrial SOD1 expressions were detected, with a decrease of 44 ± 5 % and an increase of 46 ± 6 %, respectively suggesting that changes in mitochondrial aerobic metabolism and SOD1 and cytochrome c are induced in platelets of MS patients. The author discovered CB formation in the degenerating dendrites of Purkinje neurons as a consequence of pre and postnatal nutritional stress in developing rats (Sharma and Ebadi, 2014). At the ultra-structural level, CB is composed of multi-lameller electron dense membrane stacks formed as a consequence of mitochondrial degeneration due to lipid peroxidation, nutritional stress and/or environmental neurotoxins such as Kainic acid and Domoic acid. These multi-lamellar stacks were degraded by lysosome as a result of autophagy during oxidative and nitrative stress of free radicals. Metallothioneins (MTs) inhibited CB formation by acting as free radical scavengers as the researchers and other have reported (Sogawa et al. 2001; Sharma et al., 2013a, Sharma et al., 2013b).

It is now well-established that MT-3 is significantly reduced in the hippocampal CA-3 and dentate gyrus regions of AD patients, which may promote mitochondrial degeneration, leading to CB formation, triggering pro-apoptotic events, and eventually neuronal demise. Hence therapeutic interventions to inhibit CB formation by either antioxidants and/or by pharmacological agents will be beneficial for the effective clinical management of AD and other neurodegenerative disorders of unknown etiopathogenesis. MTs are a family of low molecular weight cysteine-rich zinc-binding proteins. Although the four isoforms of MTs (MT1-4) were discovered about 40 years ago, their functional significance still remains enigmatic. MT1 and 2 are ubiquitously present in various organs including CNS, whereas MT-3 and MT-4 are present in restricted organs. MT-3 was discovered in the CNS and its isomer was recognized as a growth inhibitory factor (GIF) which is significantly reduced in AD patients and several other neurodegenerative disorders (Kojima et al., 1998). The expression of the canine MT-3 mRNA was found exclusively in the CNS, where neurons in the olfactory bulb, hippocampus and cerebral cortex showed predominant signals, suggesting its clinical significance in cognitive function (Irie et al., 2004).

Recent studies confirmed that MT-3 is also expressed in other organs. These findings not only indicate that MT-3 has a much wider tissue distribution, but also it might have other unknown functions. MT-3 gene is also expressed in the salivary gland but not in the thyroid gland (Ghazi et al., 2011). While salivary ducts showed intense immuno-reactivity with anti-MT-3, weak immunoreactivity was observed in acinar cells. This, together with the findings that some neuromodulators (i.e., NGF) exist in the salivary gland and that MT-3 may participate in the transport in renal tubules, suggests that MT-3 may have other functions than cytoprotection in the salivary gland. Several new proteins interacting with MT-3 as determined through immunoaffinity chromatography and mass spectrometry were reported (Ghaz et al., 2011). These new proteins include: Exo84p, 14-3-3 Zeta, α and β Enolase, Aldolase C, Malate dehydrogenase, ATP synthase, and Pyruvate kinase that have now been classified into three functional groups: transport and signaling, chaperoning and scaffolding, and glycolytic metabolism. These interactions support a proposed model for the regulation of the GIF activity of MT-3 in the CNS. A detailed study is required to elucidate the exact role of CB formation and Aβ as early diagnostic biomarkers of neurodegeneration and MTs as therapeutic biomarkers of regeneration in AD and other diseases.

Autoantibodies as Biomarkers in AD Recently several biomarkers have been introduced for the differential diagnosis of AD. However, most of them provide inconsistent results. The novel approach (*autoantibody*) not only explaines the discrepancy of results in previous studies, but also provide a new standard as a biomarker of AD. Compared to other biomarkers which have variable measurements on diagnosis, the autoantibody approach accurately measures Aβ level with high sensitivity for AD. It is envisaged that this technology will provide not only early diagnosis, but also therapy for AD to accomplish EBPT of AD. The titres of anti-β-amyloid antibodies in CSF was lower in AD patients compared to normal patients (Du et al., 2001).

Recent studies focused on use of an autoantibody, were directed not only for novel biomarkers development but also for future theranostic applications. However, there are concerns whether an autoantibody method provides a reliable biomarker. A number of reports showed that patients with AD have lower levels of serum anti-Aβ antibodies than healthy individuals, and others argued that the level of anti-Aβ antibody may be higher in AD (Gustaw et al., 2008). It was reported that autoantibodies are self-reactive and widely implicated as causal agents in autoimmune diseases (DeMarshall et al., 2015). These are detected in the blood of all human sera, regardless of age, gender, or the presence or absence of disease. While the underlying mechanism for their ubiquity remains unknown, it is hypothesized that they participate in the clearance of blood-borne cell and tissue debris generated in both healthy and diseased individuals. Although much evidence supports the debris clearance role, recent studies also suggest a causal role for autoantibodies in disease progression. These investigators presented examples of autoimmune diseases that emphasize a direct causal role for autoantibodies and discussed the evidence supporting their involvement in a wide variety of other diseases, including cancers and several neurological and neurodegenerative diseases. Lastly, translational strategies that take advantage of the "cause and/or effect" relationship of autoantibodies and recent advancements in their detection exploit autoantibodies as sensitive and specific biomarkers for achieving EBPT of AD and other neurodegenerative disorders of unknown etiopathogenesis. Their use in the diagnosis and staging of AD was presented, and future applications in clinical medicine and basic science were highlighted. An international study group was constituted for obtaining scientific information and developing a guide for implementing biomarkers into routine clinical practice.

α-Synuclein Index As a Biomarker in AD The discovery of α-Synuclein (α-syn) as a major component of Lewy bodies, neuropathological hallmark of PD, dementia with Lewy bodies, and of glial inclusions in MSA initiated the investigation of α-Syn as a biomarker in CSF. Due to the involvement of the periphery in PD the quantification of α-Syn in serum, plasma and saliva was investigated as well. Simonsen et al. (2015) reviewed the development of multiple assays for the quantification of α-Syn to yield novel insights into its species in the different fluids; the optimal preanalytical conditions required for quantification and the potential clinical value of α-Syn as biomarker, suggesting approaches to use of CSF α-Syn in neurodegenerative diseases including AD. The researchers discovered that human dopaminergic (SK-N-SH and SHY-5Y) neurons and primary hippocampal cultured neurons are highly sensitive to α-Synuclein nitration in response to environmental neutotoxins (KA, DOM) and hence increase the α-Synuclein Index (SI: Nitrated α-Synuclein/Native α-Synuclein) (Sharma et al., 2003, Sharma 2015; Sharma 2016). Environmental neurotoxins such as Kainic acid and Domoic acid increase α-Synuclein index, whereas MTs inhibit SI to prevent CB formation by serving as free radical scavengers. MT3 is significantly reduced in the hippopcampal CA3 and dentate gyrus regions of AD patients, which could render AD patients highly susceptible to progressive neurodegeneration. Hence SI and CB formation could be used as sensitive biomarkers for the early detection of neurodegenerative disorders such as AD and PD. Furthermore, any physiological or pharmacological intervention, augmenting brain regional MTs and inhibition of SI and CB formation will be beneficial for the effective clinical management of AD patients. In addition, consumption of sea food primarily fish, rich in PUFA, Vitamin-D and Vitamin-E can nullify the deleterious effects of Ethanol which serves as a free radical donor to cause synaptic degeneration and demyelination to accelerate early AD pathogenesis.

Natural self-reactive antibodies in the blood may play a crucial role in the control of potentially toxic proteins that may accumulate in the aging brain. Serum IgG levels to monomeric α-Synuclein in DLB and AD were explored with a sensitive ELISA assay. Antibody levels revealed differences in patients compared to healthy subjects and were dependent on diagnosis, disease duration, and age. Anti-α-Synuclein IgG levels were increased in both patient groups, but in early DLB to a greater extent than in AD. Increased antibody titer was most evident in younger patients, while with advanced age, relatively low levels were observed, similar to healthy individuals, exhibiting stable antibody levels independent of age indicating the presence of differentially altered IgG levels against α-Synuclein in DLB and AD, which may relate to a disturbed α-Synuclein homeostasis. These observations may facilitate the development of novel, preclinical biomarkers and immunotherapeutic strategies that target α-Synuclein in AD. The researchers discovered that SI is significantly increased in response to neurotoxic agents such as 1-Methyl, 4-phenyl, 1, 2,3,6-Tetrahydropyridine (MPTP), Rotenone, Salsolinol, and 1-Benzyl-Tetrahydroisoquinoilines (1-Benzyl-TIQs) in cultured human dopaminergic (SK-N-SH) cells in culture, hence it could be used an early sensitive biomarker of neurodegeneration. Usually α-Synuclein is estimated in the serum, plasma, and CSF on a routine basis for the clinical evaluation of neurodegenerative α-synucleinopathies. However direct estimates of total α-Synuclein in these fluids is nonspecific and may not provide accurate estimates of disease progression or regression. *The researchers used double radioimmunoprecipitation to estimate SI, which is time-consuming, cumbersome, and requires radioactivity. Technically-improved methods to estimate SI, by developing sensitive ELISA, high-resolution LC-MS spectrometry, or nanosensing devices can readily differentiate between native α-Synuclein vs nitrated α-Synuclein for the accurate determination of SI from normal, MCI and AD patient's serum, plasma, and CSF samples. Further studies in this direction would go a long way in the EBPT of various neurodegenerative α-synucleinopathies including AD.*

Natural self-reactive antibodies in the peripheral blood may play a significant role in the control of potentially toxic proteins that may accumulate in the aging brain. Koehler et al. (2013) recently explored serum IgG levels to monomeric α-Synuclein in DLB and AD with a highly sensitive ELISA assay. Antibody levels revealed differences in patients compared to healthy subjects and were dependent on diagnosis, disease duration, and age. Anti-α-

Synuclein IgG levels were increased in both patient groups, but in early DLB to a much greater extent than in AD. Increased antibody titer was most evident in younger patients, while with advanced age relatively low levels were observed, similar to healthy individuals, exhibiting stable antibody levels independent of age indicating the presence of differentially altered IgG levels against α-Synuclein in DLB and AD, which may relate to a disturbed α-Synuclein homeostasis by the disease process. These observations may facilitate the development of novel, preclinical biomarkers and immunotherapeutic strategies that target α-Synuclein in AD.

Biochemical Markers in AD Parameters of oxidative stress and biomarkers of endothelial dysfunction in the blood of 21 AD patients under treatment compared with 10 controls were evaluated to elucidate the contribution of AD to the oxidative stress (Gubandru et al., 2013). In addition, IL-6, TNF-α, ADMA and Homocysteine were significantly increased in AD patients. Protein carbonyls were higher in AD group, while Glutathione reductase and total antioxidant capacity were lower, suggesting decreased defense ability against the deleterious effects of ROS. Besides, a higher level of advanced glycation end-products was observed in AD patients. Depending on the treatment, a distinct inflammatory and oxidative stress was observed. In Rivastigmine-treated group, IL-6 levels were 47% lower than the remaining AD patients; Homocysteine and Glutathione reductase were unchanged in the Rivastigmine, Donepezil, and Donepezil-Memantine groups. Although the study was based on a limited population, the results could constitute the basis for further investigations regarding the effect of medication and diet on AD patients. 12/15-Lipoxygenase (12-15LO) is a lipid-peroxidizing enzyme widely expressed in the CNS where it is involved in the neurobiology of AD as it modulates Aβ and APP processing. However, its biological effect on tau protein remains unknown (Giannopoulos et al., 2013).

A study, investigated the biomarkers of AD in the aqueous humor of patients with open-angle glaucoma (OAG) (Inoue et al., 2013). Aqueous humor samples were collected from 38 patients with cataracts, 20 patients with POAG, and 32 patients with exfoliation glaucoma. The levels of Apolipoprotein (Apo-AI, Apo-CIII, Apo-E), Transthyretin (TTR), Complement factor H, Complement C3, and α2-Macroglobulin (α2M) were determined by multiplex bead immunoassay. POAG patients had significantly higher Apo AI, ApoCIII, ApoE, TTR, and α2M compared with cataract patients. Corresponding values for exfoliation glaucoma patients were also higher compared with those for cataract patients and those levels correlated positively in patients with OAG. Complement factor H and complement C3 levels did not differ among groups. Mean deviation values for the Humphrey visual field test correlated positively with levels of Apo-AI, Apo-E, TTR, and complement factor H in OAG patients, but age and IOP values were not correlated with protein levels.

In general Aβ peptides are important for the diagnosis and prognosis of AD as reliable biomarkers. A simple and sensitive electrochemical method was developed for the detection of Aβ peptides using gold nanoparticles modified with Aβ (1-16)-heme (Aβ (1-16)-heme-AuNPs) (Liu et al., 2013). Monoclonal antibody (mAb) specific to the N-terminus of Aβ was immobilized onto gold electrode for the capture of Aβ (1-16)-heme-AuNPs. The anchored Aβ (1-16)-heme-AuNPs showed electrocatalytic O_2 reduction. Pre-incubation of the mAb-covered electrode with Aβ decreased the amount of Aβ (1-16)-heme-AuNPs, resulting in the decrease of the reduction current of O_2 to H_2O_2. This assay was sensitive and selective to Aβ peptides. The voltammetric responses were proportional to the concentrations of Aβ ranging from 0.02 to 1.50 nM, with a detection limit of 10 pM. To demonstrate reprodicibility of the method for the analysis of Aβ, artificial CSF containing Aβ (1-40), Aβ (1-42) and Aβ (1-16) was tested, to quantify Aβ in a biological matrix, and in the design of new electrochemical biosensors for the detection of peptides and proteins. Furthermore, it was shown that tau increases ubiquitinated proteins and causes activation of the unfolded protein response (UPR) in the brain suggesting that tau interferes with protein quality control in the endoplasmic reticulum (ER) (Abisambra et al., 2013). Consistent with this, Ubiquitin was associated with the ER in human AD brains and tau transgenic (rTg4510) mouse brains, but was not co-localized with tau. The increased ubiquitinated protein was accompanied by increased phosphorylated protein kinase R-like ER kinase (pPERK), a biomarker that indicates UPR activation. Thus by depleting soluble tau in cells, brain could reverse UPR activation. Tau accumulation facilitated its deleterious interaction with ER membrane and associated proteins that are essential for ER-associated degradation (ERAD), including Valosin-containing protein (VCP) and Hrd1. Based on these findings, the effects of tau accumulation on ERAD efficiency were evaluated using the CD3δ reporter, an ERAD substrate. Indeed, CD3δ accumulated in both *in vitro* and *in vivo* models of tau overexpression and AD brains, suggesting that soluble tau impairs ERAD, resulting in UPR activation. However, the reversibility of this process, suggested that tau-based therapeutics could significantly delay cell death and therefore disease progression.

A study was performed to investigate whether a proteolytic fragment of the tau protein could serve as blood-based biomarker of cognitive function in AD (Henriksen et al., 2013). These investigators developed a sensitive ELISA specifically detecting Disintegrin and Metalloproteinase 10 (ADAM10)-generated fragment of Tau-A, characterized the assay for specificity and reactivity in healthy human serum, and used samples from the Tg4510 tau transgenic mice, which over-express the tau mutant P301L and exhibit a tauopathy similar to that observed in AD. Serum samples from 21 well-characterized AD patients were used, and correlated the Tau-A levels to cognitive function. The Tau-A ELISA detected the cleavage sequence at the N-terminus fragment of tau generated by ADAM10 with no cross-reactivity to intact tau or brain extracts. In brain extracts from Tg4510 mice 10X higher levels of Tau-A were detected indicating a pathological significance of this biomarker. In serum from healthy individuals reproducible levels of Tau-A were detected, indicating that the analyte is present in serum. In AD patients an inverse correlation between the cognitive assessment score (Mattis Dementia Rating Scale (MDRS) and Tau-A was observed. Based on the hypothesis that tau is cleaved proteolytically and then released into the blood, these investigators provided evidence for the presence of an ADAM10-generated tau fragment (Tau-A) in serum. In addition, Tau-A showed an inverse correlation to cognitive function, providing evidence that this serum biomarker has pathological significance for AD. It was proposed that only MCI with high Aβ amyloid is indicative of incipient AD, yet MCI with low Aβ amyloid may reflect other neurodegenerative processes. The extent to which Aβ influenced cognitive function in healthy older adults and adults with MCI was determined who underwent PET neuroimaging for Aβ and neuropsychological tests, assessing the cognitive domains of verbal and visual episodic memory, executive function, visuo-construction, attention and processing speed, and language at baseline (Lim et al., 2013). MCI with low Aβ performed worse than MCI with high Aβ on measures of executive function, attention, visuo-construction and language. No significant differences were observed between HC high and low Aβ groups. When compared with HC with low Aβ, both MCI high and low Aβ groups performed worse on episodic memory. However, only the MCI low Aβ group performed worse than HC low

Aβ on neuropsychological tests. When compared with HC with low Aβ amyloid, MCI with high Aβ amyloid present with impairments restricted to episodic memory, and the episodic memory impairments in MCI with low Aβ were accompanied by impairments in neuropsychological tests, *suggesting that MCI with high Aβ reflects prodromal AD, and that Aβ deposition accelerates gray matter atrophy at early stages of the disease even before cognitive impairment is manifested.* Hence identification of at-risk individuals at the pre-symptomatic stage has become a major research interest because it will allow early theranostic interventions before irreversible synaptic and neuronal loss.

The prognostic value of subjective memory complaints (SMCs) in the diagnosis of dementia of the AD is yet to be established. While some studies have found an association between SMCs and cognitive decline, many have found a stronger association with depression, which raises questions about their diagnostic capability. The association between SMC severity (as measured using the MAC-Q, a brief SMC questionnaire) and affect, memory, and AD biomarkers (β-amyloid deposition and the APOEε4 allele) in healthy elderly controls and individuals with MCI was examined (Buckley et al., 2013). They analyzed individuals drawn from the Australian Imaging Biomarkers and Lifestyle (AIBL) Study of Aging and noticed that SMCs were more severe in MCI patients than in HCs. SMC severity was related to affective variables and the interaction between age and group membership (HC/MCI). Within the HC group, SMC severity was related to affective variables only, while severity correlated only with age in the MCI group. SMCs were not related to cognitive variables or AD biomarkers. SMCs were related to poorer mood *(depression and anxiety)* in the cognitively healthy elderly; however mean levels were subclinical which argued for the assessment of affective symptomatology along with cognitive assessment in elderly memory complainers.

Glucose Metabolism in AD Among the pathogenic processes, altered Thiamine metabolism and Insulin resistance are characterized as major pathogenic mechanisms. Considering that AD patients exhibit cerebral Glucose hypometabolism due to impaired Insulin signaling and altered Thiamine metabolism, some potential diagnostic biomarkers for AD from abnormal glucose metabolism to develop drugs targeting at repairing insulin signaling and correcting thiamine metabolism were proposed. Thus abnormalities in Glucose metabolism play a significant role in AD pathophysiology via induction of pathogenic factors such as oxidative stress, and mitochondrial dysfunction. The causes, pathogeneses, and consequences of cerebral hypometabolism will help in finding ideal diagnostic biomarker(s) and disease-modifying therapy in AD. The following points were addressed: (1) the major challenges in the development of blood-based biomarkers of AD, such as patient heterogeneity, inclusion of the "right" control population, and the blood-brain barrier; (2) the need for a clear definition of the purpose of the individual biomarkers (e.g., prognostic, diagnostic, or monitoring therapeutic efficacy); (3) a critical evaluation of the ongoing biomarker approaches; and (4) the need for standardization of preanalytical variables and analytical methodologies (Henriksen et al., 2013).

A phenotype was characterized in a large family with a PSEN1 F177S mutation by performing clinical assessments, neuroimaging, and neuropathological analysis (Hausner et al., 2014). In two subjects, clinical and neuropsychological assessments, structural MRI, [18]FdG-PET imaging, AD biomarkers in CSF and genetic analysis were available. In three deceased subjects, medical records were reviewed. In one subject, a complete neuropathological examination was available. Cognitive impairment and neurological symptoms developed around 30 years of age and worsened rapidly. All subjects died about 7 years (range, 6-8 years) after disease onset before 40 years of age. The diagnostic information for AD, in addition to neuroimaging and CSF analysis showed, neuritic plaques and neurofibrillary tangles. Anti-dementia treatment in one subject did not alter the duration of survival. Moreover the PSEN1 F177S mutation leads to typical AD starting at age 30 and a homogeneous phenotype with rapid cognitive decline and prominent neurological symptoms. Excessive amyloid β-42 production in the cerebral cortex corresponded well with other PSEN1 mutations. Hence the development of validated and standardized biomarkers for AD that allow for an early presymptomatic diagnosis and discrimination from other types of dementia and neurodegenerative diseases is needed to accelerate the development of novel disease-modifying therapies.

Aβ1-42 Peptide in the CSF of AD Patients A study was focused on the value of Aβ1-42 peptide in the CSF as the core neurochemical biomarker for the amyloidogenic mechanisms in early-onset familial and late-onset sporadic AD (Lista, 2013). These investigators discussed the use of Aβ1-42 in combination with evolving neuroimaging biomarkers in AD diagnosis. Multimodality neuroimaging techniques, providing structural-functional-metabolic aspects of brain pathophysiology, are helpful to predict and monitor the progression of the disease. Thus advances in multimodality neuroimaging provide new insights into brain organization and enable the detection of specific proteins and/or protein aggregates associated with AD. The combination of biomarkers from different methodologies is believed to be risk-value to accurately identify asymptomatic and prodromal individuals who will progress to dementia and represent rational biomarker candidates for preventive and symptomatic pharmacological interventions.

Physiological and Neurobehavioral Biomarkers of AD The physiological biomarkers include electrophysiological and circadian rhythm biomarkers and are assessed based on the computerized EEG analysis. These biomarkers are assessed based on the analysis of different EEG frequencies. Primarily the dominance of δ and θ rhythm is noticed among AD patients and their sleep wakeful cycle is impaired due to disturbance in the 5-HTergic neurotransmission. In addition neuropsychological and epidemiological biomarkers could be used to clinically assess AD patients on a longitudinal basis. Computerized EEG analysis is very practical and noninvasive approach to assess the extent of neurodegeneration and regeneration in AD patients. Computerized EEG analysis is a noninvasive approach to longitudinally assess the extent of neurodegeneration or regeneration in AD patients. Recently how commonly prescribed pharmacologic treatments affect Event-Related Potential (ERP) biomarkers as tools for predicting AD in individuals with MCI was investigated. These investigators gathered baseline ERP data from two MCI groups (*those taking AD medications and those not*) and determined which subjects developed AD and which remained cognitively stable. They utilized a multivariate system of ERP components to measure the effects of medication among these 4 subgroups. Discriminant analysis produced classification scores as a measure of similarity to each group, and found a significant main Group effect but no main AD medications effect and no group by medications interaction suggesting that AD medications have negligible influence on ERP components as biomarkers of disease progression. Furthermore, the clinical utility of multiscale entropy (MSE) by surface EEG in patients with AD that was correlated to cognitive and behavioral dysfunction was assessed. A total of 108 AD patients, subjected to digital EEG recordings, were analyzed using MSE methods. The appropriate parameters and time scale factors from EEG signals, and within-subject consistency in different EEG epochs and correlations of MSE measures to cognitive and neuropsychiatric symptoms of AD were assessed. Increased severity of AD was associated with decreased MSE complexity as measured by short-time scales, and with increased MSE complexity as measured by long-time scales. MSE complexity in EEGs of the temporal and occipito-parietal electrodes correlated with the cognitive function. MSE complexity in various brain areas was also correlated to neuropsychiatric symptoms. The MSE analysis revealed abnormal EEG complexity across short- and long-time scale that was correlated to cognitive and neuropsychiatric assessments suggesting that the MSE-based EEG complexity analysis may provide a simple and economical method to quantify the severity of cognitive and neuropsychiatric symptoms in AD patients.

Pathological Biomarkers in AD The pathological biomarkers include Apolipoprotein E (APO-E) polymorphism, In general Aβ and C-reactive proteins are estimated from the CSF to assess the extent of neurodegeneration in AD patients. These two biomarkers can be estimated to differentiate AD from vascular dementia and other clinical conditions including pressure hydrocephalus. These biomarkers also shed some light regarding the incidence of bipolar disorders in AD patients. Aβ and C-reactive proteins are estimated from the CSF to assess the extent of neurodegeneration in AD patients. The major neuropathologic hallmarks in AD consist of neuronal loss in selected brain regions, deposition of extracellular senile plaques, and intracellular neurofibrillary tangles. In addition, neuroinflammation is a characteristic feature of AD pathology and is thought to contribute to the neurodegeneration. Inflammation occurs in pathologically vulnerable regions of the AD brain, with increased expression of acute phase proteins and proinflammatory cytokines.

IN-VIVO MOLECULAR BIOMARKERS IN AD

Diagnostic criteria for AD recognize a key role of neuroimaging biomarkers for early diagnosis. Diagnostic accuracy depends on which biomarker (i.e., amyloid imaging, [18]FdG-PET, SPECT, or MRI) and how it is measured ("metric": visual, manual, semiautomated, or automated segmentation/computation). Recently it was reported that neurons are anatomically and physiologically connected to each other, and these connections are involved in various neuronal functions (Hirano and Yamada, 2013). Multiple neural networks involved in neurodegenerative diseases can be detected using network analysis in functional neuroimaging. The basic methods and theories of voxel-based network analyses, such as principal component analysis, independent component analysis, and seed-based analysis, were introduced. Disease-and symptom-specific brain networks were identified using [18]FdG in patients with AD which evaluates individual patients and serve as diagnostic tools as well as biomarker for therapeutic interventions. Many functional MRI studies showed that posterior cingulate cortex and medial prefrontal cortex are deactivated by externally driven cognitive tasks; such brain regions construct the "default mode network" which is disrupted from the preclinical phase of AD and is associated with amyloid deposition in the brain. Default mode network is also impaired in PD, with inconsistent results due to the heterogeneous pharmacological status, differences in mesocortical dopaminergic impairment, and simultaneous amyloid deposition. Recently cerebral glucose metabolism in physiological and pathological conditions and the contribution of glucose transportation abnormality and intracellular Glucose catabolism dysfunction in AD pathophysiology were reviewed, and an hypothesis was proposed that multiple pathogenic cascades induced by impaired cerebral glucose metabolism result in neurodegeneration and consequently cognitive deficits in AD (Chen and Zhong, 2013).

Another study was performed to build outcomes for future use in clinical practice into RCT designs (Gauthier et al., 2013; Gauthier et al., 2014). The Clinical Dementia Rating Scale Sum of Boxes (CDR-SB) is the most reliable for RCT at different stages of AD, with the Relevant Outcome Scale (ROSA) for AD as a suitable alternative. The significance of current AD biomarkers for the determination of efficacy of disease-modifying drugs is yet to be established; however, amyloid-specific test is required prior to treatment with drug acting primarily on Aβ-42. In addition, serial MRI may be required to monitor adverse side effects associated with such drugs. Hence global clinical scales such as CDR-SB and ROSA should be considered at slowing disease progression.

CSF and Amyloid PET Biomarkers in AD Lumbar puncture (LP) is usually performed in memory clinics to detect the existence of various biomarkers in AD. The patient-acceptance of LP, incidence of and risk factors for post-LP complications were investigated by enroling 3868 patients (50% women, age 66 ± 11 years, mini mental state examination 25 ± 5) at 23 memory clinics (Duits et al., 2015). Regression analysis was used to evaluate risk factors for post-LP complications, such as typical post-lumbar puncture headache (PLPH) and back pain. A total of 1065 patients (31%) reported post-LP complaints; 589 patients (17%) reported back pain, 649 (19%) headache, of which 296 (9%) reported typical PLPH. Only few patients needed medical intervention: 11 (0.3%) received a blood patch, 23 (0.7%) were hospitalized. The important risk factor for PLPH was history of headache. An atraumatic needle and age >65 years were preventive. Gender, rest after LP, or volume of CSF, had no effect, indicating that the overall risk of LP complications for biomarker assessment was relatively low.

Comparative Diagnostic Accuracy of AD A study was performed to compare the diagnostic accuracy of CSF biomarkers and amyloid PET for diagnosing early-stage AD (Palmqvist et al., 2015). These investigators included 122 healthy elderly and 34 patients with MCI who developed AD dementia within 3 years (MCI-AD). Aβ deposition in 9 brain regions was examined with [^{18}F]-Flutemetamol PET. CSF was analyzed with INNOTEST and EUROIMMUN ELISAs. The results were replicated in 146 controls and 64 patients with MCI-AD. The best CSF measures for identifying MCI-AD were Aβ42/total tau (t-tau) and Aβ42/hyperphosphorylated tau (p-tau). The best PET measures performed similarly; anterior cingulate, posterior cingulate/precuneus, and global neocortical uptake). CSF Aβ42/t-tau and Aβ42/p-tau performed better than CSF Aβ42 and Aβ42/40. The CSF Aβ42/t-tau had the highest accuracy of all CSF/PET biomarkers. The combination of CSF and PET was not better than using either biomarker separately. Amyloid PET and CSF biomarkers could identify early AD with high accuracy. There were no differences between the CSF and PET measures and no improvement was noticed when combining them. Regional PET measures were not better than assessing the global Aβ deposition. The choice between CSF and amyloid PET biomarkers for identifying early AD could be based on availability, costs, and doctor/patient preferences since both had equally high diagnostic accuracy. This study provided evidence that amyloid PET as well as CSF biomarkers identify early-stage AD equally accurately.

Recent studies reported that the choice of biomarkers for early detection of AD is important for improving the accuracy of imaging-based prediction of conversion from MCI to AD (Ota et al., 2015). These authors assessed the effects of imaging modalities and brain atlases on prediction. They also investigated the influence of support vector machine recursive feature elimination (SVM-RFE) on predictive performance. Eighty patients with amnestic MCI [40 developed AD within 3 years] underwent MRI and ^{18}FdG-PET imaging. Using Automated Anatomical Labeling (AAL) and LONI Probabilistic Brain Atlas (LPBA40), they extracted features representing gray matter density and relative cerebral metabolic rate for glucose in each ROI from the baseline MRI and ^{18}FdG-PET data, respectively. The interactions between atlas and modality choices were significant. The main effect of SVM-RFE was significant, but the interactions with the other factors were not significant. Multimodal features were found to be better than unimodal features to predict AD and ^{18}FdG-PET neuroimaging proved better than MRI. Furthermore, SVM-RFE could improve the predictive accuracy when using atlas-based features.

^{11}C- Pittsburg Compound (PiB) as a PET Biomarker of AD and MCI It is now realized that the incorporation of biomarkers increases the diagnostic accuracy of AD. In a Cochrane review, the ligand ^{11}C-PiB showed a high sensitivity, but low specificity for detecting patients with MCI who would develop Alzheimer's dementia (Laeger, 2015). These investigators suggested that with presently available limited treatment options for MCI, ^{11}C-PiB-PET cannot be recommended for routine use in MCI and should be used only in selected cases where a positive scan may alter clinical management. The longitudinal relationship between Aβ deposition, gray matter atrophy, and cognitive impairment in asymptomatic individuals with AD pathology was further characterized by PIB-PET imaging (Doré et al, 2013). In a similar study, regional analysis was performed to relate cortical thickness to PIB retention and episodic memory. A total of 93 elderly normal control subjects (NCs) and 40 patients with AD from the Australian Imaging, Biomarkers, and Lifestyle Study of Aging cohort participated in this study, who underwent neuropsychological evaluation as well as MRI and PIB-PET imaging. As many as 64 NCs underwent repeated neuroimaging and neuropsychological evaluation 18 and 36 months later. There was a significant reduction in cortical thickness in the precuneus and hippocampus associated with episodic memory impairment in the NC PIB-positive (NC+) group when compared with the NC-group. Cortical thickness was also correlated negatively with neocortical PIB in the NC+ group. Longitudinal analysis showed gray matter (GM) atrophy in the temporal lobe and the hippocampi of the NC+ group. Over time, GM atrophy became more extensive in the NC+ group, especially in the temporal lobe. In asymptomatic individuals, Aβ deposition was associated with GM atrophy and memory impairment. The earliest signs of GM atrophy were detected in the hippocampus, the posterior cingulate, and precuneus regions, and with disease progression in the temporal lobes, suggesting that Aβ deposition is not a benign process and that interventions with anti-Aβ therapy at early stages could be more effective in the clinical management of AD.

In-Vivo Molecular Imaging Biomarkers in AD These biomarkers have been used extensively and successfully for the better clinical management of AD because of their increased sensitivity and specificity. Particularly PET imaging using ^{18}F and ^{11}C-labeled radiopharmaceuticals has shown great promise in the early clinical diagnosis of AD and its outcome following treatment. In addition to significant reduction in the fronto-temporal uptake of ^{18}FdG, ^{11}C or ^{18}F labeled Pittsburg compound (^{18}F-PIB) is picked up specifically by amyloid plaques. Hence PIB compound was approved by FDA and is routinely used in various labs all over the world for the differential diagnosis, prognosis and personalized clinical management of AD. Similarly MRI provides information regarding the extent of cortical atrophy, hippocampal atrophy, callosal atrophy and lateral ventricular enlargement. Simulteneously it is now possible to detect brain regional concentrations of several neurochemical agents that are influenced by AD. For example, there is significant reduction in the N-Acetyl Aspartic acid (N-AA), Phosphocreatine to Creatine ratio and Glutamate and Choline important in GABAergic neurotransmission and Ach synthesis respectively. Single biomarker analysis may not provide clear picture of AD, it is therefore highly significant to analyze several other biomarkers in combination to obtain more precise information regarding the extent of neuronal damange or repair in the AD brain. Hence multiple diagnostic biomarkers are analyzed simultaneously for the differential diagnosis and prognosis and individualized treatment of AD.

Recently postmortem brain samples were used to investigate the molecular biomarkers and their clinical significance for the diagnosis of AD (Marutle. et al, 2013). *In vitro* binding assays demonstrated increased [³H]-PIB (fibrillar Aβ) and [³H]-PK11195 (activated microglia) binding in the frontal cortex (FC) and hippocampus (HIP), as well as increased binding of [³H]-L-deprenyl (activated astrocytes) in the HIP, but a decreased [³H]-Nicotine (α4β2 nicotinic acetylcholine receptor (nAChR)) binding in the FC of AD cases compared to age-matched controls. Autoradiography was also performed to investigate the distributions of [³H]-L-deprenyl, [³H]-PIB as well as [¹²⁵I]-α-bungarotoxin (α7 nAChRs) and [³H]-Nicotine in cerebral hemispheres of a typical AD case. A distinct lamination pattern was observed with [³H]-PIB binding in all layers and [³H]-deprenyl in superficial layers of the FC. In contrast, [³H]-PIB showed low binding to fibrillar Aβ, but high binding of [³H]-deprenyl to activated astrocytes throughout the HIP. The [³H]-PIB binding was also low and the [³H]-deprenyl binding was high in all layers of the medial temporal gyrus and insular cortex in comparison to the frontal cortex. Low [³H]-Nicotine binding was observed in all layers of the frontal cortex in comparison to medial temporal gyrus layers, insular cortex and hippocampus. Immunohistochemical analyses revealed abundant GFAP+ve and α7 nAChR expressing GFAP+ astrocytes in the vicinity and surrounding Aβ neuritic plaques in the FC and HIP in AD. Although fewer Aβ plaques were observed in the HIP, some GFAP+ve astrocytes contained Aβ-positive (6 F/3D) granules within the somata, suggesting that astrocytosis shows a distinct pattern in AD brain compared to fibrillar Aβ, and that different types of astrocytes may be associated with the pathophysiology of AD. These findings provide further support to microglia as essential components of the amyloid hypothesis (Gandy et al., 2013). Furthermore, the use of PET and structural MR fusion imaging can improve the diagnostic accuracy of dementia. In other neurodegenerative dementias, each disease exhibits a specific metabolic reduction pattern. In dementia with Lewy bodies, occipital Glucose metabolism is decreased, while in fronto-temporal dementia, frontal and anterior temporal metabolism is decreased. These ¹⁸FdG-PET findings and amyloid deposits are significant biomarkers for various neurodegenerative dementias including AD. Randomized clinical trials (RCTs) for putative disease-modifying drugs in AD are using cognitive outcomes, Assessment Scale - cognitive subscale, activities of daily living scales, Cooperative Study Activities of Daily Living, and time from mild cognitive impairment to AD dementia. Cortical glucose metabolism, brain amyloid β accumulation, and hippocampal atrophy imaging suggested as potential biomarkers in predicting which patients with MCI will convert to AD.

Recently the prognostic ability of [^{11}C]PIB PET, [^{18}F] FdG PET and quantitative hippocampal volumes was estimated with MRI in predicting conversion to AD in patients with MCI (Bruck et al., 2013). The study group comprised 29 patients with MCI who underwent ^{11}C-PIB-PET and MR imaging. Of these, 22 also underwent ^{18}FdG-PET imaging. All subjects were invited for clinical evaluation after 2 years. During the follow-up, 17 patients had converted to AD while 12 continued to meet the criteria for MCI. The two groups did not differ in age, gender or education level, but the converter group tended to have lower MMSE and Word List learning than the nonconverter group. High ^{11}C-PIB retention in the fronto-temporal regions and anterior and posterior cingulate predicted conversion to AD. Also reduced ^{18}F-FdG uptake in the left lateral temporal cortex (LTC) predicted conversion, but hippocampal volumes did not. In ROC analysis the measurements that predicted the conversion were ^{11}C-PIB retention in the lateral frontal cortex and ^{18}FdG uptake in the left LTC. Both PET methods resulted in good sensitivity and specificity and neither was superior to the other.

The MCI due to AD was identified by, using amyloid imaging of Aβ deposition and ^{18}FdG imaging reflecting neuronal dysfunction as PET biomarkers (Hatashita et al., 2013). Sixty-eight MCI patients underwent cognitive testing, ^{11}C-PIB-PET and ^{18}FdG PET at baseline and follow-up. PIB distribution volume ratio (DVR) was calculated using Logan graphical analysis, and the SUVR was used as quantitative analysis for ^{18}FdG. Thirty (44.1%) of all 68 MCI patients converted to AD over 19.2 ± 7.1 months. The annual rate of MCI conversion was 23.4%. A positive Aβ PET biomarker identified MCI due to AD in individual MCI subjects with a sensitivity (SS) of 96.6% and specificity (SP) of 42.1%. The positive predictive value (PPV) was 56.8%. A positive Aβ biomarker in Apo-E ε4/4 carriers distinguished with a SS of 100%. In individual MCI subjects who had impairment in episodic memory and aged older than 75 years, Aβ biomarker identified MCI due to AD with higher SS of 100%, SP of 66.6% and PPV of 80%, compared to ^{18}FdG biomarker alone or both PET biomarkers combined. However, when assessed in precuneus, both Aβ and ^{18}FdG biomarkers had the greatest level of certainty for MCI due to AD with a PPV of 87.8%, suggesting that the Aβ PET biomarker primarily defines MCI due to AD in individual MCI subjects. Furthermore, combined ^{18}FdG biomarker in a cortical region of precuneus enhanced diagnostic value in predicting AD.

The appearance of β-amyloidosis and brain injury biomarkers in cognitively normal (CN) persons is thought to define risk for the future development of cognitive impairment due to AD, but their interaction is poorly understood. An hypothesis was tested that the existence of β-amyloidosis as well as brain injury biomarkers would lead to progressive neurodegeneration (Knopman et al., 2013). A sum of 191 CN persons (median age, 77 years; range, 71-93 years) underwent MRI, ^{18}FdG-PET, and ^{18}F-PIB-PET imaging twice over a span of 15 months. Participants were grouped based on the presence of β-amyloidosis, defined as a PIB-PET SUVr >1.5, alone (stage 1) or with brain injury (stage 2 + 3), defined as hippocampal atrophy or ^{18}FdG hypometabolism. These investigators also studied patients with MCI or dementia. There were 25 CN participants with both high PIB retention and low hippocampal volume or ^{18}FdG hypometabolism at baseline. On follow-up, participants had greater loss of medial temporal lobe volume and increased glucose hypometabolism in the medial temporal lobe compared with the other CN groups. The changes were similar to those in the cognitively impaired participants. Extratemporal regions did not show similar changes.

Higher rates of medial temporal neurodegeneration occurred in CN individuals who had abnormal levels of β-amyloid as well as brain injury biomarkers.

Although it is well established that neuroinflammation is a pathological hallmark of AD, its role in cognitive impairment and course of development during the disease progression remains uncertain (Kreisl et al., 2013). To address these questions, PET imaging with ^{11}C-PBR28 was performed to measure translocator protein 18 kDa (TSPO), a putative biomarker for inflammation. Patients with AD, MCI, and older controls were also scanned with ^{11}C-PIB to measure amyloid burden. Twenty-nine amyloid-positive patients, (19) Alzheimer's, 10 mild cognitive impairment), and 13 amyloid-negative control subjects were studied to determine whether TSPO binding is elevated in patients with AD, and to determine whether TSPO binding correlates with neuropsychological measures, grey matter volume, ^{11}C-PIB binding, or age of onset. Patients with AD, but not those with MCI, had higher ^{11}C-PBR28 binding in cortical brain regions than controls. The most significant differences were noticed in the parietal and temporal cortices, with no difference in subcortical regions or cerebellum. ^{11}C-PBR28 binding inversely correlated with performance on Folstein Mini-Mental State Examination, Clinical Dementia Rating Scale Sum of Boxes, Logical Memory Immediate (Wechsler Memory Scale Third Edition), Trail Making part B and Block Design (Wechsler Adult Intelligence Scale Third Edition) tasks, with the largest correlations observed in the inferior parietal lobule. ^{11}C-PBR28 binding also inversely correlated with grey matter volume. Early-onset (<65 years) patients had higher ^{11}C-PBR28 binding than late-onset patients, and in parietal cortex and striatum ^{11}C-PBR28 binding correlated with lower age of onset. Generally partial volume results were in agreement; however, the correlation between ^{11}C-PBR28 and ^{11}C-PIB binding was seen only after partial volume correction suggesting that neuroinflammation, indicated by increased ^{11}C-PBR28 binding to TSPO, occurs after conversion of MCI to AD and worsens with disease progression. Hence inflammation may contribute to the precipitous disease, typically observed in early-onset patients. Furthermore, ^{11}C-PBR28 may be useful in longitudinal studies to mark the conversion from MCI or to assess response to treatments of AD.

Recently, the diagnostic accuracy of biomarker vs metric in differentiating AD from healthy and prognostic accuracy to predict progression in MCI was evaluated (Frisoni et al., 2013). The outcome measure was positive (negative) likelihood ratio, LR+ (LR-), defined as the ratio between the probability of positive (negative) test outcome in patients and the probability of positive (negative) test outcome in healthy controls. Diagnostic LR+ of biomarkers was between 4.4 and 9.4 and LR- between 0.25 and 0.08, whereas prognostic LR+ and LR- were between 1.7 and 7.5, and 0.50 and 0.11, respectively. Within metrics, LRs varied up to 100-fold: LR+ from ~1 to 100; LR- from ~1.00 to 0.01. Biomarkers accounted for 11% and 18% of diagnostic and prognostic variance of LR+ and 16% and 24% of LR-. Across all biomarkers, metrics accounted for an equal or larger amount of variance than biomarkers: 13% and 62% of diagnostic and prognostic variance of LR+, and 29% and 18% of LR-. Within biomarkers, the largest proportion of diagnostic LR+ and LR- variability was within [18]FdG-PET and MRI metrics, respectively.

Diagnostic and Prognostic Accuracy of Imaging Biomarkers in AD It now realized that the diagnostic and prognostic accuracy of imaging AD biomarkers depends on how the biomarker is measured and on the biomarker itself. Hence the establishment of SOPs is extremely important to biomarker use in the clinical drug trials. Currently, no clinical or radiological techniques have been validated to distinguish AD from idiopathic normal pressure hydrocephalus (iNPH). Both share anatomical and clinical similarities: AD is a form of irreversible degenerative dementia, whereas the dementia manifested in iNPH is potentially reversible through neurosurgical interventions. Hence, it is important to find specific imaging biomarkers that distinguish the two conditions. In addition, the ability to predict the response to neurosurgery in iNPH is yet to be established. The merits and limitations of the MRI parameters currently used to distinguish AD from iNPH and to predict the response after treatment of iNPH were analyzed (Di Ieva et al., 2014). It was suggested that the combination of different neuroimaging as well as quantitative and qualitative parameters could provide new insight for better diagnosis and treatment of these two different diseases. The accumulation of Aβ plaque, as a hallmark of AD, is believed to develop many years prior to symptoms and is reflected by reduced CSF levels of the peptide Aβ1-42. An hypothesis was tested that baseline levels of CSF proteins involved in microglial activity, synaptic function and Aβ metabolism predict the development of Aβ plaques, assessed by longitudinal CSF Aβ-42 decrease in cognitively healthy people. A study was performed on 46 healthy people with three to four CSF samples (Mattsson et al., 2013a; Mattsson et al., 2013b). There was an overall reduction in Aβ-42 from a mean concentration of 211-195 pg/ml after 4 years. Linear mixed-effects models using longitudinal Aβ-42 as the response variable, and baseline proteins as explanatory variables (n = 69 proteins potentially relevant for Aβ metabolism, microglia or synaptic/neuronal function), identified 10 proteins with significant effects on longitudinal Aβ-42. *The most significant proteins were angiotensin-converting enzyme (ACE), Chromogranin A (CgA) and receptor tyrosine kinase (AXL).* ROC analysis identified 11 proteins with significant effects on longitudinal Aβ42 (overlapping with the proteins identified by linear mixed-effects models). Several proteins (including ACE, CgA and AXL) were associated with Aβ-42 reduction only in subjects with normal baseline Aβ-42, and not in subjects with reduced baseline Aβ-42 suggesting that baseline CSF proteins related to Aβ metabolism, microglial activity or synapses predict Aβ-42 reduction in cognitively healthy elders. The finding that some proteins only predict Aβ-42 reduction in subjects with normal baseline Aβ-42 suggested that they predict future development of the Aβ pathology at the earliest stages of AD, prior to widespread development of Aβ plaques in the brain.

MRI as A Biomarker in AD In a study, the association of the rate of cognitive decline in the years leading up to structural MRI with an established biomarker, hippocampal volume was examined (Fleischman et al., 2013). The sample comprised 211 participants who had an average of 5.5 years of cognitive data prior to structural MRI imaging. There was significant variability in the trajectories of cognitive change prior to imaging and that cognitive decline was associated with smaller hippocampal volumes. Domain-specific analyses suggested that this association was driven by decline in working memory. These results emphasized the importance of examining cognitive change and its association with brain structure during the years in which older persons are considered cognitively healthy. It is now realized that resting-state functional MRI has great potential for characterizing pathophysiological changes during the preclinical phase of AD. To assess the functional relationship between default mode network integrity and CSF biomarkers of AD pathology in cognitively normal older individual, a cross-sectional cohort study was performed among 207 older adults with normal cognition (Clinical Dementia Rating, 0) (Wang et al., 2013). Resting-state functional connectivity MRI measures of default mode network integrity. Decreased CSF Aβ-42 and increased phosphorylated tau-181 were associated with reduced default mode network integrity, with the decreases in functional connectivity between the posterior cingulate and medial temporal regions. The reductions in functional connectivity were not correlated to age or structural atrophy in the posterior cingulate and medial temporal areas. Similar resting-state fMRI findings in relation to CSF biomarkers were obtained using ROI analyses and voxel-based correlation mapping, suggesting that both Aβ and tau pathology affect neuronal network integrity before clinical onset of AD

Recent studies established that along with cortical abnormalities, white matter microstructural changes such as axonal loss and myelin breakdown are implicated in the pathogenesis of AD (Fieremans et al., 2013). A white matter model was introduced that relates non-Gaussian diffusional kurtosis imaging metrics to characteristics of white matter tract integrity, including the axonal water fraction, the intra-axonal diffusivity, and the extra-axonal axial and radial diffusivities. This study reported white matter tract integrity metrics in subjects with amnestic MCI, AD, and age-matched healthy controls to investigate their sensitivity, diagnostic accuracy, and associations with white matter changes through the course of AD. With tract-based spatial statistics and ROI analyses, increased diffusivity in the extra-axonal space (extra-axonal axial and radial diffusivities) in several white matter tracts sensitively and discriminated healthy controls from those with amnestic MCI, while widespread decreased axonal water fraction discriminated amnestic MCI from AD. These white matter tract integrity metrics in the corpus callosum significantly correlated with speed processing in amnestic MCI. These findings have implications for the course and spatial progression of white matter degeneration in AD, and suggest the mechanisms by which these changes occur, and demonstrate the viability of the white matter tract integrity metrics as potential neuroimaging biomarkers of the earliest stages of AD and disease progression. Previous studies have demonstrated disruption in structural and functional connectivity in the AD. However, it is unknown how these disruptions alter brain network reorganization. With the modular analysis of graph theory, and datasets acquired by the resting-state functional MRI (R-fMRI), the brain regional organization patterns between the AD group and the cognitively normal control (CN) group was compared (Zhang et al., 2013).

The largest homotopic module (defined as the insula module) in the CN group was degenerated in the AD group. Specifically, the 8 pairs of the bilateral regions (the opercular part of inferior frontal gyrus, area triangularis, insula, putamen, globus pallidus, transverse temporal gyri, superior temporal gyrus, and superior temporal pole) of the insula module had lost symmetric functional connectivity, and the gray matter concentration (GMC) was significantly lower in AD group. These investigators quantified the functional connectivity changes with an index (index A) and structural changes with the GMC index in the insula to demonstrate their potential as AD biomarkers. The results were validated with 6 additional independent datasets and demonstrated specific structural and functional reorganization from young to old, and for diseased, suggesting that by combining the structural GMC analysis and functional modular analysis in the insula, a new biomarker can be developed. In addition a study was performed to assess amyloid imaging regarding clinical utility and impact.

Overlapping Symptoms of Cognition and Movement Patients are often mistaken to suffer from PD or AD because of the overlapping clinical symptoms of cognition and movement. A literature search was conducted in several databases, searching articles between 2008 and 2013 following the Preferred Reporting Items for Systematic Reviews and Meta-Analyses (PRISMA) guidelines (Wahlster et al., 2013). The results were reported according to the clinical correlates of amyloid imaging from 33 studies. Five studies evaluated amyloid imaging for the diagnosis. Nine studies assessed the prognostic value. Twenty-two studies provided correlations to cognitive measures. Amyloid imaging provided a high reliability in the diagnosis and prognosis, but cognitive measures showed weak correlations. The evidence indicated that amyloid imaging has not arrived yet in routine clinical practice. However, it can provide benefits in diagnostic accuracy up to 10 years before clinical diagnosis. This can be a basis for early preventive treatment strategies such as anti-amyloid therapy indicating that amyloid imaging is crucial to understand the early pathologic process in AD. However, the diagnosis of DLB is difficult to differentiate from other degenerative diseases.

In a study, the differential diagnosis using CSF biomarkers was investigated (Kaerst et al., 2013). These investigators analyzed data of patients suffering from degenerative, ischemic, or inflammatory diseases and identified those with DLB, PD, and AD for further analyses. When considering the underlying pathophysiological mechanisms involved in idiopathic normal pressure hydrocephalus (iNPH), white matter is often the main locus of investigation. However, when an axon in the brain is damaged, degeneration of the neuron can occur proximally and AD, associated with cortical thinning, is a common pathologic comorbidity with iNPH. Differences in cortical thickness between CSF tap test (CSFTT) responders and non-responders in iNPH patients and patterns of cortical thickness were compared in iNPH patients with that of AD patients (Kang et al., 2013). Thirty-two iNPH patients (16 CSFTT responders and 16 CSFTT non-responders) and 16 AD patients were imaged with MRI, including 3-D volumetric analyses for cortical thickness analysis. Among the iNPH patients, CSFTT non-responders, when compared to responders, had significant cortical thinning in the left superior frontal gyrus at the level of a false discovery rate (FDR), and showed widespread cortical thinning in most areas of the brain. Relative to the CSFTT responders, AD patients showed significant cortical thinning in superior and medial frontal gyrus, left precentral gyrus, postcentral gyrus, paracentral lobule, precuneus, and superior parietal lobule after FDR correction. However, comparing patterns of cortical thinning between AD patients and CSFTT non-responders revealed no significant differences. Differences in cortical thickness correlated with CSFTT response for iNPH patients may indicate a possibility for considering patterns of cortical thinning in patients with ventriculomegaly as potential brain imaging biomarkers for the prediction of CSFTT responders suggesting that comorbid AD pathology might be related to the cortical thinning patterns found in CSFTT non-responders. Hence further studies, using normal controls and combinations of other biomarkers associated with AD, would be necessary to evaluate these hypotheses.

The structural and functional neuroimaging of dementia have evolved over the last few years. The most common forms of dementia, AD, Lewy body dementia (LBD), and fronto-temporal lobar degeneration (FTLD), have distinct patterns of cortical atrophy and hypometabolism that evolve over time, as recently reported (Haller et al., 2013). These investigators also discussed unspecific white matter alterations on T_2-weighted and fluid-attenuated inversion recovery (FLAIR) images as well as cerebral microbleeds, which often occur during normal aging and may affect cognition. The third part summarized molecular neuroimaging biomarkers to visualize amyloid deposits, tau protein deposits, and neurotransmitter systems. The fourth section reviewed the utility of advanced image techniques as predictive biomarkers of cognitive decline in individuals with early symptoms compatible with MCI. As only about half of MCI cases will progress to clinically overt dementia, whereas the other half remain stable or might even improve, the discrimination of stable versus progressive MCI is of paramount importance for both individual patient treatment and patient selection for clinical trials. The fifth and final part discussed the inter-individual variation in the neurocognitive reserve, which is a potential constraint for all proposed methods. (a) Many forms of dementia have spatial atrophy patterns detectable on neuroimaging. (b) Early treatment of dementia is beneficial, indicating the need for early diagnosis. (c) Advanced image analysis techniques detect subtle anomalies invisible on radiological evaluation. (d) Inter-individual variation explains variable cognitive impairment despite the same degree of atrophy.

In a recent study, a novel MRI-based biomarker that predicts the individual progression of MCI to AD on the basis of pathological brain aging patterns was presented (Gaser et al., 2013). By employing regression methods, the expression of normal brain-aging patterns forms the basis to estimate the brain age. If the estimated age is higher than the chronological age, a positive brain age gap estimation (BrainAGE) score indicates accelerated atrophy and is considered a risk factor for conversion to AD. The BrainAGE framework was applied to predict the individual brain ages of 195 subjects with MCI at baseline, of which a total of 133 developed AD during 36 months of follow-up (corresponding to a pre-test probability of 68%). The ability of the BrainAGE framework to correctly identify MCI-converters was compared with the performance of commonly used cognitive scales, hippocampus volume, and state-of-the-art biomarkers derived from CSF. With accuracy rates of up to 81%, BrainAGE outperformed all cognitive scales and CSF biomarkers in predicting conversion of MCI to AD within 3 years of follow-up. Each additional year in the BrainAGE score was associated with a 10% greater risk of developing AD. Furthermore, the post-test probability was increased to 90% when using baseline BrainAGE scores to predict conversion to AD. This framework allowed an accurate prediction even with multicenter data. Its fast and fully automated nature facilitates the integration into the clinical workflow. It can be used as a tool for screening as well as for monitoring treatment options.

A recent study examined the association of rate of cognitive decline as a function of hippocampal volume reduction, as an established biomarker, by performing structural MRI (Fleischman et al., 2013). The sample comprised 211 participants who had an average of 5.5 years of cognitive data prior to structural MRI. There was significant variability in the trajectories of cognitive change prior to imaging and faster cognitive decline was associated with smaller hippocampal volumes. Domain-specific analyses suggested that this association was driven primarily by decline in working memory. The results emphasize the importance of examining cognitive change and its association with brain structure during the years in which older persons are considered cognitively healthy.

MRS Biomarkers in AD In addition to MRI, Proton magnetic resonance spectroscopy (MRS) provides a window into the biochemical changes associated with the loss of neuronal integrity and other neurodegenerative pathology that involve the brain before the manifestations of cognitive impairment in patients who are at risk for AD. It is now possible to detect brain regional concentrations of several neurochemical agents that are influenced by AD. For example, there is significant reduction in the N-acetyl aspartic acid (N-AA), phosphocreatine to creatine ratio and glutamate and choline important in GABA-ergic neurotransmission and ACh synthesis respectively. Single biomarker analysis may not provide a clear picture of AD, therefore, it is highly significant to analyze several other biomarkers in combination to obtain more precise information regarding the extent of neuronal damage or repair in the AD brain. Hence multiple diagnostic biomarkers are analyzed simultaneously for the differential diagnosis and prognosis of AD. Recent MRS studies focsed on normal aging, MCI, and dementia, and how MRS metabolites may be potential biomarkers for early diagnosis of dementia-related pathologic changes in the brain (Graff-Radford et al., 2013). Significantly reduced neurochemicals were: NAA, a marker of neuronal injury, Pcr/CR ratio (markers of high-energy phosphorylated metabolites), Choline (precursor for the synthesis of the neurotransmitter, Ach, and Phosphatidyl choline for the synthesis of plasma membrane), and Glutamate (precursor for the synthesis of inhibitory neurotransmitter, GABA) were noticed in patients with AD. (*A detailed description is beyond the scope this chapter*).

Multimodality Fusion Imaging in AD Recently Trzepacz et al (2014) compared ^{18}F-PIB-PET amyloid imaging, ^{18}FdG-PET for metabolism, and MRI for structure to predict conversion from amnestic MCI to Alzheimer's dementia using data from the ADNI cohort. Numeric neuroimaging variables for each imaging modality were estimated along with Apo-E genotype. Performance of these biomarkers for predicting conversion from MCI to Alzheimer's dementia at 2 years was evaluated in 50 late amnestic MCI subjects, 20 of whom converted. Multivariate modeling revealed that among individual modalities, MRI had the highest predictive accuracy (67%) which increased by 9% to 76% when combined with ^{18}F-PIB-PET, producing the highest accuracy among any biomarker combination. Individually, ^{18}F-PIB-PET generated the best sensitivity, and ^{18}FdG-PET had the lowest. Among individual brain regions, the temporal cortex was found to be most predictive for MRI and ^{18}F-PIB-PET. A conceptual framework for simulations was presented to determine the utility of biomarker enrichment to increase statistical power to detect a treatment effect in future AD prevention trials. A limited set of simulations to illustrate aspects of this framework were included (Leoutsakos et al., 2014). These investigators simulated data based on the AD anti-inflammatory prevention trial, and sample sizes, biomarker positive predictive values, and treatment effects. They also investigated the consequences of assuming homogeneity of parameter estimates as a function of dementia outcome. Use of biomarkers to increase the sample fraction that would develop ignoring sample heterogeneity resulted in overestimation of power suggesting that biomarker enrichment can increase statistical power, but estimates of the expected increase were sensitive to a variety of assumptions.

ADNI in AD Biomarker Analyses Recent studies explained the ADNI which is a longitudinal, multicenter study designed to develop clinical, imaging, genetic, and biochemical biomarkers for the early diagnosis and tracking of AD (Weiner et al., 2013). The study aimes to enroll 400 subjects with early MCI, 200 subjects with early AD, and 200 normal control subjects. The major accomplishments of ADNI are as follows: (1) the development of standardized methods for clinical tests, *MRI, PET, and CSF biomarkers* in a multicenter setting; (2) elucidation of the patterns and rates of change of imaging and *CSF biomarkers* in control subjects, MCI patients, and AD patients. CSF biomarkers are consistent with disease trajectories predicted by Aβ cascade and tau-mediated neurodegeneration hypotheses for AD, whereas brain atrophy and hypometabolism show predicted patterns but exhibit differing rates of change depending on region and disease severity; (3) the assessment of alternative methods of diagnostic categorization. Currently, the best optimum features from *multiple modalities, including MRI, ^{18}FdG-PET, CSF biomarkers, and clinical tests*; (4) the development of methods for the early detection of AD. CSF biomarkers, Aβ-42 and tau, as well as amyloid PET may reflect the earliest steps in AD pathology in mildly symptomatic or even nonsymptomatic subjects, and are leading biomarkers for the detection of AD in its preclinical stages; (5) the improvement of clinical trial efficiency through the identification of subjects who will undergo future clinical decline and the use of more sensitive outcome measures to reduce sample sizes. Baseline cognitive and/or MRI measures generally predicted future decline better than other modalities, whereas MRI measures of change are most efficient outcome measures; (6) the confirmation of the AD risk loci CLU, CR1, and PICALM and the identification of novel candidate risk loci; (7) worldwide impact through the establishment of ADNI-like programs in Europe, Asia, and Australia; (8) understanding the biology and pathobiology of normal aging, MCI, and AD through integration of ADNI biomarker data with clinical data from ADNI to stimulate research that will resolve controversies about hypotheses on the etiopathogenesis of AD, thereby advancing efforts to find disease-modifying drugs for AD; and (9) the establishment of infrastructure to allow sharing of data to interested scientific investigators throughout the world.

Postoperative Cognitive Dysfunction Biomarkers Postoperative cognitive dysfunction (POCD) is an adverse condition characterized by declined cognitive functions following surgeries and anesthesia. POCD is associated with increased hospital stay and mortality and histological similarities to AD. Most early studies were conducted in patients receiving cardiac surgery. In a study, the incidence of POCD in patients after liver transplantation was measured to examine the correlation between neurological dysfunction and biomarkers of dementia-based diseases (Li et al., 2013). These investigators studied 25 patients who had a liver transplantation between July 2008 and February 2009. Patients with prior encephalopathy or risk factors associated with the development of POCD were excluded. The correlation between patient variables and the development of POCD was examined. Serum levels of Aβ and CRP were measured by ELISA and compared between patients with and without POCD. POCD was present in 11 (44%) of the 25 patients. Patients with POCD had significantly higher MELD scores, were more often Child-Pugh class C and received more blood transfusion during surgery. The serum β-amyloid protein and CRP concentrations were increased at 24 hours after surgery in the POCD group, indicating that the incidence of POCD in liver transplant patients was greater than that reported in other surgical patients. The increase in the serum biomarkers of dementia in the POCD patients supports the hypothesis that chronic cognitive defects are due to a process similar to that seen in AD. In addition exposure to vascular risk factors has a deleterious effect on brain MRI and cognitive measures.

Traumatic Brain Injury (TBI) and Cognitive Dysfuntion Biomarkers TBI survivors frequently suffer from deficits in cognitive functions and a reduced quality of life. Axonal injury, observed in many TBI patients, results in accumulation of APP. Post-injury enzymatic cleavage of APP can generate Aβ peptides, a hallmark of AD. At autopsy, brains of AD and a subset of TBI victims display similarities including accumulation of Aβ peptides and neurofibrillary tangles of p-tau proteins. Epidemiological evidence suggests a link between TBI and AD, implying that TBI has neurodegenerative sequelae. Hence Aβ peptides and tau may be used as biomarkers in interstitial fluid (ISF) using cerebral microdialysis and/or CSF following TBI. Recently, the literature on Aβ peptides and tau as potential biomarkers following TBI was reported (Tsitsopoulos et al., 2013). Elevated CSF and ISF tau protein levels were observed following severe TBI suggesting correlation with clinical outcome. Although Aβ peptides are produced by normal neuronal metabolism, high levels of fibrillary Aβ peptides may be neurotoxic. Increased CSF and/or ISF Aβ levels post-injury may be related to neuronal activity and/or the presence of axonal injury. However the heterogeneity of animal models, clinical cohorts, analytical techniques, and the complexity of TBI make the clinical value of tau and Aβ as biomarkers uncertain. Moreover, the link between early post-injury changes in tau and Aβ peptides and the future risk of developing AD remains unknown. Future studies using rapid biomarker sampling combined with analytical techniques and/or novel pharmacological approaches may provide more information on the importance of Aβ peptides and tau protein in both acute pathophysiology and long-term consequences of TBI. In a similar study, a cerebral microdialysis (MD) was performed to test the hypothesis that interstitial Aβ levels are altered following TBI and related to the injury type, cerebral energy metabolism, age of the patient, and the level of consciousness (Marklund et al., 2013). These investigators evaluated 10 mechanically ventilated patients with a severe TBI who had intracranial pressure and MD monitoring. Each MD sample was analyzed for hourly energy metabolic biomarkers (lactate, pyruvate, glucose and lactate/pyruvate ratio), cellular distress biomarkers (glutamate, glycerol) and urea. The remaining MD samples were analyzed for Aβ1-40 and Aβ1-42 in pooled 2-hour fractions up to 14 days post-injury using the Luminex xMAP technique allowing detection of the key Aβ peptides, Aβ40 and Aβ42. Both Aβ40 and Aβ42 were higher in patients with predominately diffuse axonal injury compared to patients with focal TBI at day 1- 6 post- injury, Aβ42 was significantly increased at 113-116 hrs post-injury. The Aβ levels did not correlate with the interstitial energy metabolism, age of the patient, or the level of consciousness suggesting that origin of potentially toxic Aβ species are related to axonal injury following TBI.

Clinical Assessment of Post-Stroke AD Risk A study explored the pattern of measures that predict stroke and AD risk (Weinstein et al., 2013). A cognitive battery was administered to 1679 dementia and stroke-free Framingham offspring between 1999 and 2004; participants were also free of other neurological conditions that could affect cognition and >90% also had MRI examination. Cognitive and MRI measures were correlated to evaluate risks of stroke and AD ≤10 years of follow-up. A total of 55 offspring participants sustained strokes and 31 developed AD. Offspring who scored <1.5 SD below predicted mean scores, for age and education, on an executive function test, had a higher risk of future stroke (hazard ratio [HR], 2.27; 95% confidence interval; additional cognitive tests also predicted AD. Participants with low (<20 percentile) total brain volume and high (>20 percentile) white matter hyper-intensity volume had a higher risk of stroke but not AD. Hippocampal volume at the bottom quintile predicted AD in the offspring and original cohorts. A stepwise increase in stroke risk was apparent with increasing numbers of these cognitive and imaging biomarkers. Specific patterns of cognitive and brain structural measures observed even in early aging predict stroke risk and may serve as biomarkers for risk prediction.

MISCELLANEOUS BIOMARKERS IN AD

Recently various miscellaneous biomarkers have been discovered to facilitate early differential diagnosis and treatment of AD. These include, mitochondrial biomarkers such as mitochondrial DNA which is significantly reduced in AD patients. Due to increased oxidative and nitrative stress the mitochondrial DNA is oxidized at the guanosine residues to synthesize 8-OH, 2-deoxy guanosine which can be detected from the CSF and urine samples of AD patients. In addition the degeneration of mitochondrial membranes enhances Charnoly Body (CB) formation. CBs are pleomorphic, multi-lamellar (usually penta or hepta lamellar) electron-dense membrane stacks that are formed as a consequence of free radical over-production during oxidative and nitrative stress. The excessive production of 8-OH, 2dG augments CB formation which is inhibited by MTs. As cysteine-rich, low molecular weight zinc-binding proteins, MTs inhibit CB formation and provide mitochondrial protection by acting as free radical scavengers. In addition polyunsaturated fatty acid (PUFA) including: Linoic acid, Linolinic acid, and Arachidonic acid provide structural fluidity to the plasma membrane. These fatty acids are destroyed as result of lipid peroxidation which induces structutural and functional breakdown of polyunsaturated fatty acids of plasma membranes. PUFA are also extremely important for the brain regional myelination particularly during intrauterine life. Nutritional stress or drug abuse (particularly Ethanol) has deleterious impact on the fetal brain development and it may impair normal myelinogenesis. In addition CB formation is augmented by environmental neurotoxins such as Kainic acid and Domoic acid which induces selective apoptosis in the hippocampal CA-3 and dentate gurus neuronal progenitor cells during early embryonic life. Selective apoptosis of hippocampal CA-3 and dentate gyrus neurons is also noticed among patients dying with AD. Thus MTs inhibit CB formation whereas the environmental neurotoxins enhance CB formation which can be used as an early and sensitive biomarkers of neurodegeneration in the aging or environmental neurotoxins exposed brain. In addition the researchers discovered that the protein, α-Synuclein is nitrated in AD patients CSF. Human DAergic neurons and primary hippocampal cultured neurons are highly sensitive to ONOO- stress to increase α-Synuclein nitration and hence α-Synuclein index (SI). In general, environmental neurotoxins increase SI, whereas MTs inhibit CB formation by serving as free radical scavengers. Earlier studies by Uchida reported significantly reduced MT3 in the hippopcampal region of AD patients, which may render the AD patients highly susceptible to progressive neurodegeneration due to enhanced SI induction and CB formation. Hence SI and CB formation can be used for the early detection of AD and other progressive neurodegenerative disorders of aging to assess compromised brain regional mitochondrial bioenergetics. *Any physiological or pharmacological approach augmenting brain regional MTs and inhibiting CB formation and SI will be clinically beneficial for the personalized clinical management of AD. To promote peripheral diagnosis of AD, these two novel biomarkers (SI and CB) can be detected in the lymphocytes, skin cells, buccal mucosa, and the cells from the vaginal smears of AD victims.* In addition consumption of foods primarily rich in PUFA can nullify to a certain extent the deleterious effects of Ethanol and other toxic substances which can induce free radical-mediated demyelination and neurodegeneration. A further study is required in this direction.

Hormones as Biomarkers in AD Although the majority of studies have focused on the association between sex hormones and dementia, emerging evidence supports the role of other hormone signals in increasing the risk of dementia. However, due to the lack of an integrated view on interactions of hormone signaling pathways associated with dementia, molecular mechanisms through which hormones contribute to the increased risk of dementia has remained unclear and translating hormone signals to potential diagnostic and therapeutic applications has not been fully investigated. Using an integrative knowledge- and data-driven approach, a global hormone interaction network in the context of dementia was constructed, which was filtered down to a model of convergent hormone signaling pathways (Younesi et al., 2013). This model was evaluated for its clinical relevance through pathway recovery test, evidence-based analysis, and biomarker-guided analysis. Translational validation of the model was performed using the novel mechanism discovery approach. The results revealed the existence of hormone interaction network underlying dementia. Seven hormone signaling pathways converge at the core of the hormone interaction network, which were linked to the risk of dementia. Amongst these pathways, Estrogen signaling pathway took the major part in the model and insulin signaling pathway was analyzed for its association to learning and memory functions. Validation of the model through off-target effects suggested that hormone signaling pathways contribute to the pathogenesis of dementia. Hence the integrated network model of hormone interactions underlying dementia may serve as an initial translational platform for identifying potential therapeutic targets and candidate biomarkers for dementia-spectrum disorders such as AD. Furthermore, a double-blind, placebo-controlled random trial was conducted in which 1537 patients with probable AD received 100 mg of Semagacestat, 140 mg of Semagacestat, or placebo daily (Doody et al., 2013). Changes in cognition from baseline to week 76, were assessed with the use the AD Assessment Scale for cognition (ADAS-cog), in which scores range from 0 to 70 and higher scores indicated increased cognitive impairment, and changes in functioning were assessed with AD. Cooperative Study-Activities of Daily Living (ADCS-ADL) scale, in which scores range from 0 to 78 and higher scores indicated better functioning. A mixed-model repeated-measures analysis was performed. The trial was terminated before completion on the basis of a recommendation by the data and safety monitoring board. At termination, there were 189 patients in the placebo group, 153 patients in the group receiving 100 mg, and 121 patients in the group receiving 140 mg of Semagacestat. The ADAS-cog scores and ADCS-ADL scores worsened in all three groups. Patients treated with Semagacestat lost more weight and had more skin cancers and infections. Lab findings included reduced levels of T lymphocytes, immunoglobulins, albumin, total protein, and Uric acid and elevated levels of eosinophils, monocytes, and cholesterol. Patients receiving the higher dose had significant worsening of functional ability. Furthermore, it was reported that hormonal changes associated with the menopausal transition and post-menopause have the potential to influence AD symptoms and pathogenesis, but effects of menopause on AD risk can be addressed only indirectly (Henderson et al., 2013). Nine randomized clinical trials of Estrogen-containing hormone therapy in AD patients were identified by a systematic literature search. *Hormone therapy did not improve cognitive symptoms of women with AD.* No clinical trials of hormone therapy address AD prevention, *but one clinical trial provided evidence that continuous, combined Estrogen plus Progesterone initiated at age 65 years or older may increase the risk of dementia.* The critical window hypothesis suggested that hormone therapy initiated at a younger age in closer temporal proximity to menopause may reduce the risk of AD. This hypothesis was supported by observational research but is not addressed by clinical trial data. Well-designed cohort studies, convergent evidence from proper lab models, and long-term clinical trials using surrogate biomarkers of brain function and neuropathology could provide relevant answers. Effects of selective Estrogen receptor modulators such as Raloxifene may differ from those of Estrogens. Moreover potential effects of Phytoestrogens have not been well worked out as yet.

Biomarkers in Vascular Dementia vs AD Vascular factors contribute to the development of disease pathology in neurodegenerative dementia such as AD. Another entity, called vascular dementia (VaD), comprises a less defined group of dementia patients having vascular diseases that especially emerge in the elderly population and requires differential diagnosis. In a retrospective study, CSF biomarkers t-tau, p-tau and Aß42 were analyzed from of a total of 131 patients with AD, MCI, VaD, and stroke (Wahlster et al., 2013). CSF profile in AD patients was altered in a similar way as in stroke patients, without statistical differences. In stroke, increases depend largely on size and duration after the initial event. Total tau levels were useful to differ between VaD and stroke. Aß42 decreased in a similar way in AD, VaD and stroke and had a trend towards lower levels in MCI but not in controls. Chronic cerebral hypoperfusion induced by permanent occlusion of the bilateral common carotid artery (BCCAO) in rats was used to explore basic cellular and molecular mechanisms of AD and VaD. Despite the apparent cognitive dysfunction in rats with BCCAO, the molecular biomarkers or pathways involved in the pathological alternation have not been clearly identified. In a similar study, the temporal changes in gene expression in the hippocampus of rats were examined after BCCAO using longitudinal microarray analysis (Bang et al., 2013). Gene Ontology (GO) and pathway analyses were performed to identify the functional involvement of temporally regulated genes in BCCAO. Two major gene expression patterns were observed in the hippocampus. One pattern, which was composed of 341 early up-regulated genes after the surgical procedure, was involved in immune-related biological functions. Another pattern composed of 182 temporally delayed down-regulated genes was involved in sensory perception such as olfactory and cognition functions. In addition to the two gene expression patterns, the temporal change of GO, and the pathway activities using all differentially expressed genes confirmed that an immune response was the major early change, whereas sensory functions were delayed responses. Moreover, FADD and SOCS3 were identified as possible core genes in the sensory functional loss using text-based mining and interaction network analysis. Hence the biphasic regulatory mechanism could provide molecular evidence of BCCAO-induced impaired memory as well as molecular mechanism of the development of VaD.

Neurobehavioral Disturbance in AD Behavioral disturbances belong to the major symptoms of dementia and are also common in MCI and AD. The identification of symptoms is clinically interesting, as interventions targeting syndromes may be more effective than the management of individual symptoms. A study was performed to compare the behavioral syndromes that underlie the symptoms in MCI and AD (Van der Mussele et al., 2014). The study population consisted of 270 MCI and 402 AD patients. Behavioral assessment was performed by means of Middelheim Frontality Score (MFS), Behave-AD, Cohen-Mansfield Agitation Inventory (CMAI), and Cornell Scale for Depression in Dementia (CSDD). Principal components analysis with Direct Oblimin rotation was carried out on the MFS score ≥5, seven cluster scores of the Behave-AD and the total scores of the CMAI and the CSDD. Three factors explained behavior in the MCI group including; *depression, psychosis, and agitation syndrome.* Similar factors were found in AD, but agitation, depression, psychosis, and the structure differed slightly among MCI and AD subjects. Diurnal rhythm disturbances and frontal lobe symptoms were associated with the depressive syndrome in MCI and in AD with the agitation syndrome. Behavioral syndromes correlated in AD, but not in MCI, and the prevalence and severity of the behavioral syndromes were higher in AD than in MCI, except for the severity of the depression suggesting that in both MCI and AD, three similar behavioral syndromes exist, but behavior in MCI is more dominated by a depression syndrome, whereas behavior in AD is more geared toward agitation syndrome.

Circadian Rhythm as a Biomarker in AD It is known that human motor activity has intrinsic fractal structure with similar patterns from minutes to hrs. The fractal activity patterns are physiologically important because the patterns persist under different environmental conditions but are significantly reduced with aging and AD. It was reported that dementia patients, known to have disrupted circadian rhythmicity, also have disrupted fractal activity and that the disruption is more pronounced in patients with amyloid plaques (biomarker of AD severity) (Hu et al., 2013). Moreover, the degree of disruption in fractal activity is associated with vasopressinergic and neurotensinergic neurons (two major circadian neurotransmitters) in suprachiasmatic nucleus (SCN), and can predict changes of the two neurotransmitters better than traditional circadian measures suggesting that the SCN impacts human activity as a function of time and that disrupted fractal activity could serve as a non-invasive biomarker of SCN neurodegeneration in AD.

Neurobehavioral Biomarkers of AD Although use of biomarkers in early AD detection is growing, it remains unknown whether sophisticated biomarker testing is more efficient than neuropsychological tests focused on memory. The predictive value of the Memory Impairment Screen (MIS), a simple and brief memory test, in elderly subjects with subjective memory loss was evaluated (Modrego and Gazulla, 2013). A prospective cohort of 105 patients with subjective memory loss was followed up from December 2007 to April 2011. At baseline, the patients underwent neuropsychological examination with Mini-Examen-Cognoscivo (Spanish adaptation of the Mini-Mental State Examination), MIS, Clinical Dementia Rating scale, Blessed Dementia Rating Scale, and Geriatric Depression Scale. The final endpoint of the study was the conversion to dementia, mostly of probable AD type according to the National Institute of Neurological and Communicative Disorders and Stroke and the AD and Related Disorders Association work group criteria. The patients were reevaluated every 6 months. After a mean follow-up of 2 years, 57 patients developed AD and 48 did not. A baseline score of 0 or 1 on the MIS predicted conversion to AD, with a sensitivity of 42.9%, a specificity of 98%, and a positive predictive value of 96%. The area under the curve was 0.76. Thus in the clinical setting in patients referred for memory complaints, the MIS score at baseline (0 and 1) was useful to predict who may develop AD within at least a year. However the MIS proved more useful when combined with higher sensitivity tests. Furthermore, novel technologies and biomarkers for early AD detection and evaluating the suitability of a new approach for early AD diagnosis were identified (López-de-Ipiña et al., 2013). These methods examine the potential of applying intelligent algorithms to speech features obtained from suspected patients in order to contribute to the improvement of diagnosis of AD and its severity. Artificial Neural Networks (ANN) were used for the automatic classification of the two classes (AD and control subjects). Two issues were analyzed for feature selection: *Spontaneous Speech and Emotional Response*. Linear features as well as non-linear ones, such as Fractal Dimension, were explored. This approach was noninvasive, economical, and without any side effects. The results were satisfactory for early diagnosis and classification of AD. It is known that dementia caregiving is associated with elevations in depressive symptoms and increased risk for cardiovascular diseases (CVD). The efficacy of the Pleasant Events Program (PEP), a 6-week Behavioral Activation intervention was designed to reduce CVD risk and depressive symptoms in caregivers (Moore et al., 2013). These investigators randomized 100 dementia family caregivers to either the 6-week PEP intervention (N = 49) or a time-equivalent Information-Support (IS) control condition (N = 51). Assessments were completed pre-and post-intervention and at 1-year follow-up. Biological assessments included CVD risk biomarkers IL-6 and D-dimer. Psychosocial outcomes included depressive symptoms, positive affect, and negative affect. Participants receiving the PEP intervention had significant reductions in IL-6, depressive symptoms, and negative affect from pre-to post-treatment. For IL-6, significant improvement was observed in

20% of PEP participants and 6.5% of IS participants. For depressive symptoms, significant improvement was found for 32.7% of PEP vs 11.8% of IS participants. Group differences in change from baseline to 1-year follow-up were insignificant. The PEP program decreased depression and improved a measure of physiological health in older dementia caregivers.

Comparative Analyses of Multimodality AD Biomarkers To examine whether the diagnostic method of neuronal dysfunction (DIMENSION), a new EEG analysis method, reflected pathological changes in the early stages of AD, a comparative study of CSF biomarkers and SPECT imaging was conducted (Kouzuki et al., 2013). Subjects included 32 patients in the early stages of AD with a Mini-Mental State Examination score ≥ 24. CSF levels of p-tau-181 and Aβ-42 were estimated using sandwich ELISA. EEG recordings were performed for 5 min with the subjects awake in a resting state with their eyes closed. The mean value of the EEG α bipolarity (Dα) and the standard deviation (Dσ) were calculated with DIMENSION. SPECT analyses were also done for comparison with DIMENSION measures. Patients with parietal hypoperfusion had increased p-tau-81 and Dσ, and decreased Dα. In addition, there was a negative correlation between Dα and p-tau181, p-tau181/Aβ42, and a positive correlation between Dσ and p-tau181/Aβ42. Hence Dα and Dσ were related to cerebral hypoperfusion and p-tau181/Aβ42. Furthermore, DIMENSION analysis could detect subtle changes in the early-stage Alzheimer's brain, suggesting its usefulness for the detection of early-stage AD. Moreover, EEG measurement is a quick and easy diagnostic test, and is useful for repeated examinations for the longitudinal analyses.

Antioxidants as Theranostic Biomarkers in AD Antioxidants including polyphenols play a key role as therapeutic agents in the brain. Numerous antioxidants are able to cross the blood brain barrier and do not produce adverse effects in human body. These antioxidants have been proposed for their role as theranostic biomarkers. The therapeutic potential of green tea and apple are linked to the phenolic compounds. Although the beneficial effects of these compounds are clear, relatively few studies have focused on their anti-inflammatory potential. Moreover these therapeutic agents may influence several other diagnostic biomarkers including Aβ, t-tau, and p-tau in the CNS of AD patients which needs further studies. A recent study tested whether daily consumption of a beverage with high antioxidants combining extracts of green tea and apple over a period of 8 months would affect biomarkers of inflammation in AD patients in initial phase, moderate phase, and a control group (Rubio-Perez and Morillas-Ruiz, 2013). The administration of the antioxidant beverage (AB) to the three groups did not produce a significant change in serum levels of the anti-inflammatory cytokines IL-4 and IL-10. In contrast, AB had effects on proinflammatory cytokines, decreasing the serum levels of cytokines IL-2, IFN-γ and TNF-α. Recently the researchers published in detail the therapeutic potential of antioxidants in neurodegenerative disorders and highlighted the theranostic potential of Melatonin, MTs, and CoQ$_{10}$ as therapeutic targets and ^{18}F or ^{11}C-labeled PET imaging radioligands (Sharma and Ebadi, 2013). *Consumption of food rich in Glutathione, N-Acetyl Cysteine, B-Vitamins (Thiamine), Vitamin-D, Vitamin-E, PUFA, Melatonin, Curcumin, various flavonoid antioxidants, and micronutrients such as Zinc and Magnesium can nullify the deleterious effects of free radicals that are generated as a byproduct of the mitochondrial oxidative phosphorylation, whereas Ethanol intake, environmental neurotoxins, and excitotoxic agents can induce progressive neurodegeneration due to free radical overproduction, microglial activation, and neuroinflammation in AD.* Furthermore, the researchers emphasized the antidepressant effect of Tryptophan-rich diet in boosting brain regional Serotonin synthesis implicated in mood alleviation and sleep regulation, both of which are impaired in AD patients (Shabbir et al., 2013). Hence it would be interesting to evaluate the clinical utility of antioxidants as theranostic biomarkers in AD and other neurodegenerative diseases.

It is well established that intracellular tau protein (τ), when released extracellularly during neurodegeneration, could evoke direct toxic effects on the cholinergic neurotransmission through muscarinic receptors and thus contribute to the pathogenesis of AD. The *in vitro* effects of six naturally occurring monomeric τ isoforms on rat hippocampal synaptosomal choline transporters CHT1 (large transmembrane proteins associated with high-affinity choline transport and vulnerable to actions of Aβ *in vitro* or *in vivo*) was evaluated (Kristofikova et al.,, 2013). Some τ isoforms inhibited choline transport at nM concentrations. Moreover, the actions of τ 352/441 were not influenced by previous depolarization of synaptosomes or by depletion of Cholesterol. Specific binding of [^{3}H] Hemicholinium-3 was not altered by τ 352/441 at higher concentrations. Results of *in vitro* tests on CHT1 transporters from Cholesterol-depleted synaptosomes supported interactions between Aβ 1-40 and τ 352. In addition, these investigators developed surface plasmon resonance biosensors to monitor complexes of Aβ 1-42 and τ 352 using a sandwich detection method and suggested that protein τ, similar to Aβ peptides, can contribute to the pathogenesis of AD through its actions on CHT1 transporters. However, the interaction mechanisms are quite different (τ probably exerts its effects through direct interactions of microtubule binding repeats with extracellular portions of the CHT1 protein without influencing the Choline recognition site, whereas Aβ through lipid rafts in the surrounding membranes). Thus N-terminal insert of τ is not necessary but the N-terminal domain plays a significant role. This biosensor could be used to detect Aβ-τ complexes in CSF to evaluate prospective biomarkers of AD in future.

Biomarkers in BPD and AD There are currently no biomarkers that are able to differentiate patients with bipolar disorder (BPD) from healthy controls. While there is evidence that peripheral gene expression differences between patients and controls can be utilized as biomarkers for psychiatric illness, it is unresolved whether use or residual effects of antipsychotic and mood stabilizer medication, drives the differential transcription. It was tested whether gene expression changes in first-episode, never-medicated BPD patients, can contribute to a biological classifier that is less influenced by medication and could potentially serve as a biomarker for BPD (Clelland et al., 2013). These investigators employed microarray technology to measure global leukocyte gene expression in first-episode and currently medicated BPD patients, and matched healthy controls. Following an initial feature selection, they developed a cross-validated 10-gene model to predict the diagnostic group of sample (26 medicated patients and 12 controls), with 89% sensitivity and 75% specificity. The 10-gene predictor was further explored on an independent cohort consisting of 3 pairs of monozygotic twins discordant for BPD, plus the original enrichment sample cohort (the 3 never-medicated BPD patients and 13 matched control subjects), and experimental replicates. 83% of the test sample was correctly predicted, with a sensitivity of 67% and specificity of 100%. In addition, 88% of sample diagnostic classes were classified correctly for both the enrichment and the replicate samples. Furthermore, these investigators developed a peripheral gene expression biomarker profile, that could classify healthy controls from patients with BPD receiving antipsychotic or mood stabilizing medication, which had both sensitivity and specificity.

Experimental Models in AD Biomarker Discovery It is now well established that preclinical models permit the evaluation of candidate biomarkers and assessment of pipeline agents before clinical trials are initiated and provide a translational opportunity to advance biomarker discovery (Sabbagh et al., 2013). Relatively fast and inexpensive data can be obtained from examination of peripheral biomarkers, though they currently lack the sensitivity and consistency of imaging techniques such as MRI or PET. Plasma and CSF biomarkers in animal models can assist in development and implementation of similar approaches in clinical populations. These biomarkers may also be useful to advance a treatment for human trials. Longitudinal studies in experimental models of AD can determine initial presentation and progression of biomarkers that may also be used to evaluate disease-modifying efficacy of drugs. Further refinement of biomarkers in preclinical systems will not only aid in drug development, but may facilitate diagnosis and disease monitoring in AD patients. Epidemiological evidence links severe or repeated TBI to the development of AD. Accumulation of APP occurs with high frequency after TBI, particularly in injured axons, and APP may be cleaved to Aβ peptides playing key pathophysiological roles in AD.

Multiple Diagnostic Biomarkers in AD Recently Cross-sectional and longitudinal studies were performed to examine regions of cortical thinning and CSF-AD biomarkers associated with apathy and hallucinations in individuals including clinically normal elderly, MCI, and mild AD dementia in 57 research sites across North America (Donovan et al., 2014). A total of 812 community-dwelling volunteers and 413 participants in the CSF sub-study participated in this study. Structural MRI data and CSF concentrations of Aβ1-42, total tau, and phosphorylated tau derived from the ADNI database were analyzed. Apathy and hallucinations were measured at baseline and over 3 years using the Neuropsychiatric Inventory-Questionnaire. General linear models and mixed effects models were used to evaluate the relationships among baseline cortical thickness in seven regions, and baseline CSF biomarkers, apathy, and hallucinations. Covariates *included diagnosis, sex, age, Apo-E genotype, premorbid intelligence, memory performance, processing speed, antidepressant use, and AD duration.* Reduced baseline inferior temporal cortical thickness was predictive of increasing apathy, and reduced supra-marginal cortical thickness was predictive of increasing hallucinations over time. There was no association with cortical thickness at baseline. CSF biomarkers were not related to severity of apathy or hallucinations suggesting that increased baseline temporal and parietal atrophy is associated with worsening apathy and hallucinations in AD spectrum cohort, while adjusting for multiple disease-related variables and localized cortical neurodegeneration may contribute to the pathophysiology of apathy and hallucinations and their adverse consequences in AD.

Diagnostic Accuracy of Equipments in Biomarker Discovery A study was performed on patients with MCI for a follow-up of 38.9 months (Richard et al., 2013). Diagnostic accuracy of individual instruments and incremental value of entorhinal cortex volume on MRI and p-τ/Aβ ratios in CSF after administration of Rey's Auditory Verbal Learning Memory Test was calculated and expressed as the 'Net Reclassification Improvement' (NRI), which is the change in the percentage of individuals that are diagnosed as AD or non-AD case. A short memory test, MRI and CSF significantly contributed to the differentiation of those MCI patients who remained stable during follow-up from those who developed AD. The memory test, MRI and CSF improved the diagnostic accuracy by 21%, 22.1%, and 18.8% respectively. After administration of a short memory test, however, the NRI of MRI was +1.1% and of CSF was -2.2%. After administration of a brief test of memory, MRI or CSF did not influence the diagnostic accuracy for predicting progression to AD in patients with

MCI, suggesting that NRI is easy to interpret for the evaluation of potential added value of new diagnostic instrument in routine clinical practice.

PUFA as Biomarker in AD PUFA are involved in the structural and functional integrity of plasma membranes and myelinogenesis. In general, Linoic acid, Linolinic acid, and Arachidonic acid provide structural fluidity to the plasma membrane, whereas Cholesterol provides membrane stability. Deficiency of PUFA or neurotoxic insult during early stages of brain development may lead to demyelination and impaired memory as myelin serves as an insulator for normal nerve conduction required for normal inter-neuronal communication. Oxidative and nitrative stress due to increased production of ROS and/or RNS may cause lipid peroxidation involving structural and functional breakdown of PUFA in the neuronal membranes. On the other hand MTs may inhibit degeneration of mitochondrial and other membranes by preventing CB formation and by acting as free radical scavengers. Hence circulating PUFA may be considered as one of the candidate biomarkers for the clinical evaluation of AD. Recently the researchers reported that maturation of the human brain may be enhanced by intake of PUFA in early adolescent life (Arain et al., 2013).

MMPs as Biomarkers in AD There is a complex relationship between MMPss (MMPs) and TIMPs in AD. MMPs and their natural tissue inhibitors (TIMPs) are involved in cell signaling and the release of extracellular matrix (ECM) and non-ECM molecules (Mroczko e al., 2013). Nonregulated MMP activity and an imbalance between MMPs and TIMPs might contribute to neurodegenerative diseases such as AD, which is the common cause of dementia. MMPs and TIMPs are localized in neuritic senile plaques and neurofibrillary tangles in the postmortem brains of patients with AD. Some MMPs induce tau aggregation and neurofibrillary tangles *in vitro*. Moreover, MMPs contribute to AD pathogenesis via the disruption of the blood-brain barrier and neurodegeneration. However, MMPs can degrade both soluble and fibrillar forms of Aβ. In addition, Aβ enhances the expression of MMPs in neuroglial cultures and induces the release of TIMP-1 by neuronal cells. Inhibition of Aβ-induced MMP activity resulted in an improvement of performance tests in mice. Examination of MMP-9, MMP-2, and TIMP-1 in the CSF contributed to differentiate between AD and other types of dementia. A recent report described the role of MMPs and TIMPs in neurodegeneration, as well as their usefulness as CSF or plasma biomarkers in the diagnosis of AD as well as other neurodegenerative disorders and vascular dementia. To identify potential biomarkers associated with AD-like neuropathologies in the murine brain, proteomic analysis was conducted from the neocortices of TgCRND8 mice and it was found that Phosphoprotein enriched in astrocytes 15kDa (PEA-15) is expressed at higher levels in the neocortical proteomes from 6-month old TgCRND8 mice, as compared to non-transgenic mice (Thomason et al., 2013). Immunostaining for PEA-15 revealed reactive astrocytes associated with the neocortical amyloid plaques in TgCRND8 mice and in post-mortem human AD brains suggesting increased PEA-15 expression in reactive astrocytes of an AD mouse model and human AD brains.

Recently the author highlighted that there is a need of early, sensitive, specific, and economical peripheral and/or central biomarker(s) for the differential diagnosis, prognosis, and treatment of neurodegenerative disorders (Sharma et al., 2013). These can be classified as clinical, biochemical, genetic, proteomic, and neuroimaging biomarkers. Novel discoveries of genetic as well as nongenetic biomarkers may be utilized for the personalized treatment during preclinical (premotor) and clinical (motor) stages. For instance premotor biomarkers in PD including hyper-echogenicity of substantia nigra, olfactory and autonomic dysfunction, depression, hyposmia, deafness, REM sleep disorder, and impulsive behavior may be noticed during preclinical stage; while neuroimaging biomarkers (PET, SPECT, MRI), and neuropsychological deficits can facilitate differential diagnosis of both PD and AD. Single-cell profiling of neurons has identified pyridoxal kinase and lysosomal ATPase as biomarker genes for PD prognosis. Promising biomarkers include: fluid biomarkers, neuromelanin antibodies, pathological forms of α-Syn, DJ-1, amyloid β and tau in the CSF, patterns of gene expression, metabolomics, urate, as well as protein profiling in the blood and CSF samples. In addition, reduced brain regional N-acetyl-aspartate is a biomarker for the *in vivo* assessment of neuronal loss using MRS and T_2 relaxation time with MRI. To confirm PD as well as AD diagnosis, the PET biomarkers include ^{18}F-DOPA for estimating DA-ergic neurotransmission, [18]FdG for mitochondrial bioenergetics, ^{18}F-BMS for mitochondrial complex-1, [11]C- (R)-PK11195 for microglial activation, SPECT imaging with ^{123}I-Flupane and ^{123}I-βCIT for dopamine transporter (DAT), and urinary salsolinol and 8-hydroxy, 2-deoxyguanosine (8-OH,2dG) for neuronal loss. In addition the researchers discussed the merits and limitations of CoQ_{10}, mitochondrial ubiquinone-NADH oxidoreductase (Complex-1), Melatonin, α-Synculein index, CB formation, and MTs as novel biomarkers to confirm diagnosis for early and effective treatment of PD as well as AD.

Peripheral Biomarkers in AD Peripheral biomarkers to diagnose AD have not been established. Donovan et al. (2013) hypothesized platelet membrane-associated protein changes may differentiate patients clinically defined with probable AD from noncognitive impaired controls. Platelets, were obtained from individuals before fractionation by ultracentrifugation. Following a comparison of individual membrane fractions by SDS-PAGE for general proteome uniformity, equal protein weight from the membrane fractions for five representative samples from AD and five samples from controls were pooled. AD and control protein pools were further divided into molecular weight regions by SDS-PAGE. Tryptic peptides were analyzed by reverse-phase liquid chromatography coupled to tandem mass spectrometry (LC-MS/MS). Ionized peptide intensities were averaged for each identified protein in the two pools to estimate relative abundance between the two membrane protein pools. Log2-transformed ratio (AD/control) of protein abundances fit a normal distribution, thereby permitting determination of significantly altered proteins in the AD pool. A total of 144 proteins were significantly altered in the platelet membrane proteome from patients with probable AD. Particularly, secretory (α) granule proteins were significantly reduced in AD. The reduction of Thrombospondin-1 (THBS1) in the AD platelet membrane proteome was confirmed by immunoblotting. There was a high connectivity of proteins in other pathways implicated by proteomic changes to the proteins that define secretory granules. Thus depletion of secretory granule proteins was consistent with a preponderance of platelets in circulation in AD. Significantly altered pathways implicated additional AD-related defects in platelet glycoprotein synthesis, lipid homeostasis, amyloidogenic proteins, and regulators of protease activity, many of which could be useful biomarkers for AD.

Bioinformatics in Biomarker Discovery of AD Recently it was reported that with the increasingly digital nature of biomedical data and as the complexity of analyses in medical research increases the need for accurate information capture, traceability and accessibility has become crucial to medical researchers to accomplish their research goals (McClatchey et al., 2013). Grid-or Cloud-based technologies, based on Service Oriented Architectures (SOA), are used for managing distributed data and algorithms paticularly for the complex image analysis, traceability of processes and collaborative study. There are few examples of medical systems based on Grids that provide research data needed to facilitate complex analyses. This report introduced the CRISTAL software to manage neuroimaging projects that have been studying biomarkers for AD. The software enables to track the evolution of workflows and datasets. It also tracks the outcomes of various analyses and provides traceability throughout the lifecycle. It can be applied as a reusable tool for supporting researchers by providing necessary tools to conduct collaborative clinical analyses. For instance early identification of persons at risk for cognitive decline in aging is critical to optimizing treatment to delay or avoid a clinical diagnosis of MCI or dementia due to AD.

Lymphocytes in AD Biomarkers Discovery Given the limitations to analyze brain cells, it is important to study whether peripheral lymphocytes can provide biomarkers for AD. A study was performed to determine whether lymphocytes of AD patients present DNA damage and repair kinetics different from those found in elderly matched controls (EC group) following *in vitro* treatment with hydrogen peroxide (Leandro et al. 2013). These investigators found that AD patient cells showed an altered DNA repair kinetics as determined by comet assay. Real-time quantitative analysis of genes associated with DNA stress response also showed that FANCG and CDKN1A are up-regulated in AD, while MTH1 is down-regulated, compared with the control group. In contrast, the expression of ATM, ATR and FEN1 genes did not differ between these groups. Interestingly, TP53 protein expression was increased in AD patients. Therefore, kinetics of the stress response in the DNA were significantly different in AD patients, supporting the hypothesis that DNA repair pathways may be compromised in AD and that peripheral lymphocytes can detect this condition.

Urinary Metabolites as Biomarkers in AD The difficulty in developing a diagnostic assay for Creutzfeldt- Jakob disease (CJD) and other transmissible spongiform encephalopathies (TSEs) arises from the fact that the infectious agent is an improperly folded form of an endogenous cellular protein. This precludes the use of gene based technologies currently applied to the detection of other infections. To circumvent this problem the research objective was to identify a set of proteins exhibiting differential abundance in response to TSE infection. A recent study assessed the disease specificity of urine proteins to identify scrapie infected mice (Lamoureux et al., 2013). 2-D gel electrophoresis was employed to analyze urine samples from both prion-infected mice and a transgenic mouse model of AD. The identity of the differentially abundant diagnostic proteins was investigated by mass spectrometry. The introduction of fluorescent dyes, that allow multiple samples to be visualized on 2-D gel, increased the accuracy for the discovery of protein biomarkers for disease. The accuracy of differentially abundant proteins to classify naïve sample set was identified. The results demonstrated that at the time of clinical presentation the differential abundance of urine proteins was capable of identifying the prion infected mice with a sensitivity of 87% and specificity of 93%.

Biomarkers to Differentiate AD vs VaD AD and vascular dementia (VaD) are the major forms of dementia affecting elderly people, in which several metabolites are altered in CSF and serum. These metabolites could be risk factors or potential biomarkers; however their significance is not clearly understood in the context of the disease progression. Ray et al (2013) measured serum levels of Homocysteine, Dihydroepiandrosterone sulphate (DHEA-S) and Lipoprotein (a) or LP (a) measured by ELISA in AD, VaD, and age matched control subjects. The serum Homocysteine was significantly elevated compared to control both in AD and VaD subjects, but to a higher extent in the latter. Lp (a) was increased only in the serum of VaD subjects compared to control. Likewise, serum DHEA-S level was lowered in AD but not in VaD compared to control, suggesting that alterations in Homocysteine and LP (a) in serum could be used as biomarkers of vascular pathology in AD or VaD, while the lowering of serum DHEA-S is a consequence of AD pathology.

Miscellaneous AD Biomarkers Miscellaneous biomarkers including α-Synuclein index (SI) and Charnoly body are recently-introduced novel biomarkers, which require further investigation for the early and accurate diagnosis of AD. The mitochondrial biomarkers such as mtDNA, is significantly reduced in AD patients. Furthermore due to increased oxidative stress the mtDNA is oxidized particularly at the guanosine residues. So the researchers notice significantly increased 8-OH, 2-dG in the CSF and urine samples of AD patients. In addition, the degeneration of mitochondrial membranes enhances CB formation as described earlier. The excessive production of 8-OH, 2dG augments CB formation which is inhibited by MTs as these low molecular weight zinc-binding proteins. MTs inhibit CB formation by acting as free radical scavengers (Sharma et al., 1993; Sharma and Ebadi, 2014; Sharma et al., 2013a). In addition, polyunsaturated fatty acid including Linoic acid, Linolinic acid, and Arachidonic acid provide structural fluidity to the plasma membrane. These fatty acids are destroyed as a result of lipid peroxidation which may induce structural and functional breakdown of plasma membrane due to damage to PUFA which form a structural and functional component of the plasma membrane. The PUFA are extremely important for the brain regional myelination particularly during intrauterine life. Nutritional stress or drug abuse *(particularly Ethanol)* may have severe impact on the fetal brain development and may even impair normal synaptogenesis and myelinogenesis. In addition, CB formation is augmented by environmental neurotoxins such as Kainic acid and Domoic acid which induce selective apoptosis in the hippocampal CA-3 and dentate gurus neuronal progenitor cells during early embryonic life as noticed in AD patients (Dakshinamurti et al., 1991; Dakshinamurti et l., 1993; Dakshinamurti et al., 2003). MTs inhibit CB formation whereas the environmental neurotoxins including Kainic acid and Domoic acid augment CB formation which is an early manifestation of neurodegeneration in the aging or environmental neurotoxins-exposed brain. Human dopaminergic neurons and primary hippocampal cultured neurons are highly sensitive to α-Synuclein nitration and hence increase the α-Synuclein index. Kainic acid and Domoic acid increase α-Synuclein index, whereas MTs inhibit CB formation by serving as free radical scavengers and via Zinc-mediated transcriptional regulation of genes involved in growth, proliferation, and differentiation. MT3 is significantly reduced in the hippopcampal region of AD patients, which could render AD patients highly susceptible to progressive neurodegeneration. Hence α-Syncuelin indices and CB formation could be used for the early detection of neurodegenerative disorders such as AD and PD (Sharma et al. 2003). Hence, any physiological or pharmacological approach augmenting brain regional MTs and/or inhibition of SI and CB formation will be beneficial for the effective clinical management of AD patients. In addition, consumption of sea food primarily fish, rich in PUFA, vitamin-D and vitamin-E can nullify the deleterious effects of Ethanol which serves as a free radical donor to cause synaptic degeneration and demyelination to enhance early AD pathogenesis as describe earlier.

Domoic Acid as a Molecular Probe in AD In earlier studies, the researchers discovered that intrauterine exposure to a rigid structural analog of Glutamate, Domoic acid causes selective damage to hippocampal CA-3 and dentate gyrus regions of the mice progeny (Sharma ad Ebadi, 1992; Sharma and Dakshinamurti, 1992; Sharma et al., 1994; Sharma and

Dhalla 2000). Neuronal loss in the CA-3 and dentate gyrus is also noticed in patients with AD. This neuronal loss leads to memory decline in AD patients. Domoic acid binds to Kainate receptors to enhance apoptosis by augmenting CB formation in experimental animals, whereas a selective 5-HT$_{1A}$ receptor agonist, 8-hydroxy-DPAT suppressed Domoic acid-induced seizure activity and protected hippocampal CA-3 neurons (Sharma and Dakshinamurti 1993). Local microinjection of GABA or systemic Vitamin B$_6$ treatment, suppressed Domoic acid, Picrotoxin, and Pentylene tatrazole-induced seizure activity as determined by computerized EEG analysis. Furthermore, Domoic acid induced apoptosis when exposed to cultured vascular smooth muscle cells. Hence it can be used as a biomarker to examine the therapeutic potential of various pharmacological agents developed for the treatment of AD and vascular dementia. Furthermore, the researchers highlighted the importance of Domoic acid as a tool to examine the molecular neurobiology of stroke and AD (Sharma and Dhalla, 2001).

AD Biomarkers for Personalized Medicine Recent research in the mental health field brings new hope to patients and promises to revolutionize the field of AD. Personalized pharmacogenetic tests that aid in diagnosis and treatment choice are now becoming available for clinical practice. Aβ peptide biomarkers in the CSF of patients with AD are available and the radiologists are now able to visualize amyloid plaques specific to AD in live patients using PET-imaging approved by the FDA. A novel blood-based assay is developed to aid in the diagnosis of depression based on activation of the HPA axis, metabolic, inflammatory, and neurochemical pathways. Serotonin reuptake inhibitors have shown increased remission in specific ethnic subgroups and cytochrome P450 gene polymorphisms can predict antidepressant tolerability among AD patients. This research will help to eradicate trial and error prescription in PM. Souslova et al (2013) recently described the novel diagnostic tests and EBPT for AD and MDD. In addition, it is proposed that MCI is a syndrome which, depending on various neurobiological, psychological, and social factors, carries a high risk of developing into dementia (Karakaya et al., 2013).

Most results reflect not only a lack of effectiveness of drug therapy but also methodological constraints in true prodromal AD based on clinical criteria. Biomarkers may help to identify MCI as a prodromal phase of dementia, so it is important to use them to improve specificity of case selection in future studies. For MCI as a prodromal syndrome of AD, clinical trials with disease modifying drugs that target underlying pathological mechanisms such as Aβ accumulation and neurofibrillary tangle formation may help develop effective treatment options in the future. Alternative pharmacological approaches are currently being evaluated in phase 1 and phase 2 studies. Nevertheless, a lack of approved pharmaco-therapeutic options has led to specific interventions that focus on patient education and life-style related factors. It was recently reported that an international task force of investigators from academia, industry, nonprofit foundations, and regulatory agencies met to review lessons learned from the Bapineuzumab and Solanezumab trials, and to incorporate insights gained from these trials into future clinical studies (Vellas et al., 2013).

Although there was consensus that AD should be treated during its earliest stages, the concept of secondary prevention need to be described accurately as treatment of preclinical, presymptomatic, or early AD. There continues to be a need for new biomarkers; however the most reliable biomarker of clinical efficacy across the entire spectrum of disease from asymptomatic to AD dementia is a measure of cognition. The task force made many recommendations that should improve the clinical success in future trials, including larger phase 2 or combined phase 2/phase 3 trials, clear evidence of target engagement in the CNS, evidence of downstream effects on biomarkers before initiating phase 3 studies, consideration of adaptive and targeted trial designs, and use of sensitive measures of cognition as the important indicators of treatment.

Clinical Significance of AD Biomarkers & Future Prospectus In general drug candidates directed against Aβ are mainstream in AD drug development (Blennow et al., 2013). Active and passive Aβ immunotherapy has come in stage of clinical trials. However, an increasing number of reports on difficulties in identifying any clinical benefit in phase II-III clinical trials on this type of anti-Aβ drug candidates have caused concern among researchers, pharmaceutical companies, and other stakeholders which provide critics of the amyloid cascade hypothesis that *Aβ deposition may be a bystander, and not the cause, of the disease or that the amyloid hypothesis may only be valid for the familial form of AD*. Most researchers argue that it is the trial design that will need refinement to allow for identifying a positive clinical effect of anti-Aβ drugs. Future trials need to be performed in an earlier stage of the disease and that specific biomarkers are essential to guide and facilitate drug development. Advances in the AD have led to the novel discoveries of both imaging (MRI and PET) and CSF biomarkers to further elucidate the exact pathogenic processes of the disease. AD biomarkers will have a key role in future clinical trials to enable early diagnosis. Moreover, Aβ biomarkers (*CSF Aβ42 and amyloid PET*) may be essential to allow for testing a drug on patients with evidence of brain Aβ pathology. Aβ and APP biomarkers will be of tremendous use to verify target engagement of a drug candidate in humans, thereby bridging the gap between mechanistic data from transgenic AD models and large phase III trials. Finally, downstream biomarker evidence (*CSF tau proteins and MRI volumetry*) that the drug ameliorates neurodegeneration with beneficial clinical effects on cognition and functioning, will be essential for labeling an anti-Aβ drug as disease modifying agents. In addition advances in blood biomarker discovery will help in identifying AD in its preclinical stage, allowing treatment to be initiated before irreversible damage occurs. Recently Gupta et al (2013) discussed some previous and current approaches being adopted in the field of AD biomarker discovery. Individual blood biomarkers have been unsuccessful in defining the disease pathology, progression and thus diagnosis. This directs the need for discovering a multiplex panel of blood biomarkers as a promising approach with high sensitivity and specificity for early diagnosis. However, it is a challenge to standardize a universal blood biomarker panel due to the innate differences in the population tested, nature of the samples, and methods utilized in different studies across the globe.

COMPARATIVE ANALYSES AND PHARMACODYNAMICS OF AD BIOMARKERS

Early differential diagnosis of AD is currently difficult and poses a significant challenge to the physician. Hence AD diagnosis is based on exclusion criteria which is not very well defined and asystematic. Assessment of biomarkers including: loss of immediate and delayed memory, acalculia, hyposmia, mood swings (*depression and anxiety*), and hypogustia may provide some vague idea regarding disease severity and/or progression, yet not quite reliable for the exact clinical diagnosis of AD. Similarly cognitive biomarkers including learning, intelligence, memory, and behavior can be assessed, however these biomarkers can alter in various other clinical conditions, such as dementia with Lewy body, HIV/AID dementia, Huntington's diseases, Amyotrophic lateral sclerosis, and Down's syndrome, hence cannot be considered specific for the early EBPT of AD. There has been an intense quest in the novel discovery of peripheral diagnostic biomarker(s) of AD as it may provide safe, noninvasive, and effective method of clinical diagnosis. Biochemical analyses of circulating ACh, Acetyl Choline esterase, β-Secretase, Amyloid Precursor Protein, Aβ, C-reactive protein (CRP) and monoamine oxidases (*those are significantly increased in AD*) have provided a lead in understanding and development of novel drugs for the effective treatment of AD. Similarly genetic biomarker, Apolipoprotein-Eξ4 (APO-E) as a risk factor could be a useful biomarker in understanding the basic molecular genetics and pathogenesis of AD. Although APO-E may have some functional correlation with Aβ, it is not highly specific as several patients with AD do not demonstrate any direct relationship with APO-E mutation and or with other biochemical biomarkers. Similarly, omic biomarkers including genomic, proteomic, matabolomic, glycomic, lipidomic, and metallomic are being explored to facilitate early and accurate differential diagnosis and successful clinical management of this devastating disease with multiple etiologies including diet, life style, and environmental neurotoxins etc. Although comparative analyses of omic biomarkers seem quite promising, it is a costly and relatively less accessible to general public at this moment. Numerous sets of genes, proteins, lipids, carbohydrates, and metal ions, may be simultaneously altered in AD patients, which makes the data interpretation more challenging. Undoubtedly, CSF analyses of Aβ1-42, tau, and phosphorylated tau provides a better estimate of AD progression/regression, however lumber tap is an invasive procedure particularly in aging persons with compromised immune system. Some physicians also determine the circulating and CSF levels of IGF-1, Cortisol, brain derived nerve growth factor (BDNF), Iron, Folic acid, Thiamine, and Vitamin B_{12} to get better idea regarding their nutritional status, general health, and well-being as a palliative treatment option. There is no doubt that pathological diagnosis of autopsy brain samples provides the definite diagnosis of AD, it is of limited use to a patient of AD for EBPT. Moreover, unlike other tissues, brain biopsy is usually contraindicated and considered highly invasive with some iatrogenic potential. However, hippocampal atrophy, frontotemporal atrophy, callosal atrophy, enlargement of lateral ventricles, existence of Aβ plaques, neurofibrillary tangles, and twisted microtubules provide the final diagnosis of AD, yet only during autopsy examination. As described earlier, the researchers discovered CB formation in the aging under-nourished rat cerebellar Purkinje cell dendrites as pleomorphic multi-lamellar electron-dense stacks of degenerated mitochondrial membranes, which can be detected in the lymphocytes, skin, cells, the cells from buccal mucosa, and vaginal smears; however it requires high resolution transmission electron microscopy, is time consuming and cumbersome procedure. Nevertheless, the rationale of investigating CBs and other subcellular biomarkers from skin cells, seems logical, as both neuronal cells as well as skin cells are derived from the same neuroectodermal plate during embryonic development. A preliminary evidence of (platelets and lymphocytes) CB formation can be obtained by estimating the mitochondrial membrane potential (ΔΨ) collapse, mitochondrial DNA oxidation product, 8-OH-2dG synthesis, and α-Synuclein index (*a ratio of nitrative α-synuclein vs native α-synuclein*) particularly to rule out parkinsonian dementia with Lewy bodies from AD. Furthermore, development of novel MAO-A and MAO-B specific CB antagonists and brain regional induction of MTs, Reserveratrol, Sirtuins, or other antioxidants may provide better therapeutic avenues for the effective clinical management of AD. Indeed *in-vivo* analyses of AD biomarkers, employing multi-modality molecular imaging has shown great promise. *In general voxel-based CT provides basic information regarding the electron density per unit area, MRI provides information regarding proton density per unit area, and PET imaging provides information regarding photon density per unit area.* Although CT and MRI can provide information regarding various pathological biomarkers *in vivo* including: *cortical atrophy, hippocampal atrophy, callosal atrophy, and enlargement of lateral ventricles,* these morphological changes may be noticed even in chronic Alcoholism and in patients suffering from other drugs of abuse, and schizopherenia, in addition to AD. Moreover CT and MRI cannot decipher a basic difference between living and nonliving brain tissue. However *in-vivo* noninvasive PET imaging employing sensitive biomarkers such as [18]FdG provides precise information regarding brain regional glucose hypometabolism and indirectly mitochondrial bioenergetics. In addition, Pittsburg compound, ^{18}F-Florbetapir provides information regarding truncated/nontrucated Aβ aggregates and is also nonspecific as several patients with AD may or may not have Aβ plaques in their CNS. Recent mass spectroscopic analyses have demonstrated truncated and poly-glutamated 4-42 Aβ as a highly predominant form the senile plaques of AD patients as compared to senile plaques in normal aging subjects. Furthermore, the microglial biomarker and TSPO localizing agent, ^{18}F or[11]C-labelled PK-11195 has proven beneficial in the early EBPT of AD with limited success. Hence more extensive research regarding peripheral and/or central biomarkers will go a long way in the early and effective clinical management to eventually accomplish the ultimate goal of EBPT in AD.

CONCLUSION

Early identification of persons at risk for cognitive decline in aging is critical to optimizing treatment to delay or avoid a clinical diagnosis of MCI or dementia due to AD. Currently, detection procedures are being improved, but once accurate and reproducible assays are developed, it will be possible to define their relationship to early diagnosis and progression of AD as discussed in this chapter. It is now realized that no single measure fulfils all the criteria for a biomarker in AD, but combinations of measures are more likely to provide synergistic benefit. Hence strategies are being developed to apply recent advances of the cause of AD to the development of biomarkers that will accurately identify at-risk individuals, enable early diagnosis, and reflect the progression of disease to EBPT of AD. The latter will be particularly important for testing disease-modifying therapies. Recent reports reflect the application of various clinical, imaging or biochemical measurements, alone or in combination, to general AD populations. The biomarker field is approaching a stage when certain combinations of clinical, imaging and biochemical measures may identify individuals at risk for developing the disease. However, their general applicability may be limited. Future neuroimaging network analysis will expose novel and interesting findings that will elucidate the detailed mechanisms of AD. With the recent developments and innovations of *in-vitro* and *in-vivo* biomarkers, it is becoming possible to differentially diagnose MCI from AD. It seems that *in-vitro* CSF biomarkers possess relatively more diagnostic accuracy as compared to *in-vivo* molecular imaging employing CT, SPECT, PET, and MRI. However in combination with omic analyses, these biomarkers promise to prove highly beneficial for effective therapeutic interventions with minimum or no adverse effects and relatively more beneficial effects to the patient. AD and PD are the most common neurodegenerative diseases (Schapira, 2013). The most promising diagnostic biomarker is the analysis of α-Synuclein in the CSF samples of PD patients. However α-Synuclein concentrations may also be modulated by certain disease-modifying agents. The author proposed that *in-vitro* estimation of SI and ex-vivo detection of CB formation may further facilitate confirming AD diagnosis at early stages of disease progression and implementing proper therapeutic interventions. Attention is now turning to stratification of AD into certain at-risk groups defined by genotype. The application of multimodality biomarker screening to these populations may be more beneficial for AD patients. Since CB formation as pre-apoptotic hallmark of compromised mitochondrial bioenergetics is now well-established; it can be used as an early diagnostic biomarker of AD progression and novel drug discovery biomarker during early phase, and enhance charnolophagy during chronic phase to facilitate early clinical management in the peripheral platelets and lymphocytes of AD patients. Recent studies emphasized the involvement of CB in the genetic predisposition to neurodegenerative disorders such as PD and cancer (Li et al., 2014), in Aβ deposition (Zhang et al., 2015), and the therapeutic potential of MTs as potent antioxidants, anti-apoptotic, and anti-inflammatory factors to prevent CB sequestration will further facilitate developing new theranostic strategies for personalized treatment of AD as well as numerous other neurodegenerative disorders of unknown etiopathogenesis (Yamamoto et al., 2015). The future discovery of novel biomarkers will eventually provide better EBPT for AD patients and better quality of life.

REFERENCES

Abisambra, J. F., Jinwal, U. K., Blair, L. J., O'Leary, J. C., 3rd., Li, Q., Brady, S., Wang, L., Guidi, C. E., Zhang, B., Nordhues, B. A., Cockman, M., Suntharalingham, A., Li, P., Jin, Y., Atkins, C. A. & Dickey, C. A. (2013). Tau accumulation activates the unfolded protein response by impairing endoplasmic reticulum-associated degradation. *J Neurosci.*, *33*, 9498-94507.

Andreasson, U., Perret-Liaudet, A., van Waalwijk, van Doorn, L. J., Blennow, K., et al., (2015). A Practical Guide to Immunoassay Method Validation. *Front Neurol.*, *6*, 179.

Bagdy, G. & Juhasz, G. (2013). Biomarkers for personalized treatment in psychiatric diseases. *Expert Opin Med Diagn.*, *7*, 417-422.

Bang, J., Jeon, W. K., Lee, I. S., Han, J. S. & Kim, B. Y. (2013). Biphasic functional regulation in hippocampus of rat with chronic cerebral hypoperfusion induced by permanent occlusion of bilateral common carotid artery. *PLoS One.*, *8*, e70093.

Bateman, R. J., Munsell, L. Y., Morris, J. C., Swarm, R., Yarasheski, K. E. & Holtzman, D. M. (2006). "Human amyloid-beta synthesis and clearance rates as measured in cerebrospinal fluid *in vivo*". *Nature Medicine*, *12* (7), 856–861.

Bekris, L. M., Lutz, F., Montine, T. J., Yu, C. E., Tsuang, D., Peskind, E. R. & Leverenz, J. B. (2013). MicroRNA in Alzheimer's disease: an exploratory study in brain, cerebrospinal fluid and plasma. *Biomarkers.*, *18*, 455-466.

Biological markers of amyloid β-related mechanisms in Alzheimer's disease. *Experimental Neurology*, *223* (2), 334–346.

Blennow, K. & Zetterberg, H. (2013). The application of cerebrospinal fluid biomarkers in early diagnosis of Alzheimer disease. *Med. Clin. North Am.*, 97, 369-376.

Braunewell, K. H. (2012). The Vicinin-line proteins VILIP-1 and VILIP-3 in Alzheimer's disease. –old wine in new bottles. *Frontiers in Molecular Neuroscience.*, 5, 1-11.

Bruck, A., Virta, J. R., Koivunen, J., Koikkalainen, J., Scheinin, N. M., Helenius, H., Någren, K., Helin, S., Parkkola, R., Viitanen, M. & Rinne, J. O. (2013). [11C]PIB, [18F]FDG and MR imaging in patients with mild cognitive impairment. *Eur J Nucl Med Mol Imaging.*, 40(10), 1567-1572.

Buckley, R., Saling, M. M., Ames, D., Rowe, C. C., Lautenschlager, N. T., Macaulay, S. L., Martins, R. N., Masters, C. L., O'Meara, T., Savage, G., Szoeke, C., Villemagne, V. L. & Ellis, K. A. (2013). Australian Imaging Biomarkers and Lifestyle Study of Aging (AIBL) Research Group. Factors affecting subjective memory complaints in the AIBL aging study: biomarkers, memory, affect, and age. *Int. Psychogeriatr.*, 25, 1307-1315.

Caraci, F., Bosco, P., Leggio, G. M., Malaguarnera, M., Drago, F., Bucolo, C. & Salomone, S. (2013). Clinical Development of new Disease-Modifying Drug Treatments For Alzheimer's Disease. *Curr. Top. Med.*, 13(15), 1853-1863.

Carboni, L., Lattanzio, F., Candeletti, S., Porcellini, E., Raschi, E., Licastro, F. & Romualdi, P. (2015). Peripheral leukocyte expression of the potential biomarker proteins Bdnf, Sirt1, and Psen1 is not regulated by promoter methylation in Alzheimer's disease patients. *Neurosci Lett.*, 1605, 44-48.

Chapman, R. M., Porsteinsson, A. P., Gardner, M. N., Mapstone, M., McCrary, J. W., Sandoval, T. C., Guillily, M. D., Reilly, L. A. & Degrush, E. (2012). The Impact of AD Drug Treatments on Event-Related Potentials as Markers of Disease Conversion. *Curr Alzheimer Res.*, 10, 732-741.

Chen, Z. & Zhong, C. (2013). Decoding Alzheimer's disease from perturbed cerebral glucose metabolism: Implications for diagnostic and therapeutic strategies. *Prog Neurobiol.*, 108, 21-43.

Cheng, L., Quek, C. Y., Sun, X., Bellingham, S. A. & Hill, A. F. (2013). The detection of microRNA associated with Alzheimer's disease in biological fluids using next-generation sequencing technologies. *Front Genet.*, 4, 150.

Choi, Y. S., Hou, S., Choe, L. H. & Lee, K. H. (2013). Targeted human cerebrospinal fluid proteomics for the validation of multiple Alzheimer's disease biomarker candidates. *J Chromatogr B Analyt Technol Biomed Life Sci.*, 930, 129-135.

Clelland, C. L., Read, L. L., Panek, L. J., Nadrich, R. H., Bancroft, C. & Clelland, J. D. (2013). Utilization of Never-Medicated Bipolar Disorder Patients towards Development and Validation of a Peripheral Biomarker Profile. *PLoS One.*, 8, e69082.

Dakshinamurti, K., Sharma, S. K., Sundaram, M. & Watanabe, T. (1993). Hippocampal changes in developing postnatal mice following intrauterine exposure to domoic acid. *J Neurosci.*, 13, 4486-4495.

Dakshinamurti, K., Sharma, S. K. & Geiger, J. D. (2003). Neuroprotective actions of pyridoxine. *Biochim Biophys Acta.*, 1647, 225-229.

Dakshinamurti, K., Sharma, S. K. & Sundaram, M. (1991). Domoic acid induced seizures activity in rats. *Neurosci. Lett.*, 127, 193-197.

Dani, M., Edison, P. & Brooks, D. J. (2015). Imaging biomarkers in tauopathies. *Parkinsonism Relat Disord. in press.*

Darreh-Shori, T., Vijayaraghavan, S., Aeinehband, S., Piehl, F., Lindblom, R. P., Nilsson, B., Ekdahl, K. N., Långström, B., Almkvist, O. & Nordberg, A. (2013). Functional variability in butyrylcholinesterase activity regulates intrathecal cytokine and astroglial biomarker profiles in patients with Alzheimer's disease. *Neurobiol Aging.*, *34*, 2465-2481

Deborah, T. J., Stephen B. P., David S. P., Giuseppe C. D., Jeffrey, B., Mark, H. G., Colin, M. L., Roberto, C. & Kevin B. J. (2008). "Stabilization of Neurotoxic Soluble β-Sheet-Rich Conformations of the Alzheimer's Disease Amyloid-β Peptide". *Biophysical Journal*, *94* (7), 2752–2266.

DeMarshall, C., Sarkar, A., Nagele, E. P., Goldwaser, E., Godsey, G., Acharya, N. K. & Nagele, R. G. (2015). Utility of Autoantibodies as Biomarkers for Diagnosis and Staging of Neurodegenerative Diseases. *Int. Rev. Neurobiol.*, *122*, 1-51.

Desikan, R. S., Rafii, M. S., Brewer, J. B. & Hess, C. P. (2013). An Expanded Role for Neuroimaging in the Evaluation of Memory Impairment. *Am J Neuroradiol.*, *34*, 2075-2082.

Di Ieva, A., Valli, M. & Cusimano, M. D. (2014). Distinguishing Alzheimer's Disease from Normal Pressure Hydrocephalus: A Search for MRI Biomarkers. *J. Alzheimers Dis.*, *38*, 331-350.

Donovan, N. J., Wadsworth, L. P., Lorius, N., Locascio, J. J., Rentz, D. M., Johnson, K. A., Sperling, R. A. & Marshall, G. A. (2014). Alzheimer Disease Neuroimaging Initiative. Regional cortical thinning predicts worsening apathy and hallucinations across the Alzheimer disease spectrum. *Am J Geriatr Psychiatry.*, *22*, 1168-1179.

Donovan, L. E., Dammer, E. B., Duong, D. M., Hanfelt, J. J., Levey, A. I., Seyfried, N. T. & Lah, J. J. (2013). Exploring the potential of the platelet membrane proteome as a source of peripheral biomarkers for Alzheimer's disease. *Alzheimers Res Ther.*, *5*, 32.

Doody, R. S., Raman, R., Farlow, M., Iwatsubo, T., Vellas, B., Joffe, S., Kieburtz, K., He, F., Sun, X., Thomas, R. G. & Aisen, P. S. (2013). Alzheimer's Disease Cooperative Study Steering Committee, Siemers E, Sethuraman G, Mohs R; Semagacestat Study Group. A phase 3 trial of semagacestat for treatment of Alzheimer's disease. *N Engl J Med.*, *369*, 341-350.

Doré, V., Villemagne, V. L., Bourgeat, P., Fripp, J., Acosta, O., Chetélat, G., Zhou, L., Martins, R., Ellis, K. A., Masters, C. L., Ames, D., Salvado, O. & Rowe, C. C. (2013). Cross-sectional and longitudinal analysis of the relationship between Aβ deposition, cortical thickness, and memory in cognitively unimpaired individuals and in Alzheimer disease. *JAMA Neurol.*, *70*, 903-911.

Du, Y., Dodel, R., Hampel, H., Buerger, K., Lin, S., Eastwood, B., Bales, K., Gao, F., et al. (2001). "Reduced levels of amyloid beta-peptide antibody in Alzheimer disease". *Neurology*, *57*, 801–805.

Duits, F. H., Martinez-Lage, P., Paquet, C., Engelborghs, S., Lleó, A., Hausner, L., et al., (2015). Performance and complications of lumbar puncture in memory clinics: Results of the multicenter lumbar puncture feasibility study. *Alzheimers Dement.*

Fieremans, E., Benitez, A., Jensen, J. H., Falangola, M. F., Tabesh, A., Deardorff, R. L., Spampinato, M. V., Babb, J. S., Novikov, D. S., Ferris, S. H. & Helpern, J. A. (2013). Novel White Matter Tract Integrity Metrics Sensitive to Alzheimer Disease Progression. *AJNR Am J Neuroradiol.*, *34*, 2105-2112.

Fiolaki, A., Tsamis, K. I., Milionis, H. J., Kyritsis, A. P., Kosmidou, M. & Giannopoulos, S. (2014). Atherosclerosis, biomarkers of atherosclerosis and Alzheimer's disease. *Int J Neurosci.*, *124*, 1-11.

Fleischman, D. A., Yu, L., Arfanakis, K., Han, S. D., Barnes, L. L., Arvanitakis, Z., Boyle, P. A. & Bennett, D. A. (2013). Faster cognitive decline in the years prior to MR imaging is associated with smaller hippocampal volumes in cognitively healthy older persons. *Frontiers in Neurosci*, *5*, 21.

Fleischman, D. A., Yu, L., Arfanakis, K., Han, S. D., Barnes, L. L., Arvanitakis, Z., Boyle, P. A. & Bennett, D. A. (2013). Faster cognitive decline in the years prior to MR imaging is associated with smaller hippocampal volumes in cognitively healthy older persons. *Front Aging Neurosci.*, *5*, 21.

Foster, J. K., Albrecht, M. A., Savage, G., Lautenschlager, N. T., Ellis, K. A., Maruff, P., Szoeke, C., Taddei, K., Martins, R., Masters, C. L. & Ames, D. (2013). AIBL Research Group. Lack of reliable evidence for a distinctive ε4-related cognitive phenotype that is independent from clinical diagnostic status: findings from the Australian Imaging, Biomarkers and Lifestyle Study. *Brain.*, *136*, 2201-2216.

Frisoni, G. B., Bocchetta, M., Chételat, G., Rabinovici, G. D., de Leon, M. J., Kaye, J., Reiman, E. M., Scheltens, P., Barkhof, F., Black, S. E., Brooks, D. J., Carrillo, M. C., Fox, N. C., Herholz, K., Nordberg, A., Jack, C. R., Jr. Jagust, W. J., Johnson, K. A., Rowe, C. C., Sperling, R. A., Thies, W., Wahlund, L. O., Weiner, M. W., Pasqualetti, P. & Decarli, C. (2013). For ISTAART's NeuroImaging Professional Interest Area. *Neurology.*, *81*, 487-500.

Frost, S. M., Kanagasingam, Y., Sohrabi, H. R., Taddei, K., Bateman, R., Morris, J., Benzinger, T., Goate, A., Masters, C. L. & Martins, R. N. (2013). Pupil Response Biomarkers Distinguish Amyloid Precursor Protein Mutation Carriers from Non-Carriers. *Curr Alzheimer Res.*, *10*, 790-796.

Gandy, S. & Heppner, F. L. (2013). Microglia as dynamic and essential components of the amyloid hypothesis. *Neuron.*, *78*, 575-577.

Gardner, R. C., Valcour, V. & Yaffe, K. (2013). Dementia in the oldest old: a multi-factorial and growing public health issue. *Alzheimers Res Ther.*, *5*, 27.

Gaser, C., Franke, K., Klöppel, S., Koutsouleris, N. & Sauer, H. (2013). Alzheimer's Disease Neuroimaging Initiative. *PLoS One.*, *8*, e67346.

Gauthier, S., Leuzy, A., Racine, E. & Rosa-Neto, P. (2013). Diagnosis and management of Alzheimer's disease: Past, present and future ethical issues. *Prog Neurobiol.*, *110*, 102-113.

Gauthier, S., Leuzy, A. & Rosa-Neto, P. (2014). How Can We Improve Transfer of Outcomes from Randomized Clinical Trials to Clinical Practice with Disease-Modifying Drugs in Alzheimer's Disease? *Neurodegener Dis.*, *13*, 197-199.

Gezen-Ak, D., Dursun, E., Hanağası, H., Bilgiç, B., Lohman, E., Araz, O. S., Atasoy, I., Alaylıoğlu, M., Onal, B., Gürvit, H. & Yılmazer, S. (2013). BDNF, TNFα, HSP90, CFH, and IL-10 Serum Levels in Patients with Early or Late Onset Alzheimer's Disease or Mild Cognitive Impairment. *J Alzheimers Dis. Isord.*, *37*(1), 185-195.

Ghani, M., Reitz, C., Cheng, R., Vardarajan, B. N., Jun, G., Sato, C., Naj, A., Rajbhandary, R., et al., (2015). Association of Long Runs of Homozygosity With Alzheimer Disease Among African American Individuals. *JAMA Neurol.*, *72*(11), 1313-1323..

Ghazi, I. E. I., Martin, B. L. & Armitage, I. M. (2011). New Proteins Found Interacting with Brain Metallothionein-3 Are Linked to Secretion. *International Journal of Alzheimer's Disease*, 2011, 1-9.

Giannopoulos, P. F., Joshi, Y. B., Chu, J. & Praticò, D. (2013). The 12-15-lipoxygenase is a modulator of Alzheimer's-related tau pathology *in vivo*. *Aging Cell.*, *12*, 1082-1090.

Glodzik, L., Rusinek, H., Pirraglia, E., McHugh, P., Tsui, W., Williams, S., Cummings, M., Li, Y., Rich, K., Randall, C., Mosconi, L., Osorio, R., Murray, J., Zetterberg, H., Blennow, K. & de Leon, M. (2014). Blood pressure decrease correlates with tau pathology and memory decline in hypertensive elderly. *Neurobiol Aging.*, *35*, 64-71.

Goutagny, R. & Krantic, S. (2013). Hippocampal Oscillatory Activity in Alzheimer's Disease: Toward the Identification of Early Biomarkers? *Aging Dis.*, *4*, 134-140.

Graff-Radford, J. & Kantarci, K. (2013). Magnetic resonance spectroscopy in Alzheimer's disease. *Neuropsychiatr Dis Treat.*, *9*, 687-696.

Gubandru, M., Margina, D., Tsitsimpikou, C., Goutzourelas, N., Tsarouhas, K., Ilie, M., Tsatsakis, A. M. & Kouretas, D. (2013). Alzheimer's disease treated patients showed different patterns for oxidative stress and inflammation markers. *Food Chem Toxicol.*, *61*, 209-214.

Guedes, J., Cardoso, A. L. & Pedroso de Lima, M. C. (2013). Involvement of microRNA in microglia-mediated immune response. *Clin Dev Immunol.*, Article ID 186872, 11 pages.

Gupta, V. B., Sundaram, R. & Martins, R. N. (2013). Multiplex biomarkers in blood. *Alzheimers Res Ther.*, *5*, 31.

Gustaw, K. A., Garrett, M. R., Lee, H. G., Castellani, R. J., Zagorski, M. G., Prakasam, A., Siedlak, S. L., Zhu, X., et al. (2008). "Antigen-antibody dissociation in Alzheimer disease: A novel approach to diagnosis". *J. of Neurochem.*, *106*, 1350–1356.

Haller, S., Garibotto, V., Kövari, E., Bouras, C., Xekardaki, A., Rodriguez, C., Lazarczyk, M. J., Giannakopoulos, P. & Lovblad, K. O. (2013). Neuroimaging of dementia in 2013: what radiologists need to know. *Eur Radiol.*, *23*(12), 3393-404.

Hansson, O., Zetterberg, H., Vanmechelen, E., Vanderstichele, H., Andreasson, U., Londos, E., Wallin, A., Minthon, L. & Blennow, K. (2010). Evaluation of plasma Abeta (40) and Abeta (42) as predictors of conversion to Alzheimer's disease in patients with mild cognitive impairment. *Neurobiology of Aging*, *31*, 357–367.

Harald, H., Yong, S., Dominic, W. M., Paul, A., Les S. M., Henrik, Z., John T. Q., Kaj, B., Hatashita, S. & Yamasaki, H. Diagnosed mild cognitive impairment due to Alzheimer's disease with PET biomarkers of beta amyloid and neuronal dysfunction. *PLoS One.*, *8*, e66877 (2013).

Hausner, L., Tschäpe, J. A., Schmitt, H. P., Hentschel, F., Hartmann, T. & Frölich, L. (2014). Clinical characterization of a presenilin 1 mutation (F177S) in a family with very early-onset Alzheimer's disease in the third decade of life. *Alzheimers Dement.*, *10*, 27-39.

Henderson, V. W. (2014). Alzheimer's disease: Review of hormone therapy trials and implications for treatment and prevention after menopause. *J. Steroid Biochem. Mol. Biol.*, *142*, 99-106.

Henriksen, K., O'Bryant, S. E., Hampel, H., Trojanowski, J. Q., Montine, T. J., Jeromin, A., Blennow, K., Lönneborg, A., Wyss-Coray, T., Soares, H., Bazenet, C., Sjögren, M., Hu, Lovestone, S., Karsdal, M. A. & Weiner, M. W. (2014). Blood-Based Biomarker Interest Group. The future of blood-based biomarkers for Alzheimer's disease. *Alzheimers Dement.*, *10*(1), 115-131.

Henriksen, K., Wang, Y., Sørensen, M. G., Barascuk, N., Suhy, J., Pedersen, J. T., Duffin, K. L., Dean, R. A., Pajak, M., Christiansen, C., Zheng, Q. & Karsdal, M. A. (2013). An enzyme-generated fragment of tau measured in serum shows an inverse correlation to cognitive function. *PLoS One.*, *8*, e64990.

Hirano, S. & Yamada, M. (2013). [Network analyses in neuroimaging studies]. *Brain Nerve*, *65*, 659-667.

Holland, D., Desikan, R. S., Dale, A. M. & McEvoy, L. K. (2013). Higher Rates of Decline for Women and Apolipoprotein E {varepsilon}4 Carriers. *AJNR Am J Neuroradiol.*, *34*, 2287-2293.

Howe, E. (2013). Clinical implications of the new diagnostic guidelines for dementia. *Innov Clin Neurosci.*, *10*, 32-38.

Hu, K., Harper, D. G., Shea, S. A., Stopa, E. G. & Scheer, F. A. (2013). Noninvasive fractal biomarker of clock neurotransmitter disturbance in humans with dementia. *Sci Rep.*, *3*, 2229.

Ibanez, C., Sim, C., Barupal, D. K., Fiehn, O., Kivipelto, M., Cedazo-Mínguez, A. & Cifuentes, A. (2013). A new metabolomic work flow for early detection of Alzheimer's disease. *J Chromatogr A.*, *1302*, 65-71.

Ibanez, C., Cifuentes, A. & Simo, C. (2015). Recent Advances and Applications of Metabolomics to Investigate Neurodegenerative Diseases. *Int Rev Neurobiol.*, *122*, 95-132.

Inarrea, P., Alarcia, R., Alava, M. A., Capablo, J. L., Casanova, A., Iñiguez, C., Iturralde, M., Larrodé, P., Martín, J., Mostacero, E. & Ara, J. R. (2014). Mitochondrial Complex Enzyme Activities and Cytochrome c Expression Changes in Multiple Sclerosis. *Mol Neurobiol.*, *49*(1), 1-9.

Inoue, T., Kawaji, T. & Tanihara, H. (2013). Elevated levels of multiple biomarkers of Alzheimer's disease in the aqueous humor of eyes with open-angle glaucoma. Invest. *Ophthalmol. Vis. Sci.*, *54*, 5353-5358.

Inoue, T., Kawaji, T. & Tanihara, H. (2013). Elevated levels of multiple biomarkers of Alzheimer's disease in the aqueous humor of eyes with open-angle glaucoma. *Invest Ophthalmol Vis Sci.*, *54*, 5353-5358.

Irie, Y., Mori, W., Keung, M., Mizushima, Y. & Wakabayashi, K. (2004). Expression of Neuronal Growth Inhibitory Factor (Metallothionein-III) in the Salivary Gland. *Physiol. Res.*, *53*, 719-723.

Ishii, K. (2014). PET Approaches for Diagnosis of Dementia. AJNR Am *J Neuroradiol.*, *35*, 2030-2038.

Jorge, P. J. & Lennart, M. (2010). Amyloid-β–induced neuronal dysfunction in Alzheimer's disease: From synapses toward neural networks. *Nature Neuroscience*, *13*, 812–818.

Kaerst, L., Kuhlmann, A., Wedekind, D., Stoeck, K., Lange, P. & Zerr, I. (2013). Cerebrospinal fluid biomarkers in Alzheimer's disease, vascular dementia and ischemic stroke patients: a critical analysis. *J Neurol.*, *260*, 2722-2727.

Kang, K., Yoon, U., Lee, J. M. & Lee, H. W. (2013). Idiopathic normal-pressure hydrocephalus, cortical thinning, and the cerebrospinal fluid tap test. *J Neurol Sci.*, *334*(1-2), 55-62.

Kapoor, S. (2013). Emerging new biomarkers of Alzheimer's disease. *Int J Geriatr Psychiatry.*, *28*, 880.

Karakaya, T, Fuber, F., Schroder, J. & Pantel, J. (2013). Pharmacological Treatment of Mild Cognitive Impairment as a Prodromal Syndrome of Alzheimer's Disease. *Curr Neuropharmacol.*, *11*, 102-108.

Kim, S., Swaminathan, S., Inlow, M., Risacher, S. L., et al., (2013). Alzheimer's Disease Neuroimaging Initiative (ADNI). Influence of genetic variation on plasma protein levels in older adults using a multi-analyte panel. *PLoS One.*, *8*, e70269.

Knopman, D. S., Jack, C. R., Wiste, H. J., Weigand, S. D., Vemuri, P., Lowe, V. J., Kantarci, K., Gunter, J. L., Senjem, M. L., Mielke, M. M., Roberts, R. O., Boeve, B. F. & Petersen, R. C. (2013). Selective Worsening of Brain Injury Biomarker Abnormalities in Cognitively Normal Elderly Persons With β-Amyloidosis. *JAMA Neurol.*, *70*, 1030-1038.

Koehler, N. K., Stransky, E., Shing, M., Gaertner, S., Meyer, M., Schreitmüller, B., et al., (2013). Altered Serum IgG Levels to α-Synuclein in Dementia with Lewy Bodies and Alzheimer's Disease. *PLoS One.*, *8*, e64649.

Kojima, S., Shimada, A., Kodan, A., Kobayashi, K., Morita, T., Yamano, Y. & Umemura, T. (1998). Molecular cloning and expression of the canine metallothionein-III gene. *Can J Vet Res.*, *62*, 148-151.

Korczyn, A. D. (2013). Is Alzheimer's disease a homogeneous disease entity? *J. Neural. Transm.*, *120*, 1475-1477.

Kouzuki, M., Asaina, F., Taniguchi, M., Musha, T. & Urakami, K. (2013). The relationship between the diagnosis method of neuronal dysfunction (DIMENSION) and brain pathology in the early stages of Alzheimer's disease. *Psychogeriatrics.*, *13*, 63-70.

Kreisl, W. C., Lyoo, C. H., McGwier, M., Snow, J., Jenko, K. J., Kimura, N., Corona, W., Morse, C. L., Zoghbi, S. S., Pike, V. W., McMahon, F. J., Turner, R. S. & Innis, R. B. (2013). Biomarkers Consortium PET Radioligand Project Team. *In vivo* radioligand binding to translocator protein correlates with severity of Alzheimer's disease. *Brain.*, *136*, 2228-2238.

Kristofikova, Z., Ripova D. Hegnerová, K., Sirova, J. & Homola, J. (2013). Protein τ-Mediated Effects on Rat Hippocampal Choline Transporters CHT1 and τ-Amyloid β Interactions. *Neurochem Res.*, *38*, 949-959.

Kuhlmann, A., Wedekind, D., Stoeck, K., Lange, P. & Zerr, I. (2013). Using Cerebrospinal Fluid Marker Profiles in Clinical Diagnosis of Dementia with Lewy Bodies, Parkinson's Disease, and Alzheimer's Disease. *Dement. Geriatr. Cogn. Disord.*, *36*, 263-278.

Kumar, P., Dezso, Z., Mackenzie, C., Oestreicher, J., Agoulnik, S., Byrne, M., Bernier, F., Yanagimachi, M., Aoshima, K. & Oda, Y. (2013). Circulating miRNA Biomarkers for Alzheimer's Disease. *PLoS One.*, *8*, e69807.

Laeger, U. (2015). [PET with amyloid ligands should not be applied routinely in early diagnostics of Alzheimer's disease]. *Ugeskrift for Laeger.*, *177*, 32.

Lamoureux, L., Simon, S. L., Plews, M., Ruddat, V., Brunet, S., Graham, C., Czub, S. & Knox, J. D. (2013). Urine proteins identified by two-dimensional differential gel electrophoresis facilitate the differential diagnoses of scrapie. *PLoS One.*, *8*, e64044.

Leandro, G. S., Lobo, R. R., Oliveira, D. V., Moriguti, J. C. & Sakamoto-Hojo, E. T. (2013). Lymphocytes of patients with Alzheimer's disease display different DNA damage repair kinetics and expression profiles of DNA repair and stress response genes. *Int J Mol Sci.*, *14*, 12380-12400.

Lee, S. L., Thomas, P. & Fenech, M. (2015). Genome instability biomarkers and blood micronutrient risk profiles associated with mild cognitive impairment and Alzheimer's disease. *Mutat Res.*, *776*, 54-83.

Leger, G. C. & Massoud, F. (2013). Novel disease-modifying therapeutics for the treatment of Alzheimer's disease. *Expert Rev Clin Pharmacol.*, *6*, 423-442.

Leidinger, P., Backes, C., Deutscher, S., Schmitt, K., Muller, S. C., Frese, K., Haas, J., Ruprecht, K., Paul, F., Stahler, C., Lang, C. J., Meder, B., Bartfai, T., Meese, E. & Keller, A. (2013). A blood based 12-miRNA signature of Alzheimer disease patients. *Genome Biol.*, *14*, R78.

Leoutsakos, J. M., Bartlett, A. L., Forrester, S. N. & Lyketsos, C. G. (2014). Simulating effects of biomarker enrichment on Alzheimer's prevention trials: Conceptual framework and example. *Alzheimers Dement.*, *10*(2), 152-161.

Leung, R., Proitsi, P., Simmons, A., Lunnon, K., Güntert, A., Kronenberg, D., Pritchard, M., Tsolaki, M., Mecocci, P., Kloszewska, I., Vellas, B., Soininen, H., Wahlund, L. O. & Lovestone, S. (2013). Inflammatory proteins in plasma are associated with severity of Alzheimer's disease. *PLoS One.*, *8*, e64971.

Li, H., Liang, Y., Chen, K., Li, X., Shu, N., Zhang, Z. & Wang, Y. (2013). Different patterns of white matter disruption among amnestic mild cognitive impairment subtypes: relationship with neuropsychological performance. *J Alzheimers Dis.*, *36*, 365-376.

Li, Z., Lin, Q., Ma, Q., Lu, C. & Tzeng, C. M. (2014). Genetic predisposition to Parkinson's disease and cancer. *Curr Cancer Drug Targets.*, *14*(3), 310-321.

Lim, Y. Y., Ellis, K. A., Harrington, K., Kamer, A., Pietrzak, R. H., Bush, A. I., Darby, D., Martins, R. N., Masters, C. L., Rowe, C. C., Savage, G., Szoeke, C., Villemagne, V. L., Ames, D. & Maruff, P. (2013). Cognitive consequences of high Aβ amyloid in mild cognitive impairment and healthy older adults: implications for early detection of Alzheimer's disease. *Neuropsychology.*, *27*, 322-332.

Lim, Y. Y., Villemagne, V. L., Laws, S. M., Ames, D., Pietrzak, R. H., Ellis, K. A., et al., (2013). Australian Imaging, Biomarkers and Lifestyle (AIBL) Research Group. BDNF Val66Met, Aβ amyloid, and cognitive decline in preclinical Alzheimer's disease. *Neurobiol Aging.*, *34*, 2457-2464.

Lim, Y. Y., Ellis, K. A., Harrington, K., Kamer, A., Pietrzak, R. H., Bush, A. I., et al., (2013). (The AIBL Research Group) Cognitive consequences of high Aβ amyloid in mild cognitive impairment and healthy older adults: Implications for early detection of Alzheimer's disease. *Neuropsychology*, *27*(3), 322-332.

Lista, S., Garaci, F. G., Ewers, M., Teipel, S., Zetterberg, H., Blennow, K. & Hampel, H. (2014). CSF Aβ1-42 combined with neuroimaging biomarkers in the early detection, diagnosis and prediction of Alzheimer's disease. *Alzheimers Dement.*, *10*(3), 381-92

Liu, L., Zhao, F., Ma, F., Zhang, L., Yang, S. & Xia, N. (2013). Electrochemical detection of β-amyloid peptides on electrode covered with N-terminus-specific antibody based on electrocatalytic O2 reduction by Aβ (1-16)-heme-modified gold nanoparticles. *Biosens Bioelectron.*, *49*, 231-235.

Liu, D. & Zhou, X. H. (2013). ROC analysis in biomarker combination with covariate adjustment. *Acad Radiol.*, *20*, 874-882.

Lopez-de-Ipina, K., Alonso, J. B., Travieso, C. M., Sole-Casals, J., Egiraun, H., Faundez-Zanuy, M., Ezeiza, A., Barroso, N., Ecay-Torres, M., Martinez-Lage, P. & Martinez de

Lizardui, U. (2013). On the selection of non-invasive methods based on speech analysis oriented to automatic Alzheimer disease diagnosis. *Sensors (Basel).*, *13*, 6730-6745.

Luo, X., Hou, L., Shi, H., Zhong, X., Zhang, Y., Zheng, D., Tan, Y., Hu, G., Mu, N., Chan, J., Chen, X., Fang, Y., Wu, F., He, H. & Ning, Y. (2013). CSF levels of the neuronal injury biomarker visinin-like protein-1 in Alzheimer's disease and dementia with Lewy bodies. *J Neurochem.*, *127*(5), 681-690.

Manzine, P. R., Barham, E. J., Vale Fde, A., Selistre-de-Araújo, H. S., Iost Pavarini, S. C. & Cominetti, M. R. (2013). Correlation between mini-mental state examination and platelet ADAM10 expression in Alzheimer's disease. *J Alzheimers Dis.*, *36*, 253-260.

Marklund, N., Farrokhnia, N., Hånell, A., Vanmechelen, E., Enblad, P., Zetterberg, H., Blennow, K. & Hillered, L. (2014). Monitoring of β-Amyloid Dynamics after Human Traumatic Brain Injury. *J Neurotrauma.*, *31*(1), 42-55.

Marutle, A., Gillberg, P. G., Bergfors, A., Yu, W., Ni, R., Nennesmo, I., Voytenko, L. & Nordberg, A. (2013). ³H-deprenyl and ³H-PIB autoradiography show different laminar distributions of astroglia and fibrillar β-amyloid in Alzheimer brain. *J Neuroinflammation.*, *10*, 90.

Marutle, A., Gillberg, P. G., Bergfors, A., Yu, W., Ni, R., Nennesmo, I., Voytenko, L. & Nordberg, A. (2013). ³H-deprenyl and ³H-PIB autoradiography show different laminar distributions of astroglia and fibrillar β-amyloid in Alzheimer brain. *J Neuroinflammation.*, *10*, 90.

Mattsson, N., Andreasson, U., Persson, S., Carrillo, M. C., Collins, S., Chalbot, S., Cutler, N., et al., (2013). Alzheimer's Association QC Program Work Group. CSF biomarker variability in the Alzheimer's Association quality control program. *Alzheimers Dement.*, *9*, 251-261.

Mattsson, N., Insel, P., Nosheny, R., Zetterberg, H., Trojanowski, J. Q., Shaw, L. M., Tosun, D. & Weiner, M. (2013). CSF protein biomarkers predicting longitudinal reduction of CSF β-amyloid42 in cognitively healthy elders. *Transl. Psychiatry.*, *3*, e293.

McClatchey, R., Branson, A., Anjum, A., Bloodsworth, P., Habib, I., Munir, K., Shamdasani, J. & Soomro, K. (2013). neuGRID Consortium. Providing traceability for neuroimaging analyses. *Int J Med Inform.*, *82*, 882-894.

Modrego, P. J. & Gazulla, J. (2013). The predictive value of the memory impairment screen in patients with subjective memory complaints: a prospective study. *Prim Care Companion CNS Disord.*, *15*(1).

Monge Argilés, J. A., Blanco Cantó, M. A., Leiva Salinas, C., Flors, L., Muñoz Ruiz, C., Sánchez Payá, J., Gasparini Berenguer, R. & Leiva Santana, C. (2014). A comparison of early diagnostic utility of Alzheimer disease biomarkers in brain brain magnetic resonance and cerebrospinal fluid. *Neurologia.*, *29*(7), 397-401.

Moore, R. C., Chattillion, E. A., Ceglowski, J., Ho, J., von Känel, R., Mills, P. J., Ziegler, M. G., Patterson, T. L., Grant, I. & Mausbach, B. T. (2013). A randomized clinical trial of Behavioral Activation (BA) therapy for improving psychological and physical health in dementia caregivers: Results of the Pleasant Events Program (PEP). *Behav Res Ther.*, *51*, 623-632.

Moran, C., Beare, R., Phan, T. G., Bruce, D. G., Callisaya, M. L. & Srikanth, V. (2015). Alzheimer's Disease Neuroimaging Initiative (ADNI). Type 2 diabetes mellitus and biomarkers of neurodegeneration. *Neurology.*

Moreth, J., Mavoungou, C. & Schindowski, K. (2013). Is abeta a sufficient biomarker for monitoring anti-abeta clinical studies? A critical review. *Front Aging Neurosci.*, *5*, 25.

Mroczko, B., Groblewska, M. & Barcikowska, M. (2013). The Role of MMPss and Tissue Inhibitors of Metalloproteinases in the Pathophysiology of Neurodegeneration: A Literature Study. *J Alzheimers Dis.*, *37*(2), 273-283.

Mukaetova-Ladinska, E. B., Abdell-All, Z., Andrade, J., da Silva, J. A., Boksha, I., Burbaeva, G., Kalaria, R. J. & O'Brien, J. T. (2013). Platelet Tau Protein as a Potential Peripheral Biomarker in Alzheimer's disease: An Explorative Study. *Curr Alzheimer Res.*, (in press)

Naudi, A., Cabre, R., Jove, M., Ayala, V., Gonzalo, H., Portero-Otín, M., Ferrer, I. & Pamplona, R. (2015). Lipidomics of Human Brain Aging and Alzheimer's Disease Pathology. *Int. Rev. Neurobiol.*, *122*, 133-89

Nutu, M., Zetterberg, H., Londos, E., Minthon, L., Nägga, K., Blennow, K., Hansson, O. & Ohrfelt, A. (2013). Evaluation of the cerebrospinal fluid amyloid-β1-42/Amyloid-β1-40 ratio measured by ELISA to distinguish Alzheimer's disease from other dementia disorders. *Dement Geriatr. Cogn. Disord.*, *36*, 99-110.

Oh, J., Yoo, G., Chang, Y. W., Kim, H. J., Jose, J., Kim, E., Pyun, J. C. & Yoo, K. H. (2013). A carbon nanotube metal semiconductor field effect transistor-based biosensor for detection of amyloid-beta in human serum. *Biosens Bioelectron.*, *50*, 345-350.

Olivieri, F., Rippo, M. R., Procopio, A. D. & Fazioli, F. (2013). Circulating inflamma-miRs in aging and age-related diseases. *Front Genet.*, *4*, 121.

Ota, K., Oishi, N., Ito, K. & Fukuyama, H. (2015). SEAD-J Study Group; Alzheimer's Disease Neuroimaging Initiative. Effects of imaging modalities, brain atlases and feature selection on prediction of Alzheimer's disease. *J. Neurosci. Methods.* 256, 168-183

Palmqvist, S., Zetterberg, H., Mattsson, N., Johansson, P., Alzheimer's Disease Neuroimaging Initiative, Minthon, L., Blennow, K. & Olsson, M. (2015). Swedish BioFINDER study group, Hansson O. Detailed comparison of amyloid PET and CSF biomarkers for identifying early Alzheimer disease. *Neurology*, *85*(14), 1240-1249.

Perrin, R. J., Payton, J. E., Malone, J. P., Gilmore, P., Davis, A. E., Xiong, C., et al. (2013). Quantitative Label-Free Proteomics for Discovery of Biomarkers in Cerebrospinal Fluid: Assessment of Technical and Inter-Individual Variation. *PLoS ONE*, *8*(5), e64314.

Plagg, B., Marksteiner, J., Kathrin, M., Kniewallner, K. M. & Humpel, C. (2015). Platelet dysfunction in hypercholesterolemia mice, two Alzheimer's disease mouse models and in human patients with Alzheimer's disease. *Biogerontology*, *16*, 543–558.

Podlesniy, P., Figueiro-Silva, J., Llado, A., Antonell, A., Sanchez-Valle, R., Alcolea, D., Lleo, A., Molinuevo, J. L., Serra, N. & Trullas, R., (2013). Low CSF concentration of mitochondrial DNA in preclinical Alzheimer's disease. *Ann Neurol.*, *74*(5), 655-568.

Portelius, E., Appelkvist, P., Stromberg, K. & Hoglund, K. (2014). Characterization of the Effect of a Novel γ-Secretase Modulator on Aβ: A Clinically Translatable Model. *Curr Pharm Des.*, *20*(15), 2484-2490.

Randall, C., Mosconi, L., de Leon, M. & Glodzik, L. (2013). Cerebrospinal fluid biomarkers of Alzheimer's disease in healthy elderly. *Front Biosci (Landmark Ed).*, *18*, 1150-1173.

Ray, L., Khemka, V. K., Behera, P., Bandyopadhyay, K., Pal, S., Pal, K., Basu, D. & Chakrabarti, S. (2013). Serum Homocysteine, Dehydroepiandrosterone Sulphate and Lipoprotein (a) in Alzheimer's Disease and Vascular Dementia. *Aging Dis.*, *4*, 57-64.

Rembach, A., Ryan, T. M., Roberts, B. R., Doecke, J. D., Wilson, W. J., Watt, A. D., Barnham, K. J. & Masters, C. L. (2013). Progress towards a consensus on biomarkers for Alzheimer's disease: a review of peripheral analytes. *Biomark Med.*, 7, 641-662.

Richard, E., Schmand, B. A., Eikelenboom, P. & Van Gool, W. A. (2013). Alzheimer's Disease Neuroimaging Initiative. MRI and cerebrospinal fluid biomarkers for predicting progression to Alzheimer's disease in patients with mild cognitive impairment: a diagnostic accuracy study. *BMJ Open.*, 3(6), pii, e002541.

Rival, T., Page, R. M., Chandraratna, D. S., Sendall, T. J., Ryder, E., Liu, B., Lewis, H., Rosahl, T., et al. (2009). "Fenton chemistry and oxidative stress mediate the toxicity of the β-amyloid peptide in a Drosophila model of Alzheimer's disease". *The European Journal of Neuroscience*, 29 (7), 1335–1347.

Rongve, A., Arsland, D. & Graff, C. (2013). [Alzheimer's disease and genetics]. *Tidsskr Nor Laegeforen.*, 133, 1449-1452.

Rosen, C., Hansson, O., Blennow, K. & Zetterberg, H. (2013). Fluid biomarkers in Alzheimer's disease - current concepts. *Mol. Neurodegener.*, 8, 20.

Ross, J., Sharma, S., Winston, J., Nunez, M., Bottini, G., Franceschi, M., Scarpini, E., et al., (2013). CHF5074 Reduces Biomarkers of Neuroinflammation in Patients with Mild Cognitive Impairment: A 12-Week, Double-Blind, Placebo- Controlled Study. *Curr Alzheimer Res.*, 10, 742-753.

Rubio-Perez, J. M. & Morillas-Ruiz, J. M. (2013). Serum Cytokines Profile in Alzheimer's Patients after Ingestion of an Antioxidant Beverage. *CNS Neurol Disord Drug Targets*, 12(8), 1233-1241.

Sabbagh, J. J., Kinney, J. W. & Cummings, J. L. Alzheimer's disease biomarkers: correspondence between human studies and animal models. *Neurobiol Dis.*, 56, 116-130.

Sabbagh, J. J., Kinney, J. W. & Cummings, J. L. (2013). Alzheimer's disease biomarkers in animal models: closing the translational gap. *Am J Neurodegener Dis.*, 2, 108-120.

Sancesario, G. M. & Bernardini, S. (2015). How many biomarkers to discriminate neurodegenerative dementia? *Crit Rev Clin Lab Sci.*, Aug 18, 1-13.

Schapira, A. H. (2013). Recent developments in biomarkers in Parkinson disease. *Curr Opin Neurol.*, 26, 395-400.

Seubert, P., Vigo-Pelfrey, C., Esch, F., Lee, M., Dovey, H., Davis, D., Sinha, S., Schlossmacher, M., et al. (1992). "Isolation and quantification of soluble Alzheimer's beta-peptide from biological fluids". *Nature*, 359, 325–327.

Sharma, S. & Ebadi, M. (2013). Antioxidant Targeting in Neurodegenerative Disorders. Ed. I. Laher, Springer Verlag. Germany. Chapter 85, p. 1-85 (in Press)

Sharma, S., Rais, A., Nel, W., Sandhu, R. & Ebadi, M. (2013a). Clinical significance of Metallothioneins in Cell Therapy and Nanomedicine. *Int. J. Nanomedicine.*, 8, 1477-1488.

Sharma, S. & Ebadi, M. (2014). Charnoly body as universal biomarker of cell injury. *Biomarkers & Genomic Medicine.*, 6, 89-98.

Sharma, S., Refaey, H. El. & Ebadi, M. (2006). Complex-1 activity and ^{18}F-DOPA uptake in genetically engineered mouse model of Parkinson's disease and the neuroprotective role of coenzyme Q$_{10}$. *Brain Res. Bull.*, 70, 22-32.

Sharma, S., Carlson, E. & Ebadi, M. (2003). The Neuroprotective Actions of Selegiline in Inhibiting 1-Methyl, 4-Phenyl, Pyridinium Ion (MPP[+])-Induced Apoptosis in Dopaminergic Neurons. *J. Neurocytology*, 32, 329-343.

Sharma, S. & Ebadi, M. (2014). Charnoly body as universal biomarker of cell injury. *Biomarkers & Genomic Medicine.*, *6*, 89-98.

Sharma, S., Moon, C. S., Khogali, A., Haidous, A., Chabenne, A., Ojo, C., Jelebinkov, M., Kurdi, Y. & Ebadi, M. (2013b). Biomarkers in Parkinson's disease (recent update). *Neurochem Int.*, *63*, 201-129.

Sharma, S., Moon, C. S., Khogali, A., Haidous, A., Chabenne, A., Ojo, C., Jelebinkov, M., Kurdi, Y. & Ebadi, M. (2013). Biomarkers in Parkinson's disease (recent update). *Neurochem Int.*, *63*, 201-129.

Sharma, S. K., Bolster, B. & Dakshinamurti, K. (1994). Picrotoxin and Pentylene tetrazole induced seizure activity in pyridoxine-deficient rats. *J. Neurol. Sci.*, *121*, 1-9.

Sharma, S. K. & Dhalla, N. S. (2000). Domoic acid as a tool in Molecular Pharmacology. Pharmacology and therapeutics in New Millenium. Ed. S.K. Gupta. Springer Verlag, Germany. pp. 130-137.

Sharma, S. K. & Ebadi, M. (1992). Seizure Activity in Pyridoxine-Deficient Adult Rats. *Epilepsia.*, *33*, 235–247.

Sharma, S. K., Selvamurthy, W. & Dakshinamurti, K. (1993). Effect of environmental neurotoxins in the developing brain. *Biometeorology.*, *2*, 447-455.

Sharma, S. K. & Dakshinamurti, K. (1993). Suppression of domoic acid induced seizures by 8-(OH)-DPAT. *J Neural Transm Gen Sect.*, *93*, 87-98.

Sherif, F. F., Zayed, N. & Fakhr, M. (2015). Discovering Alzheimer Genetic Biomarkers Using Bayesian Networks. *Adv Bioinformatics.*, 2015, 639367

Simonsen, A. H., Kuiperij, B., Ali El-Agnaf, O. M., Engelborghs, S., Herukka, S. K., Parnetti, L., Rektorova, I., Vanmechelen, E., Kapaki, E., Verbeek, M. & Mollenhauer, B. (2016). The utility of α-synuclein as biofluid marker in neurodegenerative diseases: a systematic review of the literature. *Biomark Med.*, *10*(1), 19-34

Sogawa, C. A., Asanuma, M., Sogawa, N., Miyazaki, I., Nakanishi, T., Furuta, H. & Ogawa, N. (2001). Localization, regulation, and function of metallothionein-III/growth inhibitory factor in the brain. *Acta Med.*, *55*(1), 1-9.

Soldan, A., Pettigrew, C., Li, S., Wang, M. C., Moghekar, A., Selnes, O. A., Albert, M. & O'Brien, R. (2013). BIOCARD Research Team. Relationship of cognitive reserve and cerebrospinal fluid biomarkers to the emergence of clinical symptoms in preclinical Alzheimer's disease. *Neurobiol Aging.*, *34*(12), 2827-2834.

Sood, S., Gallagher, I. J., Lunnon, K., Rullman, E., Keohane, A., Crossland, H., Phillips, B. E., Cederholm, T., Jensen, T., van Loon, L. J., Lannfelt, L., Kraus, W. E., Atherton, P. J., Howard, R., Gustafsson, T., Hodges, A. & Timmons, J. A. (2015). A novel multi-tissue RNA diagnostic of healthy ageing relates to cognitive health status. *Genome Biol.*, *16*, 185.

Sorensen, K. C., Simonsen, A. H., Holmetoft, U. B., Hasselbalch, S. G. & Heegaard, N. H. (2013). Neprilysin-Like Activity Correlates with CSF-Tau and Phospho-Tau in Patients with Alzheimer's Disease. *J. Alzheimers Dis.*, *37*(2), 379-87.

Souslova, T., Marple, T. C., Spiekerman, A. M. & Mohammad, A. A. (2013). Personalized medicine in Alzheimer's disease and depression. *Contemp Clin Trials.*, *36*(2), 616-623.

Sultana, R., Baglioni, M., Cecchetti, R., Cai, J., Klein, J. B., Bastiani, P., Ruggiero, C., Mecocci, P. & Butterfield, A. D. (2013). Lymphocyte mitochondria: toward identification of peripheral biomarkers in the progression of Alzheimer disease. *Free Radic Biol Med.*, *65*, 595-606.

Taverna, M., Straub, T., Hampel, H., Rujescu, D. & Lichtenthaler, S. F. (2013). A New Sandwich Immunoassay for Detection of the α-Secretase Cleaved, Soluble Amyloid-β Protein Precursor in Cerebrospinal Fluid and Serum. *J. Alzheimers Dis.*, *37*(4), 667-678.

Thomason, L. A., Smithson, L. J., Hazrati, L. N., McLaurin, J. & Kawaja, M. D. (2013). Reactive astrocytes associated with plaques in TgCRND8 mouse brain and in human Alzheimer brain express phosphoprotein enriched in astrocytes (PEA-15). *FEBS Lett*, *587*, 2448-2454.

Toledo, J. B., Xie, S. X., Trojanowski, J. Q. & Shaw, L. M. (2013). Longitudinal change in CSF Tau and Aβ biomarkers for up to 48 months in ADNI. *Acta Neuropathol.*, *126*(5), 659-670.

Toombs, J., Paterson, R. W., Lunn, M. P., Nicholas, J. M., Fox, N. C., Chapman, M. D., Schott, J. M. & Zetterberg, H. (2013). Identification of an important potential confound in CSF AD studies: aliquot volume. *Clin Chem Lab Med.*, *12*, 1-7.

Trushina, E. & Mielke, M. M. (2014). Recent advances in the application of metabolomics to Alzheimer's Disease. *Biochim Biophys Acta.*, *1842*(8), 1232-1239.

Trzepacz, P. T., Yu, P., Sun, J., Schuh, K., Case, M., Witte, M. M., Hochstetler, H. & Hake, A. (2014). Alzheimer's Disease Neuroimaging Initiative. Comparison of neuroimaging modalities for the prediction of conversion from mild cognitive impairment to Alzheimer's dementia. *Neurobiol Aging.*, *35*(1), 143-151.

Tsitsopoulos, P. P. & Marklund, N. (2013). Amyloid-β Peptides and Tau Protein as Biomarkers in Cerebrospinal and Interstitial Fluid Following Traumatic Brain Injury: A Review of Experimental and Clinical Studies. *Front Neurol.*, *4*, 79.

Tsuruoka, M., Hara, J., Hirayama, A., Sugimoto, M., Soga, T., Shankle, W. R. & Tomita, M. (2013). CE-MS-based metabolome analysis of serum and saliva from neurodegenerative dementia patients. *Electrophoresis.*, *34*, 2865-2872.

Van der Mussele, S., Marien, P., Saerens, J., Somers, N., Goeman, J., De Deyn, P. P. & Engelborghs, S. (2014). Behavioral Syndromes in Mild Cognitive Impairment and Alzheimer's Disease. *J Alzheimers Dis.*, *38*(2), 319-29.

Vasunilashorn, S., Glei, D. A., Lin, Y. H. & Goldman, N. (2013). Apolipoprotein e and measured physical and pulmonary function in older Taiwanese adults. *Biodemography Soc Biol.*, *59*, 57-67.

Vellas, B., Carrillo, M. C., Sampaio, C., Brashear, H. R., Siemers, E., Hampel, H., Schneider, L. S., et al., (2013). EU/US/CTAD Task Force Members. Designing drug trials for Alzheimer's disease: what we have learned from the release of the phase III antibody trials: a report from the EU/US/CTAD Task Force. *Alzheimers Dement.*, *9*, 438-444.

Wahlster, P., Niederländer, C., Kriza, C., Schaller, S. & Kolominsky-Rabas, P. L. (2013). Clinical Assessment of Amyloid Imaging in Alzheimer's Disease: A Systematic Review of the Literature. *Front Hum Neurosci.*, *7*, 456.

Wang, L., Brier, M. R., Snyder, A. Z., Thomas, J. B., Fagan, A. M., Xiong, C., Benzinger, T. L., Holtzman, D. M., Morris, J. C. & Ances, B. M. (2013). Cerebrospinal Fluid Aβ42, Phosphorylated Tau181, and Resting-State Functional Connectivity. *JAMA Neurol.*, *70*(10), 1242-1248.

Weiner, M. W., Veitch, D. P., Aisen, P. S., Beckett, L. A., Cairns, N. J., Green, R. C., Harvey, D., Jack, C. R., Jagust, W., Liu, E., Morris, J. C., Petersen, R. C., Saykin, A. J., Schmidt, M. E., Shaw, L., Shen, L., Siuciak, J. A., Soares, H., Toga, A. W. & Trojanowski, J. Q. (2013). Alzheimer's Disease Neuroimaging Initiative. The

Alzheimer's Disease Neuroimaging Initiative: A review of papers published since its inception. *Alzheimers Dement.*, S1552-5260(13)02429-1.

Weinstein, G., Beiser, A. S., Decarli, C., Au, R., Wolf, P. A. & Seshadri, S. (2013). Brain Imaging and Cognitive Predictors of Stroke and Alzheimer Disease in the Framingham Heart Study. *Stroke.*, *44*(10), 2787-94.

White, M. T. & Xie, S. X. (2013). Adjustment for measurement error in evaluating diagnostic biomarkers by using an internal reliability sample. *Stat Med.*, *32*, 4679-58.

Xiang, Y., Lam, S. M. & Shui, G. (2015). What can lipidomics tell us about the pathogenesis of Alzheimer disease? *Biol Chem.*, Jul 31.

Yamamoto, T., Uchiyama, T., Higuchi, Y., Asahina, M., Hirano, S., Yamanaka, Y. & Kuwabara, S. (2015). Subthalamic nucleus deep brain stimulation modulate catecholamine levels with significant relation to clinical outcome after surgery in patients with Parkinson's disease. *PLOS*, Sep 22.

Yang, A. C., Wang, S. J., Lai, K. L., Tsai, C. F., Yang, C. H., Hwang, J. P., Lo, M. T., Huang, N. E., Peng, C. K. & Fuh, J. L. (2013). Cognitive and neuropsychiatric correlates of EEG dynamic complexity in patients with Alzheimer's disease. *Prog Neuropsychopharmacol Biol Psychiatry.*, *47*, 52-61.

Yarchoan, M., Louneva, N., Xie, S. X., Swenson, F. J., Hu, W., Soares, H., Trojowski, J. Q., Lee, V. M., Kling, M. A., Shaw, L. M., Chen-Plotkin, A., Wolk, D. A. & Arnold, S. E. (2013). Association of plasma C-reactive protein levels with the diagnosis of Alzheimer's disease. *J Neurol Sci.*, *333*(1-2), 9-12.

Yon, J. M., Lin, C., Oh, K. W., Baek, H. S., Lee, B. J., Yun, Y. W. & Nam, S. Y. (2013). Emodin prevents Ethanol-induced developmental anomalies in cultured mouse fetus through multiple activities. *Birth Defects Res B Dev Reprod Toxicol.*, *98*, 268-275.

Younesi, E. & Hofmann-Apitius, M. (2013). A network model of genomic hormone interactions underlying dementia and its translational validation through serendipitous off-target effect. *J Transl Med.*, *11*, 177.

Zetterberg, H., Andreasson, U., Hansson, O., Wu, G., Sankaranarayanan, S., Andersson, M. E., Buchhave, P., Londos, E., et al., (2008). "Elevated cerebrospinal fluid BACE1 activity in incipient Alzheimer disease". *Archives of Neurology*, *65*(8), 1102–1107.

Zhang, H. Y., Xie, C., Chen, G., Zhang, Z. J., Gao-Jun Teng, G. J. & Li, S. J. (2013). Modular reorganization of brain resting state networks and its independent validation in Alzheimer's disease patients. *Front Hum Neurosci*, *7*, 456.

Zhang, A. H., Sun, H. & Wang, X. J. (2013). Recent advances in metabolomics in neurological disease, and future perspectives. *Anal Bioanal Chem.*, *405*(25), 8143-8150.

Zhang, S., Lei, C., Liu, P., Zhang, M., Tao, W., Liu, H. & Liu, M. (2-15). Association between variant amyloid deposits and motor deficits in FAD-associated presenilin-1 mutations: A systematic review. *Neuroscience & Biobehavioral Reviews*, *56*, 180–192.

Zhou, F. C., Balaraman, Y., Teng, M., Liu, Y., Singh, R. P. & Nephew, K. P. (2011). Alcohol alters DNA methylation patterns and inhibits neural stem cell differentiation. *Alcohol Clin Exp Res.*, *35*, 735-746.

Zhou, X. & Xu, J. (2015). Identification of Alzheimer's disease-associated long noncoding RNAs. *Neurobiol Aging.*, *36*(11), 2925-2031.

Chapter 11

BIOMARKERS IN PERSONALIZED THERANOSTICS OF VASCULAR DEMENTIA

ABSTRACT

Vascular dementia (VaD) affects millions of patients with various manifestations of cognitive decline, which could be attributed to cerebrovascular or cardiovascular diseases. Theranostics of VaD depends on the identification of environmental and genetic risk factors including; cerebral autosomal-dominant arteriopathy with subcortical infarcts and leukoencephalopathy (CADASIL). Mitochondrial oxidative stress, hypoxic-ischemia, inflammation, accumulation of advanced glycation products, and pro-inflammatory cytokines were held responsible in the pathogenesis of VaD. Hence it is exceedingly prudent to determine the risk factors and molecular pathology by investigating specific biomarkers which can be classified as: biochemical, molecular, genetic, endocrinological, anatomical, imaging, and neuropathological; for the early EBPT of VaD. The biomarkers of VaD in the serum and CSF samples include; β-amyloid, phosphorylated tau, matrix metalloproteases (MMPs), sulfatids, albumin, and pro-inflammatory C-reactive proteins. In addition, Charnoly Body (CB) formation and microRNAs can be detected as pre-apoptotic biomarkers of compromised mitochondrial bioenergetics to further authenticate VaD theranostics. CB formation occurs in response to nutritional stress and/or neurotoxic insult in the most vulnerable hippocampal neurons due to cerebrovascular insufficiency, which can be attenuated by dietary interventions, physiological Zinc, and metallothioneins (MTs). MTs provide ubiquinone (CQ_{10})-mediated neuroprotection by serving as free radical scavengers, by maintaining the mitochondrial redox balance, by inhibiting CB formation, and by inhibiting progressive neurodegenerative α-synucleinopathies. MTs also activate Zinc-mediated transcriptional regulation of genes involved in cell growth, proliferation, differentiation, and development; hence may be utilized as novel biomarkers of VaD. In addition to genetic analysis of MTs, NOTCH 3, APOE 4, NOS, and CADASIL; omics and microRNA analyses may provide novel biomarkers to accomplish EBPT of VaD. This chapter provides recent update on *in-vitro* biomarkers from the serum and CSF and *in-vivo* neuroimaging biomarkers for the differential diagnosis and effective EBPT of VaD.

Keywords: neuroimaging, Charnoly body, evidence-based personalized theranostics (EBPT), cerebral autosomal-dominant arteriopathy with subcortical infarcts and leukoencephalopathy (CADASIL).

INTRODUCTION

Dementia is defined as a progressive neurodegenerative disease characterized by loss of cognition and functional disability in day to day life (Mills et al., 2007; Kirshner, 2009). It is currently considered as a major public health problem affecting >20 million people and the number is alarmingly increasing in industrially-developed countries (Shoji (2011). The prevalence of two major types of dementia, Alzheimer Disease (AD) and vascular dementia (VaD) is ~4.4% and 1 to 2% respectively in the industrially-developed countries; however its prevalence is lower in the developing countries (Ray et al., 2013). AD accounts for 70-75% cases of dementia in elderly whereas, VaD comprises a small but significant group accounting to ~20% cases, the second most common form of dementia after AD (Simonsen et al., 2012). Vascular co-morbidity may exist in >30% patients with AD and >50% patients with VaD may exhibit pathology associated with AD, suggesting a 3.4 to 73% overlap between AD and VaD (Formichi et al., 2010). Hence, the diagnosis of dementia is challenging as in many elderly patients both the entities may coexist with other neurodegenerative diseases (*often termed as mixed dementia*). The original term '*multi infarct dementia*' is now replaced by an updated term *vascular cognitive impairment* (VCI) which refers to any cognitive impairment caused by or associated with vascular risk factors and ranges from mild cognitive impairment to overt dementia (Legge and Hachinski, 2010).

Generally VaD may be caused by hemorrhagic, ischemic, and hypoxic injury to brain. VaD is a group of heterogeneous disorders in which the presence of ischemia/infarction may cause cognitive decline however, the degree of such impairment is directly proportional to the extent of neuronal damage and location of the lesion (Chui et al., 2006; Giannakopoulos et al. 2007; Grinberg et al., 2010). The National Institute of Neurological Disorders and Stroke and Association internationale pour la Recherche et l'Enseignement en Neurosciences (NINDS-AIREN) state that small vessel disease such as microvascular angiopathy (*lacunar infarction*), periventricular ischemia, and large vessel athero-embolic disease causing territorial infarction can result in cognitive impairment and may be included as a criteria of VaD theranostics (Roman et al., 1993). Numerous possible pathogenic factors including: accumulation of advanced glycation end-products (AGE) and activation of pro-inflammatory cytokines (i.e., IL1β, TNFα, IL-6, C-reactive protein, and NFκβ), including experimental studies on animals and cultured neurons demonstrated that oxidative stress, mitochondrial dysfunction, inflammatory response and accumulation of abnormal β- amyloid are involved in the etiopathogenesis of VaD (Ray et al., 2013). According to California criteria; theranostics of VaD requires neuropathological assessment, Computed tomography (CT), Positron emission tomography (PET), Magnetic resonance imaging (MRI), and Magnetic resonance spectroscopy (MRS) (Chui et al., 1992; Wetterling et al., 1996; Erkinjuntti and Gauthier, 2009). Generally, the risk factors for stroke are also the risk factors for dementia. Clinically-evident hypertension has a significant association with dementia while hyperlipidemia and metabolic syndrome could be predictive of dementia risk (Forette et al., 1998; Shumaker et al., 2003; Rapp et al., 2003; Kirshner 2009). Transient ischemic attacks (TIA) also predispose to increased risk of stroke and 30% of the patients who suffer stroke develop dementia within 6 to 12 months. Although the exact etiopathogenesis of VaD remains unknown, diabetes mellitus, hormone replacement therapy for post-menopausal women, obesity, improper dietary habits including; food rich in trans saturated fats and lacking omega-3 fatty acids

(Docohexanoic acid: DHA, and Eicosapentanoic acid: EPA) and polyunsaturated fatty acids (Linoeic acid, Linolinic acid and Arachidonic acid), various environmental neurotoxins, drug addiction, aging, and unhealthy life style including sedentary life style, tobacco and alcohol intake, lack of exercise, physical and mental stress, overmedication and late night sleep have been proposed in the etiopathogenesis of VaD and can aggravate the disease process. Several of these risk factors excluding genetic may be prevented by dietary manipulations, moderate exercise, and healthy life style modifications. Age of onset of stroke and lack of education are also associated with higher risk of dementia (Kirshner 2009). CADASIL, an inherited disorder, manifested as syndrome of migraine, mood disorder, recurrent TIA, stroke, and early development of dementia; the root cause of which is primarily microvascular disease, is an independent age-related pathogenesis of AD and VaD. Owing to the diversified risk factors, further studies are needed to understand the exact etiopathogenesis of VaD.

In this chapter, recent update on various *in-vitro* biomarkers from the serum and CSF samples and *in-vivo* multimodality neuroimaging biomarkers for the effective EBPT of VaD are described systematically. It is envisaged that the information in this chapter will be of considerable interest to medical students, clinicians, and basic researchers interested in learning more about this devastating progressive neurodegenerative disorder of unknown etiopathogenesis.

Classification of Biomarkers in VaD Indeed accurate classification of dementia would significantly impact the theranostics of dementia. Currently, there is no approved drug for the treatment of VaD. Hence, it is exceedingly important to reduce the risk factors and provide adequate treatment with proper vascular agents for preventing and/or prolonging the onset of VaD. The major risk factors, hypertension, and hyperlipidemia can be controlled only with conventional treatment to reduce the risk of VaD. Therefore there is a dire need to classify and determine the specific etiology of dementia based on the biomarkers analyses. These biomarkers must be easily measurable to facilitate early theranostics. In this regard, the surrogate biomarkers of VaD, based on functional neuroimaging, CSF and blood based analysis have gained importance as these are noninvasive and easy to perform as compared to pathological analysis on postmortem brain samples. Moreover pre-mortem analysis of these biomarkers would enhance the thranostic capability of VaD (Quinn et al., 2010). The most significant VaD biomarkers which could be used for the early theranostics of VaD can be broadly classified as: clinical biomarkers (neurobehavioral assessment), pathological biomarkers (identifying cellular/histological changes), biochemical biomarkers (serum, plasma, CSF biomarkers), neuroimaging biomarkers including: multimodality fusion imaging with CT, MRI/MRS, PET, and SPECT imaging to acquire structural as well as functional information simultaneously regarding the diseases process, genetic biomarkers (identifying genes involved in cerbrovascular disease), omics and microRNA biomarkers (identifying subcellular components of VaD).

There are various *risk factors involved in the pathogenesis of VaD.* Various risk factors including hypertension, hyperlipidemia, obesity, drugs of abuse, overmedication, hormone replacement therapy, and environmental factors could lead to the pathogenesis of VaD. Activation of pro-inflammatory cytokines, abnormal accumulation of amyloid–β, accumulation of advanced glycation products, inflammation, and mitochondrial oxidative stress are caused by hypoxia, hemorrhage, and ischemia, resulting in the pathogenesis of VaD. Various biomarkers in VaD such as: Omics/microRNA, genetic biomarkers, neuroimaging biomarkers, CSF and serum biochemical biomarkers, pathological biomarkers, and clinical biomarkers, which can be used for the differential diagnosis, prognosis, and effective treatment of VaD. These biomarkers possess moderate diagnostic utility. Apolipoprotein-A1, dimers of apolipoprotein-A2, albumin, and immunoglobulin-G have higher levels in the CSF samples of VaD compared to AD patients, whereas integral membrane 2B-C, terminal fragment, C3a peptide lacking c-terminal arginine, cystatin-C, ubiquitin-3a from CT, neuroendocrine protein 7B2 (secretogranin V), and C4a peptide des-Arg levels are lower in VaD as compared to AD patients. Several *candidate biomarkers of VaD in plasma/serum are:* C-reactive protein, homocysteine, lipoprotein-A, malondialdehyde, total –SH, calcium, magnesium, thyroid stimulating hormone (TSH) β sceratase, and neprilysin levels are increased in VaD as compared to normal control and AD patients. DHEA-S levels remain unaltered in VaD but are reduced in AD patients. Folate and vitamin B_{12} and s-RAGE are lowered in VaD as compared to AD patients. Genes predisposing to cerebrovascular disease are ACE, AGT, eNOS, PON, and MTHFR, MEF2A, ALOX5, LTA, APOM, and PDE4D. Genes which influence the brain tissue responses include neurotropic factors brain-derived growth factor (BDNF), nerve growth factor (NGF), and vascular endothelial-derived growth factor (VEGF), apo-E, and MMPss, glutamate and GABA receptors, adhesion molecules, transcription factors, ion channels, NOS pathways genes. The genes known to alter risk of cerebro-vascular diseases in community are: PDE4D, ALOX-5AP, LTA4H, chromosome-9 p21, 4q25, APO-4 in CADASIL, Specific pathways genes such as APP, PPAR-γ, LPL and LIPC. *Omega-3 fatty acids and PUFA* can regulate the function of various VaD biomarkers. Various risk factors including altered circadian rhythms, drug abuse, environmental and psychological stress, and lack of exercise can induce CB formation, and obesity due to abnormal microRNA and abnormal adipogenesis as a consequence of leptin and orexin gene dysregulation. Omega-3 fatty and PUFA prevent vascular dementia by providing new membrane synthesis and stabilization.

Several methods of collection, detection, and analysis of proteins in the CSF and plasma samples of VaD patients have been described including; purification of candidate biomarkers (*chromatographic and electrophoresis*) and protein profiling employing multiplex enzyme-linked immunosorbent assay (ELISA), surface enhanced laser desorption/ionization time of flight mass spectrometry (SELDI-TOF), and peptide mass fingerprinting (Formichi et al., 2010; Simonsen et al., 2012). Various statistical methods to calculate probability, sensitivity, and specificity were described to determine the theranostic utility of these biomarkers. Although several biomarkers were correlated with underlying pathological processes at the cellular and molecular level; the biochemical biomarkers were directly correlated with clinical and imaging findings in dementia. However, their pathological correlation is yet to be established (Pluta et al., 2009; Kaerst et al., 2013). Humpel (2011) highlighted that the detection of biomarkers in CSF can only support the clinical diagnosis of VaD. Recent studies on biomarkers emphasized on inflammation, hemostasis, oxidative stress, hypoxia-ischemia, accumulation of biochemical substances, complex proteins and other metabolites in the hypertensive-atheromatous disease and hyperlipidemia in tissue and CSF (Pantoni et al., 2006; Ray et al., 2013).

CSF Biomarkers of VaD Although, biomarkers can be quantitatively estimated in various body fluids such as saliva, blood, urine and tissue; CSF has been studied extensively because it drains the ventricular system of the brain and concentration of various metabolites may directly reflect various pathological processes in the brain providing a lead to develop sensitive and specific biomarkers to differentially diagnose various etiological types of dementia (Humpel 2011). CSF biomarkers in dementia have been reported extensively in AD and have shown promise as sensitive theranostic tool however, limited studies are yet available in this direction and the candidate CSF biomarkers studied so far exhibit conflicting results and lack specificity due to heterogenous nature of VaD. Similarly protein biomarkers are not specific to VaD; nevertheless when used in combination can increase the theranostic certainty of VaD (Pantoni and Sarti, 2006). In this context, CSF serum albumin ratio, CSF index and CSF total protein are biomarkers having high diagnostic value as these can accurately identify structural and functional integrity of the blood-brain barrier and microvascular damage. An increased albumin level and increased index is well established, however they are unspecific and may not distinguish VaD from AD (Wardlaw et al., 2006; (Leblanc et al., 2006). Sulfatide a biomarker for demyelination, is used to identify the extent of demyelination in the white matter and is elevated in VaD. The cytoskeletal organelle, neurofilament is estimated to evaluate axonal degeneration and white matter damage, is increased in CSF samples of VaD patients, but not in patients with AD pathology; indicating axonal damage as a characteristic feature of VaD (Tullberg et al., 2000; Tullberg et al., 1992; Wallin et al., 2001). Furthermore, the matrix metalloproteases (MMPs) in the CSF, have been estimated to identify changes in the extracellular matrix associated with vascular diseases with inflammation. MMPs attack the myelin and are considered as biomarkers of demyelination. Various studies have shown that MMPs are increased in patients with VaD (Glavin et al., 2011; Rosenberg et al., 2001; Liuzzi et al., 2002). Several CSF biomarkers were used for evaluating their theranostic utility in AD. Conflicting results were reported and their potential utility lies in differentiating VaD from AD and the other neurodegenerative diseases. These studies showed significant overlap between VaD and AD (Simonsen et al., 2012; Formichi et al., 2010). However, serum to CSF Folate ratio can be used to differentiate VaD from AD. This ratio is significantly reduced in VaD. The reduced folate ratio is a characteristic of VaD (Hagnelius et al., 2008; Simonsen et al., 2012). In addition, AD is characterized by Aβ plaque deposition irrespective of its etiopathogenesis. Aβ (1-42) is peptide formed after Aβ is cleaved from Amyloid Precursor Protein by secretases. A significant reduction of Aβ 42 in patients with AD as well as VaD suggests a significant overlap making it difficult to distinguish AD from VaD. Amyloid β (1-42), total tau & phosphorylated tau (p-tau) are extensively studied in AD and there are numerous reports on their theranostic utility in AD. Increased CSF levels of tau and decreased levels of Aβ 42 were detected in AD as well as VaD; but more specifically in AD. Hence a combined analysis of these CSF biomarkers is recommended for the differential theranostics of VaD (Kaerst et al., 2013; Paraskevas et al., 2009; Thaweepoksomboon et al., 2011; Pluta et al., 2011; Schoonenboom etal., 2012).

The protein biomarkers represent various physiological processes such as degradation (*ubiquitin*), protease inhibition (*Cystatin C and α-1 Anti-Chymotrypsin*), inflammation (*C3a, C4a*) are associated with neurodegenerative diseases including all forms of dementia. However their theranostic utility is enhanced when used along with Folate ratio, Amyloid β (1-42), total tau, or p-tau levels. However, these biomarkers lack specificity and need to be validated and investigated in large prospective multicentric trials. A biomarker of neuronal death, heart fatty acid binding protein (HFABP) is elevated in CSF from patients with various neurodegenerative diseases. Although HFABP can be detected in VaD and AD, it lacks specificity (Olsson et al., 2013).

Serum and Plasma Biomarkers of VaD Apart from CSF, certain biomarkers have been identified in the serum and plasma samples of patients with VaD, AD, and other neurodegenerative diseases. C-reactive protein is inflammatory biomarker and its levels are elevated in VaD. Hyperhomocysteinemeia is a well established vascular risk factor and its increased levels authenticate causal relationship with vascular lesion and thereby VaD (Chacon et al., 2004; Malaguarnera et al., 2004). Elevated levels of serum Homocysteine were also observed in AD patients and are implicated in the vascular pathogenesis of AD. Recently several studies revealed that elevated serum Homocysteine is associated with hippocampal and cortical atrophy in patients with VaD (Den et al., 2003). Although deficiency of Vitamin B_{12} and Folate causes Hyperhomocysteinemia, the supplementation of these vitamins failed to produce any improvement in patients with dementia. Hence the theranstic role of Homocysteine in VaD remains controversial (Aisen et al., 2008). Elevated Lipoprotein a [Lipo (a)] is considered as an independent genetic risk factor for VaD, but not in AD, which facilitates understanding the pathogenesis of atherogenic processes in VaD (Berglund et al., 2004; Tsimikas et al., 2012).

Dehydroepiandrosterone (DHEA) and its metabolite, Dehydroepiandrosterone Sulphate (DHEA-S) have neuroprotective effects. Their levels in CNS are increased in neurodegenerative diseases. However it remains uncertain whether altered levels of DHEA-S in circulation is a cause or effect of VaD (Kurata et al., 2004; Naylor et al., 2008; Aldred et al., 2010). Serum level of DHEA-S remained unaltered as reported by a few studies on patients with VaD. A detailed study is needed to determine the exact clinical significance of these and other biomarkers in the differential theranostics of VaD, as several factors may influence their levels in blood. Furthermore, these biomarker studies should be correlated and confirmed with imaging and histopathological studies to authenticate VaD theranostics. Similarly oxidative stressors such as Malondialdehyde (MDA), Thyroid Stimulating Hormone (TSH), Calcium and Magnesium are nonspecifically elevated in patients with dementia suggesting their involvement in the vascular etiopathogenesis of dementing illnesses (Forti et al., 2012).

The receptor for advanced glycation end products (RAGE) is cell-bound and belongs to immunoglobulin superfamily, which may be activated by pro-inflammatory ligands including advanced glycol-oxidation end products and β-amyloid peptide. Clinical studies showed that higher plasma levels of RAGE are associated with reduced risk of coronary artery disease, hypertension, metabolic syndrome, arthritis, and AD (Hamaguchi and Yamada, 2008). Similarly atherosclerotic cerebrovascular disease is a significant cause of VaD. So, protective nature of this biomarker requires further validation. It was demonstrated that only RAGE and Beta-site APP cleaving enzyme 1 (BACE-1) are predictor of cognitive impairment after stroke, however, there was no association with Neprilysin (NEP) or Apolipoprotein E (APOE) (Geroldi et al., 2008). Whether these biomarkers may help in distinguishing VaD from vascular cognitive impairment after acute ischemic stroke, remains unknown. Increased levels of Thrombin, D-Dimer, and Thrombin fragment 1+2, and biomarkers of endothelial dysfunction; Von Willebrand factor, and Plasminogen Activator Inhibitor are associated with cerebrovascular thrombosis and thereby VaD. This association may be secondary to chronic inflammation. These mechanisms may underlie prothrombotic state, cerebral microinfarction, and eventually subcortical small vessel infarction. Most of the cases of dementia have mixed etiopathogenesis contributing a variable amount of vascular pathology (Neuropathology group of the Medical Research Council Cognitive Function and Aging Study) (Casserly and Topol, 2004; MRC-CFAS, 2001).

Genetic Biomarkers of VaD It is now recognized that identifying new risk factors for ischemic stroke could help improve prevention strategies and identify new theranostic targets in VaD. Genetic risk factors are particularly interesting, because they confer a direct clue to the biological pathways involved. Ischemic stroke is a heterogeneous disorder, and must be considered for genetic susceptibility factors. In Western countries, most ischemic strokes can be attributed to large-artery atherosclerosis (*atherothrombotic stroke*) and small-artery occlusion (*lacunar stroke*) (Debette and Seshadri, 2009). The genes underlying VCI are of two exclusive classes: (a) genes that predispose individuals to cerebrovascular disease, and (b) genes that determine tissue responses to cerebrovascular disease (e.g., genes conveying ischemic tolerance or susceptibility, or the ability to recover from ischemic insult) (Forti et al., 2010). In the first category, genes that confer susceptibility to hypertension and atherosclerosis were identified with some monogenic forms of disease such as CADASIL, induced by mutations in NOTCH 3 gene. In the the the second category; genes that modify tissue responses to injury were also identified and at least three sets of genes in the AD pathway, the Presenilins, Amyloid Precursor Protein (APP), and APOE interact with the VCI disease pathway. The Presenilins mutations causing AD, interact directly with Notch proteins, including Notch 3 (*mutations of which cause CADASIL*) (Haritunians et al., 2005; Gridley, 2007; Marchesi, 2014). There is direct evidence from both human and animal studies for specific non-AD genes that play a significant role in tissue responses to ischemia. Earlier studies in humans suggest that variants in the genes for platelet glycoprotein and α-Fibrinogen affect post stroke outcomes without affecting stroke risk.

Animal studies suggested glutamate and γ-aminobutyric acid receptors, acid-sensing ion channels, proteases, growth factors and their receptors, and transcription factors as the major molecules involved in influencing brain responses to cerebro-vascular injury (Lo et al., 2003; Rosenstein et al., 2004). In addition, chromosome 9p21.3 genotype is associated with VaD and AD (Emanuele et al. (2011). Linkage and association analyses (including single nucleotide polymorphism EDN1, MHTFR, and NOS3, APOE 4) and AGTR1, AGTR2 of renal angiotensin system) have association of these genes with the pathogenesis of small vessel disease, CVD, and VaD. The genes/molecules are studied extensively in relation to the cardiovascular disease and attempts are being made to determine predisposition to cerebrovascular disease and VaD (Debette and Seshadri, 2009; Visvikis-Siest and Marteau., 2006). Genetic diseases such as Sickle Cell disease, Fabry disease, and Homocysteinuria, and genes involved in inflammation (LTC4S, IL-6), thrombosis (TGB3, factor VIII), lipid metabolism (APOE, PON 1 PON2, PON3, APOA5, LPL, LDL), endothelial function and oxidative stress (NOS3, MTHFR) and genes identified through linkage analysis in an Icelandic population (ALOX5, PDE4d) are all candidate biomarkers to establish association with cerebrovascular disease, ischemia-stroke, and VaD (Debette and Seshadri, 2009). There are limited studies available regarding the genetic biomarkers in VaD. Hence potential genetic and molecular biomarkers of VaD such as genes responsible for cerebrovascular disease, genes influencing the native tissue response and molecules such as soluble receptor levels for various metabolites and enzymes in VaD have been proposed as potential biomarkers to correlate and confirm pathogenesis of VaD. Further studies are needed to establish their clinical significance (Hamaguchi and Yamada, 2008; Battistin and Cagnin 2010). The proposed biomarker genes predisposing to cerebrovascular disease are ACE,

AGT, eNOS, PON and MTHFR, MEF2A, ALOX5, LTA, APOM, PDE4D. Certain genes can influence the brain tissue response to VaD such as: Neurotrophic Factors: BDNF, NGF, vascular growth factors (VEGF), APOE, MMPss, Glutamate, and GABA receptors, Adhesion Molecules, Transcription Factors, Ion Channels, NOS pathway genes, and genes/loci those alter risk of VaD in a community are PDE4D, ALOX5AP, LTA4H, 9p21, 4q25, APOE 4 in CADASIL, Specific Pathway Genes, APP, PPAR-γ, LPL and LIPC (Visvikis-Siest and Marteau, 2006; Debette et al., 2009).

miRNA Biomarkers in VaD Various types of microRNAs are impaired due to abnormal adipogenesis in obesity to influence the genetic predisposition of VaD. A further study is required to determine their exact significance in the theranostic management of VaD. Further studies employing omics biotechnology and microRNA analysis would provide precise knowledge regarding the exact etiopathogenesis and theranostic management of VaD in future. Early mild cognitive impairment (MCI) syndrome *in vitro* can be estimated by quantitative estimation of brain-enriched cell-free miR (microRNAs) in the blood is possible by RT-qPCR method. As miRNAs are important epigenetic regulators of numerous cellular processes including neurodegenerative diseases, specific miRNAs such as the miR-132 and miR-134 families paired with miR-491-5p and miR-370, respectively have proven most suitable for detecting MCI of varied etiology and AD. In addition, the use of brain-enriched neurites/synapses miRNA enables detection of early pathologic events occurring in degenerating neurons (Munekazu, 2012). Numerous miRNAs including guardian of endothelial cells, miR 126 and others are found in vascular inflammatory processes could serve as biomarkers of early detection of vascular cognitive impairment. Also, theranostic potential of miRNAs is a future challenge. The invention of novel modifications of RNA bases and the synthesis of artificial antisense miRNA or antagomir, may be used as novel therapeutic tools to manipulate miRNA and control vascular inflammatory diseases (Munekazu, 2012). Although free radicals can induce inflammation by activating redox-sensitive pro-inflammatory transcription factors, the endothelial dysfunction induced by oxidative stress can release VEGFs and prostanoids promoting vascular leakage, protein extravasation, and cytokine production. Inflammation enhances oxidative stress by upregulating the expression of ROS–producing enzymes and downregulating antioxidant defenses. miRNAs of these transcription factors can act as potential biomarkers in circulation for VaD. A study suggests Dicer1 (*Ribonuclease III*) as a key enzyme of the miRNA machinery, which is responsible for synthesis of mature functional miRNAs (Ungvari et al., 2013). There is evidence that Dicer1 in endothelial cells may regulate angiogenic processes, a biomarker to be explored as theranostic target in VaD. Role of dysregulation of Dicer1 in age-related impairment of angiogenesis identified a number of miRNAs that are downregulated in CMVECs in dementia. Aging induces cerebromicrovascular rarefaction and impaired cerebral angiogenesis in response to hypoxia or VEGF administration. This plays a predominant role in impairment of regional cerebral blood flow and the occurrence of VCI as a function of aging. Because the role of miRNA regulation and function in the 'aging vascular system' is an emerging area, further investigations are needed to determine the contribution of individual miRNAs or miRNA familes in gene expression that underlie microvascular aging and hence, VaD.

Biomarkers of Cell-Based Therapy for VaD There are limited studies as yet available on the therapeutic potential of cell-based therapy in VaD. Laboratory studies showed that transplanted bone marrow stem cells improve neurological diseases of the CNS by generating neural cells or myelin-producing oligodendroglial cells and by enhancing neural plasticity (Brenneman et al., 2010; Sharma and Ebadi, 2011a; Sharma and Ebadi, 2011b; Sharma et al., 2011; Yang et al., 2010). However there has been lack of objective data providing evidence for clinical improvement. Autologous bone marrow derived mononuclear cells were administered intrathecally to a 61 year old woman who was diagnosed with VaD (Sharma et al., 2012). After follow up of 2 years she showed clinical signs of improvements as assessed by MMSE and FIM along with PET/CT neuroimaging. Improved metabolic activity in this patient provided evidence of benefits of cell-based therapy and suggestion to investigate various stem cell biomarkers employing omics biotechnology in future studies on VaD. Recently significant efforts were made to explore the basic molecular mechanisms of atherosclerosis *(the underlying cause of cerebrovascular and cardiovascular disease)*, which remains a major cause of morbidity and mortality worldwide. Because of the complex pathophysiology of cardiovascular disease, different research methods have been combined to unravel genetic aspects, molecular pathways, and cellular functions involved in atherogenesis, vascular inflammation, and dyslipidemia to gain a multifaceted picture addressing this complexity. Recent evolution of high-throughput technologies can generate data at the DNA, RNA, and protein levels with sophisticated bioinformatic technology. These data sets are integrated to enhance information and are being used as regulated networks. Various genomics, transcriptomics, proteomics, and epigenomics—and systems biology data were acquired to explore pathomechanisms of vascular inflammation and atherosclerosis (Doring et al., 2012).

Cerebrolysin, a naturally occurring substance represents a therapeutic strategy for neurological disorders like dementia, stroke, and traumatic brain injury (Chen et al., 2013). It is a neuro-peptide mimicking the action of neurotrophic factors that enhances neurogenesis, sustaining the brain's self-repair, promotes neural progenitor cell migration, synaptic density rebuilding neuronal cytoarchitecture, restorative processes, decreases the infarct volume and edema formation, and augments neuronal recovery. Since mitochondrial redox balance is impaired as a consequence of brain regional cerebrovascular insufficiency, antioxidants such as Quercetin and Isoquercitrin as natural flavonoids may help to provide mitochondrial neuroprotection in VaD. Similarly Melatonin reduces free radical generation by enhancing Glutathione levels. Neurotrophic factors such as Nerve Growth Factor (NGF), Glial Cell-Derived Neurotrophic Factor (GDNF) and Brain-Derived Neurotrophic Factor (BDNF) have already been implicated as targets for the theranostic management of various neurodegenerative diseases. These neurotropic factors are generally present in significantly high amounts in the bone marrow-derived mononuclear cells. A recombinant DNA vaccine is composed of domains of NOIs (Neurite Outgrowth Inhibitors). The immunological mechanism inducing effective antibodies against the specific domains and the modulation of mRNA expression regarding NOIs could help in repair/regeneration of neural and oligodendrocytic damage. Stem cells might be an alternative to brain regeneration. In experimental models of acute ischemic stroke (AIS) using Q-dot labeled MNCs, the researchers established that these cells exhibit preferential chemotaxis in the periinfarcted region and are exponentially eliminated as a function of time (Brenneman et al., 2009). Although the exact molecular mechanism of neuroprotection by MNCs remains enigmatic, it is assumed that it could be through autocrine and paracrine mechanism by local release of neuroprotective biomarkers such as; Insulin Like Growth Factor (IGF-1), Endothelial Derived Growth Factor (EDGF), von Wilebrand Factor (VWF), and Granulocyte Colony Stimulating

Factor (G-CSF), and IL-4 and IL-10 as an anti-inflammatory cytokines. Naive human chorionic villi and amniotic fluid derived cells release significant amounts of BDNF, as well as VEGF. In addition, Nimodipine as an L-type voltage-dependent Ca^{2+} channel antagonist and an anti hypertensive agent can also reduce ischemic nerve cell death in VaD. Further studies in this direction promise to discover sensitive and specific biomarkers to accomplish EBPT of VaD.

Neuroimaging Biomarkers Neuro-imaging has been studied extensively in various types of dementia including VaD. Particularly CT and MRI specific changes have been identified as potential biomarkers demonstrating mechanisms of vascular injury and their effects in the parenchyma, which can be detected in all the stages of VaD. Phase contrast MRI and the analyses of hemodynamics in the brain were regarded as potential biomarkers, however their sensitivity and specificity needs further evaluation. Neuroimaging findings correlate very well with the underlying pathological processes and hence have gained significance in research and theranostic investigation on VaD. It has been confirmed that T_2 weighted MRI sequences alone or in combination with CT can identify Leukoaraiosis (*white matter lesions*), Microvascular Angiopathy, Lacunar Infarction, Dilation of Virchow –Robin Spaces, Pulse Wave Encephalopathy, parameters of cerebral embolic disease, which were correlated with post mortem findings of vascular pathology of dementia. However, there is still a need for the development of imaging parameters having diagnostic utility but also having capacity of determining etiopathogenesis, differentiating VaD from AD and other neurodegenerative diseases. *Ligand Specific Positron Emission Tomography (PET)* and Single Photon Emission Computed Tomography (SPECT) will serve as future theranostic methods when these ligands are developed for different proteins detected in VaD e.g., *Tau, Aβ 40* and several others. Arterial Spin Labeling, which measures absolute blood flow though cerebral vessels, confers better results than SPECT in detecting hypoperfused areas. Moreover it is cost effective and avoids use of radioactive substances. *Functional MRI (fMRI)* can assess neuronal function through blood oxygen level-dependent (BOLD) changes. Although the neurovascular mechanism underlying BOLD changes is still poorly understood, fMRI is used in neurological research. Furthermore, T_2-T_2'-T_2 Relaxometry and susceptibility-weighted magnetic resonance imaging takes into account not only the magnitude but also the phase and signals for gradient echo MRI sequence. The ability of susceptibility-weighted MRI which is able to differentiate Calcium, Iron and hemorrhagic products, can be promising biomarkers in differentiating the aging brain from VaD (Vitali et al., 2008).

Pathological Biomarkers of VaD The exact diagnosis of VaD depends on the histopathological analysis of post mortem brain samples or animal models; which not only confirm the specificity of biomarkers but also facilitate classifying the disease process at the cellular, molecular, and genetic level. The characteristic pathology like microvascular angiopathy (MVA), CADASIL, hypertensive vasculopathy, cerebral amyloid angiopathy (CAA) and athero-embolic or thrombotic diseases have been identified (Mills et al., 2007; Legge and Hachinski, 2010; Hachinski, 2007). These biomarkers can be divided into six major categories including: (i) biomarkers of cerebral autosomal arteriopathy with subcortical infarcts and leukoencephalopathy (CADASIL), (ii) biomarkers of microvessel angiopathy (MVA), (iii) biomarkers of hypertensive vasculopathy, (iv) biomarkers of cerebral amyloid angiopathy, (v) biomarkers of atherosclerosis or thrombotic disease, and (vi) Charnoly Body (CB) formation due to mitochondrial degeneration and eventually apoptosis of the most vulnerable cells in the hippocampal dentate gyrus and CA-3 regions due to cerebrovascular insufficiency in VaD (Erkinjuntti and Gauthier, 2009; Sharma et al. 2010; Sharma and Ebadi, 2014a; Sharma and Ebadi 2014b; Sharma et al., 2013a; Sharma et al., 2013b; Sharma, 2013, Sharma et al., 2014c; Sharma, 2014).

Clinical Biomarkers in VaD Clinical assement of VaD is based on neurobehavioral biomarkers which are assessed by performing mental status examination (MSE). MSE evaluates the extent of intellectual deterioration and personality change. This is followed by language performance test to acquire high yield results for the clinical assessment of VaD (O'Bryant et al., 2008). Among the different types of MSEs, Mini MSE of Folstein, HIS scale and WAIS (Wechsler Adult intelligent scale) are most useful. These tests use evaluation of attention span, temporal & spatial orientation and retentive (declarative) memory. A score < 23 on Mini MSE of Folstein is usually diagnostic of dementia. Further typing is based on identification of risk factors as in VaD (Oosterman et al., 2006; Donnella et al., 2007). Furthermore, the Hachinski Ischemic Score Scale (HIS) is a simple bed-side clinical biomarker and is used for differentiating types of dementia (*primary degenerative, vascular, multi infarct, mixed type*). A cut-off score ≤ 4 for dementia of other types and ≥ 7 for VaD has a sensitivity of 89% and a specificity of 89%. (Pantoni and Inzitari, 1997; Moroney 1997). Wetterling et al. DSM-IV Criteria for VaD takes into account memory impairment, one of the cognitive disturbances such as aphasia, apraxia, agnosia & laborator imaging findings in support of vascular etiology (Wetterling et al., 1996). ICD-10 Research Criteria (DCR-10) for VaD is similar to DSM IV criteria with additional evaluation of consciousness, and decline in emotional & social behavior. ADDTC (Alzheimer's Disease Diagnostic and Treatment Centers) Criteria for the Diagnosis of Probable Ischemic VaD takes into consideration memory decline, history of vascular risk factors, neurological signs, and neuroimaging findings, relatively early appearance of gait disturbance and urinary incontinence to favor diagnosis of dementia with probable ischemic etiology. Ischemic scores classified as VD by different diagnostic guidelines set by Hachinski are as follows: Score indicating VaD ≥7; ADDTC criteria: 10.3±3.4; DSM-IV criteria: 6.5±4.4; ICD-10 criteria: 7.9±4.0; NINDSAIREN criteria: 12.5±2.6. Orthostatic circulatory disturbances such as alteration in mean arterial pressure, postural hypotension are associated with development of VaD and in some other neurodegenerative diseases (Risberg et al., 1993; Passant et al., 1997; Passant et al 1996).

Limitations in Biomarker studies Although biomarkers have been studied extensively, there is no consensus on the definitions of standard procedures, uniqueness of processing and storage, analysis and interpretation of results, and their diagnostic utility. It is important to identify biomarker that is not only specific but also stable. In routine clinical practice it is desirable to use stable biomarkers due to time constraints and handling of specimens. Moreover, RNA stabilizers or exclusion of RNA chips, use of anticoagulants may give rise to variable results. Hence large multi-centric trials are needed to compare diagnostic accuracy of different labs all over the world (Humpel, 2011).

There are limitations in use of different analytical methods. For instance ELISA, used routinely may differ from xMAP-luminex technology when CSF and plasma samples are analyzed which also affects the cut off values. Hence, standardization of international values is required. Validation of biomarkers in body fluids need standardization with universal and valid criteria for clinical diagnosis, defining healthy controls, reproducibility in multiple centers and correlated with post mortem diagnosis. CSF diagnosis of dementia supports only clinical and not post mortem diagnosis. Novel potential biomarkers of VaD such as ADMA

(*Asymmetrical Dimethylarginine*) which is a biomarker of endothelial dysfunction, adhesion molecule P-Selectin may contribute to vascular processes and thereby dementia need further studies and validation. Currently CSF Isoprostane, a biomarker of oxidative stress, Aβ Oligomer, α Synuclein, TDP-43, CSF DJ-1, TDP- 43 are investigated in AD. As dementia is defined as mixed etiology, there is a dire need to consider all these biomarkers along with newer biomarkers of vascular injury in determining causal relationship to VaD. Innovative neuroimaging techniques such as DTI, MR spectroscopy, functional MRI, β-amyloid PET imaging may provide newer insights in the etiopathogenesis of VaD (Atwood et al., 2004). Gadolinium Diethylene Triamine Penta Acetic acid (DTPA) also shows promise in detecting vascular pathology on dementia; however all these imaging biomarkers need further validation through multicentric trials. Dysfunction in autonomic regulation of cerebral blood flow is also associated with VaD where imaging biomarkers may provide theranostic utility (Legge and Hachinski. 2010). As yet there is no consensus on criteria, definitions and analysis of VaD in neuropathological assessment. Though numerous gross and microscopic changes have been identified, there is a need of multidisciplinary team performing large multicenter clinico-pathological studies to harmonize the diagnostic approach and validate the biomarkers under investigation; e.g., abandonment of term lacunae which is a source of confusion and reducing inter-observer variability (Leblanc et al., 2006). Genetics and molecular biology may show a definitive avenue towards diagnosis and behavior of VaD. Although genome wide association studies are technically feasible, these are still expensive.

CSF Biomarkers With High Diagnostic Capability Certain biomarkers are significantly and specifically elevated in the CSF samples of patients suffering from VaD. In general, elevated CSF total protein and CSF to serum albumin ratio may be used to detect blood brain barrier breakdown due to damage in the microvasculature. Significantly elevated CSF sulfated levels facilitate early identification of dmyelination in the white matter. The existence of neurofilaments can be utilized to detect axonal degeneration and as a biomarker of white matter damage. MMPss (MPs) can be estimated to detect changes in the extracellular matrix associated with cardiovascular diseases (CVD) and inflammation. Lower serum to CSF Folate ratio is found in VaD patients. Furthermore increased CSF levels of total tau, phosphorylated tau, and decreased Aβ-42 could be utilized to differentiate VaD from AD and other neurodegenerative diseases.

Imaging Biomarkers in VaD Various non-invasive *in-vivo* imaging systems can be utilized for the personalized theranostics and hence effective treatment of VaD. For instance, T1 and T2 weighted MRI and FLIR imaging provide basic information about deep white matter hyperintensities (DWMH), which significantly correlate with small vessel CVD, embolic disease, and VaD (Mills, 2009). Periventricular hyperintensities (PVH) are associated with CVD, and ischemic disease. Infarction (lacunar, site specific such as basal ganglia -cystic lesions, number & size) is significantly associated with CVD and VaD. High signals in basal ganglia are implicated in atherosclerotic arteries and VaD. Dilated Virchow Robin Space (VRS) is related to VaD on autopsy studies. Pulse wave encephalopathy seen as lacunar infarction and white matter hyperintensity (WMH) are associated with abnormal pulse pressure and Windkessel effect leading to CVD. Hemorrhage (number, size, and location) is associated with CVD. Similarly, brain atrophy can be used to estimate age and site related changes and vascular pathology. By using CT imging, ventricular size, medial temporal atrophy, acute or chronic hemorrhage, hypodensities defining infarction as per size, location can be detected; however, these data have not been validated and its association with

VaD is yet to be established. In addition, transcranial Doppler imaging can be utilized to detect spontaneous cerebral emboli related to embolic infarct and VaD.

Neuropathological Biomarkers Recently several neuropathological biomarkers of VaD have been proposed. Clinically most significant pathological biomarkers are described below: Biomarkers of CADASIL, CRV, and RNS proved highly significant to diagnose familial small vessel diseses. Biomarkers of MVA are represented as thickening of small vessel wall, luminal narrowing, degeneration of tunica media, fibrinoid necrosis, and inflammation, which can be used for the clinical assessment of microvascular angiopathy. In addition, vasculitides may have diagnostic utility in noncerebral amyloid angiopathy (CAA) associated angiopathy. The biomarkers of hypertensive vasculopathy can be used to assess *Circle of Willis*, presence of aneurysms, and stenosis of vessels to assess atherosclerosis. Biomarkers of CAA can be used to assess amyloid deposition in vessels on routine H & E staining and Congo red positive Aβ antibody staining, as an indicator of CAA. Similarly biomarkers of atherosclerotic or thrombotic diseases due to ischemia or hemorrhage can be evaluated to assess cerebrovascular injury. The existence of infarcts: *number, size, location, acute or chronic, cyctic, warershed, lacunar* (white matter, grey matter, brain stem), laminar necrosis, hippocampal injury, cribriform change, can be used as parameters of CVD and VaD to correlate clinically with imaging observations. Incomplete ischemic injury is associated with CVD. The loss of myelin on H&E and special stain such as LFB is associated with Leukoencephalopathy. Furthermore, Charnoly Body (CB) formation can be used as an early diagnostic biomarker of hippocampal CA-3 and dentate gyrus lesions, which require further validation and distinction form lesions in AD (*CB is a pleomorphic, preapoptotic biomarker of compromised mitochondrial bioenergetics, which is induced due to free radical overproduction during nutritional stress and/or environmental toxic exposure in a highly vulnerable cell*). In addition, mixed multiple pathology is noticed in cardiovascular disease (CVD). Furthermore, the author discovered that bone marrow-derived mononuclear cells provide neuroprotection by modulating proinflammatory microglia an *in-vitro* cultured model of cerebral ischemia (Sharma et al., 2011).

CONCLUSION

In this chapter recent knowledge on the development of VaD biomarkers is described for the information of a basic scientist as well as physician. Diagnosis of VaD depends on the detection of vascular risk factors. In general, MTs, NOTCH 3, APOE 4, NOS, and CADASIL genes are involved in VaD. Oxidative and nitrative stress can also induce VaD. *In-vitro* and *in-vivo* molecular biomarkers facilitate diagnosis of VaD. Charnoly Body (CB) formation may serve as a pre-apoptotic biomarker of comromized mitochondrial bioenergetics in VaD. In addition, omics and microRNA analysis may provide novel biomarkers for VaD. A variety of candidate biomarkers of VaD have been identified in CSF, blood, by performing neuro-imaging methods, on neuropathological examination, and genetic analyses. These diagnostic biomarkers have shown promise in their utility for etiological diagnosis and behavior of vascular cognitive impairment in VaD; however, lack of specificity and criteria to identify and define these biomarkers of VaD prompts further large scale study to evaluate their exact theranostic significance. Particularly, recent discovery of CB formation as a pre-apoptotic biomarker of oxidative stress and compromised mitochondrial bioenergetics may serve as a novel biomarker of VaD. In addition, biomarkers of oxidative and nitrative stress in the serum and CSF samples can be detected for the early EBPT of VaD. A further study in this direction will go a long way in the successful personalized clinical management of VaD.

REFERENCES

Aisen, P. S., Schneider, L. S., Sano, M., et al. (2008). High-dose B vitamin supplementation and cognitive decline in Alzheimer disease: a randomized controlled trial. *JAMA.*, *300*, 1774–1783.

Aldred, S. & Mecocci, P. (2010). Decreased dehydroepiandrosterone (DHEA) and dehydroepiandrosterone sulfate (DHEAS) concentrations in plasma of Alzheimer's disease (AD) patients. *Arch. Gerontol. Geriatr.*, *51*, e16–e18.

Atwood, L. D., Wolf, P. A., Heard-Costa, N. L., et al. (2004). Genetic variation in white matter hyperintensity volume in the Framingham Study. *Stroke.*, *35*, 1609-1613.

Battistin, L. & Cagnin, A. (2010). Vascular cognitive disorder. A biological and clinical overview. *Neurochem. Res.*, *35*, 1933-1938.

Berglund, L. & Ramakrishnan, R. (2004). Lipoprotein(a): an elusive cardiovascular risk factor. *Arterioscler. Thromb. Vasc. Biol.*, *24*, 2219–2226.

Brenneman, M., Sharma, S., Harting, M., et al. (2010). Autologous bone marrow mononuclear cells enhance recovery after acute ischemic stroke in young and middle-aged rats. *J. Cereb. Blood Flow. & Metab.*, *30*, 140-149.

Casserly, I. & Topol, E. (2004). Convergence of atherosclerosis and Alzheimer's disease: inflammation, cholesterol and misfolded proteins. *Lancet.*, *363*, 1139–1146.

Chacón, I. J., Molero, A. E., Pino-Ramírez, G., et al. (2009). Risk of dementia associated with elevated plasma homocysteine in a latin American population. *Int. J. Alzheimers Dis.*, 2009, 632489.

Chen, N., Yang, Mi., Guol, J., Zhoul, M., Zhu, C. & He, Li. The Cochrane Collaboration. Published by John Wiley & Sons, Ltd. Jan 2013.

Chui, H. C., Victoroff, J. I. & Margolin, D. (1992). Criteria for the diagnosis of ischemic vascular dementia proposed by the State of California Alzheimer's Disease Diagnostic and Treatment Centers. *Neurology.*, *42*, 473-480

Chui, H. C., Zarow, C., Mack, W. J., et al. (2006). Cognitive impact of subcortical vascular and Alzheimer's disease pathology. *Ann Neurol.*, *60*, 677-687.

Debette, S. & Seshadri, S. (2009). Genetics of Atherothrombotic and Lacunar Stroke. *Circ Cardiovasc Genet.*, *2*, 191–198.

Den, H. T., Vermeer, S. E., Clarke, R., et al., (2003). Homocysteine and brain atrophy on MRI of non-demented elderly. *Brain.*, *126*, 170–175.

Donnella, A. J., Pliskina, N., Holdnackb, J., et al., (2007). Rapidlyadministered short forms of the Wechsler Adult Intelligence Scale—3rd edition. *Arch. Clin. Neuropsychol.*, *22*, 917–924.

Doring, Y., Noels, H. & Weber, C. (2012). The Use of High-Throughput Technologies to Investigate Vascular Inflammation and Atherosclerosis. *Arterioscler Thromb Vasc Biol.*, *32*, 182-195.

Emanuele, E., Lista, S., Ghidoni, R., et al., (2011). Chromosome 9p21.3 genotype is associated with vascular dementia and Alzheimer's disease. *Neurobiol. Aging.*, *32*, 1231-1235.

Erkinjuntti, T. & Gauthier, S. (2009). The concept of vascular cognitive impairment. *Front Neurol Neurosci.*, *24*, 79-85.

Forette, F., Seux, M., Staessen, J. A., et al., (1998). Prevention of dementia in randomized double-blind placebo-controlled Systolic Hypertension in Europe (Syst-Eur) trial. *Lancet.*, *352*, 1347–1351.

Formichi, P., Parnetti, L., Radi, E., et al., (2010). CSF Biomarkers Profile in CADASIL—A Model of Pure Vascular Dementia: Usefulness in Differential Diagnosis in the Dementia Disorder. *Int J Alzheimers Dis.*, 959257.

Forti, P., Pisacane, N., Rietti, E., et al., (2010). Metabolic syndrome and risk of dementia in older adults. *J. Am. Geriatr. Soc.*, *58*(3), 487-492.

Forti, P., Olivelli, V., Rietti, E., et al., (2012). Thyroid-Stimulating hormone as a predictor of cognitive impairment in an elderly cohort. *Gerontology.*, *58*, 41–49.

Fredman, P., Wallin, A., Blennow, K., et al., (1992). Sulfatide as a biochemical marker in cerebrospinal fluid of patients with vascular dementia. *Acta Neurol. Scand.*, *85*, 103–106.

Galvin, J. E. (2011). Dementia screening, biomarkers and protein misfolding. Implications for public health and diagnosis. *Prion.*, *5*, 16-21.

Geroldi, D., Falcone, C. & Emanuele, E. (2006). Soluble receptor for advanced glycation end products: from disease marker to potential therapeutic target. *Curr. Med. Chem.*, *13*, 1971-1978.

Giannakopoulos, P., Gold, G., Kovari, E., et al., (2007). Assessing the cognitive impact of Alzheimer disease pathology and vascular burden in the aging brain: the Geneva experience. *Acta Neuropathol.*, *113*, 1–12.

Gridley, T. (2007). Notch signaling in vascular development and physiology. *Development*, *134*, 2709-2718.

Grinberg, L. T. & Heinsen, H. (2010). Toward a Pathological Definition of Vascular Dementia *J Neurol Sci.*, *299*, 136–138.

Hachinski, V. (2007). The 2005 Thomas Willis Lecture: Stroke and vascular cognitive impairment: A transdisciplinary, translational and transactional approach. *Stroke.*, *38*, 1396.

Hagnelius, N., Wahlund, L. & Nilsson, T. (2008). CSF/serum folate gradient: physiology and determinants with special reference to dementia. *Dement Geriatr Cogn. Disord*, *25*, 516–523.

Hamaguchi, T. & Yamada, M. (2008). Genetic factors for cerebral amyloid angiopathy. *Brain Nerve.*, *60*, 1275-1283.

Haritunians, T., Chow, T., De Lange, R. P. J., et al., (2005). Functional analysis of a recurrent missense mutation in Notch3 in CADASIL. *J. Neurol. Neurosurg. Psychiatry*, *76*, 1242-1248.

Humpel, C. (2011). Identifying and validating biomarkers for Alzheimer's disease. *Trends Biotechnol.*, *29*, 26-32.

Kaerst, L., Kuhlmann, A., Wedekind, D., et al., (2013). Cerebrospinal fluid biomarkers in Alzheimer's disease, vascular dementia and ischemic stroke patients: a critical analysis. *J Neurol.*, *260*, 2722–2727.

Kirshner, H. S. (2009). Vascular dementia: A review of recent evidence for prevention and treatment. *Curr. Neurol. Neurosci. Rep.*, *9*, 437-442.

Kurata, K., Takebayashi, M., Morinobu, S., et al., (2004). β-estradiol, dehydroepiandrosterone, and dehydroepiandrosterone sulfate protect against N-methyl-D-aspartate-induced neurotoxicity in rat hippocampal neurons by different mechanisms. *J. Pharmacol. Exp. Ther.*, 2004, *311*, 237–245.

Leblanc, G. G., Meschia, J. F., Stuss, D. T., et al., (2006). Genetics of Vascular Cognitive Impairment. The Opportunity and the Challenges. *Stroke.*, *37*, 248-255.

Legge, S. D. & Hachinski, V. (2010). Vascular cognitive impairment (VCI) Progress towards knowledge and treatment. *Dement Neuropsychol.*, 2010, *4*, 4-13.

Liuzzi, G. M., Trojano, M., Fanelli, M., et al. (2002). Intrathecal synthesis of MMPs-9 in patients with multiple sclerosis: Implication for pathogenesis. *Mult. Scler.*, *8*, 222–228.

Lo, E. H., Dalkara, T. & Moskowitz, M. A. (2003). Mechanisms, challenges and opportunities in stroke. *Nat. Rev. Neurosci.*, *4*, 399–415

Malaguarnera, M., Ferri, R., Bella, R., et al., (2004). Homocysteine, vitamin B12 and folate in vascul Wetterling dementia and in Alzheimer disease. *Clin. Chem. Lab. Med.*, *42*, 1032–1035.

Marchesi, V. T. (2014). Alzheimer's disease and CADASIL are heritable, adult-onset dementias that both involve damaged small blood vessels. *Cell Mol. Life Sci.*, *71*(6), 949-55.

Mills, S., Cain, J., Purandare, N., et al., (2007). Biomarkers of cerebrovascular disease in dementia. *Br. J. Radiol.*, *80*, S 128 – S 145.

Moroney, J. T. (1997). Meta-analysis of the Hachinski Ischemic Score in pathologically verified dementias. *Neurology.*, *49*, 1096 – 1105.

Munekazu, Y. (2012). MicroRNAs in vascular biology *Int. J. Vasc. Med.* 794898,

Naylor, J. C., Hulette, C. M., Steffens, D. C., et al., (2008). Cerebrospinal fluid dehydroepiandrosterone levels are correlated with brain dehydroepiandrosterone levels, elevated in Alzheimer's disease, and related to neuropathological disease stage. *J. Clin. Endocrinol. Metab.*, *93*, 3173–3178.

Neuropathology group of the Medical Research Council Cognitive Function and Ageing Study (MRC-CFAS). Pathological correlates of late-onset dementia in a multicentre, community-based population in England and Wales. *Lancet.*, 2001, *357*, 169–175.

O'Bryant, S. E., Humphreys, J. D., Smith, G. E., et. al., (2008). Detecting dentia with the Mini- Mental State Examination (MMSE) in highly educated individuals. *Arch. Neurol.*, *65*, 963–967.

Olsson, B., Hertze, J., Ohlsson, M., et al., (2013). Cerebrospinal fluid levels of heart fatty acid binding protein are elevated prodromally in Alzheimer's disease and vascular dementia. *J Alzheimers Dis.*, *34*, 673-679.

Oosterman, J. M. & Scherder, E. J. (2006). Distinguishing between vascular dementia and Alzheimer's disease by means of the WAIS: a meta-analysis. *J. Clin. Exp. Neuropsychol.*, *28*, 1158-1175.

Pantoni, L. & Inzitari, D. (1993). Hachinski's ischemic score and the diagnosis of vascular dementia: a review. *Ital. J. Neurol. Sci.*, *14*, 539-546.

Pantoni, L., Sarti, C., Alafuzoff, I., et al., (2006). Postmortem examination of vascular lesions in cognitive impairment: a survey among neuropathological services. *Stroke.*, *37*, 1005-1009.

Paraskevas, G. P., Kapok, E., Papageorgiou, S. G., et al., (2009). CSF biomarker profile and diagnostic value in vascular dementia. *Euro. J. Neurol.*, *16*, 205–211.

Passant, U., Warkentin, S. & Gustafson, L. (1997). Orthostatic hypotension and low blood pressure in organic dementia: a study of prevalence and related clinical characteristics. *Int. J. Geriatr. Psychiatry.*, *12*, 395-403.

Passant, U., Warkentin, S., Karlson, S., et al., (1996). Orthostatic hypotension in organic dementia: relationship between blood pressure, cortical blood flow and symptoms. *Clin. Auton. Res.*, *6*, 29–36.

Pluta, R., Jolkkonen, J., Cuzzocrea, S., et. al., (2011). Cognitive impairment with vascular impairment and degeneration. *Curr. Neurovasc. Res.*, *8*, 342–350.

Pluta, R., Ulamek, M. & Jablonski, M. (2009). Alzheimer's mechanisms in ischemic brain degeneration. *Anat. Rec. (Hoboken)*, *292*, 1863–1881.

Quinn, T. J., Gallacher, J., Deary, I. J., et al., (2011). Association between circulating hemostatic measures and dementia or cognitive impairment: systematic review and meta-analyzes. *J. Thromb. Haemost.*, *9*, 1475–1482.

Rapp, S. R., Espeland, M. A. & Shumaker, S. A. (2003). Effect of estrogen plus progestin on global cognitive function in post menopausal women. The Women's Health Initiative Memory Study: a randomized controlled trial. *JAMA.*, *289*, 2663–2672.

Ray, L., Khemka, V., Behera, P., et al., (2013). Serum Homocysteine, Dehydroepiandrosterone Sulphate and Lipoprotein (a) in Alzheimer's Disease and Vascular Dementia. *Aging Dis.*, *4*(2), 57–64.

Risberg, J., Passant, U., Warkentin, S., et al., (1993). Regional cerebral blood flow in frontal lobe dementia of non-Alzheimer type. *Dementia.*, *4*, 186-187.

Román, G. C., Tatemichi, T. K., Erkinjuntti, T., et. al., (1993). Vascular dementia: diagnostic criteria for research studies. Report of the NINDS-AIREN International Workshop. *Neurology.*, *43*, 250-260.

Rosenberg, G. A., Sullivan, N. & Esiri, M. M. (2001). White matter damage is associated with MMPss in vascular dementia. *Stroke.*, *32*, 1162–1168.

Rosenstein, J. M. & Krum, J. M. (2004). New roles for VEGF in nervous tissue– beyond blood vessels. *Exp. Neurol.*, *187*, 246–253.

Schoonenboom, N., Reesink, F., Verwey, N., et. al., (2012). Cerebrospinal fluid markers for differential dementia diagnosis in a large memory clinic cohort, *Neurology.*, *78*, 47–54.

Sharma, A., Badhe, P., Gokulchandran, N., et al., (2012). Autologous Bone Marrow Derived Mononuclear Cell Therapy for Vascular Dementia. *J. Stem Cell. Res. Ther.*, *2*, 129.

Sharma, S., Bing, Y., Brenneman, M., et al., (2010). Bone Marrow Mononuclear Cells Protect Neurons and Modulate Microglia in Cell Culture Models of Ischemic Stroke. *J. Neurosci. Res.*, *88*, 2869-2876.

Sharma, S. & Ebadi, M. (2014). Antioxidant targeting in neurodegenerative disorders. Ed. I. Laher, Springer Verlag. Germany. Chapter 85, pp.1-30.

Sharma, S. & Ebadi, M. (2011a). Metallothioneins As Early & Sensitive Biomarkers of Redox Signaling in Neurodegenerative Disorders. *Journal of Institute of Integrative Omics & Applied Biotechnonogy (IIOAB Journal)*, *2*, 98-106.

Sharma, S. & Ebadi, M. (2014b). Significance of Metallothioneins in Aging Brain. *Neurochem Int.*, *65*, 40-48.

Sharma, S. & Ebadi, M. (2011b). Therapeutic Potential of Metallothioneins as Antiinflammatory Agents in Polysubstance Abuse. *IIOAB Journal.*, *2*, 50-61.

Sharma, S., Moon, C. S., Khogali, A., et al., (2013b). Biomarkers of Parkinson's disease (Recent Update). *Neurochem. Int.*, *63*, 201-229.

Sharma, S., Nepal, B., Moon, C. S., et. al., (2014c). Psychology of Craving. *Open Jr of Medical Psychology.*, *3*, 120-125.

Sharma, S., Rais, A., Sandhu, R., et al., (2013). Clinical significance of metallothioneins in cell therapy and nanomedicine. *Int. J. Nanomedicine.*, *8*, 1477–1488.

Sharma, S., Yang, B., Xi, X., et al., (2011). IL-10 Directly Protects Cortical Neurons by Activating PI-3 Kinase and STAT-3 Pathways. *Brain Res*, *1373*, 189-194.

Sharma, S. (2013). Charnoly Body as a Sensitive Biomarker in Nanomedicine. (Invited Speaker) International Translational Nanomedicine Conference. Boston, U.S.A. July 25-27.

Sharma, S. (2014). Molecular Pharmacology of Environmental Neurotoxins. In Kainic Acid: Neurotoxic Properties, Biological Sources, and Clinical Applications. Nova Science Publishers. New York Chapter 4, pp. 46-93.

Sheinerman, K. S., Tsivinsky, V. G., et al., (2012). Plasma microRNA biomarkers for detection of mild cognitive impairment. *Aging.*, *4*, 590- 605.

Shoji, M. (2011). Biomarkers of Dementia. *Int. J. Alzheimers. Dis.*, 564321.

Shumaker, S. A., Legault, C., Rapp, S. R., et. al., (2003). Estrogen plus progestin and the incidence of dementia and mild cognitive impairment in postmenopausal women. The Women's Health Initiative Memory Study: a randomized controlled trial. *JAMA.*, *289*, 2651–2652.

Simonsen, A. H., Hagnelius, N. O., Waldemar, G., et al., (2012). Protein Markers for the Differential Diagnosis of Vascular Dementia and Alzheimer's Disease. *Int. J. Proteomics.*, 824024.

Thaweepoksomboon, J., Senanarong, V., Poungvarin, N., et al., (2011). Assessment of cerebrospinal fluid (CSF) beta-amyloid (1–42), phosphorylated tau (ptau-181) and total Tau protein in patients with Alzheimer's disease (AD) and other dementia at Siriraj Hospital, Thailand. *J. Med. Assoc. Thai.*, *94*, S77–S83.

Tsimikas, S. & Hall, J. L. (2012). Lipoprotein (a) as a potential causal genetic risk factor of cardiovascular disease: a rationale for increased efforts to understand its pathophysiology and develop targeted therapies. *J. Am. Coll. Cardiol.*, *60*, 716–721.

Tullberg, M., Mansson, J. E., Fredman, P., et. al., (2000). CSF sulfatide distinguishes between normal pressure hydrocephalus and subcortical arteriosclerotic encephalopathy. *J. Neurol, Neurosurg Psychiatry.*, *69*, 74–81.

Ungvari, Z., Tucsek, Z., Sosnowska, D., et. al., (2013). Aging induced dysregulation of dicer1-dependent microRNA expression impairs angiogenic capacity of rat cerebromicrovascular endothelial cells. *J. Gerontol. Biol. Sci. Med. Sci.*, *68*(8), 877–891.

Visvikis-Siest, S. & Marteau, J. B. (2006). Genetic variants predisposing to cardiovascular disease. *Curr. Opin. Lipidol.*, *17*, 139-151.

Vitali, P., Migliaccio, R., Agosta, F., et al., (2008). Neuroimaging in Dementia. *Semin Neurol.*, *28*, 467-483.

Wallin, A. & Sjogren, M. (2001). Cerebrospinal fluid cytoskeleton proteins in patients with subcortical white-matter dementia. *Mech. Aging Dev.*, *122*, 1937– 1949.

Wardlaw, J. M., Sandercock, P. A., Dennis, M. S., et al., (2003). Is breakdown of the bloodbrain barrier responsible for lacunar stroke, leukoaraiosis, and dementia? *Stroke.*, *34*, 806–812.

Wetterling, T., Kanitz, R. D. & Borgis, K. J. (1996). Comparison of Different Diagnostic Criteria for Vascular Dementia (ADDTC, DSM-IV, ICD-10, NINDS-AIREN). *Stroke.*, *27*, 30-36.

Yang, B., Strong, R., Sharma, S., et al., (2010). Therapeutic Time Window and Dose-Response of Autologous Bone Marrow Mononuclear Cells for Ischemic Stroke. *J. Neurosci. Res.*, *89*, 833-839.

Chapter 12

BIOMARKERS IN PERSONALIZED THERANOSTICS OF AMYTROPIC LATERAL SCLEROSIS

ABSTRACT

Amyotropic lateral sclerosis (ALS) is a progressive and fatal neurodegenerative disease of motoneurons. Usually patients suffering from ALS expires within 2-5 years following the disease onset. The exact molecular mechanism of motor neuron degeneration is unknown and different causal hypotheses including; genetic, viral, traumatic and environmental mechanisms have been proposed. Theranostic strategies based on mechanistic insights are more or less ineffective in the clinical management of ALS. Hence the novel discovery of reliable biomarkers of ALS is exceedingly important to understand the ALS pathogenesis and assessment of disease prognosis. Recently various biomarkers including: omics and imaging approaches have been employed to understand the basic molecular mechansims of disease process and how to treat ALS more effectively. CSF is currently the most promising body fluid, followed by blood (*serum*, *plasma*), urine, and saliva for the omic analyses and differential diagnosis of ALS. This chapter provides an overview about peptide/protein biomarker candidates that demonstrate significantly altered levels in body fluids of ALS patients. Furthermore, limitations and advantages of omics and other approaches for ALS biomarker discovery in body fluids and validation of biomarker candidates are addressed for the successful EBPT of ALS.

Keywords: proteomics, evidence based personalized theranostics

INTRODUCTION

Amyotropic lateral sclerosis (ALS) is a severe neurodegenerative disease that causes progressive muscle weakness, eventually resulting in death, because of respiratory failure. Usually, genetic variants are thought to predispose to this devastating condition. Sporadic ALS is one of the most common neurological diseases; most patients die within 3-4 years after symptoms onset. ALS is a complicate and progressive neurodegenerative disease. Its pathogenic mechanisms remain uncertain and there is no specific test for its diagnosis. For years, scientists have been searching for specific biomarkers associated with ALS to assist clinical diagnosis and monitor disease progression. Some specific inflammatory events in the CNS participate in the pathogenesis of ALS. Oxidative stress is a disturbance in the pro-oxidative/antioxidative balance favoring the pro-oxidative state. Autopsy and lab findings indicate that oxidative stress and astrocyte dysfunction play a key role in motor neuron degeneration in ALS. Oxidative stress biomarkers in CSF, plasma, and urine are elevated, suggesting that *abnormal oxidative stress occurs even outside the CNS. It is generally held that agricultural chemicals, heavy metals, military service, professional sports, excessive physical exertion, chronic head injury, and certain foods might be associated with ALS risk*, with an intimate association with smoking. At the cellular level, these risk factors may be involved in generating oxidative stress. Experimental studies have indicated that a combination of insults that induce oxidative stress can exert additive deleterious effects on motor neurons, suggesting that multiple exposures in the hostle environments are important. As the disease progresses, nutritional deficiency, cachexia, psychological stress, and impending respiratory failure may further increase oxidative stress. Moreover, ALS is possibly a systemic disease. Laboratory, pathologic, and epidemiologic evidence supports the hypothesis that oxidative stress is central in the ALS pathogenic process, particularly in genetically susceptive individuals. Grossman, (2013) provided a brief description to improve diagnostic accuracy in cases with similar presentations that are due to distinct histopathologic abnormalities. These authors proposed a staged approach to diagnosis, beginning with a screening assessment of specific, quantitative neuropsychological measures, followed by assessments of imaging and fluid biomarkers. Their goal of this study was to determine the specific histopathologic abnormalities contributing to an individual's neurodegenerative condition.

The expansion of a noncoding hexanucleotide repeat (GGGGCC) in the chromosome 9 open reading frame (C9orf72) gene has been identified as the most common cause of familial *and* sporadic *ALS in Caucasian populations.* The role of the C9orf72 repeat expansion in Korean ALS patients, however, was not reported. Therefore, Jang et al. (2013) investigated the frequency of the C9orf72 repeat expansion in 254 Korean patients with familial (n = 8) and sporadic (n = 246) ALS and found that none of the patients had this expansion. The number of hexanucleotide repeats ranged from 2 to 11 in the 254 ALS patients without the expansion suggesting that the C9orf72 repeat expansion is not the primary cause of ALS in the Korean population. Recently D'Amico et al. (2013) highlighted that if the researchers are to improve ALS treatment; well-designed biochemical and genetic epidemiological studies, combined with a multidisciplinary research, are needed that will provide basic knowledge of ALS etiology, pathophysiology, and prognosis. Kruger et al. (2013) reported that ALS is a progressive neurodegenerative disorder of motor neurons leading to death of the patients, mostly within 2-5 years after disease onset. The molecular mechanism of motor neuron degeneration is only partially understood and therapeutic strategies based on mechanistic insights are ineffective. The discovery of reliable biomarkers of ALS diagnosis and progression is exceedingly important to understand the ALS pathogenesis and the assessment of disease prognosis. Proteomic approach is an important pillar in ALS biomarker discovery. CSF is the most promising body fluid for the differential proteome analyses, followed by blood (*serum, plasma*), and even urine and saliva.

In this chapter, a brief description of biomarkers of ALS is provided for the successful EBPT of ALS. The chapter provides an overview about peptide/protein biomarker candidates that demonstrate significantly altered levels in certain body fluids of ALS patients. These findings are discussed according to proposed pathomechanisms to identify modifiers of ALS progression and to pave the way for the development of theranostic strategies. Furthermore, limitations and advantages of proteomic and other approaches for ALS biomarker discovery in different body fluids and validation of biomarker candidates are addressed.

Intronic Hexanucleotide (GGGGCC)-Repeat Expansion in C9ORF72 in ALS It is well known that ALS is a fatal motor neuron disease, and is most common among European populations. ALS is characterized by the absence of reliable diagnostic biomarkers. The expansion of a noncoding hexanucleotide repeat (GGGGCC) in the chromosome 9 open reading frame (C9orf72) gene has been identified as the most common cause of familial and sporadic ALS in Caucasian populations and was identified as a major cause of ALS and FTD. Some ALS patients exhibit signs of Parkinsonism, and many Parkinsonism patients develop dementia. In a study Akimoto et al. (2013) examined if the hexanucleotide repeat expansion was present in Parkinsonism patients, to clarify if there exists a relationship between the repeat expansion and disease. These investigators studied the size of the hexanucleotide repeat expansion in 135 PD patients and 39 patients with atypical Parkinsonism and compared with 645 Swedish control subjects. No correlation between PD or atypical parkinsonism and the size of the GGGGCC repeat expansion in C9ORF72 was observed, indicating that GGGGCC-repeat expansion in C9ORF72 is not a cause of Parkinsonism. In a similar study, Huye et al., (2013) detected a hexanucleotide repeat expansion in C9ORF72 to cause frontotemporal lobar degeneration, frontotemporal dementia (FTD)-ALS, and ALS. Patients with frontotemporal lobar degeneration with the C9ORF72 repeat expansion were more likely than those without to present with psychosis. These investigators screened DNA samples from 192 unrelated subjects with schizophrenia for the C9ORF72 repeat expansion. None of the subjects with schizophrenia had the pathogenic expansion. C9ORF72 repeat expansions either did not cause schizophrenia. Recently, a hexanucleotide repeat expansion in the C9ORF72 gene was identified to account for a significant portion of Caucasian families affected by FTD and ALS. Given the clinical overlap of FTD with AD, these investigators hypothesized that C9ORF72 expansions might contribute to AD. In Caucasians, they found C9ORF72 expansions in the pathogenic range of FTD/ALS (>30 repeats) at a proportion of 0.76% in AD cases versus 0 in control subjects. In contrast, no large expansions were detected in African Americans. However, in the range of normal variation of C9ORF72 expansions, they detected significant differences in distribution and mean repeat counts between Caucasians and African Americans. Clinical and pathological re-evaluation of C9ORF72 expansion carriers revealed 9 clinical autopsy confirmed AD and 2 FTD final diagnoses, suggesting that large C9ORF72 expansions lead to a phenotypic spectrum of neurodegenerative disease including AD (Kohli et al., 2013).

Serum HMGB1 AutoAb as a Biomarker of ALS As high mobility group box 1 (HMGB1) is elevated in spinal cord tissues of patients with ALS, therefore, Huye et al., (2013) hypothesized that serum autoantibody against HMGB1 (HMGB1 autoAb) might represent an effective biomarker for ALS. Patients with ALS, AD, PD, and healthy age-matched controls were recruited for this study. ALS group consisted of 61 subjects, the other groups each consisted of 40 subjects. A polyclonal antibody was raised against HMGB1 to develop an ELISA-based methodology for screening serum samples. All samples were coded for masked comparison. For statistic analyses, two-tailed Student's t-test, ANOVA, Bonferroni multiple comparison test, Spearman correlation, and ROCs were applied. The level of HMGB1 autoAb significantly increased in patients with ALS as compared with AD,

PD, and healthy control subjects. Particularly, higher HMGB1 autoAb level was found in more severe disease status, confirming that serum HMGB1 autoAb may serve as a biomarker for the diagnosis of ALS and can be used to monitor disease progression (Hwang et al;. 2013; Jin et al., 2013).

MS biomarkers can be broadly classified as (i) *In-vivo* and (ii) *in-vitro* biomarkers as well as (i) invasive and (ii) non-invasive biomarkers to facilitate early and accurate diagnosis of MS. In addition the researchers can perform conventional (CT and structural) and advanced neuroimaging (including fMRI, DTI, and PET imaging with specific radioligand) to authenticate the diagnosis and prognosis. For example, Gadolinium enhanced MRI can provide information regarding the structural and functional integrity of the blood brain barrier, which is compromised in MS patients. Various diagnostic biomarkers of MS are used in combination to correlate and confirm the diagnosis which includes a combination of medical history, MRI, CT, PET, and CSF examination. In addition the researchers can detect the existence of autoantibodies. The detection of Neopterin protein as well as oligoclonal bands further authenticate and confirm MS diagnosis. The CSF and urine biomarkers can also be used for the diagnosis of MS. The MS diagnosis can be confirmed by measuring CSF and urine biomarkers including, kappa (κ) and lambda (λ) light chain, Neopterin, and ubiquitin C-terminal hydrolase. Various CSF biomarkers can be detected for confirming the diagnosis of MS. These biomarkers include, Feutin-A, spinal PKCγ, peptidyl arginine deaminase (PADs) for prognosticating MS. Neurofilament, monomeric and dimeric κ and γ FLCs can help in the differential diagnosis of MS. In addition, CSF SOD, reduced CSF amyloid-β, and soluble AAP can facilitate MS diagnosis. CSF, Iso-P can also be used as a biomarker of tissue damage. Abnormal myelin hypercitrulination and reduced BNDF can also confirm MS diagnosis in combination with other diagnostic biomarkers. Various biomarkers of MS can be detected in blood, plasma, serum, and urine samples in addition to CSF. However detection limits will vary depending on the biological source. As many as 12 biomarkers have been discovered so far which can be used on a routine basis. For example, oligoclonal bands, CD-44 deficiency, elevated sCD-144, vitamin-D, 24-S-hydroxycholesterol in plasma, low serum LPRs, low CD-70, increased myelin basic proteins (MBPs), increased α-integrins, HLA-DRB-1 gene polymorphism, urinary metabolites, and CD-20 have been discovered. The renin angiotensin system is impaired in MS. It is represented by significant reductions in Angiotensin-II and Angiotensin Converting Enzyme-II, and increase in Angiotensin Converting Enzyme (ACE). The most important genetic biomarkers in MS include TOB-1 polymorphism, epigenetic changes in DNA (DNA sequences, DNA methylation, histone modification, and miRNA-associated silencing) can be determined for the MS patients. Furthermore there is experimental evidence that kit/kit mice exhibit extensive neurodegeneration as noticed in MS patients. Response gene to complement (RGC-32) is also impaired in MS patients, hence can be used for the diagnosis, clinical management, and prognosis of MS.

The microRNAs can be used as biomarkers for the differential diagnosis and confirmation of MS. Out of 17 miRNAs that are altered in MS; *Let-7e, CD-226, and Gly-307 SER* have been directly implicated in multiple immune diseases including MS. Various immunological biomarkers those are important in the differential diagnosis and treatment of MS include; induction of autoimmune T cells, increased synthesis of immunoglobulin-γ (IgG), cytotoxic NKG 2C+, CD4 T cells, and FASL expression of astrocytes. Various inflammatory biomarkers can be employed for the early diagnosis, prognosis, and treatment of MS. During the progression of MS, most common clinical manifestation is the existence of idiopathic intermediate uveitis, B7-H3 plays a diverse role in the regulation of T cell responses, Muc-1 which plays an anti-inflammatory role in experimental allergic encephalomyelitis (EAE) (an experimental model of MS), enhanced mB7-H3 expression, over activation of CD4 (+) T cells (Th1 and Th17 subpopulation), Muc-1 a member of the tethered glycoproteins, reduced sB7-H3 levels in MS, B7-H3 which plays a diversified role in regulating T cell response. In addition, APRIL (a proliferation-inducing ligand), and trans locator protein (18 kDa: TSPO) expression are significantly enhanced in MS. Hence 18KDa, TSPO proteins is radiolabeled with ^{18}F or ^{11}C, in PET biomarkers to evaluate the extent of neuro-inflammation in MS as discussed in the text. Several diversified biomarkers that can be used for the clinical management of MS have been proposed. For example, β-1,4-GalT-I as an inflammatory mediator regulating adhesion and migration of inflammatory cells in EAE, Oxidative Stress Biomarker Isoprostanes (IsoP) are sensitive biomarkers of oxidative stress, PET Biomarkers, TSPO (18 KD Proteins), ^{18}FdG Imaging, Modification of galactosylated carbohydrate chains to modulate selectin-ligand biosynthesis, *In-Vivo* Gd-enhancement MRI to determine BBB integrity, interaction with E-Selectin. NFL, GFAP and β-Tub II proteins are significantly increased in MS patients.

CD70: Therapeutic Target in Human MS and ALS In addition, CD70, MRS Biomarker (Reduced NAA), invasive Investigations, noninvasive investigations, MTs, α-Synuclein index (SI), and the existence of Charnoly body can be used as biomarkers of neurodegeneration/regeneration in MS and ALS. α-Synuclein index (SI) is the ratio of nitrated α-Synuclein vs native α-Synuclein (Sharma et al., 2003); MTs are neuroprotective anti-inflammatory, low molecular weight, metal (Zn^{2+})-binding, -SH rich antioxidant proteins, which prevent various neurodegenerative α-synucleinopathies by preventing Charnoly body formation and by acting as free radical scavengers. Charnoly bodies are formed due to mitochondrial degeneration as a consequence of free radical overproduction as the researchers have reported in our recent publications (Sharma et al., 2013a; Sharma et al., 2013b).

Protein Disulfide Isomerase (PDI) as Biomarker of ALS Protein disulfide isomerase (PDI) is an oxidoreductase assisting oxidative protein folding in the endoplasmic reticulum of all types of cells, including neurons and glia. In neurodegenerative disorders, such as ALS, up-regulation of PDI is an important part of unfolded protein response (UPR) that represents an adaption reaction and thereby protects the neurons. Particularly, studies on animal models of familial ALS with mutant Cu/Zn superoxide dismutase 1 (SOD1) have shown that the mutant SOD1 in astrocytes or microglia regulates the progression of the disease. Jaronen et al. (2013) discovered an early up-regulation of PDI in microglia of transgenic (tg) mutant SOD1 mice, indicating that in addition to neurons, UPR takes place in glial cells in ALS. This observation was supported by the observation that the expression of a UPR marker GADD34 (*growth arrest and DNA damage-inducible protein*) is induced in the spinal cord glia of tg mutant SOD1 mice. Because mutant SOD1 can cause sustained activation of NADPH oxidase (NOX), these investigators investigated the role of PDI in UPR-induced NOX activation in microglia. In BV-2 microglia, UPR resulted in NOX activation with increased production of superoxide and increased release of TNF-α, which was recapitulated in primary rat microglia, murine macrophages and human monocytes. In addition, pharmacological inhibition of PDI or its down-regulation by short interfering RNAs prevented NOX activation in microglia and subsequent production of superoxide, confirming that UPR, caused by protein misfolding, may lead to PDI-dependent NOX activation and contribute to neurotoxicity in neurodegenerative diseases including ALS.

ALS Biomarkers. Turner et al. (2013) reported that the last 30 years have seen a major advance in the understanding of the clinical and pathological heterogeneity of ALS, and its overlap with FTD. Multiple biochemical pathways converge on a common clinical syndrome characterized by progressive loss of upper and lower motor neurons. *Pathogenic themes in ALS include excitotoxicity, oxidative stress, mitochondrial dysfunction, neuroinflammation, altered energy metabolism, and RNA mis-processing.* The transgenic rodent, overexpressing mutant SOD-1, is currently one of several models of ALS pathogenesis. The nematode, fruit fly and zebrafish all offer better insight, and the development of induced pluripotent stem cell-derived motor neurons holds promise for the screening of novel biomarkers and candidate therapeutics. The lack of useful biomarkers in ALS contributes to diagnostic delay, and the inability to stratify patients by prognosis may be an important factor in the failure of therapeutic trials. Biomarkers sensitive to disease activity might lessen reliance on clinical measures and survival as trial endpoints and reduce the length of study. Emerging proteomic biomarkers of neuronal loss and glial activity in CSF, a cortical signature derived from structural and functional MRI, and the development of more sensitive measurements of lower motor neuron physiology are leading a new phase of biomarker-driven theranostic discovery.

Oxidative Stress and ALS D'Amico et al. (2013) reported that oxidative stress is a disturbance in the pro-oxidative/antioxidative balance favoring the pro-oxidative state. Autopsy and laboratory studies in ALS indicate that oxidative stress plays a significant role in motor neuron degeneration and astrocyte dysfunction. Oxidative stress biomarkers in CSF, plasma, and urine were elevated in these patients, suggesting that abnormal oxidative stress is generated outside of the CNS. *Agricultural chemicals, heavy metals, military service, professional sports, excessive physical exertion, chronic head trauma, and certain foods might be associated with ALS risk, with a stronger association between risk and smoking. At the cellular level, these factors are involved in generating oxidative stress.* Experimental studies indicate that a combination of insults that induce modest oxidative stress can exert deleterious effects on motor neurons, suggesting that multiple exposures in environments are important. *As the disease progresses, nutritional deficiency, cachexia, psychological stress, and impending respiratory failure may further increase oxidative stress.* Moreover, accumulating evidence suggests that ALS is possibly a systemic disease. Laboratory, pathologic, and epidemiologic evidence supports the hypothesis that oxidative stress is central in the pathogenic process, particularly in genetically susceptive individuals. If the researchers are to improve ALS treatment, well-designed biochemical and genetic epidemiological studies, combined with a multidisciplinary research approach, are needed that will provide knowledge crucial to our understanding of ALS etiology, pathophysiology, and prognosis, in addition to novel biomarker(s) discovery.

SOD1 as ALS Biomarker Therapies designed to decrease the level of SOD1 are currently in a clinical trial for patients with SOD1-linked familial ALS. Winer et al. (2013) determined whether the SOD1 protein in CSF may be a pharmacodynamic marker for antisense oligonucleotide therapy and a biomarker for ALS. Antisense oligonucleotides targeting human SOD1 were administered to rats expressing SOD1G93A. The human SOD1 protein levels were measured in the brain and CSF samples. In human CSF samples, the following proteins were measured: SOD1, tau, phosphorylated tau, VILIP-1, and YKL-40. Ninety-three participants with ALS, 88 healthy controls, and 89 controls with a neurological disease (55 with dementia of the Alzheimer type, 19 with MS, and 15 with peripheral neuropathy). Antisense oligonucleotide-treated SOD1G93A rats had decreased human SOD1 mRNA and decreased protein levels in the brain. The rats' CSF samples showed a similar decrease in hSOD1 levels after additional measurements. The CSF SOD1 levels were higher in the ALS participants, which did not correlate with disease characteristics in ALS or controls with dementia of the Alzheimer type, but they did correlate with tau, phosphorylated tau, VILIP-1 and YKL-40 levels in controls with dementia of the Alzheimer type. These studies suggested that SOD1 in CSF may be an excellent pharmacodynamic marker for SOD1-lowering therapies, because antisense oligonucleotide therapy lowered protein levels in the rat brain and rat CSF samples and because SOD1 levels in CSF samples from humans remained stable as a function of time.

Mutation Screening of SOD1 in ALS A study reported genetic analysis and mutation screening of SOD1 in 60 Iranian ALS patients (Alavi et al. 2013). Linkage analysis in 4 families identified a disease-linked locus that included the known ALS gene, SOD1. Screening of SOD1 identified homozygous p. Asp90Ala causing mutations in all the linked families. Haplotype analysis suggested that the p.Asp90Ala alleles in these patients might share a common founder with the Scandinavian recessive p.Asp90Ala allele. Subsequent screening in all the patients resulted in 3 other mutations in SOD1, including p.Leu84Phe in the homozygous state. These investigators presented the phenotypic features of the mutation-bearing patients. SOD1 mutations were found in 11.7% of the cohort, 38.5% of the familial ALS probands, and 4.25% of the sporadic ALS cases, indicating that SOD1 mutations contribute significantly to ALS.

CSF Metabolomics in ALS A study was performed to (a) devise an untargeted metabolomics methodology that could compare CSF from ALS patients and controls by liquid chromatography coupled to high-resolution mass spectrometry (LC-HRMS); (b) ascertain a metabolic signature of ALS; (c) identify metabolites as diagnostic or pathophysiologic biomarkers (Blasco et al., 2013). An innovative procedure was developed to analyze CSF components by UPLC coupled with a Q-Exactive mass spectrometer that utilizes electrospray ionization. These researchers created a metabolomic profiles of the CSF from ALS patients and patients with other neurological conditions and performed multivariate and univariate analyses (OPLS-DA) to assess the contribution of individual metabolites and compounds in other studies. Metabolomic analysis of 66 CSF samples from ALS patients and 128 from controls accurately predicted the diagnosis of ALS in >80% of cases. OPLS-DA identified 4 features that discriminated diagnostic group and revealed that untargeted metabolomics with LC-HRMS is a robust procedure to generate a specific metabolic profile for ALS from CSF and could facilitate development of disease-specific biomarkers.

pNF-H As a Phosphorylated Neurofilament in ALS It is currently recognized that the phosphorylated neurofilament heavy subunit (pNF-H), a major structural component of motor axons, is a promising biomarker in ALS, but has been studied primarily in CSF. Boylan et al. (2013) examined pNF-H concentrations in plasma, serum, and CSF as a biomarker for disease progression and survival in ALS. These researchers measured pNF-H concentration by ELISA in plasma (n=43), serum and CSF (n=20) in ALS patients. They included plasma of an ALS cohort (n=20) from an earlier study to evaluate baseline pNF-H levels in relation to disease progression using the ALS Functional Rating Scale (ALSFRS-R), survival and anatomical region of ALS onset. Higher pNF-H levels in plasma, serum and CSF showed evidence of association with faster decline in ALSFRS-R. There was evidence of higher serum and plasma pNF-H levels with shorter survival rates, although this evidence was weaker for CSF. The pNF-H concentration in plasma (n=62) was higher in patients with bulbar onset than in patients with spinal onset. Increased pNF-H concentration in plasma, serum and CSF was associated with excelerated ALS progression, suggesting that factors affecting pNF-H levels or their detection in serum and plasma in relation to disease may differ from those in CSF and that site of ALS onset (*bulbar vs spinal*) may influence pNF-H levels in peripheral blood; hence further study on pNF-H in CSF, serum and plasma samples may confirm its theranostic potential as an ALS biomarker.

miRNA As a Blood Biomarker of ALS/MS Recently mutations in the profilin 1 (PFN1) gene, encoding a member of the profilin family of actin-binding proteins, were reported in patients with familial ALS. Daoud et al. (2013) determined the prevalence of PFN1 mutations by sequencing the coding region of this gene in 94 familial ALS patients from France and Quebec. No mutations were identified, suggesting that PFN1 gene mutations are a rare cause of familial ALS among patients with European ancestry. It is known that microRNAs (miRNAs) are single-stranded, small noncoding RNAs that regulate gene expression. Because they are stable in serum, they can be developed as biomarkers for various diseases. In MS, miRNAs were studied in cell populations but not in the circulation. In MS, a major challenge is to develop immune biomarkers to monitor disease. These investigators explored whether circulating miRNAs could be identified in MS and whether they are linked to disease progression and/or disability. A total of 368 miRNAs were measured in plasma in 10 relapsing-remitting MS (RRMS) patients, 9 secondary progressive MS (SPMS) patients, and 9 healthy controls (HCs) using miRCURY LNA™ Universal RT microRNA PCR (Gandhi et al., 2013). These investigators validated 19 miRNAs on an independent set of 50 RRMS patients, 51 SPMS patients, and 32 HCs and found that circulating miRNAs are differentially expressed in RRMS and SPMS versus HCs and in RRMS versus SPMS patients. The miRNAs were also linked to Expanded Disability Status Scale (EDSS). Particularly, hsa-miR-92a-1* was identified in the largest number of comparisons. It was different in RRMS versus SPMS, and RRMS versus HCs, and showed an association with EDSS and disease duration. miR-92 has target genes involved in cell cycle regulation and cell signaling. The let-7 family of miRNAs differentiated SPMS from HCs and RRMS from SPMS. It is now known that let-7 miRNAs regulate stem cell differentiation and T cell activation, activates Toll-like receptor-7, and are linked to neurodegeneration. hsa-miR-454 differentiated RRMS from SPMS, and hsa-miR-145 differentiated RRMS from HCs and RRMS from SPMS. The circulating miRNAs (let-7 and miR-92) that were differentially expressed in RRMS versus SPMS also differentiated ALS from RRMS patients, but were not different between SPMS and ALS, suggesting that similar molecular events may occur in SPMS and ALS; hence circulating miRNAs may be used as blood biomarkers to monitor ALS as well as MS.

pNfH as a Biomarker in ALS It is now realized that a diagnostic biomarker for ALS would permit early intervention with disease-modifying therapies while a biomarker for disease activity could accelerate novel drug discovery by facilitating shorter, cost-effective drug trials in a smaller number of patients. Neurofilaments are the most abundant cytoskeletal proteins. Ganesalingam et al. (2013) determined whether pNfH was a biomarker for ALS. pNfH levels were determined using an ELISA for 150 ALS subjects and 140 controls. A 7-fold elevation in the CSF levels of phosphorylated neurofilament heavy subunit (pNfH) in ALS was observed. There was a 10-fold elevation of pNfH compared to ALS mimics and other neurodegenerative and inflammatory conditions. pNfH achieved a diagnostic sensitivity of 90% and specificity of 87% in distinguishing ALS from controls. These researchers also detected an inverse correlation between CSF pNfH levels and disease duration and suggested that pNfH represents a promising theranostic biomarker of ALS.

CD133 (+) Stem Cells Transplantation in ALS Improvements in quality of life and life expectancy was observed in ALS patients transplanted with CD133 (+) stem cells into their frontal motor cortices. However, there are concerns regarding the capacity of cells from these patients to engraft and differentiate into neurons. Gonzalez et al. (2013) evaluated the *in vitro* capacity of CD133(+) stem cells to differentiate into neuron lineage from 13 ALS patients. Stem cells were obtained through leukapheresis and cultured in a control medium or neuroinduction medium for 2-48 hrs. The neuronal genes expression was analyzed by RT-PCR and immunohistochemical techniques. Fluorescence microscopic analysis demonstrated that CD133(+) stem cells from ALS patients incubated for 48 hrs in a neuroinduction medium increased neuronal proteins such as N*estin, β-Tubulin III, Neuronal-Specific Enolase, and Glial Fibrillary Acidic Protein. Although a*n increase in the expression of β-Tubulin III, Nestin, Olig2, Islet-1, Hb9, and Nkx6.1 was noticed, no correlation was found between age, sex, or ALS functional scale and the CD133(+) stem cell response to the neuroinduction medium, suggesting that CD133(+) stem cells from ALS patients, like stem cells of healthy subjects, are able to differentiate into preneuron cells.

Keratan Sulfate (KS) Expression in ALS In general, biopolymers consist of 3 major classes, i.e., polynucleotides (*DNA, RNA*), polypeptides (*proteins*) and polysaccharides *(sugar chains)*. It is now well-accepted that polynucleotides and polypeptides play central roles in the pathogenesis of neurodegenerative diseases. But, sugar chains have been poorly studied in this process, and their biological/clinical significance remains uncertain. Hirano et al. (2013) investigated the role of Keratan Sulfate (KS), a long sugar chain of proteoglycan, in ALS pathogenesis. They employed ALS model SOD1 (G93A) mice and GlcNAc6ST-1(-/-) mice, which are KS-deficient in the CNS. SOD1 (G93A) GlcNAc6ST-1(-/-) mice exhibited a shorter lifespan than SOD1 (G93A) mice and an accelerated appearance of clinical symptoms (body weight loss and decreased rotarod performance). KS expression was induced exclusively in a subpopulation of microglia in SOD1 (G93A) mice, and became detectable around motoneurons in the ventral horn during the early disease phase before body weight loss. During this phase, the expression of M2 microglial biomarkers was augmented in SOD1 (G93A) mice, and was attenuated in SOD1 (G93A) GlcNAc6ST-1(-/-) mice. M2 microglia were less during the early disease phase in SOD1 (G93A) GlcNAc6ST-1(-/-) mice. KS expression in microglia was also detected in some ALS cases, suggesting that KS plays a suppressive role in the early phase pathogenesis and may represent a novel target for therapeutic intervention of ALS.

MRI Analyses of ALS Bastin et al. (2013) investigated brain-wide white matter structural changes associated with ALS using an automatic single seed point tractography-based segmentation method, probabilistic neighborhood tractography (PNT), which provides estimates of both tract integrity and shape. Diffusion MRI data were acquired from 30 patients with ALS and 30 matched controls. PNT was used to segment 12 major projection, commissural and association fibers, and assess differences in how the shape of an individual subject's tract compares to that of a predefined reference tract, in addition to providing tract-average mean diffusivity ($\langle D \rangle$) and fractional anisotropy (FA) data. Across all 12 tracts, group-averaged $\langle D \rangle$ was larger, while group-averaged FA was equal to or smaller in value for patients than controls. These differences were significant for right cingulum ⟨D⟩ , and left and right corticospinal tract (CST) ⟨D⟩ and FA. There were greater topological differences from the reference tract in left and right CST, and right uncinate fasciculus for patients than controls. The rate of disease progression was negatively correlated with bilateral CST FA. These researchers concluded that ALS, although affecting CST, is associated with subtle changes in white matter tract integrity and shape in several other fibers within the brain. Correlations between CST integrity and disease progression suggested that quantitative tractography may provide useful biomarkers of disease evolution in ALS.

Kolind et al., (2013) applied a novel MRI sequence (mcDESPOT) sensitive to water pools within myelin and intra- and extra-cellular spaces to 23 ALS patients, seven PLS patients and 12 healthy controls, with interval follow-up in 15 ALS and four PLS patients. PLS patients were distinguished by widespread cerebral myelin water fraction reductions, independent of disease duration and clinical upper motor neuron burden. ALS patients showed a significant increase in intra- and extra-cellular water, indirectly linked to neuroinflammatory activity. Limited measures of cognitive impairment in the ALS group were associated with myelin changes within the anterior corpus callosum and frontal lobe projections. Longitudinal changes were only significant in the PLS group. Myelin imaging had potential to distinguish PLS from ALS, and value as a biomarker of extramotor involvement. PLS may be a more active cerebral pathological process than its rate of clinical deterioration. Koppers et al. (2013) identified two loci in a recent, large, genome-wide association study (GWAS) that increase susceptibility to ALS. These 2 loci on chromosomes 9 and 19 consist of 4 genes: UNC13a, IFNK, MOBKL2b, and C9ORF72. A hexanucleotide repeat expansion in the noncoding region of C9ORF72 was identified as the cause of chromosome 9-linked ALS-FTD (*frontotemporal dementia*). It was determined whether the coding regions of these genes harbor rare, nonsynonymous variants that play a role in ALS pathogenesis. In DNA from 1019 sporadic ALS patients and 1103 control subjects of Dutch descent, these invsetigators performed a mutation screening analysis in the coding region of these 4 genes by resequencing the exons. A total of 16 amino acid-changing rare variations were identified, 11 in UNC13a and 5 on chromosome 9. Some of these were unique to ALS, but were detected in a single patient. None of the genes showed significant enrichment of rare variants in the coding sequence, sugesting that rare variants in the coding region of UNC13a, IFNK, MOBKL2b, and C9ORF72 are unlikely to be a genetic cause of ALS.

Minocycline-Induced Inhibition of Microglial Activation Minocycline is generally used to inhibit microglial activation. It is accepted that activated microglia exert pro-inflammatory (M1) and anti-inflammatory (M2) functions. The *in vivo* status of activated microglia is probably on a continuum between these two extreme states. However, the mechanisms regulating microglial polarity remain uncertain. Kobayashi et al., (2013) addressed this question focusing on Minocycline. They used SOD1 (G93A) mice which exhibit the motor neuron-specific neurodegenerative disease, ALS. Minocycline attenuated the induction of the expression of M1 microglia markers during the progressive phase, whereas it did not affect the transient enhancement of expression of M2 microglia markers during the early pathogenesis phase. This selective inhibitory effect was confirmed using primary cultured microglia stimulated by lipopolysaccharide (LPS) or IL-4, which induced M1 or M2 polarization, respectively. Furthermore, Minocycline inhibited the upregulation of NF-κB in the LPS-stimulated primary cultured microglia and in the spinal cord of SOD1 (G93A) mice.

IL-4 did not induce upregulation of NF-κB, indicating that Minocycline selectively inhibits the microglia polarization to a proinflammatory state, and provides a basis for understanding pathogeneses of many diseases accompanied by microglial activation including ALS.

ALS is a fatal neurodegenerative disorder of motor neurons. Although most cases of ALS are sporadic (sALS) and of unknown etiology, there are also inherited familial ALS (fALS) cases that share a phenotype similar to sALS pathological and clinical phenotype. In this study, the researchers identified two new potential genetic ALS biomarkers in human bone marrow mesenchymal stem cells (hMSC) obtained from sALS patients, namely the TDP-43 (TAR DNA-binding protein 43) and SLPI (secretory leukocyte protease inhibitor). Together with the previously discovered ones-CyFIP2 and RbBP9, they investigated whether these four potential ALS biomarkers may be differentially expressed in tissues obtained from mutant SOD1^{G93A} transgenic mice, a model that is relevant for at least 20% of the fALS cases. Quantitative real-time PCR analysis of brain, spinal cord and muscle tissues of the mSOD1^{G93A} and controls at various time points during the progression of the neurological disease showed differential expression of the four identified biomarkers in correlation with (i) the tissue type, (ii) the stage of the disease and (iii) the gender of the animals, creating thus a novel spatiotemporal molecular signature of ALS. The biomarkers detected in the fALS animal model were homologous to those that were identified in hMSC of our sALS cases. These results support the possibility of a molecular link between sALS and fALS and may indicate common pathogenetic mechanisms involved in both types of ALS. Moreover, these results may pave the path for using the mSOD1^{G93A} mouse model and these biomarkers as molecular beacons to evaluate the effects of novel drugs/treatments in ALS (Liloet al., 2013). Recent advances in our understanding of some of the genetic causes of ALS, such as mutations in SOD1, TARDBP, FUS and VCP have led to the generation of rodent models of the disease, as a strategy to help our understanding of the pathophysiology of ALS and to assist in the development of therapeutic strategies. McGoldrick et al. (2013) provided detailed descriptions of TDP-43, FUS and VCP models of ALS, and summarised potential therapeutics which were recently trialled in rodent models of the disease.

Human induced pluripotent stem cells (iPSCs) offer hope for personalized regenerative cell therapy in amyotrophic lateral sclerosis (ALS). Popescu et al. (2013) analyzed the fate of human iPSC-derived neural progenitors transplanted into the spinal cord of wild-type and transgenic rats carrying a human mutated SOD1(G93A) gene. The aim was to follow survival and differentiation of human neural progenitors until day 60 post-transplantation in two different *in vivo* envIronments, one being ALS-like. iPSC-derived neural progenitors efficiently engrafted in the adult spinal cord and survived at high numbers. Different neural progenitor, astroglial, and neuronal markers indicated that, over time, the transplanted nestin-positive cells differentiated into cells displaying a neuronal phenotype in both wild-type and transgenic SOD1 rats. Although a transient microglial phenotype was detected at day 15, astroglial staining was negative in engrafted cells from day 1 to day 60. At day 30, differentiation toward a neuronal phenotype was identified, which was further established at day 60 by the expression of the neuronal marker MAP2. A specification process into motoneuron-like structures was evidenced in the ventral horns in both wild-type and SOD1 rats. These results demonstrated proof-of-principle of survival and differentiation of human iPSC-derived neural progenitors in *in vivo* ALS environment, offering perspectives for the use of iPSC-based therapy in ALS.

ITIH4 and Gpx3 as Potential Biomarkers in ALS The diagnosis of ALS is difficult due to lack of definitive biomarkers. Tanaka et al. (2013) identified characteristic serum protein patterns that could provide candidate biomarkers for ALS. These investigators divided mutant superoxide dismutase-1 (SOD1) (H46R) rats into three groups based on disease progression: pre-symptom (90 days), onset, and end-stage. After separation of serum proteins using 2-D electrophoresis, they selected clear protein spots and identified two candidate proteins-inter-α-trypsin inhibitor heavy chain H4 (ITIH4) and Glutathione Peroxidase 3 (Gpx3). The 120 kDa ITIH4 increased at the onset of the disease and the 85 kDa ITIH4, a cleaved form, at the end-stage in the sera of the SOD1 (H46R) rats. Expression of the 85 kDa ITIH4 was substantial in ALS compared with controls or patients with muscular dystrophy, AD, or PD. The Gpx3 protein levels in the sera of SOD1(H46R) rats were upregulated pre-symptom and gradually decreased as the disease progressed. The Gpx3 protein levels were lower in the sera of the patients with ALS than in other diseases, indicating that ITIH4 and Gpx3 are potential biomarkers for ALS.

TARDBP and ANG Genes Mutations in ALS In ALS, the analysis of CSF is usually performed to exclude inflammatory processes of the CNS. Although in a small subset of patients an intrathecal synthesis of IgG is detectable, usually there is no clear explanation for this evidence. Ticozzi et al. (2013) investigated the occurrence of oligoclonal bands (OCBs) in the CSF of a large series of ALS patients, attempting a correlation with genotype data. CSF was collected from 259 ALS patients. CSF parameters were measured according to standard procedures, and detection of OCBs performed by isoelectric focusing. The patients were screened for mutations in SOD1, FUS, TARDBP, ANG, OPTN, and C9ORF72. These investigators observed the presence of OCBs in the CSF of 9/259 ALS patients (3.5%), and of disease-associated mutations in 12 cases. OCBs were more frequent in mutation carriers compared to the remaining cohort. Among patients with OCBs, two patients had the TARDBP p.A382T mutation (one of which in homozygous state), and one the ANG p.P-4S variant. Both patients carrying the p.A382T mutation had an atypical phenotype, one of them manifesting signs suggestive of a cerebellar involvement, and the other presenting neuroradiological findings suggestive of an inflammatory disorder of the CNS, suggesting that ALS patients with OCBs may harbor mutations in disease-causing genes and that mutations in both TARDBP and ANG genes may disrupt the blood-brain barrier (BBB), promoting local immune responses and neuroinflammation. Hence the role of mutant TARDBP and ANG genes on BBB integrity of ALS patients warrants further investigation.

The last 30 years have seen a major advance in the understanding of the clinical and pathological heterogeneity of ALS, and its overlap with frontotemporal dementia. Multiple, seemingly disparate biochemical pathways converge on a common clinical syndrome characterized by progressive loss of upper and lower motor neurons. Pathogenic themes in ALS include excitotoxicity, oxidative stress, mitochondrial dysfunction, neuroinflammation, altered energy metabolism, and most recently RNA mis-processing. The transgenic rodent, overexpressing mutant superoxide dismutase-1, is now only one of several models of ALS pathogenesis. The nematode, fruit fly and zebrafish all offer fresh insight, and the development of induced pluripotent stem cell-derived motor neurons holds promise for the screening of candidate therapeutics. The lack of useful biomarkers in ALS contributes to diagnostic delay, and the inability to stratify patients by prognosis may be an important factor in the failure of therapeutic trials. Biomarkers sensitive to disease activity might lessen reliance on clinical measures and survival as trial endpoints and reduce study length.

Emerging proteomic markers of neuronal loss and glial activity in cerebrospinal fluid, a cortical signature derived from advanced structural and functional MRI, and the development of more sensitive measurements of lower motor neuron physiology are leading a new phase of biomarker-driven therapeutic discovery (Turner et al., 2013).

Mutations in TAR DNA-binding protein (TARDBP) are associated with heterogenic phenotypes, including amyotrophic lateral sclerosis, frontotemporal dementia, and Parkinson's disease. In this study, the researchers investigated the presence of TARDBP mutations in a cohort of 429 Dutch patients with Parkinson's disease. Although these investgators detected 1 silent mutation, p.S332S, no missense mutations were present in their cohort. These findings, demonstrated that TARDBP mutations do not appear to contribute to the pathogenesis of Parkinson's disease in The Netherlands (van Blitterswijk et al., 2013).

The H63D polymorphism in HFE has frequently been associated with susceptibility to ALS. Regarding the role of HFE in Iron homeostasis, Iron accumulation is considered an important process in ALS. Furthermore, novel therapeutic strategies are being developed targeting this process. Evidence for this genetic association is, however, limited to several small studies. For this reason H63D polymorphism was studied in a large European cohort including 3962 ALS patients and 5072 control subjects from 7 countries. After meta-analysis of previous studies and current findings these researchers concluded that the H63D polymorphism in HFE is not associated with susceptibility to ALS, age at disease onset, or survival (van Reneenan et al., 2013).

Exposure to selenium, and particularly to its inorganic forms, has been hypothesized as a risk factor for ALS, a fast progressing motor neuron disease with poorly understood etiology. However, no information is known about levels of inorganic and some organic selenium species in the CNS of ALS patients, and recent observations suggest that peripheral biomarkers of exposure are unable to predict these levels for several Se species including the inorganic forms. Using a hospital-referred case-control series and advanced selenium speciation methods, the researchers compared the chemical species of selenium in CSF from 38 ALS patients to those of 38 reference neurological patients matched on age and gender. They found that higher concentrations of inorganic selenium in the form of selenite and of human serum albumin-bound selenium were associated with increased ALS risk (relative risks 3.9 (95% confidence interval 1.2-11.0) and 1.7 (1.0-2.9) for 0.1µg/L increase). Conversely, lower concentrations of selenoprotein P-bound selenium were associated with increased risk (relative risk 0.2 for 1µg/L increase, 95% confidence interval 0.04-0.8). The associations were stronger among cases age 50 years or older, who are postulated to have lower rates of genetic disease origin. These results suggested that excess selenite and human serum albumin bound-selenium and low levels of selenoprotein P-bound selenium in the CNS, which may be related, may play a role in ALS etiology (Vinceti et al., 2013).

Mutations in ALS Mutations in the optineurin (OPTN) gene have been associated with normal tension glaucoma and with ALS. Here, the researchers screened German familial ALS cases for OPTN mutations to gain additional insight into the spectrum and pathogenic relevance of this gene for ALS. One hundred familial German ALS cases and 148 control subjects were screened for OPTN mutations by sequence analysis of the complete OPTN coding sequence, and phenotypes of OPTN mutant patients were described. The researchers identified a novel heterozygous truncating OPTN mutation p.Lys440Asnfs*8 in 1 ALS family with an aggressive ALS disease phenotype. This mutation abolishes protein domains crucial for nuclear factor κB signaling. Moreover, they detected 3 different nonsynonymous sequence variants, which have been described previously as risk factors for primary retinal ganglion cell degeneration in normal tension glaucoma. Two of them were detected on the same allele in a family that also carries a p.Asn352Ser disease mutation in the ALS gene TARDBP. All OPTN mutant patients presented with typical spinal onset ALS. Taken together, they detected a novel truncating OPTN mutation associated with an aggressive form of ALS and confirmed that OPTN mutations are a rare cause of ALS. In addition their data suggested that in some cases plausibly more than 1 mutation in OPTN or another ALS gene might be needed to cause ALS. Finally, these findings showed that motoneurons and retinal ganglion cells, which are both projecting CNS neurons, might share common susceptibility factors (Weishaupt et al., 2013).

Therapies designed to decrease the level of SOD1 are currently in a clinical trial for patients with superoxide dismutase (SOD1)-linked familial ALS. To determine whether the SOD1 protein in CSF may be a pharmacodynamic marker for antisense oligonucleotide therapy and a disease marker for ALS, antisense oligonucleotides targeting human SOD1 were administered to rats expressing SOD1G93A. The human SOD1 protein levels were measured in the rats' brain and CSF samples. In human CSF samples, the following proteins were measured: SOD1, tau, phosphorylated tau, VILIP-1, and YKL-40. Ninety-three participants with ALS, 88 healthy controls, and 89 controls with a neurological disease (55 with dementia of the Alzheimer type, 19 with multiple sclerosis, and 15 with peripheral neuropathy). Antisense oligonucleotide-treated SOD1G93A rats had decreased human SOD1 messenger RNA levels (mean [SD] decrease of 69% [4%]) and decreased protein levels (mean [SD] decrease of 48% [14%]) in the brain. The rats' CSF samples showed a similar decrease in hSOD1 levels (mean [SD] decrease of 42% [14%]). In human CSF samples, the SOD1 levels varied a mean (SD) 7.1% (5.7%) after additional measurements, separated by months, were performed. The CSF SOD1 levels were higher in the participants with ALS (mean [SE] level, 172 [8] ng/mL; $P < .05$) and the controls with a neurological disease (mean [SE] level, 172 [6] ng/mL; $P < .05$) than in the healthy controls (mean [SE] level, 134 [4] ng/mL). Elevated CSF SOD1 levels did not correlate with disease characteristics in participants with ALS or controls with dementia of the Alzheimer type, but they did correlate with tau, phosphorylated tau, VILIP-1 and YKL-40 levels in controls with dementia of the Alzheimer type. SOD1 in CSF may be an excellent pharmacodynamic marker for SOD1-lowering therapies because antisense oligonucleotide therapy lowers protein levels in the rat brain and rat CSF samples and because SOD1 levels in CSF samples from humans are stable over time (Winer et al., 2013).

FUS Gene Mutation in Juvenile ALS Juvenile ALS is a rare form of motor neuron disease and occurs before 25 years of age. Only very few sporadic cases of juvenile-onset ALS have been reported. Rare SOD1 mutations and several FUS mutations have been identified in juvenile-onset ALS patients. To define the genetics of juvenile-onset sporadic ALS (SALS) of Chinese origin, Zou et al. (2013 sequenced all 5 exons of SOD1, exons 3-6 and 12-15 of FUS in 11 juvenile-onset SALS patients, 105 adult-onset ALS patients (including 6 familial ALS [FALS] pedigrees), and 245 healthy controls. For the 11 juvenile-onset SALS and 6 FALS cases, the other 7 exons of FUS were also screened. A heterozygous de novo missense mutation c.1574C > T (p.P525L), a heterozygous de novo 2-base pair deletion c.1509_1510delAG (p.G504Wfs*12), and a nonsense mutation c.1483C > T (p.R495X) was each identified in 1 juvenile SALS patient. A heterozygous missense mutation c.1561C > G (p.R521G) was identified in a FALS proband. In the Chinese population, the frequency of FUS mutation in FALS is 11.4% (95% confidence interval [CI], 0.9%-22.0%), higher than the Japanese (10%; 95% CI, 0.7%-19.3%), and Caucasians (4.9%; 95% CI, 3.9%-6.0%). The frequency of FUS mutation in SALS patients is 1.5% (95% CI, 0.2%-2.9%), which is similar to Koreans (1.6%; 95% CI, 0%-3.2%), but higher than in Caucasians (0.6%; 95% CI, 0.4%-0.8%), suggesting that de novo FUS mutations are associated with juvenile-onset SALS of Chinese origin and that this gene should be screened in ALS patients with a young age of onset, aggressive progression, and sporadic occurrence.

Mutations in Valosin-Containing Protein (VCP) in ALS Mutations in valosin-containing protein (VCP) gene was recently detected in familial and sporadic ALS. To define the frequency of VCP mutations in ALS patients in Chinese population, Zou et al. (2013) sequenced all 17 exons of the VCP gene in a cohort of both familial and sporadic ALS patients of Chinese origin. No nonsynonymous coding variants were identified. This indicated that VCP mutations are not a common cause of familial or sporadic ALS in Chinese population. Mutations in the profilin 1 (PFN1) gene, encoding a member of the profilin family of small actin-binding proteins, have been recently reported in patients with familial ALS. In this study the researchers aimed to determine the prevalence of PFN1 mutations by sequencing the coding region of this gene in a cohort of 94 familial ALS patients from France and Quebec. No mutations were identified in their cohort suggesting that PFN1 gene mutations are a very rare cause of familial ALS among patients with predominantly European ancestry (Daaud et al. 2013). Mutations in PFN1, a gene encoding the actin monomer-binding protein profilin 1, were recently reported in 1% to 2% of familial ALS patients. *In vitro* functional studies suggested that PFN1 mutations lead to ubiquitin-positive inclusions and impairment of cytoskeletal pathways. In this study, mutation analysis of PFN1 was performed in an Australian cohort of 110 ALS families and 715 sporadic ALS patients. No PFN1 mutations were identified in familial ALS patients. Two rare non-synonymous variants (E117D and E117G) were found in sporadic ALS patients at similar incidences to that reported in public SNP databases. Immunostaining of PFN1 in sporadic ALS and familial ALS patients, including those with mutations in SOD1, FUS, UBQLN2 and C9ORF72, found no PFN1-positive inclusions in spinal motor neurons. These data suggested that PFN1 mutations and pathology are not common in an Australian ALS cohort of predominantly European ancestry (Yang et al..2013). Mutations in the profilin 1 (PFN1) gene, encoding a protein regulating filamentous actin growth through its binding to monomeric G-actin, were recently identified in familial ALS. Functional studies performed on ALS-associated PFN1 mutants demonstrated aggregation propensity, alterations in growth cone, and cytoskeletal dynamics. Previous screening of PFN1 gene in sporadic ALS (SALS) cases led to the detection of the p.E117G mutation, which represents a less pathogenic variant according to both frequency data in control subjects and cases, and functional experiments. To determine the effective contribution of PFN1 mutations in SALS, Tiloka et al. (2013) analyzed a large cohort of 1168 Italian SALS patients and also included 203 frontotemporal dementia (FTD) cases because of the great overlap between these 2 neurodegenerative diseases. These researchers detected the p.E117G variant in 1 SALS patient and the novel synonymous change p.G15G in another patient, but none in a panel of 1512 control subjects, suggesting that PFN1 mutations in sporadic ALS and in FTD are rare, particularly in the Italian population.

REFERENCES

Akimoto, C., Forsgren, L., Linder, J., Birve, A., Backlund, I., Andersson, J., Nilsson, A. C., Alstermark, H. & Andersen, P. M. (2013). No GGGGCC-hexanucleotide repeat expansion in C9ORF72 in parkinsonism patients in Sweden. *Amyotroph Lateral Scler Frontotemporal Degener.*, *14*(1), 26-29.

Alavi, A., Nafissi, S., Rohani, M, Zamani, B., Sedighi, B., Shamshiri, H., Fan, J. B., Ronaghi, M. & Elahi, E. (2013). Genetic analysis and SOD1 mutation screening in Iranian amyotrophic lateral sclerosis patients. *Neurobiol Aging.*, 2013 May, *34*(5), 1516. e1-8.

Bastin, M. E., Pettit, L. D., Bak, T. H., Gillingwater, T. H., Smith, C. & Abrahams, S. (2013). Quantitative tractography and tract shape modeling in amyotrophic lateral sclerosis. *J Magn Reson Imaging.*, 2013 Feb 28.

Blasco, H., Corcia, P., Pradat, P. F., Bocca, C., Gordon, P. H., Veyrat-Durebex, C., Mavel, S., Nadal-Desbarats, L., Moreau, C., Devos, D., Andres, C. R. & Emond, P. (2013). Metabolomics in Cerebrospinal Fluid of Patients with Amyotrophic Lateral Sclerosis: An Untargeted Approach via High-Resolution Mass Spectrometry. *J. Proteome Res.*, *12*, 3746-3754.

Boylan, K. B., Glass, J. D., Crook, J. E., Yang, C., Thomas, C. S., Desaro, P., Johnston, A., Overstreet, K., Kelly, C., Polak, M. & Shaw, G. (2013). Phosphorylated neurofilament heavy subunit (pNF-H) in peripheral blood and CSF as a potential prognostic biomarker in amyotrophic lateral sclerosis. *J. Neurol. Neurosurg. Psychiatry.*, *84*, 467-472.

D'Amico, E., Factor-Litvak, P., Santella, R. M. & Mitsumoto, H. (2013). Clinical perspective on oxidative stress in sporadic amyotrophic lateral sclerosis. *Free Radic Biol Med.*, *65C*, 509-527.

Daoud, H., Dobrzeniecka, S., Camu, W., Meininger, V., Dupré, N., Dion, P. A. & Rouleau, G. A. (2013). Mutation analysis of PFN1 in familial amyotrophic lateral sclerosis patients. *Neurobiol Aging.*, *34*(4), 1311.e1-2. doi:

Franco, M. C., Ye, Y., Refakis, C. A., Feldman, J. L., Stokes, A. L., Basso, M., Melero Fernández de Mera, R. M., Sparrow, N. A., Calingasan, N. Y, Kiaei, M., Rhoads, T. W., Ma, T. C., Grumet, M., Barnes, S., Beal, M. F., Beckman, J. S., Mehl, R. & Estévez, A. G. (2013). Nitration of Hsp90 induces cell death. *Proc Natl Acad Sci U S A.*, *110*(12), E1102-1111.

Gandhi, R., Healy, B., Gholipour, T., Egorova, S., Musallam, A., Hussain, M. S., Nejad, P., Patel, B., Hei, H., Khoury, S., Quintana, F., Kivisakk, P., Chitnis, T. & Weiner, H. L. (2013). Circulating MicroRNAs as biomarkers for disease staging in multiple sclerosis. *Ann. Neurol.*, *73*(6), 729-740.

Ganesalingam, J., An, J., Bowser, R., Andersen, P. M. & Shaw, C. E. (2013). pNfH is a promising biomarker for ALS. *Amyotroph Lateral Scler Frontotemporal Degener.*, *14*(2), 146-149.

González-Garza, M. T., Martínez, H. R., Caro-Osorio, E., Cruz-Vega, D. E., Hernández-Torre, M. & Moreno-Cuevas, J. E. (2013). Differentiation of CD133+ stem cells from amyotrophic lateral sclerosis patients into preneuron cells. *Stem Cells Transl. Med.*, *2*(2), 129-135.

Grossman, M. (2013). Multimodal comparative studies of neurodegenerative diseases. *Journal of Alzheimer's Disease*, 33, S379-S383.

Harms, M. B., Neumann, D., Benitez, B. A., Cooper, B., Carrell, D., Racette, B. A., Perlmutter, J. S., Goate, A. & Cruchaga, C. (2013). Parkinson disease is not associated with C9ORF72 repeat expansions. *Neurobiol Aging.*, *34*(5), 1519, e1-2.

Hirano, K., Ohgomori, T., Kobayashi, K., Tanaka, F., Matsumoto, T., Natori, T., Matsuyama, Y., Uchimura, K., Sakamoto, K., Takeuchi, H., Hirakawa, A., Suzumura, A., Sobue, G., Ishiguro, N., Imagama, S. & Kadomatsu, K. Ablation of keratan sulfate accelerates early phase pathogenesis of ALS. *PLoS One.*, *8*(6), e66969.

Hof, D., Jung, H. H. & Bloch, K. E. (2013). Troponin T elevation in amyotrophic lateral sclerosis without cardiac damage. *Amyotroph Lateral Scler Frontotemporal Degener.*, *14*(1), 75-77.

Huey, E. D., Nagy, P. L., Rodriguez-Murillo, L., Manoochehri, M., Goldman, J., Lieberman, J., Karayiorgou, M. & Mayeux, R. (2013). C9ORF72 repeat expansions not detected in a group of patients with schizophrenia. *Neurobiol Aging.*, *34*(4), 1309, e9-10.

Hwang, C. S., Liu, G. T., Chang, M. D., Liao, I. L. & Chang, H. T. (2013). Elevated serum autoantibody against high mobility group box 1 as a potent surrogate biomarker for amyotrophic lateral sclerosis. *Neurobiol Dis.*, *58*, 13-18.

Jang, J. H., Kwon, M. J., Choi, W. J., Oh, K. W., Koh, S. H., Ki, C. S. & Kim, S. H. (2013). Analysis of the C9orf72 hexanucleotide repeat expansion in Korean patients with familial and sporadic amyotrophic lateral sclerosis. *Neurobiol Aging.*, *34*(4), 1311, e7-9.

Jaronen, M., Vehviläinen, P., Malm, T., Keksa-Goldsteine, V., Pollari, E., Valonen, P., Koistinaho, J. & Goldsteins, G. (2013). Protein disulfide isomerase in ALS mouse glia links protein misfolding with NADPH oxidase-catalyzed superoxide production. *Hum Mol Genet.*, *22*(4), 646-655.

Kobayashi, K., Imagama, S., Ohgomori, T., Hirano, K., Uchimura, K., Sakamoto, K., Hirakawa, A., Takeuchi, H., Suzumura, A., Ishiguro, N. & Kadomatsu, K. (2013). Minocycline selectively inhibits M1 polarization of microglia. *Cell Death Dis.*, *4*, e525.

Kohli, M. A., John-Williams, K., Rajbhandary, R., Naj, A., Whitehead, P., Hamilton, K., Carney, R. M, Wright, C., Crocco, E., Gwirtzman, H. E., Lang, R., Beecham, G., Martin, E. R., Gilbert, J., Benatar, M., Small, G. W., Mash, D., Byrd, G., Haines, J. L., Pericak-Vance, M. A. & Züchner, S. (2013). Repeat expansions in the C9ORF72 gene contribute to Alzheimer's disease in Caucasians. *Neurobiol Aging.*, *34*(5), 1519. e5-12.

Kolind, S., Sharma, R., Knight, S., Johansen-Berg, H., Talbot, K. & Turner, M. R. (2013). Myelin imaging in amyotrophic and primary lateral sclerosis. *Amyotroph Lateral Scler Frontotemporal Degener.*, *14*(7-8), 562-573.

Koppers, M., Groen, E. J., van Vught, P. W., van Rheenen, W., Witteveen, E., van Es, M. A., Pasterkamp, R. J., van den Berg, L. H. & Veldink, J. H. (2013). Screening for rare variants in the coding region of ALS-associated genes at 9p21.2 and 19p13.3. 2013. *Neurobiol Aging.*, *34*(5), 1518, e5-7.

Krüger, T., Lautenschläger, J., Grosskreutz, J. & Rhode, H. (2013). Proteome analysis of body fluids for amyotrophic lateral sclerosis biomarker discovery. *Proteomics Clin Appl.*, *7*(1-2), 123-135.

Lilo, E., Wald-Altman, S., Solmesky, L. J., Ben Yaakov, K., Gershoni-Emek, N., Bulvik, S., Kassis, I., Karussis, D., Perlson, E. & Weil, M. (2013). Characterization of human sporadic ALS biomarkers in the familial ALS transgenic mSOD1G93A mouse model. *Hum Mol Genet.*, *22*(23), 4720- 4725.

Maxmen, A. (2013). RNA: The genome's rising stars. *Nature.*, *496*, 127-129.

McGoldrick, P., Joyce, P. I., Fisher, E. M. & Greensmith, L. (2013). Rodent models of amyotrophic lateral sclerosis. *Biochim Biophys Acta.*, *1832*(9), 1421-1436.

Mutation analysis of PFN1 in familial amyotrophic lateral sclerosis patients. *Neurobiol Aging.*, 2013 May, *34*(5), 1516. e9-15.

Li, H. F. & Wu, Z. Y. (2016). Genotype-phenotype correlations of amyotrophic lateral sclerosis. *Translational Neurodegeneration*, *5*, 3.

Popescu, I. R., Nicaise, C., Liu, S., Bisch, G., Knippenberg, S., Daubie, V., Bohl, D. & Pochet, R. (2013). Neural progenitors derived from human induced pluripotent stem cells survive and differentiate upon transplantation into a rat model of amyotrophic lateral sclerosis. *Stem Cells Transl Med.*, *2*(3), 167-174.

Roos, P. M., Vesterberg, O., Syversen, T., Flaten, T. P. & Nordberg, M. (2013). Metal concentrations in cerebrospinal fluid and blood plasma from patients with amyotrophic lateral sclerosis. *Biol. Trace. Elem Res.*, *151*, 159-170.

Sharma, S., Moon, C. S., Khogali, A., Haidous, A., Chabenne, A., Ojo, C., Jelebinkov, M., Kurdi, Y. & Ebadi, M. (2013). Biomarkers in Parkinson's disease (recent update). *Neurochem Int.*, *63*(3), 201-229.

Tanaka, H., Shimazawa, M., Takata, M., Kaneko, H., Tsuruma, K., Ikeda, T., Warita, H., Aoki, M., Yamada, M., Takahashi, H., Hozumi, I., Minatsu, H., Inuzuka, T. & Hara, H. 2013. ITIH4 and Gpx3 are potential biomarkers for amyotrophic lateral sclerosis. *J Neurol.*, *260*(7), 1782-1797.

Ticozzi, N., Tiloca, C., Mencacci, N. E., Morelli, C., Doretti, A., Rusconi, D., Colombrita, C., Sangalli, D., Verde, F., Finelli, P., Messina, S., Ratti, A. & Silani, V. (2013). Oligoclonal bands in the cerebrospinal fluid of amyotrophic lateral sclerosis patients with disease-associated mutations. *J Neurol.*, *260*(1), 85-92.

Tiloca, C., Ticozzi, N., Pensato, V., Corrado, L., Del Bo, R., Bertolin, C., Fenoglio, C., Gagliardi, S., Calini, D., Lauria, G., Castellotti, B., Bagarotti, A., Corti, S., Galimberti, D., Cagnin, A., Gabelli, C., Ranieri, M., Ceroni, M., Siciliano, G., Mazzini, L., Cereda, C., Scarpini, E., Sorarù, G., Comi, G. P., D'Alfonso, S., Gellera, C., Ratti, A., Landers, J. E., Silani, V. & SLAGEN, Consortium. (2013). Screening of the PFN1 gene in sporadic amyotrophic lateral sclerosis and in frontotemporal dementia. *Neurobiol Aging.*, *34*(5), 1517. e9-10.

Turner, M. R., Bowser, R., Bruijn, L., Dupuis, L., Ludolph, A., McGrath, M., Manfredi, G., Maragakis, N., Miller, R. G., Pullman, S. L., Rutkove, S. B., Shaw, P. J., Shefner, J. & Fischbeck, K. H. (2013). Mechanisms, models and biomarkers in amyotrophic lateral sclerosis. *Amyotroph Lateral Scler Frontotemporal Degener.*, May, 14 Suppl *1*, 19-32.

van Blitterswijk, M., van Es, M. A., Verbaan, D., van Hilten, J. J., Scheffer, H., van de Warrenburg, B. P., Veldink, J. H. & van den Berg, L. H. (2013). Mutational analysis of TARDBP in Parkinson's disease. *Neurobiol Aging.*, *34*(5), 1517, e1-3.

van Rheenen, W., Diekstra, F. P., van Doormaal, P. T., Seelen, M., Kenna, K., McLaughlin, R., et al., (2013). H63D polymorphism in HFE is not associated with amyotrophic lateral sclerosis. *Neurobiol Aging.*, *34*(5), 1517, e5-7.

Vinceti, M., Solovyev, N., Mandrioli, J, Crespi, C. M., Bonvicini, F., Arcolin, E., Georgoulopoulou, E. & Michalke, B. (2013). Cerebrospinal fluid of newly diagnosed amyotrophic lateral sclerosis patients exhibits abnormal levels of selenium species including elevated selenite. *Neurotoxicology.*, *38C*, 25-32.

Weishaupt, J. H., Waibel, S., Birve, A., Volk, A. E., Mayer, B., Meyer, T., Ludolph, A. C. & Andersen, P. M. (2013). A novel optineurin truncating mutation and three glaucoma-associated missense variants in patients with familial amyotrophic lateral sclerosis in Germany. *Neurobiol Aging.*, *34*(5), 1516, e9-15.

Winer, L., Srinivasan, D., Chun, S., Lacomis, D., Jaffa, M., Fagan, A., Holtzman, D. M., Wancewicz, E., Bennett, C. F., Bowser, R., Cudkowicz, M. & Miller, T. M. (2013). SOD1 in cerebral spinal fluid as a pharmacodynamic marker for antisense oligonucleotide therapy. *JAMA Neurol.*, *70*(2), 201-207.

Yang, S., Fifita, J. A., Williams, K. L., Warraich, S. T., Pamphlett, R., Nicholson, G. A. & Blair, I. P. Mutation analysis and immunopathological studies of PFN1 in familial and sporadic amyotrophic lateral sclerosis. *Neurobiol Aging.*, 2013 Sep, *34*(9), 2235, e7-10.

Zou, Z. Y., Cui, L. Y., Sun, Q., Li, X. G., Liu, M. S., Xu, Y., Zhou, Y. & Yang, X. Z. (2013). De novo FUS gene mutations are associated with juvenile-onset sporadic amyotrophic lateral sclerosis in China. *Neurobiol Aging.*, 2013 Apr, *34*(4), 1312, e1-8.

Zou, Z. Y., Liu, M. S., Li, X. G. & Cui, L. Y. (2013). Screening of VCP mutations in Chinese amyotrophic lateral sclerosis patients. *Neurobiol Aging.*, *34*(5), 1519, e3-4.

Chapter 13

BIOMARKERS IN PERSONALIZED THERANOSTICS OF MULTIPLE SCLEROSIS (RECENT UPDATE)

ABSTRACT

Currently there is no single, specific, and sensitive biomarker for the differential diagnosis and EBPT of relapse-remitting multiple sclerosis (RRMS). Several biomarkers including: TOB-1 polymorphisms; up-regulated microRNAs (miR0145) and down-regulated CD44; CNS demylination and lesions in the veins, myelin basic proteins, neurofilaments, oligoclonal bands, Neopterin, Fetuin-A, Osteopontin, sulfatides, α-4 integrin, ubiquitin C-terminal hydrolase-L1, HLA-DRB1, and autoantibodies to NH_2-terminal α-enolase are detected in the CSF and serum samples of RRMS patients. Cytotoxic NKG2C+ CD4 T cells, spinal PKCγ-regulating pain sensitivity and locomotion, inflammatory uveitis, monomeric and dimeric κ- and λ-free light chains, urinary metabolites; CD20, sCD146 and CD44 in OPCs migration and $CD4^+$ (Th1 and Th17) cells are induced in MS. Although low density lipoprotein receptor-related protein-1 and Muc1 have anti-inflammatory role, light neurofilament subunits, enhanced β2-microglobulin, oligo-adenylate synthetase-1, and Neopterin induce immune response in MS patients. Differential lymphocyte reconstitution after Alemtuzumab treatment and MRI brain volumetry, IgG, and proliferation-inducing ligand may also be used as potential RRMS biomarkers. Progressive neurodegeneration in MC-deficient Kit/Kit mice is associated with induction in Muc1, a membrane tethered glycoprotein. In addition, E-selectin, O-mannosyl glycans, NFL, GFAP, β-Tub II proteins, NKG2C+ CD4 T cell activation, CD70, DNA methylation, histone acetylation, and miRNA-associated gene silencing were detected in MS patients. 24S-Hydroxycholesterol and Vitamin D in plasma, FasL in astrocytes, CSF Aβ, soluble APP, SOD, metallothioneins (MTs), α-Synuclein index, and Charnoly body are emerging biomarkers of RRMS. In addition, Gd-enhanced MRI can determine structural and functional intactness of blood brain barrier, myelin hypercitrullination and peptidylarginine deiminases activation. However, the mechanism of APP metabolism and whether it is affected by disease-modifying treatment remains uncertain and warrants further novel biomarker(s) discovery to precisely evaluate proinflammatory neurodegeneration and demyelination/ remyelination in RRMS. MicroRNAs are short, noncoding RNAs with gene regulatory functions whose expression may serve as MS biomarkers. This chapter highlights several emerging biomarkers and their future prospects for the personalized clinical management of RRMS with minimum or no adverse effects.

Keywords: disease-specific biomarkers, omics biomarkers, microRNA, metallothioneins, α-
synuclein index, Charnoly body, neuroimaging

INTRODUCTION

Multiple sclerosis (MS) is the most common genetically mediated autoimmune, CNS-demyelinating disease, exhibiting diverse genetic, clinical, and pathological heterogeneity and resistance to therapeutic interventions. In progressive multiple sclerosis (PMS), disease-modifying therapies have not been shown to reduce disability progression. It is a multifactorial autoimmune disease mediated by T cells in which interaction of external factors and structural features of various genes plays a pivotal role. MS is an autoimmune, chronic inflammatory, demyelinating disease, and myelin-derived glycolipids and axonal degeneration are the primary targets in this progressive neurodegenerative disorder. Nevertheless, specific biomarker(s) to progressive neurodegeneration, therapeutic responsiveness, and underlying molecular mechanism of the RRMS remain unknown. Fernández et al. (2013) recently highlighted that MS is the most frequent disabling neurological disease in young adults. Its development includes inflammation, demyelination, neurodegeneration, gliosis and repair, is responsible for the heterogeneity and individual variability in the expression and its prognosis and response to treatment. Particularly, B7-H3 has a primary role in regulating T cell responses with involvement of both humoral and cell-mediated immune systems and variable therapeutic response (Koziolek et al., 2013). As a part of PM, the search for new biomarkers identified promising candidates that may be useful for the early diagnosis of the disease for detecting prognostic and developmental profiles of the disease, and for monitoring the response to treatment.

Reently, B cells have emerged as major contributors to disease pathogenesis, but the mechanisms responsible for the loss of B cell tolerance in patients with MS are unknown. In healthy individuals, developing autoreactive B cells are removed from the repertoire at 2 tolerance checkpoints during early B cell development. Both of these central and peripheral B cell tolerance checkpoints are defective in patients with rheumatoid arthritis (RA) and type 1 diabetes (T1D). Kinnunen et al. (2013) found that only the peripheral, but not the central, B cell tolerance checkpoint is defective in patients with MS. This specific defect is accompanied by increased activation and homeostatic proliferation of mature naive B cells. Interestingly, all of these MS features parallel defects observed in FOXP3-deficient IPEX patients, who harbor nonfunctional Tregs. In contrast to patients with RA or T1D, bone marrow central B cell selection in MS appeared normal in most patients. In contrast, patients with MS suffer from a specific peripheral B cell tolerance defect that is potentially attributable to impaired Treg function and that leads to the accumulation of autoreactive B cell clones in their blood.

The development of MS involves inflammation, demyelination, neurodegeneration, gliosis and repair, that are responsible for the heterogeneity and individual variability in its progression, prognosis, and response to treatment. Accordingly, MS treatment should be tailored to address disease traits pertinent to each patient. It is now realized that dendritic cells (DC) play an important role in the development of inflammatory response in MS. However, its expression and clinical significance remains unknown. *In general, oligoclonal bands (OCBs) unique to the CSF are used in the diagnosis of MS.* However a definitive diagnostic test for MS does not exist; instead *doctors use a combination of medical history, MRI, and CSF examination to confirm its diagnosi*s. Although significant efforts have been made to identify biomarkers from CSF to facilitate diagnosis, none of these biomarkers have been successful for the personalized treatment of MS. However, at the center of personalized management is the emergence of new knowledge, enabling optimized treatment and disease-modifying therapies.

The use of plasma exchange (PE) in steroid-refractory relapses has become an important part for the treatment of steroid-resistant relapses of MS with an efficacy of 40-70%. So far, 6 studies of immunoadsorption (IA) treatment in different forms of MS have been published, 4 of them in steroid-refractory MS relapses. These studies revealed clinical improvement in 73-85% of patients. However in MS patients with non-active relapsing-remitting or secondary progressive course, there was no significant improvement, suggesting similar efficacy of IA in the treatment of steroid-refractory MS relapses compared to PE.

Urine is a source of metabolite biomarkers and can be used as a potential rapid, noninvasive, inexpensive, and efficient diagnostic tool in MS. However, urinary metabolites have not been fully explored as a source of biomarkers for MS. Gebregiworgis et al. (2013) demonstrated that urinary metabolites can be used to monitor disease-progression, and response to treatment in MS patients. NMR analysis of urine identified metabolites that differentiate experimental autoimmune encephalomyelitis (EAE)-mice (*model for MS*) from healthy and drug-treated EAE mice. Pravica et al. (2013) analyzed genetic and nongenetic biomarkers in decision-making algorithms to assist diagnosis and in predicting the disease course and therapeutic response in MS patients.

Although our understanding of dementia in the oldest old has advanced dramatically in recent years, more research is needed, particularly among varied racial, ethnic, and socioeconomic groups, and with respect to biomarkers such as neuroimaging, modifiable risk factors, and therapy. *This chapter provides an update on the emerging biomarkers in MS that have been validated so far and are thus potential candidates, as well as evaluating the diagnosis, prognosis, and development of the disability caused by the disease and the response to therapy. The chapter highlights the recent update in MS-specific biomarkers for updating the knowledge of physicians, scientists, and students interested in novel biomarker(s) discovery, early differential diagnosis, prognosis, and effective personalized treatment of RRMS with currently limited therapeutic success.*

It is now realized that the diagnosis and prognosis of initial demyelinating event (IDE) in RRMS are not straightforward. Hence novel discovery of diagnostic biomarkers is exceedingly important. Some studies suggest that oxidative stress may be one of the sources, or a consequence of the disease, due to redox imbalance. During the last decades, the effort of establishing satisfactory biomarkers for MS has proven challenging due to the clinical and pathophysiological complexities of the disease. Recent knowledge from genomics-immunogenetics, neuroimmunology, and neuroimaging, provided an extensive list of biomarkers which leads to confusion in the decision making concerning EBPT of MS.

A critical problem in MS is failure of remyelination, which is important for protecting axons against degeneration and restoring conduction deficits. The underlying mechanism of demyelination/remyelination remains unclear. N-Acetylglucosaminyltransferase-IX (GnT-IX; also known as GnT-Vb) is a brain-specific glycosyltransferase that catalyzes the branched formation of O-mannosyl glycan structures. O-Mannosylation of α-dystroglycan is critical for its function as an extracellular matrix receptor, but the biological significance of its branched structures, is unclear. Kanekiyo et al. (2013) discovered that GnT-IX formed branched O-mannosyl glycans on receptor protein tyrosine phosphatase β (RPTPβ) *in vivo*. Since RPTPβ plays a regulatory role in demyelinating diseases, GnT-IX-deficient mice were subjected to Cuprizone-induced demyelination. Cuprizone feeding for 8 weeks promoted demyelination in wild-type mice. In GnT-IX-deficient mice, the myelin content in the corpus callosum was reduced after 4 weeks of treatment, but increased at 8 weeks, suggesting enhanced remyelination under GnT-IX deficiency. Furthermore, astrocyte activation in the corpus callosum of GnT-IX-deficient mice was significantly attenuated, and an oligodendrocyte cell lineage analysis indicated that more oligodendrocyte precursor cells are differentiated into mature oligodendrocytes. Hence branched O-mannosyl glycans in the corpus callosum in the brain are a necessary component of remyelination inhibition in the Cuprizone-induced demyelination model, and that modulation of O-mannosyl glycans is a candidate for EBPT strategies.

Platelets were proposed as biomarkers in studies of mitochondrial function and aging-related and neurodegenerative diseases. Defects in mitochondrial function were found not only in the substantia nigra of PD patients but also in their platelets. Similarly, it was described in the platelet mitochondria of AD patients. Iñarrea et al. (2013) investigated mitochondrial aerobic metabolism and protein expression in platelets of MS patients and control subjects. These investigators estimated mitochondrial aconitase, superoxide dismutases 1 and 2 (SOD1 and SOD2), and respiratory complex enzyme activities in platelets, in addition to mitochondrial lipid peroxidation, SOD1, and cytochrome c expressions of MS patients and control subjects. Mitochondrial aconitase activity was higher in MS patients than in controls. A significant increase on all respiratory complexes in MS patients was observed. Mitochondrial lipid peroxidation was higher in MS patients than in controls. Significant changes of cytochrome c and SOD1 expressions were detected, with a decrease of $44 \pm 5\%$ and an increase of $46 \pm 6\%$, respectively, indicating that significant changes in aerobic metabolism and SOD1 and cytochrome c expressions are produced in platelets of MS patients.

MS As an Autoimmune Disease In T-cell-mediated autoimmune diseases of the CNS, apoptosis of Fas(+) T cells by FasL contributes to diagnosis of disease. However, the apoptosis-inducing cell population still remains to be identified. To address the role of astrocytic FasL in the regulation of T-cell apoptosis in EAE, Wang et al. (2013) immunized C57BL/6 glial fibrillary acid protein (GFAP)-Cre FasL (fl/fl) mice lacking FasL in astrocytes with MOG (35-55) peptide. GFAP-Cre FasL (fl/fl) mice were unable to resolve EAE and suffered from demyelination and paralysis, while FasL (fl/fl) control mice recovered. In contrast to FasL (fl/fl) mice, GFAP-Cre FasL (fl/fl) mice failed to induce apoptosis of Fas (+) activated CD4 (+) T cells and to increase numbers of Foxp3 (+) Treg cells beyond day 15 post immunization. The persistence of activated and GM-CSF-producing CD4 (+) T cells in GFAP-Cre FasL (fl/fl) mice also caused an increased IL-17, IFN-γ, TNF, and GM-CSF mRNA expression in the CNS. *In vitro*, FasL(+) but not FasL(-) astrocytes induced caspase-3 expression and apoptosis of activated T cells, suggesting that, FasL expression of astrocytes plays an important role in the control and elimination of autoimmune T cells from the CNS, thereby determining recovery from EAE. A type I interferon (IFN) gene signature shared by systemic lupus erythematous (SLE) and systemic sclerosis (SSc) was used to evaluate an anti-type I IFN-α receptor (IFN-αR) monoclonal antibody, MEDI-546, in a phase I trial in SSc. MEDI-546 suppressed IFN signature in blood and skin of SSc patients in a dose-dependent manner. To bridge clinical indications to SLE, Wang et al. (2013) developed a model incorporating (i) PKs and PDs in SSc patients, (ii) internalization kinetics of MEDI-546/IFN-αR complex, and (iii) the different IFN signatures between SSc and SLE. Simulations predicted that i.v. administration of MEDI-546 at 300- or 1,000-mg monthly doses could suppress IFN in blood to levels of healthy subjects in 53 and 68% of SLE patients, respectively. An innovative approach utilizing a novel biomarker characterized the PD of MEDI-546 by modeling and simulation and allowed rapid progression of MEDI-546 from a phase I study in SSc to a randomized, multiple-dose phase II trial. Activated leukocyte cell adhesion molecule (ALCAM) is involved in leukocyte migration across the BBB which is a key stage in MS pathogenesis. This study reported association of rs6437585 ALCAM polymorphism with risk and progression of MS. Wagner et al. (2013) discovered that rs6437585CT individuals had higher risk of MS and over 2 years earlier age of onset and that two ALCAM polymorphisms, rs11559013 and rs34926152, although not associated with MS itself, could modify HLA-DRB1*1501 effect. The regression analysis revealed 5-fold lower risk for MS for both rs11559013GA/HLA-DRB1*1501+ and rs34926152GT/HLA-DRB1*1501+ individuals suggesting protective role against MS for both rs11559013GA and rs34926152GT genotypes in HLA-DRB1*1501 positive patients.

Recently Katsavos and Anagnostouli (2013) provided important characteristics that a biomarker must possess to be considered as a reliable new biomarker. In general MS biomarkers may be divided into following subgroups including, (i) genetic-immunogenetic, (ii) laboratorial, and (iii) imaging. The representatives of each category were presented in a workable table, estimating their theranostic potential and efficacy to correlate with phenotypical expression, neuroinflammation, neurodegeneration, disability, and therapeutical response. Special emphasis was given to the "gold standards" of each category, like HLA-DRB1 polymorphisms, oligoclonal bands, vitamin D, and neuroimaging. Moreover, recently characterized biomarkers, like TOB-1 polymorphisms, were further discussed. Methner et al. (2013) witnessed important developments for MS, including successful phase III trials of novel oral therapeutics and identification of the potassium channel KIR4.1 as an autoimmune target. Additionally, the lung was propsed as an important site for immune-cell programming, and the relevance of a TNF receptor variant in MS paients was highlighted.

In general, MS biomarkers can be broadly classified as (i) In-vivo and (ii) in-vitro biomarkers as well as (i) invasive and (ii) non-invasive biomarkers to facilitate early and accurate EBPT of MS. In addition conventional (CT and structural) and neuroimaging (including fMRI, DTI, and PET imaging with specific radioligand) can be performed to authenticate the diagnosis and prognosis. Particularly, Gadolinium enhanced MRI provides information regarding the structural and functional integrity of the blood brain barrier, which is compromised in MS patients as illustrated in Figure 40.

Broad Classification of Biomarkers

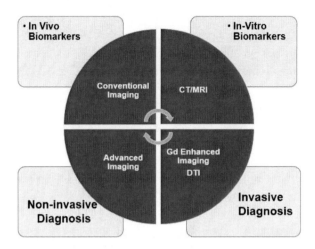

Figure 40. *Broad Classification of MS Biomarkers*: A diagram illustrating MS biomarkers which can be broadly classified as (i) *In-vivo* and (ii) *in-vitro* biomarkers as well as (i) invasive and (ii) non-invasive biomarkers to facilitate early and accurate diagnosis of MS. The researchers can perform conventional (CT and structural) and advanced neuroimaging (including fMRI, DTI, and PET imaging with specific radioligand) to authenticate the diagnosis and prognosis. For example, Gadolinium enhanced MRI can provide information regarding the structural and functional integrity of the blood brain barrier, which is compromised in MS patients.

Clinical, Neurophysiological, MRI, and CSF Biomarkers in MS Romme Christensen et al. (2013) studied CSF biomarkers and clarified whether inflammation and axonal damage are associated in progressive MS. Using ELISA, these investigators analyzed CSF from 40 secondary progressive (SPMS), 21 primary progressive (PPMS), and 36 relapsing-remitting (RRMS), and 20 non-inflammatory neurological disease (NIND) patients. Twenty-two of the SPMS patients participated in an MBP8298 peptide clinical trial and had CSF followup after one year. Compared to NIND patients, inflammatory biomarkers Osteopontin and matrix MMP9 were increased in all MS patients while CXCL13 was increased in RRMS and SPMS patients. Biomarkers of axonal damage (NFL) and demyelination (MBP) were increased in all MS patients. In progressive MS patients CSF Osteopontin and CXCL13 correlated with NFL, while Osteopontin and MMP9 correlated with MBP. MBP8298 treatment did not affect the biomarkers after one year of treatment. All biomarkers were increased after one year of follow-up except MBP, which decreased. CSF biomarkers of inflammation, axonal damage and demyelination increased in progressive MS patients, suggesting the importance of a relationship between inflammation, axonal damage, and demyelination and the significance of CSF biomarkers in MS. Ferraro et al. (2013) reviewed the records of 391 patients who had presented with a clinically isolated syndrome and selected 205 patients who were performed a baseline spinal tap and MRI scan and CSF and serum IgM oligoclonal bands (IgMOB) detection using agarose gel isoelectric focusing and analyzed the impact of baseline clinical, MRI and CSF variables on the risk of conversion to clinically definite MS, i.e., on the risk of a clinical relapse. At survival analysis, a lower age at onset, an onset with optic neuritis and the presence of CSF-restricted IgMOB increased the risk of a relapse. Only the presence of CSF-restricted IgMOB predicted a relapse within one year. Osteopontine, Sulfatides were used as biomarkers in RRMS. Serum autoantibodies (Abs) against the NH2-terminal of α-enolase (NAE) as a theranostic biomarker for HE. Body fluid miRNAs as diagnostic biomarkers including miR-145 was 3-fold up-regulated in MS patients. Neurofilament light and heavy subunits, NfL was superior over NfHSMI 35 as biomarker and is a promising candidate to estimate neuroaxonal damage and miRNAs as biomarkers of inflammation and new EBPT tools for the modulation of microglial behavior in the CNS. Branched O-mannosyl glycans in astrocytes and mitochondrial aconitase activity were higher in MS patients than in controls. A significant increase on all respiratory complex activities in MS patients was observed. Mitochondrial lipid peroxidation was significantly higher in MS patients than in controls. Significant changes of cytochrome c and mitochondrial SOD1 expressions were detected, with a decrease of $44 \pm 5\%$ and an increase of $46 \pm 6\%$, respectively. Increased IL12p40 level characterizes the CSF of MS MRI biomarkers. MANBA, CXCR5, SOX8, RPS6KB1 and ZBTB46 are genetic risk loci for MS. Potentially disease-associated autoimmunity signatures of protein microarrays. CSF biomarkers of axonal damage (*neurofilament light protein, NFL*), astrogliosis (*GFAP*), and B-cell regulation (*CXCL13*). IL-7 pathway and IL-7Rα SNPs in HCT, TNFRSF1A polymorphisms and MS, Myelin basic protein (MBP), proteolipid protein, myelin-associated oligodendrocyte basic glycoprotein, and α-B-crystallin may be detected in the CSF of MS patients.

Gajofatto et al. (2013) clinically isolated syndrome cases (i.e., subjects with an IDE compatible with MS onset and no alternative explanation) with at least 1.5 years' follow-up. All cases underwent clinical, neurophysiological, MRI, and CSF assessment, including tau, 14-3-3, and Cystatin C testing. CIS recovery, conversion to MS, and long-term neurological disability as outcome measures. Patients with neuromyelitis optica spectrum disorders, idiopathic acute transverse myelitis (IATM), Creutzfeldt-Jacob disease, and non-inflammatory/non-neurodegenerative disorders served as controls for CSF analysis. Forty-six CIS cases were included. Severe presentation was associated with incomplete recovery, while the presence of at least 3 periventricular lesions on baseline MRI correlated with MS conversion. Initial pyramidal tract involvement, incomplete CIS recovery, and number of relapses predicted neurological disability. CSF tau, 14-3-3, and Cystatin C did not correlate with any outcome measure. CIS cases had reduced tau and Cystatin C levels compared to IATM, indicating that an extensive diagnostic evaluation of patients with an IDE is beneficial for prognostication; hence novel EBPT biomarkers are needed for MS.

CSF and Blood Biomarkers of MS Ouallet et al. (2013) presented guidelines concerning serum tsts for the diagnosis of MS. A working group performed a systematic analysis of the literature, taking into consideration both previous recommendations and original articles, and then drafted guidelines, which were subjected to the critical review. Three written drafts, followed by rating of the guidelines were submitted for review to a second independent reading group. Each recommendation was presented with its grade according to the level of proof or its degree of consensus in the absence of scientific proof. Axonal degeneration was implicated in the pathogenesis of unremitting disability of MS. Madeddu et al. (2013) evaluated levels of cytoskeletal proteins including; neurofilament light protein (NFL), glial fibrillary acidic protein (GFAP), and β-tubulin (β-Tub) isoforms II and III in the CSF of MS patients and their correlation with clinical indices. CSF cytoskeletal proteins were determined in 51 patients: 33 with MS and 18 with other neurological diseases (OND). Particularly, NFL, GFAP and β-Tub II proteins were significantly increased in MS than in OND group; no significant difference was observed between MS and OND with regard to β-Tub III. The levels of β-Tub III and NFL were higher in progressive than in remitting MS. Significantly higher levels of β-Tub II and GFAP were noticed in RRMS. However, with the exception of β-Tub III, all proteins decreased in CSF concomitantly with the increasing disability (EDSS) score, indicating β-Tub II as a potential biomarker for diagnostic and β-Tub III as a prognostic biomarker of MS. Moscarello et al. (2013) discovered that abnormal myelin hypercitrullination, even in normal-appearing white matter, by peptidylarginine deiminases (PADs) correlates with disease severity and might have an important role in MS progression. Hypercitrullination promotes focal demyelination through reduced myelin compaction. These investigators reported that 2-Chloroacetamidine (2CA), a small-molecule, PAD active-site inhibitor, attenuates disease in neurodegenerative and autoimmune MS mouse models. Indeed 2CA reduced PAD activity and protein citrullination to pre-disease status suppressed T cell autoreactivity clearing brain and spinal cord infiltrates through selective removal of newly activated T cells. Moreover, 2CA prevented disease when administered before disease onset or before autoimmune induction, making hypercitrullination and PAD enzymes, therapeutic target in MS models and hence in MS patients. In the autoimmune models, disease progression induced hypercitrullination with Citrulline+epitopes targeted frequently. Hamann et al. (2013) characterized Natural killer (NK) cells from paired CSF and blood samples of patients with MS, other neuroinflammatory diseases (IND), and non-inflammatory neurological diseases (NIND) using flow cytometry. NK cell frequency in CSF was decreased compared to blood, particularly in MS patients. In contrast to blood NK cells, during neuroinflammation, CSF NK cells displayed an immature phenotype with enhanced expression of CD56 and CD27 and reduced CX3CR1 expression suggesting that for central memory T cells, CSF may represent an intermediary compartment for NK cell trafficking and differentiation before entering the CNS parenchyma.

PKCγ as a Clinically-Significant Kinase in MS In the spinal cord, PKCγ is an important kinase found in a specific subset of excitatory interneurons in the superficial dorsal horn and in axons of the corticospinal tract (CST). The major interest in spinal PKCγ has been its influences on regulating pain sensitivity but its presence in the CST indicates that it has a significant role in locomotor function. A hallmark of the animal model commonly used to study MS, EAE are motor impairments associated with the disease. It has been recognized that EAE is associated with significant changes in pain sensitivity. Given its role in generating pain hypersensitivity and its presence in a major tract controlling motor activity, Lieu et al. (2013) characterized whether EAE was associated with changes in PKCγ levels in the spinal cord. EAE initiates a significant reduction in the levels of PKCγ, primarily in the CST. These investigators did not observe any significant changes in PKCγ levels in the superficial dorsal horn but the levels tended to be below control levels in this region. They assessed the levels of PKCγ in the spinal cord of EAE mice that had recovered gross locomotor function and compared this to the levels observed in EAE mice with chronic deficits and demonstrated that PKCγ levels are dynamic and that in later stages of the disease, its expression is dependent on the degree of motor function, suggesting that PKCγ may be a useful biomarker in the disease to monitor the status of the CST. In adition, zymosan has previously been reported to have both pro-inflammatory and anti-inflammatory effects. Li et al. (2013) demonstrated that low dose zymosan prevents or reverses chronic and relapsing paralysis in EAE. In suppressing CNS autoimmune inflammation, zymosan not only regulated APC costimulator and MHC class II expression, but also promoted differentiation of T regulatory cells. Following adoptive transfer of zymosan-primed CD4(+) T cells, recipient mice were protected from EAE. In contrast, a MAPK inhibitor and a blocker of β-glucan, reversed the effects of zymosan, suggesting that zymosan may be beneficial for MS. Usually a combination of the biomarkers are used to correlate and confirm the MS diagnosis which includes medical history, MRI, CT, PET, and CSF examination. Various CSF and urinary biomarkers are illustrated in Figure 41. In addition the researchers can detect the existence of autoantibodies in MS patients. The detection of Neopterin protein as well as oligoclonal bands further confirms MS diagnosis.

Amyloid Precursor Protein and Amyloid β Peptides in MS Amyloid Precursor Protein (APP) and amyloid β (Aβ) peptides are extensively studied and their CSF measurements may be used to determine the metabolic pathways of APP *in vivo*. Reduced CSF levels of Aβ and soluble APP (sAPP) fragments are reported in inflammatory diseases, but the precise pathway of APP metabolism and whether it can be affected by disease-modifying treatments in MS remains unclear. To characterize the CSF biomarkers of APP degradation in MS, including the effects of disease-modifying therapy, Augutis et al. (2013) analyzed CSF samples from 87 MS patients (54 relapsing-remitting (RR) MS; 33 secondary progressive (SP) MS and 28 controls for sAPP and Aβ peptides by immunoassays, plus a subset of samples was analyzed by immunoprecipitation and mass spectrometry (IP-MS). Patients treated with Natalizumab or Mitoxantrone were examined at baseline, and after 1-2 years of treatment. CSF sAPP and Aβ peptide levels were reduced in MS patients; but they increased again towards normal, after Natalizumab treatment. IP-MS-measured Aβ species separated the SPMS patients from controls, with RRMS patients having intermediate levels confirming their previous observations of altered CSF sAPP and Aβ peptide in MS patients. Hence Natalizumab therapy may counteract the altered APP metabolism in MS. The CSF Aβ isoform distribution was distinct in SPMS patients, as compared to controls.

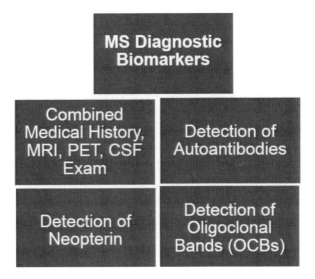

Figure 41. *MS Diagnostic Biomarkers:* A diagram illustrating diagnostic biomarkers of MS. These biomarkers are used in combination to correlate and confirm the diagnosis which includes a combination of medical history, MRI, CT, PET, and CSF examination. The researchers can also detect the existence of autoantibodies. The detection of Neopterin protein as well as oligoclonal bands further authenticates and confirms MS diagnosis.

Mast Cells Neuroprotection in MS Mast cells (MCs) are found in the brain and the meninges and play an intricate role in neuroinflammatory diseases, such as stroke and MS. Hendrix et al., (2013) showed that MC-deficient Kit/Kit mice exhibit progressive neurodegeneration in the lesioned area after brain trauma. Furthermore, these genotypes exhibit neuroinflammation, accompanied with increased macrophages/microglia, as well as increased T-cell infiltration at days 4 and 14 after injury, combined with astrogliosis at day 14 following injury. The number of proliferating Ki67 macrophages/microglia and astrocytes around the lesion area is doubled in MC-deficient mice. In parallel, MC-deficient Kit mice exhibit increased macrophages/microglia at day 4, and persistent astrogliosis at day 4 and 14 after brain trauma. Further analysis of mice deficient in one of the most relevant MC proteases, i.e., mouse mast cell protease 4 (mMCP-4), revealed that astrogliosis and T-cell infiltration are increased in mMCP-4-knockout mice. Treatment with an inhibitor of mMCP-4 increased macrophage/microglia numbers and astrogliosis, suggesting that MCs exert protection after trauma, via mMCP-4, by suppressing inflammation via their proteases.

Brain Cholesterol in MS *Brain cholesterol is primarily involved in maintaining the structural and functional integrity of the cell membrane, in signal transduction, neurotransmitter release, synaptogenesis, and membrane trafficking. Impaired brain cholesterol metabolism is noticed in various neurodegenerative diseases, such as MS, AD and HD.* Leoni and Caccia (2013) reported that since the blood-brain barrier prevents cholesterol uptake from the circulation into the brain, *de novo* synthesis is responsible for the cholesterol present in the CNS. Cholesterol is converted into 24S-hydroxycholesterol (24OHC) by cholesterol 24-hydroxylase (CYP46A1) expressed in neural cells. Plasma concentration of 24OHC depends upon the balance between cerebral production and hepatic elimination and is related to the number of metabolically active neurons in the brain. Factors affecting brain cholesterol turnover and liver elimination of oxysterols, together with the metabolism of plasma lipoproteins, genetic background, nutrition, and lifestyle habits affect its plasma levels. Either increased or decreased plasma 24OHC are seen in patients with neurodegenerative diseases. There is also evidence to suggest that reduced 24OHC is related to the loss of metabolically active cells and the extent of brain atrophy. Inflammation, dysfunction of BBB, increased cholesterol turnover might counteract this tendency resulting in increased changes. The study of plasma 24OHC may offer an insight about brain cholesterol turnover with a limited diagnostic potential.

Pro-Inflammatory Biomarkers in MS Inflammatory infiltration has been recently emphasized in the demyelinating diseases of the CNS including MS. In general biomarkers such as autoantibodies, Neopterin, and oligoclonal bands (OCBs) are used for the diagnosis of inflammatory CNS disorders including MS. Sinclair et al. (2013) investigated the correlation between the results of OCB testing and clinical diagnoses in children with neurological conditions. CSF and serum from 200 children were tested for OCBs using isoelectric focusing. The patients were divided into those with inflammatory and non-inflammatory CNS disorders. Intrathecal OCBs (*OCBs restricted to the CSF*) were found in 11 out of 58 (19%) of those with inflammatory CNS disorders compared with none of the 142 patients with non-inflammatory CNS disorders. *Diseases associated with intrathecal OCB were MS, Rasmussen encephalitis, N-Methyl-D-Aspartate receptor (NMDAR) encephalitis, voltage-gated potassium channel (VGKC) encephalopathy, herpes (HSV) encephalitis, 'other' encephalitides, acute cerebellar ataxia, and aseptic meningitis.* Mirrored OCBs (identical OCBs in the serum and CSF) were less specific but were still found in 14 out of 58 (24%)

children with inflammatory CNS disorders compared to only 6 out of 142 (4%) children with non-inflammatory CNS disorders. Diseases associated with OCBs included acute *disseminated encephalomyelitis (ADEM), VGKC encephalopathy, West nile syndrome, NMDAR encephalitis, 'other' encephalitides, polio-like illness, Rasmussen encephalitis, cerebral vasculitis, metachromatic leukodystrophy, and bacterial meningitis. Intrathecal OCBs and mirrored OCBs had a positive predictive value for inflammatory CNS disease.* Intrathecal OCBs were restricted to patients with inflammatory CNS disorders. They are a useful, but unspecific, biomarker of CNS inflammation of multiple causes. Mirrored OCBs were less specific, but still supported inflammatory CNS disorder. These investigators emphasized that the presence of either intrathecal or mirrored OCBs should raise suspicion of an inflammatory CNS disorder. Furthermore, Jiang et al. (2013) analyzed the expression of membrane B7-H3 (mB7-H3) and levels of soluble B7-H3 (sB7-H3) in MS patients to determine its clinical significance. Peripheral blood (PB) or CSF samples from healthy controls, other noninflammatory neurological disorders, viral encephalitis, and MS patients were collected. Expression of mB7-H3 on immune cells was detected by flow cytometry. Levels of sB7-H3 in serum or CSF samples were measured by ELISA. mB7-H3 expression was up-regulated in CSF from MS patients compared to PB. However, serum or CSF levels of sB7-H3 in MS patients were lower than those in controls. RMS patients had higher CSF mB7-H3 expression than the remitting subgroup. RMS patients had decreased serum and CSF sB7-H3 levels compared with the remitting subgroup. Neurological deficits showed negative correlations with serum or CSF sB7-H3 levels, but a positive correlation with CSF mB7-H3 expression. Methylprednisolone therapy elevated sB7-H3 levels and reduced mB7-H3 expression. sB7-H3 levels did not correlate with mB7-H3 expression. Enhanced mB7-H3 expression and reduced sB7-H3 levels in MS patients correlated with the clinical characteristics of MS patients, suggesting that B7-H3 may be a promising biomarker and associated with the pathogenesis of MS. In addition, β-1, 4-Galactosyltransferase I (β-1, 4-GalT-I) is a major galactosyltransferase responsible for selectin-ligand biosynthesis, mediating rolling of the inflammatory lymphocytes. Zhao et al. (2013) showed that expression of β-1,4-GalT-I was low in normal or complete Freund's adjuvant (CFA) control rats' spinal cords, and it began to increase since early stage and peaked at E4 stage of experimental autoimmune encephalomyelitis (EAE) and restored to normal level in the recovery stage. The upregulation of β-1,4-Gal T-I was primarily distributed in the white matter of spinal cord, while there was also increased staining of β-1,4-GalT-I in the grey matter. Meanwhile, the expression of E-Selectin, the substrate of β-1, 4-GalT-I, was increased, with a peak at E4 stage of EAE, and gradually decreased thereafter. Lectin blot showed that the 65 kDa-25 kDa protein bands reacted an increase at the peak stage of EAE when compared with the normal and CFA control. Ricinus Communis Agglutinin-I (RCA-I)-positive signals were intense in white matter of lumbosacral spinal cord at the peak stage of EAE (E4). β-1, 4-GalT-I and CD62E, a marker for E-Selectin located in ED1 (+) macrophages in perivascular or in the white matter in EAE lesions, and a co-localization of ED1 (+) cells with CD62E, suggesting that β-1, 4-GalT-I might serve as an inflammatory mediator regulating adhesion and migration of inflammatory cells in EAE, through the modification of galactosylated carbohydrate chains to modulate selectin-ligand biosynthesis and interaction with E-selectin.

Translocator protein in MS It is well established that TSPO (18 kDa) is a biomarker of inflammation in the brain. PET imaging exhibited increased expression of TSPO in many neuropathologic conditions. However, TSPO expression in the periphery and its correlation to CNS inflammation was not studied. In a study, PBR28, a recently synthesized ligand for TSPO that has 80-fold higher specific binding than its predecessor PK11195, was used to quantify peripheral TSPO. Harberts et al. (2013) showed that monocytes account for the majority of TSPO in peripheral blood mononuclear cells (PBMC), and that TSPO expression is stable in healthy individuals. Regions of increased PBR28 binding in the brains of MS patients correlate with active demylinating lesions observed in MRI. To measure peripheral TSPO expression in an inflammatory disease of the CNS, PBR28 can be used in an *in vitro* radioligand binding assay to estimate the amount of TSPO in the PBMC of MS and healthy donor cohorts. Surprisingly, MS patients have significantly lower amount of peripheral TSPO than healthy donors, suggesting that its expression could be used as a peripheral biomarker of MS. A further research is needed to determine if peripheral TSPO expression may also be altered in other neuroinflammatory conditions.

Blood Biomarkers in MS Several blood biomarkers have been developed for the early diagnosis, screening and follow-up of non CNS cancers. However, there is lack of knowledge on biochemical blood alterations in brain tumor patients. Ilhan-Mutlu et al. (2013) collected plasma samples of 105 adult brain tumor patients with diffuse low-grade glioma (WHO) II, n = 7), anaplastic glioma (WHO III, n = 10), glioblastoma multiforme (WHO IV, glioblastoma multiforme (GBM)) (n = 34), meningioma (WHO I, n = 8), atypical meningioma (WHO II, n = 5), and intracerebral metastasis (ICM; n = 41). These investigators measured plasma concentrations of neuropeptide Y, BDNF, GDNF, placental growth factor (PIGF), S100B, Secretagogin, IL-8, and GFAP using ELISA. Plasma biomarker concentrations were correlated to neuropathological diagnosis and neuroradiological findings. Most of the biomarkers were detectable in all diagnostic categories in variable concentrations. GFAP plasma detectability was associated with a diagnosis of GBM. Plasma GFAP and placental growth factor demonstrated potential in the differential diagnosis of unifocal GBM versus unifocal supratentorial ICM and suggested that none of the investigated biomarkers is suitable to substitute histological diagnosis. However, measurement of circulating GFAP and PIGF may support neuroradiological diagnosis of GBM versus ICM.

CSF Biomarkers in MS As CSF constitutes a specific immune micro-environment to the CSF, it may contain specific biomarkers involved in the pathogenesis of MS. Diagnosis of MS requires the exclusion of other possible diagnoses. Hence, the CSF should be routinely analyzed in patients with a first clinical event suggestive of MS. However CSF analysis is no longer mandatory for the diagnosis of RRMS, as long as MRI diagnostic criteria are fulfilled. A caution is required in diagnosing MS in patients with negative MRI findings or in the absence of CSF analysis, as CSF investigation is useful to eliminate other causes of disease. The detection of oligoclonal IgG bands in CSF has potential prognostic value and is helpful for clinical decision-making. In addition, CSF analysis is important for investigating the pathogenesis of MS. Pathophysiological and neurodegenerative findings of inflammation in MS have been derived from CSF investigations. Novel CSF biomarkers, though not yet validated, have been identified for diagnosis of MS and for ascertaining disease activity, prognosis and response to treatment, and are likely to increase in number with modern detection techniques.

Recently Stangel et al. (2013) summarized CSF findings that shed light on the differential diagnosis of MS, and highlighted the potential of novel biomarkers for this disease that could advance understanding of its pathophysiology. Although oligoclonal bands (OCBs) unique to the CSF are used in the diagnosis of MS, the precise prevalence of OCBs in MS and clinically isolated syndrome (CIS) remains uncertain. Dobson et al. (2013) used a systematic review and meta-analysis approach, the proportion of OCB-positive MS and CIS and the influence of OCBs on clinical outcomes were calculated. The relationship between latitude and OCB prevalence was calculated using linear regression. Overall, 87.7% of 12 253 MS and 68.6% of 2685 CIS patients were OCB positive. OCB-positive MS patients had an OR of 1.96 of reaching disability outcomes, although negative studies did not provide data. OCB-positive CIS patients had an OR of 9.88 of conversion to MS. Latitude predicted OCB status in MS patients but not in CIS patients. OCB positivity predicted conversion from CIS to MS. The relationship between latitude and OCBs was confirmed which requires further investigation. *The MS diagnosis can be confirmed by measuring CSF and urine biomarkers including, kappa (κ) and lambda (λ) light chain, Neopterin, and ubiquitin C-terminal hydrolase as illustrated in Figure 42.* Various other CSF biomarkers for confirming the diagnosis of MS include, *Feutin-A, spinal PKCγ, peptidyl arginine deaminase (PADs) for prognosticating MS. Neurofilament, monomeric and dimeric κ and γ FLCs.* In addition, SOD, reduced amyloid-β, and soluble AAP can facilitate MS theranostics. Moreover CSF, Iso-P can be used as a biomarker of tissue damage. Abnormal myelin hypercitrulination and reduced BNDF can also confirm MS diagnosis in combination with other diagnostic biomarkers as presented in Figure 43. However the detection limits may vary depending on the biological source. Till date, as many as 12 biomarkers have been discovered which can be used on a routine basis. For example, *oligoclonal bands, CD-44 deficiency, elevated sCD-144, Vitamin-D, 24-S-Hydroxycholesterol in plasma, low serum LPRs, low CD-70, increased myelin basic proteins (MBPs), increased α-Integrins, HLA-DRB-1 gene polymorphism, urinary metabolites, and CD-20. Various biomarkers that can be easily detected in blood, plasma, serum, and urine samples in addition to CSF are illustrated in Figure 44.*

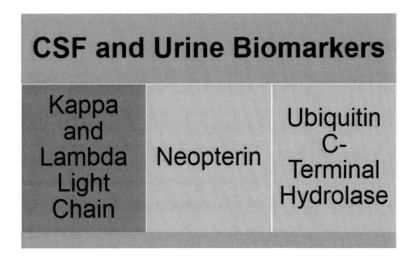

Figure 42. *CSF and Urine Biomarkers in MS:* A diagram demonstrating CSF and urine biomarkers for the diagnosis of MS. The MS diagnosis can be confirmed by measuring CSF and urine biomarkers including, kappa (κ) and lambda (λ) light chain, Neopterin, and ubiquitin C-terminal hydrolase as illustrated in this figure.

CSF Biomarkers

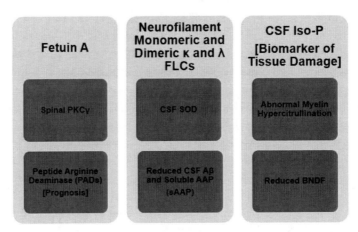

Figure 43. *CSF Biomarkers in MS:* This diagram illustrates various CSF biomarkers that can be detected for confirming the diagnosis. These biomarkers include, Feutin-A, spinal PKCγ, peptidyl arginine deaminase (PADs) for prognosticating MS. Neurofilament, monomeric and dimeric κ and γ FLCs can help in the differential diagnosis of MS. In addition, CSF SOD, reduced CSF amyloid-β, and soluble AAP can facilitate MS diagnosis. CSF, Iso-P can also be used as a biomarker of tissue damage. Abnormal myelin hypercitrulination and reduced BNDF can also confirm MS diagnosis in combination with other diagnostic biomarkers.

Blood/Plasma/Serum/Urine Biomarkers

Oligoclonal Bands	Vitamin-D	Low CD-70	HLA DRB-1 *MS Biomarkers* Polymorphism
CD-44 Deficiency	24-S Hydroxycholestrol in Plasma	Increased Myelin Basic Proteins (MBPs)	Urinary Metablolites
Elevated sCD144	Low Serum LPRs	Increased α-Integrins	CD-20

Figure 44. *Blood/Plasma/Serum/Urine Biomarkers in MS*: This diagram illustrates various biomarkers which can be detected in blood, plasma, serum, and urine samples in addition to CSF. However detection limits will vary depending on the biological source. As many as 12 biomarkers have been discovered so far which can be used on a routine basis. For example, oligoclonal bands, CD-44 deficiency, elevated sCD-144, vitamin-D, 24-S-hydroxycholesterol in plasma, low serum LPRs, low CD-70, increased myelin basic proteins (MBPs), increased α-integrins, HLA-DRB-1 gene polymorphism, urinary metabolites, and CD-20 have been discovered as illustrated in this figure.

Renin Angiotensin System in MS It is well known that the RAS is significantly impaired in MS. It is represented by reductions in Angiotensin-II and Angiotensin Converting Enzyme-II, and increase in Angiotensin converting enzyme (ACE) as shown in Figure 45. Mogi and Horiuchi (2013) reviewed the role of RAS in cognitive impairment and neurodegenerative disease, mainly in experimental studies on the angiotensin II type 2 (AT(2)) receptor. Ischemic brain damage was increased in mice with overexpression of angiotensin II, with reduced cerebral blood flow in the penumbra and an increase in oxidative stress in the ischemic area. Angiotensin II binds two types of receptors, type 1 (AT (1)) and type 2 (AT (2)). AT (1) receptor signaling has a harmful effect, and AT (2) receptor signaling has a protective effect on the brain after stroke. AT (2) receptor signaling in bone marrow stromal cells or hematopoietic cells prevented ischemic brain damage after middle cerebral artery occlusion. In contrast, AT (2) receptor signaling also affected cognitive function. Direct stimulation of the AT (2) receptor by AT (2) receptor agonist, Compound 21 (C21), enhanced cognitive function in wild-type (C57BL6) mice and an AD mouse model with intracerebroventricular injection of amyloid β (1-40). Finally, clinical research was conducted by investigating the levels of RAS components in patients with neurodegenerative diseases. A reduction of Ang-II and ACE-2 levels, and an increase in ACE level in CSF from patients with MS suggested that RAS is involved in neurodegenerative disease. Therefore, regulation of RAS might be a therapeutic target to protect neurons from neurodegeneration.

Vascular Abnormalities in MS Venous abnormalities have been associated with different neurological conditions, and the presence of a vascular involvement in MS has long been anticipated. In view of the recent debate regarding the existence of cerebral venous outflow impairment in MS due to abnormalities of the azygos or internal jugular veins (IJVs), Coen et al. (2013) studied the morphological and biological features of IJVs in MS patients. These investigators examined (a) IJVs specimens from MS patients who underwent surgical reconstruction of the IJV and specimens of the great saphenous vein used for surgical reconstruction, (b) different vein specimens from an MS patient died of an unrelated cause, and (c) autoptical and surgical IJV specimens from patients without MS. Collagen deposition was assessed by means of Sirius red staining followed by polarized light examination. The expression of collagen type I and III, cytoskeletal proteins (α-smooth muscle actin and smooth muscle myosin heavy chains), and inflammatory markers (CD3 and CD68) was investigated. The extracranial veins of MS patients showed focal thickenings of the wall characterized by a yellow-green birefringence (corresponding to thin, loosely packed collagen fibers) correlated to a higher expression of type III collagen. No differences in cytoskeletal protein and inflammatory marker expression were observed. The IJVs of MS patients presenting a focal thickening of the vein wall are characterized by the prevalence of loosely packed type III collagen fibers in the adventitia. These invesigators suggested further studies to determine whether the observed venous alterations play a role in MS pathogenesis.

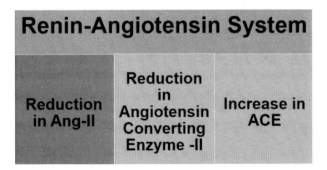

Figure 45. *Renin-Angiotensin System (RAS) in MS*: A diagram illustrating impaired renin angiotensin system in MS. The renin-angiotensin system (RAS) is significantly impaired in MS. It is represented by significant reductions in Angiotensin-II and Angiotensin Converting Enzyme-II, and increase in Angiotensin Converting Enzyme (ACE).

Personalized Diagnosis of Dementia in MS and other Neurodegenerative Diseases
Gardner et al. (2013) reported that the population of oldest old, or people aged 85 and older, is growing rapidly. Hence a better understanding of dementia in this population is of global importance. These investigators described the epidemiological studies, prevalence, clinical presentation, neuropathological and imaging features, risk factors, and treatment of dementia in the oldest old. Prevalence estimates for dementia among those aged 85+ ranged from 18 to 38%. The most common clinical syndromes are Alzheimer's dementia, vascular dementia, and mixed dementia from multiple etiologies. The rate of progression was slower than in the younger old. Single neuropathological entities such as Alzheimer's dementia and Lewy body pathology appear to have lesser relevance to cognitive decline, while mixed pathology with AD, vascular disease (especially cortical microinfarcts), and hippocampal sclerosis have increasing relevance. *Risk factors for dementia in the oldest old include a low level of education, poor mid-life general health, low level of physical activity, depression, and delirium, whereas Apo-E genotype, late-life hypertension, hyperlipidemia, and elevated peripheral inflammatory biomarkers have less relevance.* Treatment approaches require further study, but the oldest old may be more prone to negative side effects compared with younger patients and targeted therapies may be less efficacious since single pathologies are less frequent. The difficulty of defining functional decline, for a dementia diagnosis, the lack of normative neuropsychological data, and other shortcomings inherent in existing diagnostic criteria are also involved in MS.

Wimmer et al. (2013) presented a 49-year-old woman with fever, weight loss, night sweats, hematochezia, and acid reflux symptoms. Two large, firm cecal lesions were seen at colonoscopy, but multiple biopsies were inconclusive. The patient underwent a right hemicolectomy for a clinical diagnosis of colon cancer. Noncaseating granulomatous inflammation with BKg lymphocytes, plasma cells, and histiocytes exhibiting emperipolesis were identified. With these histologic features and immunoreactivity for S-100 protein and CD68, a diagnosis of Rosai-Dorfman disease was rendered. Other areas had storiform fibrosis mixed with immunoglobulin G4 (IgG4)-positive plasma cells. Although a few preliminary reports noted an increased number of IgG4-positive plasma cells in Rosai-Dorfman disease, the relationship between these 2 conditions is unclear. This was the first case report of a possible association of colonic Rosai-Dorfman disease with an increased number of IgG4-positive plasma cells.

Schulze-Topphoff (2013) reported that low expression of the antiproliferative gene TOB1 in CD4$^+$ T cells of individuals presenting with an initial CNS demyelinating event, correlated with high risk for progression to MS. EAE in Tob1$^{-/-}$ mice was associated with augmented CNS inflammation, increased infiltrating CD4$^+$ and CD8$^+$ T cell counts, and increased myelin-reactive Th1 and Th17 cells, with reduced numbers of regulatory T cells. Reconstitution of Rag1$^{-/-}$ mice with Tob1$^{-/-}$ CD4$^+$ T cells recapitulated the aggressive EAE phenotype observed in Tob1$^{-/-}$ mice. Severe spontaneous EAE was observed when Tob1$^{-/-}$ mice were crossed to myelin oligodendrocyte glycoprotein–specific T cell receptor transgenic (2D2) mice, indicating a critical role of Tob1 in adaptive T cell immune responses that drive development of EAE, its role as a biomarker for demyelinating disease activity.

OMIC BIOMARKERS IN MS

At present, specific biomarkers reflecting pathology of MS remain uncertain. The risk of developing MS depends on genetic susceptibility and environmental factors. The interaction of environmental factors with epigenetic mechanisms could affect the transcriptional and translational level. In the last decade, emerging 'omics' studies shed light on the MS mechanisms and proposed potential biomarker targets. To understand MS pathophysiology and discover a subset of biomarkers, it is becoming important to integrate the findings of the different fields of 'omics' into a systems biology network. Malekzadeh et al. (2013) discussed the recent findings of the genomic, transcriptomic and proteomic for MS to construct a unifying model. A genome-wide association study (GWAS) reported 5 loci for which there was strong, but sub-genome-wide evidence for association with MS risk. Lill et al. (2013) evaluated the role of these potential risk loci in a data set of ≈ 20,000 subjects. These investigators tested 5 SNPs: *rs228614 (MANBA), rs630923 (CXCR5), rs2744148 (SOX8), rs180515 (RPS6KB1), and rs6062314 (ZBTB46) for association with MS risk in a total of 8499 cases with MS*, 8765 unrelated control subjects and 958 trios of European descent. In addition, they assessed the evidence for association by combining newly generated data with the results from the original GWAS by meta-analysis. All 5 SNPs showed association with MS in the validation data sets. Combining these data with results from the previous GWAS, the evidence for association was strengthened further, surpassing the threshold for genome-wide significance in each case, authenticating that these 5 loci are genuine MS susceptibility loci which may lead to a better understanding of the underlying disease pathophysiology. In addition, a mutation in the IL7Rα locus was identified as a risk factor for MS, a neurodegenerative autoimmune disease characterized by inflammation, demyelination, and axonal damage.

McDonald (2005) included a total of 326 patients with MS. Single nucleotide polymorphisms in the CD40 gene (rs6074022, rs1883832, rs1535045 and rs11086998) and the KIF1B gene (rs10492972 and rs3135388) were genotyped using TaqMan technology. Korobko et al. (2013) found association of rs1883832 and rs3135388 with the risk of MS in the Novosibirsk region population. The study demonstrated effect of genetic factors on phenotypic expression of MS: a C allele of rs6074022 polymorphism (CD40) was associated with a higher rate of MS progression, and the TT genotype of rs1535045 was associated with a slower progression of MS and early MS onset. A more benign course and a higher frequency of an T allele of rs3135388 was found in familial cases compared to sporadic cases. Furthermore, Sokolova et al. (2013) conducted the association study of CD40 gene's polymorphisms and MS among residents of the Russian Federation. Their results demonstrated the need to combine data from different researchers in clinical studies to increase the power of the study. Response gene to complement (RGC)-32 is a novel molecule that plays an important role in cell proliferation. Tegla et al. (2013) investigated the expression of RGC-32 in MS brain and in peripheral blood mononuclear cells (PBMCs) obtained from patients with RRMS and that CD3 (+), CD68 (+), and GFAP (+) cells in MS plaques co-localized with RGC-32. These results showed a significant decrease in RGC-32 mRNA expression in PBMCs during relapses as compared to stable MS patients. This decrease might be useful in predicting disease activity in patients with RRMS. RGC-32 expression was also correlated with that of FasL mRNA during relapses. FasL mRNA expression was reduced after RGC-32 silencing, indicating a role for RGC-32 in the regulation of FasL expression. In addition, the expression of Akt1, cyclin D1, and IL-21 mRNA was increased during MS relapses when compared to healthy controls. Furthermore, these researchers investigated the role of RGC-32 in TGF-β-induced extracellular matrix expression in astrocytes. Blockage of RGC-32 using small interfering RNA inhibited TGF-β induction of procollagen I, fibronectin and of the reactive astrocyte marker α-smooth muscle actin (α-SMA) suggesting that RGC-32 plays a dual role in MS, both as a regulator of T-cells mediated apoptosis and as a promoter of TGF-β-mediated profibrotic effects in astrocytes.

IL7Rα has well-established roles in lymphocyte development and homeostasis, but its involvement in MS is understudied. In a study, Ashbaugh et al. (2013) used the EAE model of MS to show that a less severe form of the disease results when IL7Rα expression is restricted to thymic tissue in IL7RTg(IL7R-/-) mice. Compared with wild-type (WT) mice, IL7RTg (IL7R-/-) mice exhibited reduced paralysis and myelin damage that correlated with dampened effector responses, namely decreased TNF production. Treatment of diseased WT mice with neutralizing anti-IL7Rα Ab also resulted in improvement of EAE. In addition, chimeric mice were generated by bone marrow transplant to limit expression of IL7Rα to cells of either hematopoietic or nonhematopoietic origin. Mice lacking IL7Rα only on hematopoietic cells develop severe EAE, suggesting that IL7Rα expression in the nonhematopoietic compartment contributes to disease. Moreover, novel IL7Rα expression was identified on astrocytes and oligodendrocytes endogenous to the CNS. Chimeric mice that lack IL7Rα only on nonhematopoietic cells also develop severe EAE, which further supported the role of IL7Rα in T cell effector function. Conversely, mice that lack IL7Rα throughout both compartments are protected from disease, indicating that multiple cell types use IL7Rα signaling in the development of EAE, and inhibition of this pathway should be considered as a novel theranostic strategy for MS.

Recently, there has been evidence that a non-synonymous exchange (Gly307Ser/rs763361) of the CD226 gene on chromosome 18q22 is linked to several autoimmune diseases (ADs) including: type 1 diabetes (T1D), celiac disease (CED), rheumatoid arthritis (RA), MS, Grave's disease, Wegener's granulomatosis (WG), psoriasis, and primary sicca syndrome (pSS). Taking into consideration that different autoimmune diseases may share some common pathogenic pathways and in order to assess the overall relationship between CD226 Gly307Ser (rs763361) polymorphism and multiple autoimmune diseases, Qiu et al. (2013) searched all studies in the US National Library of Medicine's PubMed and Embase database. Crude odds ratios (OR) with 95% confidence intervals (CI) were conducted to assess the association. 7876 cases and 8558 controls from 7 published studies were selected from 149 articles. The total OR for ADs associated with the T allele was 1.19 by random effects model. Increased risks were also observed in the South American, Asian, and European population. Similarly, significant associations were observed in two genetic models in a codominant model; This meta-analysis provided evidence that CD226 Gly307Ser (rs763361) is associated with the risk of multiple autoimmune diseases.

Deficiency of the Golgi N-glycan branching enzyme Mgat5 in mice promotes T cell hyperactivity, endocytosis of CTLA-4 and autoimmunity, including MS-like disease. Multiple genetic and environmental MS risk factors lower N-glycan branching in T cells. These include variants in IL-2 receptor-α (IL2RA), IL-7 receptor-α (IL7RA), and MGAT1, a Golgi branching enzyme upstream of MGAT5, as well as vitamin D3 deficiency and Golgi substrate metabolism. Li el (2013) described linked intronic variants of MGAT5 that are associated with reduced N-glycan branching, CTLA-4 surface expression and MS, the latter additive with the MGAT1, IL2RA and IL7RA MS risk variants. The most important genetic biomarkers in MS including TOB-1 polymorphism, epigenetic changes in DNA (*DNA sequences, DNA methylation, histone modification, and miRNA-associated silencing*) can be determined for the MS theranostics. Furthermore there is evidence that *kit/kit* mice exhibit extensive neurodegeneration as noticed in MS patients. Response gene to complement (*RGC-32*) is also impaired in MS patients, hence can be used for the EBPT of MS as illustrated in Figure 46.

   Proteomics in MS Kroksveen et al. (2013) aimed to discover CSF proteins with significant difference between early MS patients and controls, and performed verification of these proteins using selected reaction monitoring (SRM). iTRAQ and Orbitrap MS were used to compare the CSF proteome of patients with clinically isolated syndrome (CIS), patients with RRMS that had CIS at the time of lumbar puncture, and controls with other neuroinflammatory disease. Of >1200 proteins, 5 proteins were identified with significant abundant difference between the patients and controls. In the initial verification using SRM a larger patient and control cohort were analyzed and also included proteins reported as differentially induced in MS. A significant difference for 11 proteins after verification, of which the 5 proteins *α-1-Antichymotrypsin, Contactin-1, Apolipoprotein D, Clusterin, and Kallikrein-6 were differentially abundant.*

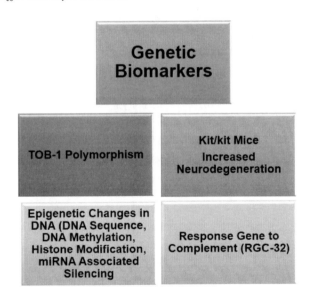

Figure 46. *Genetic Biomarkers in MS:* A diagram illustrating most important genetic biomarkers in MS including TOB-1 polymorphism, epigenetic changes in DNA (DNA sequences, DNA methylation, histone modification, and miRNA-associated silencing) can be determined for the MS patients. Furthermore there is experimental evidence that kit/kit mice exhibit extensive neurodegeneration as noticed in MS patients. Response gene to complement (RGC-32) is also impaired in MS patients, hence can be used for the diagnosis, clinical management, and prognosis of MS.

   Protein MicroArray Analysis of MS Profiling the autoantibody repertoire with large antigen collections is emerging as a powerful tool for the identification of biomarkers for autoimmune diseases. A systematic and undirected approach was taken to screen for profiles of IgG in plasma from 90 individuals with MS related diagnoses. Reactivity pattern of 11,520 protein fragments were generated on protein microarrays built within the Human Protein Atlas. For more than 2,000 antigens IgG reactivity was observed, among which 64% were found only in single individuals. These investigators used reactivity distributions among MS subgroups to select 384 antigens, which were re-evaluated on microarrays, corroborated with suspension bead arrays in a larger cohort and confirmed for specificity in inhibition assays. Among the heterogeneous pattern within and across MS subtypes, differences in recognition frequencies were found for 51 antigens, which were enriched for proteins of transcriptional regulation. Using protein fragments and complementary high-throughput protein array platforms facilitated an alternative route to discovery and verification of potentially disease-associated autoimmunity biomarkers that are currently proposed for large-scale validation studies across MS biobanks.

CYTOKINES AS BIOMARKERS IN MS

The origin of pathogenic autoantibodies remains unknown. Idiopathic pulmonary alveolar proteinosis is caused by autoantibodies against GM-CSF. Wang et al. (2013) generated 19 monoclonal autoantibodies against GM-CSF from six patients with idiopathic pulmonary alveolar proteinosis. The autoantibodies used multiple V genes, excluding preferred V-gene use as an etiology, and targeted at least 4 nonoverlapping epitopes on GM-CSF, suggesting that it is driving the autoantibodies and not a B-cell epitope on a pathogen cross-reacting with GM-CSF. The number of somatic mutations in the autoantibodies suggests that the memory B cells have been helped by T cells and re-entered germinal centers. All autoantibodies neutralized GM-CSF bioactivity, with correlations to affinity and off-rate. The binding of certain autoantibodies was changed by point mutations in GM-CSF that reduced binding to the GM-CSF receptor. Those monoclonal autoantibodies that neutralize GM-CSF may be useful in treating inflammatory disease, such as *rheumatoid arthritis, MS, cancer, and pain*. IL-17, a Th17 cell-derived proinflammatory molecule plays an important role in the pathogenesis of autoimmune diseases, including MS and its animal model, EAE. While IL-17 receptor (IL-17R) is expressed in many immune-related cells, microglia, and astrocytes, it is unknown whether IL-17 exerts a direct effect on neural stem cells (NSCs) and oligodendrocytes, thus inducing inflammatory demyelination in the CNS. Li et al. (2013) detected IL-17 receptor expression in NSCs with immunostaining and real time PCR, and cultured NSCs with IL-17 and determined NSC proliferation by neurosphere formation capability and cell count, differentiation by immunostaining neural specific biomarkers, and apoptosis of NSCs by flow cytometry. NSCs express IL-17R, and when the IL-17R signal pathway was activated by adding IL-17 to NSC culture medium, the number of NSCs was reduced and their ability to form neurospheres was diminished. IL-17 inhibited NSC proliferation, but did not induce cytotoxicity or apoptosis. IL-17 impaired the differentiation of NSCs into astrocytes and oligodendrocyte precursor cells (OPCs). The effects of IL-17 on NSCs can be blocked by p38 MAPK inhibitor. IL-17 blocked proliferation of NSCs, resulting in reduced numbers of astrocytes and OPCs. Thus, in addition to its proinflammatory role in the immune system, IL-17 may also block remyelination and neural repair in the CNS. Human soluble IL-7 receptor (sIL7R)α circulates in high molar excess compared with IL-7, but its biology remains uncertain. Lundström et al. (2013) demonstrated that sIL7Rα has affinity for IL-7 but does not bind thymic stromal lymphopoietin. Functionally, sIL7Rα competes with cell-associated IL-7 receptor to diminish IL-7 consumption and, thus, enhances the bioactivity of IL-7 when the cytokine is limited, as it is presumed to be *in vivo*. IL-7 signaling in the presence of sIL7Rα also reduces the expression of CD95 and suppressor of cytokine signaling 1, both regulatory molecules. Murine models confirm diminished consumption of IL-7 in the presence of sIL7Rα and demonstrate a potentiating effect of sIL7Rα on IL-7-mediated homeostatic expansion and EAE exacerbation. In MS and several other autoimmune diseases, IL7R genotype influences susceptibility. These investigators detected increased sIL7Rα levels, as well as increased IL-7 levels, in MS patients with the predisposing IL7R genotype, consistent with diminished IL-7 consumption *in vivo*, suggesting that sIL7Rα potentiates IL-7 activity and provides a basis to explain the increased risk of autoimmunity in individuals with genotype-induced increase in sIL7Rα.

It is known that serum and intracytoplasmic cytokines are required in host defense against microbes, but also play a pivotal role in the pathogenesis of autoimmune diseases by initiating various cellular and humoral autoimmune processes. The intricate interaction and intricate balance of pro- and anti-inflammatory processes drive, whether inflammation and eventually organ damage will occur, or the inflammatory cascade quenches. In the early and late, as well as inactive and active stages of autoimmune diseases, different cellular and molecular patterns can dominate in MS patients. However, the simultaneous assessment of pro- and anti-inflammatory biomarkers aids to define the immunological state of a patient. The most useful inflammatory biomarkers are cytokines, and their role has been well-defined in patients with autoimmune diseases and immunodeficiencies. Multiple pathological processes drive the development of autoimmunity and immunodeficiencies, most of which involve quantitative and qualitative disturbances in regulatory cells, cytokine synthesis and signaling pathways. The assessment of these biomarkers does not aid only in the mechanistic description of autoimmune diseases and immunodeficiencies, but helps to categorize diseases and evaluate therapeutic responses. Osnes et al. (2013) provided an overview, how monitoring of cytokines and regulatory cells aid in the diagnosis and follow-up of patients with autoimmune diseases and immunodeficiencies. Furthermore, these investigators pinpointed novel cellular and molecular diagnostic possibilities in these diseases.

It is known that NO-hybridization of the HIV protease inhibitor Saquinavir generates a new chemical entity named Saq-NO, that retains the anti-viral activity and exerts lower toxicity. Petković et al. (2013) showed that Saq-NO inhibits the generation of various cytokines in ConA-stimulated unfractionated murine spleen cells and rat lymph nodes stimulated with ConA as well as in purified CD4(+) T cells *in vitro* and reduced the circulating levels of cytokines in mice challenged with anti-CD3 antibody. Furthermore, Saq-NO reduced IL-17 and IFN-γ production in myelin basic protein (MBP)-specific cells isolated from rats immunized with MBP. These findings translated well into the *in vivo* setting as Saq-NO ameliorated the course of the disease in two preclinical models of MS. These results demonstrated that Saq-NO exerts immunomodulatory effects that warrants further studies on its application in autoimmune diseases. In addition, CRYAB, a small heat shock protein, has been shown to decrease neuroinflammation in EAE. Oyebamiji et al. (2012) investigated whether the expression of cell adhesion molecules and chemokine receptors on peripheral and spinal cord T cells, that could possibly affect their migration to the CNS, was altered following EAE CRYAB treatment. Less LFA-1+ lymphocytes and lower levels of iTAC, MCP-5 and MIG were observed in spinal cords of CRYAB-injected EAE animals. In addition, fewer blood T cells expressed CCR6, CXCR4 and CCR7 and *in vivo*-derived CRYAB EAE CD4+ lymphocytes were less migratory towards a MIP-3α gradient *in vitro.* Schirmer et al. (2013) investigated the expression of CD161 (KLRB1) and CCR6 on human γδ T cells in blood and CSF of patients with a clinically isolated syndrome (CIS) and MS in relapse. Flow cytometry analysis of CD161 and CCR6 expression and intracellular cytokine staining for IL-17 and interferon-γ on human γδ T cells in blood and CSF samples. Twenty-six patients with CIS/MS in active relapse, 10 patients with other autoimmune disorders, 12 patients with infectious diseases, and 15 patients with inflammatory neurological diseases were included in this study. Frequencies of CD161high and CCR6+ γδ T cells in blood and CSF samples of patients with CIS/MS in relapse and control patients. γδ T cells were increased in both blood and CSF of patients with CIS/MS in relapse as compared with controls with noninflammatory disease. The fraction of CD161high CCR6+ γδ T cells was significantly higher in the CSF of patients with CIS/MS in relapse than of those with systemic autoimmune disorders or controls with noninflammatory disease. The CD161high CCR6+ double-positive γδ T-cell population was further enriched in the CSF in relation to blood in patients with CIS/MS in relapse but not in patients with infectious disease or the other control groups. The CD161high CCR6+ γδ T-cell population was characterized by its capacity to produce IL-17. IL-17–producing CD161 high CCR6+ γδ T cells might contribute to the compartmentalized inflammatory process in the CNS of patients with MS.

Autoantibodies in MS Generaly autoantibodies and complement opsonization have been implicated in the CNS demyelinating disease, MS, but scavenger receptors (SRs) may also play pathogenetic roles. Hendrickx et al. (2013) characterized SR mRNA and protein expression in postmortem brain tissue from 13 MS patients in relation to demyelination. CD68, chemokine (C-X-C motif) ligand 16 (CXCL16), class A macrophage SR (SR-AI/II), LOX-1 (lectin-like oxidized low-density lipoprotein receptor 1), FcγRIII, and LRP-1 (low-density lipoprotein receptor-related protein 1) mRNA were upregulated in chronic MS lesions. CD68 and CXCL16 mRNA were also upregulated around chronic MS lesions. By immunohistochemistry, CD68, CXCL16, and SR-AI/II were expressed by foamy macrophages in the rim and by ramified microglia around chronic active MS lesions. CXCL16 and SR-AI/II were also expressed by astrocytes in MS lesions and by primary human microglia and astrocytes *in vitro* suggesting that SRs are involved in myelin uptake in MS, and that upregulation of CD68, CXCL16, and SR-AI/II is one of the initial events in microglia as they initiate myelin phagocytosis. As demyelination continues, additional upregulation of LOX-1, FcγRIII, and LRP-1 may facilitate this process. Hence various immunological biomarkers are important in the differential diagnosis and treatment of MS. *These include; induction of autoimmune T cells, increased synthesis of immunoglobulin-γ (IgG), cytotoxic NKG 2C+, CD4 T cells, and FASL expression of astrocytes as illustrated in Figure 47.*

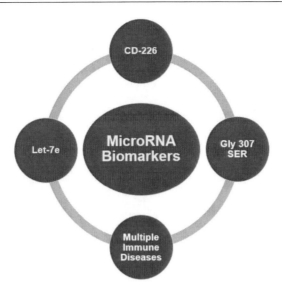

Figure 47. *MicroRNA Biomarkers in MS:* A diagram exhibiting significantly important microRNA biomarkers for the differential diagnosis and confirmation of MS. Out of 17 miRNAs that are altered in MS; Let-7e, CD-226, and Gly-307 SER have been directly implicated in multiple immune diseases including MS as illustrated in this picture.

Retinal Periphlebitis as a Biomarker of MS Ortiz-Pérez et al. (2013) assessed the association of primary retinal inflammation, namely retinal periphlebitis (RP) and microcystic macular edema, with clinical, brain, and retinal imaging biomarkers of MS severity. A total of 100 patients with MS underwent a neurologic and ophthalmic examination, MRI, and optical coherence tomography. Disability was assessed using the *Expanded Disability Status Scale* at baseline and after a 1-year follow-up. The brain volume, the gray matter volume, and T1 lesion volume were assessed at baseline as radiologic biomarkers of disease severity. Retinal nerve fiber layer thickness and macular volume at baseline were used as biomarkers of axonal damage. Five patients showed RP, 2 showed microcystic macular edema, and the retina was normal in the remaining 93. Patients with RP had a tendency toward a higher adjusted-mean *Expanded Disability Status Scale* score at baseline and disability progression after a 1-year follow-up compared with patients without primary retinal inflammation. These patients also had a higher adjusted-mean T1 lesion volume. Patients with RP had a lower adjusted-mean retinal nerve fiber layer thickness and a trend toward lower macular volume suggesting the role of RP as a biomarker of MS severity.

Riddell et al. (2013) reported that the biomarker-adaptive threshold design (BATD) allows researchers to simultaneously study the efficacy of treatment in the overall group and to investigate the relationship between a hypothesized predictive biomarker and the treatment effect on the primary outcome. It was developed for survival outcomes for Phase III clinical trials where the biomarker of interest is measured on a continuous scale. In a study, the generalizations of the BATD to accommodate count biomarkers and outcomes were developed and then studied in the MS context where the number of relapses is a commonly used outcome. Through simulation studies, these authors discovered that the BATD has - increased power compared with a traditional fixed procedure under varying scenarios for which there exists a sensitive patient subgroup. They appled the procedure for two biomarkers, baseline enhancing lesion count and disease duration at baseline, using data from a completed trial. MS duration appeared to be a predictive biomarker for this dataset, and the procedure indicated that the treatment effect is strongest for patients who have had MS for less than 7.8 years. This procedure holds promise of statistical power when the effect of treatment is significantly high in a sensitive patient subgroup.

MICRO-RNAS AS BIOMARKERS IN MS

MicroRNAs are an abundant class of small, single-stranded, noncoding RNAs that regulate gene expression post-transcriptionally by targeting mRNAs for translational repression or degradation. MicroRNA, as an important regulator of gene expression, is associated with several diseases. MicroRNAs play important roles in the regulation of immune responses. There is evidence that miRNAs also participate in the pathogenesis of MS, but how they regulate the pathogenesis of MS remains unknown. Because they are stable in serum, they are being developed as biomarkers for cancer and other diseases. In MS, miRNAs have been studied in cell populations but not in the circulation. A major challenge is to develop immune biomarkers to monitor disease. Recent studies addressed the role of miRNAs in the differentiation of progenitor cells into microglia and in the activation process, aiming at clarifying the origin of adult microglia cells and the contribution of the CNS environment to microglial phenotype, in health and disease. The identification of new members of the miRNA family associated with the pathogenesis of MS could facilitate early diagnosis and treatment. *Due to their ability to simultaneously modulate the fate of different genes, these molecules act as key regulators during immune cell differentiation and activation, and their dysfunction can contribute to pathological conditions associated with neuroinflammation.* With the recent detection of miRNAs in body fluids, the possibility for using them as diagnostic biomarkers emerged. MiRNAs can regulate the expression of the genome at the post-transcriptional level. They play an important regulatory role in autoimmunity and inflammation, and demonstrate potential as theranostic targets in many diseases. They have roles in immunity, from regulation of cell development to activation and function in immune responses.

Recent evidence suggests the involvement of miRNAs in the pathogenesis of autoimmune diseases as well as MS. Guan et al. (2013) showed that miRNA let-7e is upregulated in EAE, an animal model of MS using miRNA array and QPCR. The expression of let-7e was primarily in CD4 (+) T cells and infiltrated mononuclear cells of CNS, and correlated with the development of EAE. These investigators discovered that let-7e silencing *in vivo* inhibited encephalitogenic Th1 and Th17 cells and attenuated EAE, with reciprocal increase of Th2 cells; overexpression of let-7e enhanced Th1 and Th17 cells and aggravated EAE. They also identified IL-10 as one of the targets of let-7e and proposed that let-7e is a new miRNA involved in the regulation of encephalitogenic T-cell differentiation and the pathogenesis of EAE. MicroRNA expression profiles were identified in *several autoimmune diseases, such as rheumatoid arthritis, systemic lupus erythematosus, and MS. However, the expression profile in peripheral blood mononuclear cells (PBMCs) from primary biliary cirrhosis (PBC) patients and its role in PBC remains uncertain.* Qin et al. (2013) explored abnormal microRNA regulation in PBC of MS patients. MicroRNA array was performed in PBMCs obtained from patients versus healthy controls. Six of the 17 differentially expressed microRNAs were confirmed using QPCR. Based on bioinformatics analysis, the potential biological processes and significant signaling pathways affected by these microRNAs were identified, and generated the microRNA-gene network. According to microRNA array, a total of 17 microRNAs were differentially expressed. Six microRNAs were validated using QPCR, and the results were consistent with microRNA array analysis. The bioinformatics revealed that the potential target genes of these microRNAs were involved in *cell proliferation, cell differentiation, apoptosis, signal transduction, endocytosis, mitogen-activated protein kinase signaling pathway, transforming growth factor-β signaling pathway, Wnt signaling pathway, calcium signaling pathway, etc.* 17 microRNAs were differentially expressed in PBMCs from PBC patients. Functional bioinformatics demonstrated that prediction genes targeted by these microRNAs were involved in multiple biological processes and signaling pathways. This study confered new perspectives on the involvement of microRNA in PBC, but the precise mechanisms need to be validated in future to establish their exact role in MS theranostics.

A serial assessment of biomarkers related to disease activity could be clinically useful in some autoimmune diseases. Neuromyelitis optica (NMO) is a severe inflammatory disease of the optic nerves and spinal cord that can be associated with lupus erythematosus, Sjögren syndrome or myasthenia gravis. Chanson et al.; (2013) described the data on the use of biomarkers of disease activity in NMO. A specific and pathogenic antibody (Ab) directed against aquaporin 4 (AQP4) was discovered in this disease. The relapses were accompanied by a rise and immunosuppressive therapy by a decrease in serum anti-AQP4 Ab concentrations. However, this association was not sufficient to justify treatment changes based on anti-AQP4 Ab variations. This parameter might be helpful as a biomarker but only if a threshold inducing a relapse and justifying a switch in therapy is established. A link between disease severity and serum cytotoxicity against AQP4-expressing cells was proposed but has not yet been confirmed. Finally, the assessment of T cell immunity against AQP4 and specific cytokines could be investigated in future.

Recently Zare-Shahabadi et al. (2013) provided emerging knowledge of miRNA biogenesis, their roles in cells involved in the disease process, and potential theranostic applications. It is now recognized that the miRNAs in CNS lesions and peripheral blood can be used as potential biomarkers for the diagnosis and prognosis of various chronic diseases including MS. Also, miRNA mimics, small-molecule inhibitors of specific miRNAs, and antisense oligonucleotides can be used as therapeutic agents to combat the disease. The impaired expression of miRNAs is associated with the initiation and progression of pathophysiologic processes in several human diseases. Scleroderma (*systemic sclerosis; SSc*) is a heterogeneous autoimmune disease that includes the progressive fibrotic replacement of normal tissue architecture in multiple organs. Xhu et al. (2013) suggested that SSc skin tissues display a different miRNA expression than that found in normal controls. miRNAs with pro- or antifibrotic properties are dysregulated in SSc skin fibrosis. Serum miRNA levels are associated with SSc activity and severity. miRNAs can be used as therapeutic targets and serve as biomarkers for SSc diagnosis and assessment of disease state and severity. Hence SSc miRNA expression and the roles of dysregulation of miRNAs in SSc tissues and serum and examines the therapeutic potential of targeting miRNAs in the management of SSc patients.

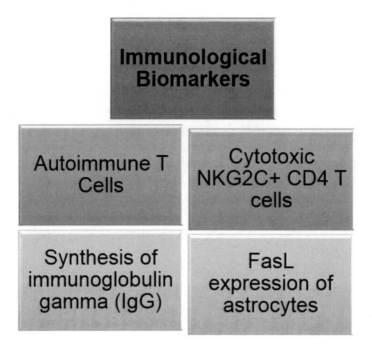

Figure 48. *Immunological Biomarkers in MS*: This diagram illustrates various immunological biomarkers important in the differential diagnosis and treatment of MS. These include; induction of autoimmune T cells, increased synthesis of immunoglobulin-γ (IgG), cytotoxic NKG 2C+, CD4 T cells, and FASL expression of astrocytes.

Keller et al. (2013) performed a comprehensive analysis of miRNA expression profiles in blood of patients with a clinically isolated syndrome (CIS) or RRMS including NGS. miRNA expression was analyzed in blood samples from treatment-naïve patients with CIS (n = 25) or RRMS (n = 25) and 50 healthy controls by NGS, microarray analysis, and qRT-PCR. In patients with CIS/RRMS, NGS and microarray analysis identified 38 and 8 significantly deregulated miRNAs, respectively. Three of these miRNAs were up- (hsa-miR-16-2-3p) or downregulated (hsa-miR-20a-5p, hsa-miR-7-1-3p) by both methods. Another 5 of the miRNAs deregulated in the NGS screen showed the same direction of regulation in the microarray analysis. qRT-PCR confirmed the direction of regulation for all 8 and was significant for 3 miRNAs. This study identified a set of miRNAs deregulated in CIS/RRMS and confirmed the underexpression of hsa-miR-20a-5p in MS. Hence hsa-miR-20a-5p and the other validated miRNAs may represent promising candidates for future evaluation as biomarkers for MS theranostics and could be of relevance in the pathophysiology of this disease.

Circulating miRNAs in MS and other Neurodegenerative Diseases Altered expression of several miRNAs has been associated with AD, MS, and ischemic injury, hence advocating the use of these small molecules as disease biomarkers and new therapeutic targets. AD is the most common form of dementia but the identification of reliable, early and non-invasive biomarkers remains a major challenge. Guedes et al. (2013) summarizes the recent advances in miRNA-mediated regulation of microglia development and activation and discussed the role of specific miRNAs in the maintenance and switching of microglial activation states and illustrated the potential of this class of nucleic acids both as biomarkers of inflammation and new therapeutic tools for the modulation of microglia behavior in the CNS. These investigators focused on the characteristics of circulating miRNAs and their values as potential biomarkers in CNS diseases, particularly in AD, HD, MS, schizophrenia, and bipolar disorder. As a class of important endogenous small noncoding RNAs that regulate gene expression at the posttranscriptional level, miRNAs play a critical role in many physiological and pathological processes. It is currently believed that miRNAs contribute to the *development, differentiation, and synaptic plasticity of the neurons*, and their dysregulation is linked to a series of diseases. MiRNAs exist in the tissues and as circulating miRNAs in several body fluids, including plasma or serum, CSF, urine, and saliva. There are significant differences between the circulating miRNA expression profiles of healthy individuals and those of patients. Consequently, circulating miRNAs may become a novel class of noninvasive and sensitive biomarkers for MS theranostics. Although little is known about the origin and functions of circulating miRNAs at present, their roles in the clinical diagnosis and prognosis of diseases make them fascinating biomarkers, particularly for tumors and cardiovascular diseases. However, there is limited data regarding the roles of circulating miRNAs in CNS diseases. Leidinger et al. (2013) presented a novel miRNA-based biomarker for detecting AD from blood samples. These investigators applied next-generation sequencing (NGS) to miRNAs from blood samples of 48 AD patients and 22 controls, yielding a total of 140 unique mature miRNAs with changed expression levels. Of these, 82 had higher and 58 had lower abundance in AD patient samples. These investigators selected 12 miRNAs for an RT-qPCR analysis on a larger cohort of 202 samples, comprising not only AD patients and healthy controls but also patients with other CNS illnesses including MCI, which represented a transitional period before the development of *AD, as well as MS, PD, major depression, bipolar disorder, and schizophrenia.* The miRNA target enrichment analysis of the selected 12 miRNAs indicated their involvement in CNS development, neuron projection, neuron projection development and morphogenesis. Using this 12-miRNA signature, these investigators differentiated between AD and controls with an accuracy of 93%, a specificity of 95% and a sensitivity of 92%. The differentiation of AD from other neurological diseases such as MS was possible with accuracies between 74% and 78%. The differentiation of the other CNS disorders from controls yielded higher accuracies indicating that deregulated miRNAs in blood might be used as biomarkers in the diagnosis of AD or other neurological diseases.

Epigenetic Changes and miRNA as Biomarkers for MS Diagnosis Currently it is being explored whether circulating miRNAs could be identified in MS and whether they are linked to disease stage and/or disability. Koch et al. (2013) reported the risk of developing MS depends on both genetic and environmental factors. Although the genetic susceptibility to MS has been investigated in detail, reports regrding epigenetic changes have only recently developed. Epigenetic changes to DNA influence gene expression without altering the DNA sequence. *DNA methylation, histone modification, and miRNA-associated silencing are the 3 most important epigenetic mechanisms that influence gene expression.* These investigators summarized recent studies on epigenetic changes and miRNA as biomarkers for diagnosing MS and predicting disease course or treatment response. Out of 17 miRNAs that were altered in MS; Let-7e, CD-226, and Gly-307 SER were directly implicated in multiple immune diseases including MS as illustrated in Figure 48. These microRNA biomarkers can now be used for the EBPT of MS. Søndergaard et al (2013) assessed whether miRNAs contribute to the altered immune activation state in RRMS patients and investigated the use of miRNAs as theranostic biomarkers in MS. They performed global miRNA expression profiling in peripheral blood mononuclear cells (PBMCs) and selected miRNAs were measured in plasma, detected expression of miRNAs by real-time qPCR and compared results with cytokines related to inflammation and disease activity. Selected miRNAs were analyzed in PBMC subpopulations, after isolating them by magnetic bead separation. Among validated miRNAs, let-7d correlated with the pro-inflammatory cytokine IL-1β. The miR-145 was 3-fold up-regulated in MS patients; its possible use as a theranostic biomarker in PBMCs, plasma and serum was confirmed by ROC-curve analysis. Thus RRMS patients in remission had altered expression of miRNAs and miR-145 was detected as a potential biomarker for the EBPT of MS in blood, plasma, and serum.

MRI BIOMARKERS IN MS

MRI Biomarkers in MS Nielsen et al. (2013) evaluated the contribution of focal cortical lesion (CL) subtypes at ultra-high-field MRI and traditional MRI metrics of brain damage to neurologic disability and cognitive performance in a heterogeneous MS cohort. Thirty-four patients with disease including clinically isolated syndrome, RRMS, and secondary progressive MS were scanned on a 7-tesla scanner to acquire fast low-angle shot (FLASH) T2*-weighted images for characterization of white matter and deep gray matter lesion volume, and CL types. Patients also underwent anatomical 3T MRI for cortical thickness estimation, and neuropsychological testing within 1 week of the 7T scan. Neurologic disability was measured using the Expanded Disability Status Scale. Type III-IV CLs had the relationship to physical disability. White matter lesion volume and type I CLs were associated with 6 of 11 neuropsychological test variables. Type III-IV CLs correlate with 4 of 11 neuropsychological tests whereas type II CLs, deep gray matter lesion volume, and cortical thickness metrics were less frequently associated with cognitive performance suggesting that Leukocortical (type I) and subpial (III-IV) CLs identified on 7T FLASH-T2* sequences can be potential biomarkers of cognitive and neurologic status in MS.

MRI, Diffusion Tensor Imaging and MS Pediatric inflammatory demyelinating diseases of the CNS are clinically heterogeneous with their mode of presentation, clinical severity, rate of progression, and prognosis. Tenembaum (2013) reported that the advent of MRI has increased our awareness regarding childhood white matter disorders. Acute disseminated encephalomyelitis (ADEM) is an immune-mediated inflammatory disorder of the CNS, typically transitory and self-limiting. The highest incidence of ADEM is observed during childhood. It is characterized by an acute encephalopathy with multifocal neurological deficits. In the absence of specific biomarkers the diagnosis of ADEM is still based on clinical presentations and MRI evidence of widespread demyelination, after ruling out other possible explanations for an acute encephalopathy. Over the past decade, many retrospective studies have focused on clinical and neuroimaging features to define specific diagnostic criteria. The occurrence of relapses in children with ADEM poses diagnostic challenge in its differentiation from MS and neuromyelitis optica (NMO). With the use of high-dose steroids, the long-term prognosis of ADEM to functional and cognitive recovery was favorable. In MS, physical and cognitive deficits not only reflect structural damage, but also functional imbalance in and between neuronal networks. Resting-state fMRI has allowed to investigate intrinsic, synchronized brain activity across the whole brain to measure the degree of functional correlation between different cortical regions. Filipi et al. (2013) described their findings obtained in MS patients at different clinical stages and discussed how fMRI may facilitate identifying novel biomarkers for EBPT of MS. Furthermore, Marschallinger et al. (2013) developed a method for the quantitative, spatial, and spatiotemporal analysis and noninvasive characterization of MS lesions from MRI with geostatistics. These investogators worked on a data set involving 3 synthetic and 3 real-world MS lesions. MS lesions were extracted ater brain normalization and the binary 3-D models of MS lesions were subjected to geostatistical indicator variography. They were able to describe the 3-D spatial structure of MS lesions. Fitting a model function to the empirical variograms, spatial characteristics of the MS lesions could be quantified by two parameters. An orthogonal plot of these parameters enabled comparison of the MS lesions suggesting that this method is a promising candidate to complement image-based statistics by incorporating spatial quantification. Sunwoo et al. (2013) determined whether the apparent diffusion coefficient (ADC) values correlate with O (6)-methylguanine DNA methyltransferase (MGMT) promoter methylation analyzed by methylation-specific multiplex ligation-dependent probe amplification (MS-MLPA) in patients with glioblastoma. The methylation status of MGMT promoter was assessed by methylation-specific PCR (MSP) and by MS-MLPA. MS-MLPA is a semiquantitative method that determines the methylation ratio. The Ki-67 labeling index was also analyzed. The mean and 5th percentile ADC values were correlated with MGMT promoter methylation status and Ki-67 labeling index using a linear regression model. Progression-free survival (PFS) was also correlated with the ADC values using Kaplan-Meier survival analysis. The mean methylation ratio was 0.21 ± 0.20. By MSP, there were 5 methylated and 21 unmethylated tumors. The mean ADC revealed a positive relationship with MGMT promoter methylation ratio and was different according to MSP-determined methylation status. Median PFS was related with methylation ratio and MSP-derived methylation status. A positive relationship was demonstrated between PFS and the mean ADC value. The 5th percentile ADC values showed a negative relationship with Ki-67 labeling index. The ADC values were correlated with PFS as well as with MGMT promoter methylation status indicating that ADC values may be investigated as a biomarker for predicting prognosis.

Tourdias and Dousset (2013) reported that MRI is an established tool in the management of MS. Loss of blood brain barrier integrity assessed by Gadolinium (Gd) enhancement is the standard biomarker of MS. To explore the cascade of the inflammatory events, other MRI, but also PET biomarkers have been reviewed which are being developed to address active neuroinflammation with increased sensitivity and specificity. Alternative MRI contrast agents, PET radiotracers and imaging techniques could be more sensitive than Gd to detect early BBB alteration, assess the inflammatory cell recruitment, and/or the edema accumulation. These biomarkers of neuroinflammation could find great relevance to augment Gd information and thereby increase our understanding of acute lesion pathophysiology and its noninvasive follow-up, especially to monitor prognosis. Furthermore, these biomarkers of inflammation combined with those of neurodegeneration may provide a complete picture of MS, which will be of great help for future EBPT strategies.

Rimkus et al. (2013) characterized the microscopic damage to the corpus callosum RRMS with diffusion tensor imaging (DTI) to investigate the correlation of this damage with disability. The DTI parameters of fractional anisotropy and mean diffusivity provide information about the integrity of cell membranes, offering two more specific indices, namely the axial and radial diffusivities, which are useful for discriminating axon loss from demyelination. Brain MRI of 30 RRMS patients and 30 age- and sex-matched healthy controls were acquired in a 3T scanner. The axial diffusivities, radial diffusivities, fractional anisotropy, and mean diffusivity of 5 segments of the corpus callosum, were correlated to the Expanded Disability Status Scale score. All corpus callosum segments showed increased radial diffusivities and mean diffusivity, decreased fractional anisotropy, in the RRMS group. The axial diffusivity was increased in the posterior midbody and splenium. The *Expanded Disability Status Scale* scores correlated with axial diffusivities and mean diffusivity, with an isolated correlation with radial diffusivities in the posterior midbody of the corpus callosum. There was no significant correlation with lesion loads, suggesting that neurological dysfunction in RRMS can be influenced by commissural disconnection, and the diffusion indices of DTI can be used as biomarkers of disability for follow up patients.

Filippi et al. (2013) reported that in MS, MRI is an important tool to confirm diagnosis and for monitoring disease progression or remission. The increased availability of ultra-high-field magnets *(7 Tesla or higher)* gives rise to questions about the benefits of their use in patients with MS. *The main advantages of ultra-high-field MRI are the improved signal-to-noise ratio, greater chemical shift dispersion, and improved contrast due to magnetic susceptibility variations, which lead to increased sensitivity.* At present, ultra-high-field MRI is primarily used to improve understanding of MS pathogenesis, better visualization of white matter lesions and their morphological characteristics; ability to visualize grey matter lesions and their exact location; the quantification of 'novel' metabolites involved in axonal degeneration; and sensitivity to Iron accumulation. In addition, the spinal cord is a site of predilection for MS lesions. While DTI is used for the study of anisotropic systems such as WM tracts, it is of limited value in tissues with more isotropic microstructures such as gray matter. In contrast, diffusional kurtosis imaging (DKI), which measures both Gaussian and non-Gaussian properties of water diffusion, provides more precise informartion of both anisotropic and isotropic structural changes. Raz et al. (2013) investigated the cervical spinal cord of patients with MS to characterize lesional and normal-appearing gray matter and WM damage by using (DKI). Nineteen patients and 16 controls underwent MR imaging of the cervical spinal cord on a 3T scanner. Fractional anisotropy, mean diffusivity, and mean kurtosis were measured in normal-appearing gray matter and WM. Spinal cord T2-hyperintense lesions were identified in 18 patients. Whole fractional anisotropy and mean kurtosis, WM fractional anisotropy, and gray matter mean kurtosis were decreased, and mean diffusivity was increased in patients compared with controls. Mean spinal cord area was lower in patients, indicating that DKI can provide better characterization of lesions in patients with MS as it provides additional and complementary information to DTI on spinal cord pathology.

Plasma Sulfatides As Biomarkers in MS Moyano et al. (2013) examined the plasma distribution of sulfatide isoforms. Sulfatides with long-chain (C24: 0 or C24: 1) and short-chain (C16: 0 or C18: 0) fatty acids were quantified in plasma of RRMS patients by ultra-high-performance liquid chromatography tandem mass spectrometry. C18: 0 and C24: 1 sulfatide plasma levels positively correlated with the Expanded Disability Status Scale. C16/C1: 0 and C16/C24: 0 ratios also correlated with the age and the time since last relapse. Healthy women showed higher levels of C16: 0 sulfatide than healthy men; however, this gender difference disappeared in MS patients indicating the potential use of sulfatides as biomarkers in relapsing-remitting MS and points to a possible association with the higher susceptibility of women to develop MS.

Hashimoto's encephalopathy (HE) is a treatable disease based on autoimmune mechanisms associated with Hashimoto's thyroiditis. Kishitani et al. (2013) recently discovered the serum autoantibodies (Abs) against the NH2-terminal of alpha-enolase (NAE) as a diagnostic biomarker for HE. The serum anti-NAE Abs were not detected in normal individuals and other disorders such as infections, collagen diseases, MS and other autoimmune conditions. The specificity of the serum anti-NAE Abs was 91% for HE whereas the sensitivity was 50%. In this clinical study of 80 cases of HE with anti-NAE Abs, the acute encephalopathic form was the most common clinical feature, and followed by chronic psychiatric form and progressive ataxia. The common neuropsychiatric features were disturbed consciousness, psychosis (*especially delirium and hallucination*), seizures, and dementia. Abnormalities on EEG and decreased blood flow on SPECT were common while abnormalities on brain MRI were rare. The early diagnosis and treatment for HE could lead to good recovery from the disease, suggesting that serum anti-NAE Abs are a useful theranostic biomarker for HE.

The newly recognized entity IgG4-related disease (IgG4-RD) is characterized by an elevated IgG4 serum concentration and tissue infiltration by IgG4-positive plasma cells. Ohyama et al. (2013) described the clinical features and nerve biopsy findings of a patient with IgG4-RD who presented with peripheral neuropathy. A 55-year-old man had histopathologically defined IgG4-RD that manifested as sensory-motor neuropathy. The neuropathic features were multiple mononeuropathies with electrophysiological findings suggestive of axonal neuropathy. Marked thickening with abundant collagen fibers and infiltration of IgG4-positive plasma cells were observed in the epineurium of the biopsied sural nerve. A moderate degree of myelinated fiber loss without evidence of segmental demyelination was present, whereas necrotizing vasculitis was not found. Oral Prednisolone treatment ameliorated the neuropathic symptoms. This case of IgG4-RD presented as sensory-motor neuropathy with pain and sclerosis of the skin in the extremities, indicating that the differential diagnosis of neuropathy should include IgG4-RD.

Podojil et al. (2013) reported that the primary focus on T(h)1 autoreactive effector cell function in autoimmune diseases, such as rheumatoid arthritis and MS, has shifted towards the role of T(h)17 autoreactive effector cells and the ability of regulatory T cells (T(reg) to modulate the pro-inflammatory autoimmune response. Therefore, the currently favored hypothesis is that a delicate balance between T (h) 1/17 effector cells and T (reg) cell function is critical in the regulation of inflammatory autoimmune disease. An intensive area of research with regard to the T (h) 1/17: T (reg) cell balance is the utilization of blockade and/or ligation of various co-stimulatory or co-inhibitory molecules, respectively, during ongoing disease to skew the immune response toward a more tolerogenic/regulatory state. Currently, FDA-approved therapies for MS patients are aimed at the suppression of immune cell function. The other favored method of treatment is a modulation or deletion of autoreactive immune cells via short-term blockade of activating co-stimulatory receptors via treatment with fusion proteins such as CTLA4-Ig and CTLA4-FasL. Based on the initial success of CTLA4-Ig, there are additional fusion proteins that are currently under development. Examples of the recently identified B7/CD28 family members are PD-L1, PD-L2, inducible co-stimulatory molecule-ligand (ICOS-L), B7-H3, and B7-H4, all of which may emerge as potential theranostic agents. The expression of both stimulatory and inhibitory B7 molecules seems to play an essential role in modulating immune cell function through a variety of mechanisms, which is supported by findings that suggest each B7 molecule has developed its own indispensable niche in the immune system. As more data are generated, the diagnostic and therapeutic potential of the B7 family-member-derived fusion proteins becomes more apparent. Besides defining the biology of these B7/CD28 family members *in vivo*, additional difficulty in the development of these therapies lies in maintaining the normal immune functions of recognition and reaction to non-self-antigens following viral or bacterial infection in the patient. Further complicating the translation of these therapies, the mechanism of action identified for a particular reagent may depend upon the method of immune-cell activation and the subset of immune cells targeted in the study.

GIroni et al. (2013) recently reported that MS is a multi-factorial disease, where a single biomarker unlikely can provide comprehensive information. Due to the non-linearity of biomarkers, traditional statistic is unsuitable to dissect their relationship. Patients affected with primary (PP=14), secondary (SP=33), benign (BB=26), relapsing-remitting (RR=30) MS, and 42 sex and age matched healthy controls were studied. These investigators performed immune-phenotypic and functional analysis of peripheral blood mononuclear cell (PBMCs) by flow-cytometry. Semantic connectivity maps (AutoCM) were applied to find the associations among immunological markers. AutoCM is a special kind of Artificial Neural Network able to find consistent trends and associations among variables. The matrix of connections, visualized through minimum spanning tree, keeps non linear associations among variables and captures connection schemes among clusters. Complex immunological relationships were related to different disease courses. Low CD4IL25+ cells level was related to SP MS. This phenotype was also associated to high CD4ROR+ cells levels. BB MS was related to high CD4+IL13 cell levels, as well as to high CD14+IL6 cells percentage. RR MS was related to CD4+IL25 high cell levels, as well indirectly to high percentages of CD4+IL13 cells. In this latter strong association could be confirmed the induction activity of the former cells (CD4+IL25) on the latter (CD4+IL13). Another interesting topographic data was the isolation of Th9 cells (CD4IL9) from the main part of the immunological network related to MS, suggesting secondary role of this new cell phenotype in MS disease. This novel application of non-linear mathematical techniques suggests peculiar immunological signatures for different MS phenotypes. Notably, the immune-network displayed by this new method, rather than a single biomarker, might be viewed as the right target of immunotherapy. Furthermore, this new statistical technique could be employed to increase the knowledge of other age-related multifactorial disease in which complex immunological networks play a substantial role. Various immunological biomarkers important in the differential EBPT of MS are presented in Figure 48. *These include; induction of autoimmune T cells, increased synthesis of immunoglobulin-γ (IgG), cytotoxic NKG 2C+, CD4 T cells, and FASL expression of astrocytes.*

Neurofilament As Biomarker of MS Neurofilaments are promising biomarkers in MS and increased levels in CSF indicate axonal damage or degeneration. Kuhle et al. (2013) compared two highly sensitive assays to measure two subunits of the neurofilament (neurofilament light (NfL) and neurofilament heavy chain (NfH) protein. These investigators evaluated the analytical and clinical performance of the UmanDiagnostics NF-light® ELISA in the CSF of a group of 148 patients with clinically isolated syndrome (CIS) or MS, and 72 controls. They compared their results with referring levels of previously-developed CSF NfHSMI35 assay. Exposure to room temperature (up to 8 days) or repetitive thawing (up to 4 thaws) did not influence measurement of NfL concentrations. Values of NfL were higher in all disease stages of CIS/MS, in comparison to controls. NfL levels correlated with the Expanded Disability Status Scale (EDSS) score in patients with relapsing disease, spinal cord relapses and with CSF markers of acute inflammation. The ability of NfL to distinguish patients from controls was greater than that of NfHSMI35 in both CIS patients and all MS stages grouped together. Thus NfL proved to be a stable protein, an important prerequisite for a reliable biomarker, and the NF-light® ELISA performed better in discriminating patients from controls, compared with the ECL-NfHSMI35 immunoassay. These investogators confirmed and expanded upon previous findings regarding neurofilaments as quantitative biomarkers of neurodegeneration to measure for neuroprotective treatment in MS studies. In a similar study, neurofilament light chain (NfL) levels in CSF of patients with RRMS were normalized by Natalizumab treatment. Kuhle et al. (2013) compared the coherence between NfL and neurofilament heavy chain (NfHSMI 35) levels in CSF samples in these patients. In 30 patients with RRMS, CSF was obtained prior to and following 12 months of Natalizumab treatment. NfHSMI 35 was measured by an electrochemiluminescence-based immunoassay. NfL levels were determined by the UmanDiagnostics NF-light® assay. NfHSMI 35 decreased in 73.3% and NfL in 90% of the patients following Natalizumab treatment. Patients experiencing a relapse showed higher NfHSMI 35 levels compared with patients in remission. This difference was less obvious for NfL. In patients in remission, NfL levels were lower following Natalizumab treatment, whereas the same comparison failed significance for NfHSMI 35, confirming reduced axonal damage under Natalizumab treatment by measuring NfHSMI 35. In comparison with NfHSMI 35, NfL changes were more pronounced and the treatment effect also included patients in remission suggesting that NfL is superior over NfHSMI 35 as therapeutic biomarker and is a promising candidate to measure neuroaxonal damage in MS treatment trials. Axelsson et al. (2013) explored the impact from immunosuppressive therapy in PMS by analyzing CSF biomarkers of axonal damage (*neurofilament light protein, NFL*), astrogliosis (*glial fibrillary acidic protein, GFAP*), and B-cell regulation (CXCL13). CSF was obtained from 35 patients with PMS before and after 12-24 months of Mitoxantrone or Rituximab treatment, and from 14 age-matched healthy control subjects. The levels of NFL, GFAP, and CXCL13 were determined by immunoassays. The mean NFL level decreased by 51%, the mean CXCL13 reduction was 55%, while GFAP levels remained unaffected. Subgroup analysis showed that the NFL reduction was confined to previously untreated patients and patients with Gd-enhancing lesions on MRI prior to study baseline. These data imply that 12-24 months of immunosuppressive therapy reduces axonal damage in PMS, particularly in patients with ongoing disease activity. Determination of NFL levels in CSF is a potential biomarker for treatment efficacy and as endpoint in phase II trials of MS.

Orbach et al. (2013) studied an array of inflammatory CSF biomarkers in patients with suspected MS to recognize potential early EBPT. CSF samples were obtained from 115 patients who presented with neurological symptomatology suggestive of MS as follows: clinically isolated syndrome (CIS) = 49, RRMS = 29, and other neurologic disorders (OND) = 37. Protein expression profiles of 30 inflammatory biomarkers were measured by multiplex Luminex bead assay and further analyzed by group comparison statistics, correlation studies and ROC analysis. IL-12 subunit p40 (IL12p40) demonstrated a differential expression between the groups, with higher levels in CIS and RRMS patients. ROC analysis demonstrated excellent diagnostic performance of IL12p40 for discrimination between CIS and OND patients. No associations were found with disease activity or severity measures. An increased IL12p40 level characterized the CSF of MS patients in identifying CIS and OND patients early in the clinical diagnostic assessment.

BDNF in MS Dhib-Jalbut et al. (2013) measured immune biomarkers in subjects with MS treated with IFNβ-1b for 12 months. IL-17 levels were significantly higher at Month 6 in relapsing subjects while BDNF levels were higher at Month 3 in relapse-free subjects. Change from baseline in IL-4 levels inversely correlated with disability score whereas change from baseline in IL-10/IFN-γ ratio inversely correlated with occurrence of relapses. CXCR3+CD8+ T-cells tended to be higher but declined with treatment in relapse-free compared with relapsing subjects, indicating the potential of cytokine and neurotrophic factors as biomarkers of clinical response to IFNβ-1b in MS.

Osteopontin as Biomarker of MS Osteopontin (OPN) is a pleiotropic protein with important roles in inflammation and immunity as a candidate biomarker for disease activity in MS. Szalardy et al. (2013) examined if proteins associated with axonal and neuronal degeneration (Tau, p-Tau and β-amyloid (1-42)) and T-cell-mediated autoimmunity (Osteopontin) are altered in the CSF of MS patients, and assessed their potential in reflecting the severity and predicting the progression and evolution of early MS. The CSF samples from patients presenting with different clinical forms of MS were evaluated by ELISA. The patients were followed-up and their clinical status was re-evaluated 5 years after sampling. While CSF levels of Tau, p-Tau and β-amyloid (1-42) did not differ between MS and Control groups, Osteopontin levels were elevated in MS patients which was associated with a relapse and correlated with clinical severity. These findings were independent of age and blood-CSF barrier function. However, none of the examined protein levels differed between groups with different clinical evolutions and no positive correlations with progression could be detected *suggesting that Tau, p-Tau and β-amyloid (1-42) are inappropriate as biomarkers in MS. This was the first study on CSF Osteopontin as biomarker of clinical severity in MS patients.* In addition, Kivisäkk et al. (2013) evaluated plasma levels of OPN in a cohort of MS patients, as a biomarker in a regular clinical setting. These investigators analyzed OPN plasma levels in 492 consecutive MS patients, using a commercial ELISA. OPN levels were higher in RRMS and secondary progressive MS, compared to healthy controls. Treatment with Natalizumab or Glatiramer acetate was associated with lower OPN levels. There was no significant association between the OPN levels and disease activity, as measured by clinical or radiological criteria. One-third of patients with high OPN levels had concurrent disorders that may also be associated with increased OPN expression, and which may mask a modest effect of MS disease activity on OPN levels. These data did not support a role for circulating OPN levels as a biomarker for disease activity in a heterogeneous clinical setting, but did not rule out a potential role in the CSF, in clinical trial, or in conjunction with other biomarkers as a theranostic biomarker in MS.

Inflammatory Biomarkers in MS Inflammatory mediators have crucial roles in leukocyte recruitment and CNS neuroinflammation. The extent of neuronal injury and axonal loss are associated with severity of CNS inflammation and determine physical disability in MS. Khademi et al. (2013) explored the associations between selected CSF biomarkers and clinical and demographic parameters in a large cohort of patients with MS and controls using data-driven multivariate analysis. Levels of MMP9, chemokine (C-X-C motif) ligand 13 (CXCL13), Osteopontin (OPN) and neurofilament-light chain (NFL) were measured by ELISA in 548 subjects comprising different MS subtypes (*relapsing-remitting, secondary* *progressive and primary progressive*), clinically isolated syndrome and persons with other neurological diseases with or without signs of inflammation/infection. There was a significant association between increased patient age and lower levels of CXCL13, MMP9 and NFL. CXCL13 levels correlated with MMP9 in the younger age groups, but less so in older patients, and after approximately 54 years of age the levels of CXCL13 and MMP9 were low. CXCL13 and MMP9 levels also correlated with both NFL and OPN in younger patients. A strong effect of age on both inflammatory and neurodegenerative biomarkers in MS patients was noticed supporting an early use of adequate immunomodulatory disease modifying drugs, in younger patients, and may provide a biological explanation for the relative inefficacy of such treatments in older patients at later disease stages. Various inflammatory biomarkers can be used for the early diagnosis, prognosis, and treatment of MS. During the progression of MS, most common clinical manifestation is the existence of idiopathic intermediate uveitis, B7-H3 plays a diverse role in the regulation of T cell responses, Muc-1 plays an anti-inflammatory role in EAE (an experimental model of MS), enhanced mB7-H3 expression, over activation of CD4 (+) T cells (Th1 and Th17 subpopulation), Muc-1 a member of the tethered glycoproteins, reduced sB7-H3 levels in MS, B7-H3 which plays a diversified role in regulating T cell response. In addition, APRIL (*a proliferation-inducing ligand*), and translocator protein (18 kDa: TSPO) expression were significantly enhanced in MS. Hence 18KDa, TSPO protein is radiolabeled with ^{18}F or ^{11}C, in PET biomarkers to evaluate the extent of neuro-inflammation in MS as explained in the text.

Myelin Basic Proteins in MS In MS, myelin basic protein (MBP), critical for the maintenance of myelin compaction and protecting against degradation, contain noncoded amino acid, "Citrulline", in abnormal proportions. Peptidyl arginine deiminase (PAD) catalyzes the post-translational citrullination of proteins via the deimination of Arg residues. In the CNS, specifically PAD2 and PAD4, are the enzymes responsible for the citrullination. Wei et al. (2013) used in silico screening of commercial libraries to find small molecules that would inhibit PAD4. An initial set of 10 diverse compounds was selected from the screen, and from these compounds, 3, 4, 6, and 8 showed inhibitory activities against PAD4 with Ki in the range of 115-153 μM. Compound 4 was selected in an *in vivo* MOG EAE mouse model study to evaluate its effect in MS-like conditions. Results from the 24 day pilot mouse study showed an improved clinical outcome for mice being administered compound 4 compared to the control group. In brain, 4 treated mice showed reduction in the CD3 +ve T cells, suggesting that compound 4 may have potential utility and confirmed that noncovalent inhibitors of PAD enzymes can be developed as potential agents targeting MS pathology.

Teunissen et al. (2013) proposed consensus definitions and nomenclature for the following groups: healthy controls (HCs), spinal anesthesia subjects (SASs), inflammatory neurological disease controls (INDCs), peripheral inflammatory neurological disease controls (PINDCs), non-inflammatory neurological controls (NINDCs), symptomatic controls (SCs). Furthermore, these investigators discussed the application of these control groups for diagnostic biomarker studies, prognostic biomarker studies, and therapeutic response studies. Clinicians treating MS patients need biomarkers in order to predict an individualized prognosis for every patient, that is, characteristics that can be measured in an objective manner, and that give information over normal or pathological processes, or about the response to a given therapeutic intervention. Fernández (2013) reported that pharmacogenetics/genomics in the fields of MS by now can be considered a promise. There are some clinical biomarkers of good prognosis (female sex, young age of onset, optic neuritis or isolated sensory symptoms at debut, long interval between initial and second relapse, no accumulation of disability after 5 years of disease evolution, normal or near normal MRI at onset). Some biomarkers in biological samples are considered as potential prognostic like IgM and neurofilaments in CSF or antimyelin and chitinase 3-like 1 in blood (plasma/sera). Baseline MRI lesion number, lesion load and location have been closely associated with a worse evolution, as well as MRI measures related to axonal damage (black holes in T1, brain atrophy, grey matter atrophy (GMA) and white matter atrophy (WMA), magnetization transfer measures and intracortical lesions). Functional measures (OCT, evoked potentials) have a potential role in measuring neurodegeneration in MS and could be very useful for prognosis. Several mathematical approaches to estimate the risk of short term use early clinical and paraclinical biomarkers to predict the evolution of the disease.

Endothelial cells (EC) form the inner lining of blood vessels and are positioned between circulating lymphocytes and tissues. It is hypothesized that EC may act as antigen presenting cells based on the intimate interactions with T cells, which are seen in diseases like MS, cerebral malaria (CM), and viral neuropathologies. Wheway et al. (2013) investigated how human brain microvascular EC (HBEC) interact and support the proliferation of T cells. HBEC express MHC II, CD40 and ICOSL for antigen presentation and co-stimulation and to take up fluorescently labeled antigens via macropinocytosis. In co-cultures, HBEC support and promote the proliferation of CD4(+) and CD8(+) T cells, which both are key in CM pathogenesis, particularly following T cell receptor activation and co-stimulation providing evidence that HBEC can trigger T cell activation, thereby providing a novel mechanism for neuroimmunological complications of infectious diseases.

IL-7 is essential for T cell development in the thymus and maintenance of peripheral T cells. The α-chain of the IL-7R is polymorphic with the existence of SNPs that give rise to non-synonymous amino acid substitutions. Shamim et al. (2013) previously found an association between donor genotypes and increased treatment-related mortality (TRM) (rs1494555G) and acute graft versus host disease (aGvHD) (rs1494555G and rs1494558T) after hematopoietic cell transplantation (HCT). Some studies have confirmed an association between rs6897932C and MS. The investigators evaluated the prognostic significance of IL-7Rα SNP genotypes in 590-recipient/donor pairs that received HLA-matched unrelated donor HCT for hematological malignancies. Consistent with the primary studies, the rs1494555GG and rs1494558TT genotypes of the donor were associated with aGvHD and chronic GvHD in the univariate analysis. The Tallele of rs6897932 was suggestive of an association with increased frequency of relapse by univariate analysis and multivariate analysis. This study provided further evidence of a role of the IL-7 pathway and IL-7Rα SNPs in HCT.

Inflammatory perivascular cuffs are comprised of leucocytes that accumulate in the perivascular space around post-capillary venules before their infiltration into the parenchyma of the CNS. Inflammatory perivascular cuffs are commonly found in the CNS of patients with MS and in the animal model, EAE. Leucocytes that accumulate in the perivascular space secrete MMPss that aid their transmigration into the neural parenchyma. Agrawal et al. (2013) described that the upstream inducer of MMPs expression, extracellular MMPs inducer (CD147), was elevated in EAE, and that its inhibition reduced leucocyte entry into the CNS. These researchers investigated whether the expression of extracellular MMP inducer varies with the temporal evolution of lesions in murine EAE, whether it was uniformly upregulated across MS specimens, and whether it was a feature of inflammatory perivascular cuffs in MS lesions. In EAE, elevation of extracellular MMPs inducer was correlated with the appearance and persistence of clinical signs of disease. In both murine and human samples, extracellular MMPs inducer was detected on endothelium in healthy and disease states but was dramatically increased in and around inflammatory perivascular cuffs on leucocytes, associated with MMPs expression, and on resident cells including microglia. Leucocyte populations that express extracellular MMPs inducer in MS lesions included CD4+ and CD8+ T lymphocytes, B lymphocytes and monocyte/macrophages. The extra-endothelial expression of extracellular MMPs inducer was a biomarker of the activity of lesions in MS, being present on leucocyte-containing perivascular cuffs but not in inactive lesions. By using a function-blocking antibody, these investigators implicate extracellular MMPs inducer in the adhesion of leucocytes to endothelial cells and determined that its activity was more crucial on leucocytes than on endothelium in leucocyte-endothelial cell engagement *in vitro*. Extracellular MMPs inducer activity regulated the level of α-4 integrin on leucocytes through a mechanism associated with NFκB signalling. Blocking extracellular MMPs inducer attenuated the transmigration of monocytes and B lymphocytes across a model of the blood-brain barrier in culture, suggesting the prominence of extracellular MMPs inducer in CNS and its significant role in inflammatory perivascular cuffs, in MMPs induction and, leucocyte adhesion. In addition, elevation of extracellular MMPs inducer may serve as an orchestrator of the infiltration of leucocytes into the CNS parenchyma.

Pediatric demyelinating diseases are important not just because 3-5% of MS cases are diagnosed in childhood, but also because their pathogenesis may provide unique insights into the earliest events and triggers of acquired demyelinating diseases. Fernández Carbonell and Chitnis (2013) provided an update into pediatric DD for the general pediatrician and child neurologist. Current evidence on epidemiology, pathology, diagnosis, management and prognosis were reviewed for both monophasic (ADEM and CIS) and polyphasic/chronic DD (MS and NMO).

To analyze Aquaporin-4 (AQP4) antibody-positive patients who do not fulfill the current diagnostic criteria of neuromyelitis optica (NMO) and NMO spectrum disorders (NMOSD), Sato et al. (2013) used a cell-based assay (CBA) with AQP4-transfected cells to detect AQP4 antibody in 298 consecutive patients with inflammatory CNS disorders. The patients were diagnosed as NMO, NMOSD, MS, or others using the respective current diagnostic criteria. The seropositive samples by CBA were also tested using a commercial ELISA. Seventy-two patients were AQP4 antibody positive. Among them, 18.1% did not meet the NMO or NMOSD criteria (7 with monophasic optic neuritis, 2 with attacks restricted to the brainstem, and 4 with myelitis with less than 3 vertebral segments) and 84.6% of these had only a single attack. The ELISA results were negative in 38.4% of those patients, and they had lower antibody titers by CBA than patients with NMO/NMOSD. Although these patients had a shorter follow-up and few attacks, they shared some clinical features with NMO/NMOSD patients such as onset age, female predominance, presence of other autoantibodies, severe optic neuritis attacks, centrally located spinal cord lesions, persisting hiccups, and nausea, or vomiting episodes.

To optimize Aquaporin-4 (AQP4) antibody (Ab) detection and to assess the influence of the increased sensitivity of the assay on the demographic and disease-related characteristics of a group of AQP4-Ab-negative patients, Marignier et al. (2013) obtained the serum samples from patients included in the French NOMADMUS database with a definite diagnosis of neuromyelitis optica (NMO) and were compared with controls. They were tested by indirect immunofluorescence and cell-based assays (CBAs) in various conditions and with several plasmids. These investigators identified the CBA on live cells transfected with the untagged AQP4-M23 isoform as the best method, with a sensitivity of 74.4% and a specificity of 100%. These investigators demonstrated a direct relationship between improvement of the sensitivity of the detection method and the distinctiveness and characteristics of the AQP4-Ab-negative NMO group. Whereas with the classic indirect immunofluorescence or current AQP4-M1 CBA these investigators found only slight differences between the 2 populations, using the AQP4-M23 CBA, and demonstrated that patients with AQP4-Ab-negative NMO expressed specific demographic and disease-related features. They were characterized by an equal male/female ratio, a Caucasian ethnicity, and an overrepresentation of simultaneous optic neuritis and transverse myelitis at first episode. In terms of disability, they experienced a better visual acuity at last follow-up compared with seropositive NMO. This raised the question of a distinct physiopathology for patients with AQP4-Ab-negative NMO and of their place in the spectrum of the disease.

Prolyl oligopeptidase (PREP) has been considered as a drug target for the treatment of neurodegenerative diseases. In plasma, PREP has been found altered in several disorders of the CNS including MS. Oxidative stress and the levels of an endogenous plasma PREP inhibitor have been proposed to decrease PREP activity in MS. In this work, the circulating levels of PREP were measured in patients suffering from relapsing remitting (RR), secondary progressive (SP), primary progressive (PP) MS, and in subjects with clinically isolated syndrome (CIS). Tenorio-Laranga et al. (2013) found a significantly lower PREP activity in plasma of RRMS as well as in PPMS patients and a trend to reduced activity in subjects diagnosed with CIS, compared to controls. No signs of oxidative inactivation of PREP, and no correlation with the endogenous PREP inhibitor, identified as activated α-2-Macroglobulin (α2M), were observed in any of the patients studied. However, a significant decrease of α-2M was recorded in MS. In cell cultures, PREP specifically stimulates immune active cells by modifying the levels of Fibrinogen β, Thymosin β4, and Collagen.

Cerebral amyloid angiopathy-related inflammation (CAA-ri) is characterized by vasogenic edema and multiple cortical/subcortical microbleeds, sharing several aspects with the recently defined amyloid-related imaging abnormalities (ARIA) reported in AD passive immunization therapies. Piazza et al. (2013) investigated the role of anti-amyloid β (Aβ) autoantibodies in the acute and remission phases of CAA-ri. These investigators used ultrasensitive technique on patients from a retrospective multicenter case-control study, and evaluated the anti-Aβ autoantibody concentration in the CSF of 10 CAA-ri, 8 CAA, 14 MS, and 25 control subjects. Levels of soluble Aβ40, Aβ42, tau, P-181 tau, and APOE genotype were also investigated. During the acute phase of CAA-ri, anti-Aβ autoantibodies were specifically increased and directly correlated with Aβ mobilization, together with augmented tau and P-181 tau. Following clinical and radiological remission, autoantibodies returned to control levels, and both soluble Aβ and axonal degeneration markers decreased in parallel, supporting the hypothesis that the pathogenesis of CAA-ri may be mediated by a selective autoimmune reaction against cerebrovascular Aβ, directly related to autoantibody concentration and soluble Aβ. The CSF dosage of anti-Aβ autoantibodies can thus be proposed as a valid alternative tool for the diagnosis of CAA-ri. Moreover, given the similarities between ARIA developing spontaneously and those observed during immunization trials, anti-Aβ autoantibodies can be considered as novel potential biomarkers in future amyloid-modifying therapies for the treatment of AD and CAA.

Comabella et al. (2013) investigated the roles of 2 polymorphisms of the TNF receptor superfamily member 1A (TNFRSF1A) gene, rs1800693 (a common variant) and rs4149584 (a coding polymorphism that results in an amino acid substitution-R92Q), as genetic modifiers of MS, and to evaluate their potential functional implications in the disease. The effects of rs1800693 and rs4149584 on 2 measures of disease severity, age at disease onset and MS Severity Score, were analyzed in 2,032 patients with MS. In a subgroup of patients, serum levels of the soluble form of TNF-R1 (sTNF-R1) were measured by ELISA; mRNA expressions of the full-length TNF-R1 and Δ6-TNF-R1 isoform were investigated in peripheral blood mononuclear cells (PBMC) by real-time PCR; cell surface expression of the TNF-R1 was determined in T cells by flow cytometry. For rs4149584, R92Q carriers were younger at disease onset and progressed slower compared to noncarriers. However, no association with disease severity was observed for rs1800693. Serum sTNF-R1 and mRNA expression of the full-length receptor were increased in patients with MS carrying the R92Q mutation, but distributed among rs1800693 genotypes; cell surface TNF-R1 expression in T cells did not differ between rs4149584 and rs1800693 genotypes. The truncated soluble Δ6-TNF-R1 isoform was identified in PBMC from patients carrying the risk allele for rs1800693, suggesting that both rs1800693 and rs4149584 TNFRSF1A polymorphisms have functional consequences in the TNF-R1 (Weinshenker et al., 2013). Variou proinflammatory biomarkers of MS are illustrated in **Figure 49**.

Inflammatory Biomarkers

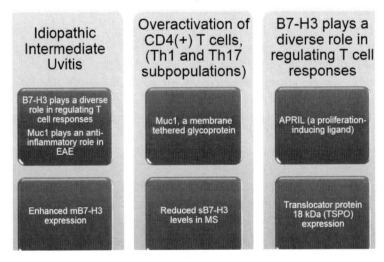

Figure 49. *Inflammatory Biomarkers in MS:* This diagram illustrates various inflammatory biomarkers for the early diagnosis, prognosis, and treatment of MS. During the progression of MS, most common clinical manifestation is the existence of idiopathic intermediate uveitis, B7-H3 plays a diverse role in the regulation of T cell responses, Muc-1 which plays an anti-inflammatory role in experimental allergic encephalomyelitis (EAE) (an experimental model of MS), enhanced mB7-H3 expression, over activation of CD4 (+) T cells (Th1 and Th17 subpopulation), Muc-1 a member of the tethered glycoproteins, reduced sB7-H3 levels in MS, B7-H3 which plays a diversified role in regulating T cell response. In addition, APRIL (a proliferation-inducing ligand), and trans locator protein (18 kDa: TSPO) expression are significantly enhanced in MS. Hence 18KDa, TSPO proteins is radiolabeled with ^{18}F or ^{11}C, in PET biomarkers to evaluate the extent of neuro-inflammation in MS as discussed in the text.

In-Vivo Imaging Biomarkers in MS

MRI and MR Spectroscopy in MS MRI-based brain volumetry is being used to assess brain volume changes from structural MRI in a range of neurologic conditions. Measures of brain volumes have been shown to be valid biomarkers of the clinical state and progression by offering high reliability and robust inferences on the underlying disease-related mechanisms. Giorgio and De Stefano (2013) examined MRI-based brain volumetry in neurology: 1) supporting disease diagnosis, 2) understanding mechanisms and tracking clinical progression of disease, and 3) monitoring treatment effect. Filippi et al. (2013) reported that MRI is sensitive in detecting MS-related abnormalities and it has become an established tool to diagnose the disease and to monitor its evolution. In patients at presentation with clinically isolated syndromes suggestive of MS, MRI has been included in the diagnostic work up and ad hoc criteria have been proposed and are updated on a regular basis. However, in patients with definite MS, the strength of the relationship between conventional MRI findings and subsequent clinical manifestations of the disease remains modest due to the relatively lack of specificity of conventional MRI to the heterogeneous pathological substrates of the disease and its inability to provide accurate estimates of such a damage outside focal lesions as well as to define the mechanisms through which the CNS recovers after tissue injury has occurred. Non-conventional MRI techniques offer new biomarkers more closely linked to the pathological features of the disease, which are likely to contribute to overcome, at least partially, these limitations. This review summarizes how MRI has improved MS diagnosis and to predict its course, as well as how it is changing our understanding of the factors associated with the accumulation of irreversible disability in this condition. A meta-analysis of randomized trials in RRMS showed a quantitative relation between the treatment effects detected on MRI lesions and clinical relapses. Sormani et al. (2013) validated that relation using data from a large and independent set of clinical trials in MS. These investigators searched for clinical trials that assessed disease-modifying drugs for RRMS and extracted data for the treatment effects on MRI lesions and on relapses from each trial, and the correlation of relative measures of these treatment effects with a weighted linear regression analysis. The R (2) value was estimated to quantify the strength of the correlation, and an interaction test to test for a difference in slope from the previously estimated equation. They identified 31 eligible trials, which provided data for 18 901 patients with RRMS. The regression equation derived using data from these studies showed a relation between the concurrent treatment effects on MRI lesions and relapses, much the same as was previously estimated. Analysis of trials that tested the same drugs in phase 2 and phase 3 studies showed that the effects on MRI lesions over short follow-up periods (6-9 months) can also predict the effects on relapses over longer follow-up periods (12-24 months), with reported effects on relapses that were within the 95% prediction intervals in eight of nine trials. These findings indicate that the effect of a treatment on relapses can be accurately predicted by the effect of that therapy on MRI lesions, implying that the use of MRI biomarkers as primary endpoints in future clinical trials of treatments for MS can be considered, in specific situations, such as in trials testing generics or biosimilars of drugs with a well-known mechanism of action or in pediatric trials testing drugs already approved for adults.

Brain MRI is widely used as a diagnostic tool in MS and provides a non-invasive, sensitive and reproducible way to track the disease. Topological characteristics relating to the distribution and shape of lesions are recognized as important neuroradiological biomarkers in the diagnosis of MS, although these have been much less well characterized quantitatively than have traditional measures such as T2 hyperintense or T1 hypointense lesion volumes. Gourraud et al. (2013) used voxel-level 3 T MRI T1-weighted scans to reconstruct the 3D topology of lesions in 284 subjects with MS and tested whether this is a heritable phenotype. To this end, they extracted the genotypes from a published genome-wide association study on these same individuals and searched for genetic associations with lesion load, shape and topological distribution. Lesion probability maps were created to identify frequently affected areas and to assess the distribution of T1 lesions in the subject population as a whole. They developed an original algorithm to cluster adjacent lesional voxels (cluxels) in each subject and tested whether cluxel topology was associated with any single-nucleotide polymorphism in the data set. To focus on patterns of lesion distribution, the first 10 principal components were computed. Although principal component 1 correlated with lesion load, none of the remaining orthogonal components correlated with any other known variable. These investigators then conducted genome-wide association studies and found 31 significant associations with principal component 8, which represents a mode of variation of lesion topology in the population. The majority of the loci can be linked to genes related to immune cell function and to myelin and neural growth; some (SYK, MYT1L, TRAPPC9, SLITKR6 and RIC3) have been previously associated with the distribution of white matter lesions in MS. Finally, a bioinformatics approach was used to identify a network of 48 interacting proteins showing genetic associations with cluxel topology in MS. This network also contained proteins expressed in immune cells and is enriched in molecules expressed in the CNS that contribute to neural development and regeneration. These results showed how quantitative traits derived from brain MRI of patients with MS can be used as dependent variables in a genome-wide association study. With the widespread availability of powerful computing and the availability of genotyped populations, integration of imaging and genetic data sets is likely to become a mainstream tool for understanding the complex biological processes of MS and other brain disorders.

Proton magnetic resonance spectroscopy (^{1}H-MRS) is capable of noninvasively detecting metabolic changes that occur in the brain tissue *in vivo*. Its clinical utility has been limited so far, however, by analytic methods that focus on metabolites and require prior knowledge about which metabolites to examine. Vingara et al. (2013) applied advanced metabolomics computational methodologies, specifically partial least squares discriminant analysis and orthogonal partial least squares, to *in vivo* (^{1}H-MRS from frontal lobe white matter of 27 patients with RRMS and 14 healthy controls). These investigators chose RRMS, a chronic demyelinating disorder of the CNS, because its complex pathology and variable disease course make the need for reliable biomarkers of disease progression more pressing. *In vivo* MRS data, when analyzed by multivariate statistical methods, can provide reliable, distinct profiles of MRS-detectable metabolites in different patient populations. Specifically, brain tissue in RRMS patients deviates in its metabolic profile from that of healthy controls. Using statistical means, the metabolic signatures of certain clinical features common in RRMS, such as disability score, cognitive impairments, and response to stress. This approach to human *in vivo* MRS data may promote understanding of the specific metabolic changes accompanying disease pathogenesis, and could provide biomarkers of disease progression that would be useful in clinical trials.

Mistry et al. (2013) performed prospective longitudinal cohort study. The reference standard was a clinical diagnosis that was arrived at (after a mean follow-up of 26 months) by the treating neurologist with a specialist interest in MS. The 7-T MRI scans were analyzed at baseline, by physicians blinded to the clinical data, for the presence of visible central veins. A consecutive sample of 29 patients referred with possible MS who had brain lesions detected on clinical MRI scans but whose condition remained undiagnosed despite expert clinical and radiological assessments. The proportion of patients whose condition was correctly diagnosed as MS or as not MS, using 7-T MRI at study onset, compared with the eventual diagnosis reached by treating physicians blinded to the result of the MRI. Of the 29 patients enrolled and scanned using 7-T MRI, 22 received a clinical diagnosis. All 13 patients whose condition was eventually diagnosed as MS had central veins visible in the majority of brain lesions at baseline. All 9 patients whose condition was not diagnosed as MS had central veins visible in a minority of lesions. T2*-weighted 7-T MRI had 100% positive and negative predictive value for the diagnosis of MS.

DTI in MS Although DTI and the magnetization transfer ratio (MTR) have been extensively studied in MS, it is still unclear if they are more effective biomarkers of disability than conventional MRI. Harrison et al. (2013) performed MRI on 117 participants with MS in addition to 26 healthy volunteers. Mean values were obtained for DTI indices and MTR for supratentorial brain and three white matter tracts of interest. DTI and MTR values were tested for correlations with measures of atrophy and lesion volume and were compared with conventional indices for prediction of disability. All DTI and MTR values correlated to an equivalent degree with lesion volume and cerebral volume fraction (CVF). Thalamic volumes correlated with all indices in the optic radiations and with mean and perpendicular diffusivity in the corpus callosum. Nested model regression analysis demonstrated that, compared with CVF, DTI indices in the optic radiations were correlated with Expanded Disability Status Scale and were also more correlated than both CVF and lesion volume with low-contrast visual acuity. Abnormalities in DTI and MTR were equally linked with brain atrophy and inflammatory lesion burden, suggesting that they are markers of MS pathology. These findings that some DTI and MTR indices are more strongly linked with disability than conventional MRI measures justifies their potential use as targeted, functional system-specific clinical trial outcomes in MS.

Hong et al. (2013) investigated whether anti-CD40 Ab and 8-oxo-dG attenuate mast cell migration and EAE development. Anti-CD40 Ab and 8-oxo-dG reduced EAE scores, mast cell numbers, expression of adhesion molecules, OX40L and Act1, levels of TNF-α, LTs, expression of cytokines, and co-localization of Treg cells and mast cells, all of which are increased in EAE-brain tissues. Each treatment enhanced Treg cells, expression of OX40, and cytokines related to suppressive function of Treg cells in EAE brain tissues. Act-BMMCs with Treg cells reduced expression of OX40L and CCL2/CCR2, VCAM-1, PECAM-1, $[Ca^{2+}]i$ levels, release of mediators, signaling molecules, Act1 related to IL-17a signals versus those in act-BMMCs without Treg cells, suggesting that IL-10- and IL-35-producing Foxp3+-Treg cells, enhanced by anti-CD40 Ab or 8-oxo-dG, suppress migration of mast cells through down-regulating the expression of adhesion molecules, and suppress mast cell activation through cell-to-cell cross-talk via OX40/OX40L in EAE development.

Ohayon et al. (2013) reported the development of CNS vasculitis in a patient with MS treated with Dacluzimab. This report included clinical, MRI, immunologic, and pathology data and CSF analysis. After completing a phase II Dacluzimab monotherapy study with an optimal response as evidenced by significant decrease in MRI disease and stable clinical examinations, the patient elected to continue Dacluzimab therapy outside of NIH study. Dacluzimab was discontinued after 21 doses due to the onset of new clinical symptoms and evidence of a vascular pattern of contrast enhancement on brain and spine MRI. Because of continued clinical deterioration, stereotactic brain biopsy was performed, showing small-vessel CNS vasculitis. Treatment was initiated with IV methylprednisolone followed by a regimen of cyclophosphamide. Immunologic studies suggest that unexpected lack of expansion of CD56 (bright) NK cells and predictable decline in FoxP3+ T-regs combined with a transient interruption in Dacluzimab dosing may have contributed to this serious side effect. Only safety data from larger phase III studies and potentially postmarketing experience may define the exact risk of Dacluzimab-induced immunopathologies. Nevertheless, these cases provide plausible hypothesis and potential biomarker that may be used to screen susceptible patients and implement preventive safety measures during potentially vulnerable periods.

Schneider et al. (2013) presented the first assessment of T lymphocytes chemotaxis rate in two Natalizumab-exposed newborns. Pregnancies in women with severe RRMS treated with Natalizumab constitute a major challenge, because withdrawal of the drug may cause relapses but continuation might have unknown effects on the infantile immune system. To identify the impact of maternal Natalizumab treatment during pregnancy on basic immune functions of the newborn. Basic immunological testing and assessment of the chemotaxis rate of freshly isolated T lymphocytes in the presence and absence of CXCL12 was performed in two neonates, whose mothers were treated with Natalizumab until the 34th week of pregnancy (pw). Both children had an uneventful birth. However, a reduction in the CXCL12-induced T-cell chemotaxis was found in both children. In contrast, the chemotaxis rate of unstimulated T lymphocytes remained unaltered. The distribution of the lymphocyte subpopulations was investigated only in case 1 and was normal. A significant reduction in the CXCL12-induced chemotaxis rate of T lymphocytes was observed and may compromise host defense function in early life. Alemtuzumab is potentially a highly effective treatment for RRMS acting via complement-mediated lysis of circulating lymphocytes. Variability in posttreatment lymphocyte recovery time was observed, with some patients showing striking durability in the efficacy of treatment. Cossburn et al. (2013) performed a study to establish whether this variation affects clinical and imaging parameters of disease. A total of 56 patients were followed for a median of 39.5 months post Alemtuzumab treatment with interval clinical assessments, lymphocyte immunophenotyping, and MRI. Timing and degree of CD4+, CD8+, and CD19+ recovery were correlated with the re-emergence of disease activity defined as clinical relapse, increasing disability, and new T2/enhancing lesions on MRI. New disease activity was recorded in 14% of patients. Mean time to CD19+, CD8+, and CD4+ reconstitution was 6, 10, and 36 months. No differences were observed in CD8+ and CD19+ reconstitution between patients with active disease and those in remission. Patients with active disease showed an accelerated recovery of CD4+ cells with a difference in absolute CD4+ counts at 24 months. CD4+ counts $<388.5 \times 10(6)$ cells/mL predicted MRI stability. Differential lymphocyte recovery in MS following Alemtuzumab may be a biomarker for relapse and also inform monitoring and treatment protocols. This study provided Class IV evidence that differential lymphocyte reconstitution after Alemtuzumab treatment may be a biomarker for relapse.

The development of therapeutics that interfere with the migration of leukocytes has revolutionized the treatment of MS and holds great promise for the treatment of a wide range of inflammatory diseases. As the molecules essential for the multi-step adhesion cascade that mediates cellular migration have been elucidated, the number of potential targets available to modulate leukocyte trafficking has increased exponentially. Griffith and Luster (2013) reviewed current understanding of these molecular targets and how these targets vary by tissue and leukocyte subset with emphasis on T cells. These investigators described the two approved therapeutics that target cell migration, Natalizumab and Fingolimod, and discussed how an improved understanding of their function could pave the way for the development of safer and more efficacious theranostics for inflammatory and autoimmune diseases.

Karlström et al. (2013) developed two parallel series, A and B, of CX3CR1 antagonists for the treatment of MS. By modifying the substituents on the 7-Amino-5-Thio-thiazolo [4, 5-Dipyrimidine core structure, these investigators achieved compounds with high selectivity for CX3CR1 over the closely related CXCR2 receptor. The structure-activity relationships showed that a leucinol moiety attached to the core-structure in the 7-position together with α-methyl branched benzyl derivatives in the 5-position displayed affinity, selectivity, as well as physicochemical properties, as exemplified by compounds 18a and 24h. Zhou et al. (2013) characterized the expression and distribution of the fibroblast surface protein (FSP), the chemokine CC-ligand 21 (CCL21) secondary lymphoid tissue chemokine CC-chemokine receptor 7 (CCR7) in renal allograft biopsy specimens obtained from patients after transplantation. These investigators recruited 165 patients who received renal transplants for this study. Histological examination of the renal allograft biopsy specimens was performed using Hematoxylin-Eosin, Periodic acid-Schiff, and Masson's Trichrome staining. Distribution and expression of FSP, CCL21, and CCR7 were determined using immunohistochemistry staining. Serum Creatinine levels were evaluated using an enzymatic Sarcosine Oxidase method. FSP was mainly localized in the cytoplasm and nucleus of renal interstitial fibroblasts and tubular epithelial cells. Compared with the normal group, an elevated number of FSP-positive fibroblasts were observed in patients with acute/active cellular rejection and chronic/sclerosing allograft nephropathy. Patients with chronic/sclerosing allograft nephropathy also showed increased total fibroblasts as compared with borderline changes. In a multiple regression analysis, CCR7-positive expression was a strong protective factor for acute/active cellular rejection and recurrent nephropathy. In contrast, CCL21-positive expression led to a high susceptibility to recurrent nephropathy among renal transplant patients. Moreover, FSP and CCL21, or CCL21 and CCR7 were localized in the interstitial fibroblasts and renal tubular epithelium cells. In addition, FSP and CCL21 expression correlated with serum Creatinine levels suggesting that the CCL21/CCR7 signaling is involved in renal fibrosis in kidney transplant patients. An increased number of FSP-positive fibroblasts may be a risk factor for acute/active cellular rejection and chronic/sclerosing allograft nephropathy after renal transplantation. These findings may help understanding of renal allograft fibrosis.

Neural precursor (NPC) based therapies are used to restore neurons or oligodendrocytes and/or provide neuroprotection in a large variety of neurological diseases. In MS models, intravenously (i.v)-delivered NPCs reduced clinical signs via immunomodulation. Deboux et al. (2013) demonstrated that NPCs were able to cross cerebral endothelial cells *in vitro* and that the multifunctional signaling molecule, CD44 involved in trans-endothelial migration of lymphocytes to sites of inflammation, plays a crucial role in extravasation of syngeneic

NPCs. In view of the role of CD44 in NPCs trans-endothelial migration *in vitro*, questioned the benefit of CD44 overexpression by NPCs *in vitro* and *in vivo*, in EAE mice. These investigators showed that overexpression of CD44 by NPCs enhanced over 2 folds their trans-endothelial migration *in vitro*, without influencing the proliferation or differentiation potential of the transduced cells. Moreover, CD44 overexpression by NPCs improved their elongation, spreading and number of filopodia over the extracellular matrix protein laminin *in vitro*. The effect of CD44 overexpression after i.v. delivery in the tail vein of EAE mice was tested. CD44 overexpression was functional *in-vivo* as it accelerated trans-endothelial migration and facilitated invasion of HA expressing perivascular sites suggesting that CD44 may be crucial not only for NPC crossing the endothelial layer but also for facilitating invasion of extravascular tissues.

Transforming growth factor β (TGFβ) is a profibrotic cytokine, and its impaired function is implicated in several fibrotic pathologies including scleroderma (systemic sclerosis [SSc]). Increased TGFβ signaling contributes to progressive fibrosis in SSc by promoting fibroblast activation, excessive extracellular matrix (ECM) deposition, and dermal thickening. Vorstenbosch et al. (2013) identified CD109 as a TGFβ coreceptor and showed that it antagonizes TGFβ signaling and TGFβ-induced ECM expression *in vitro* in human keratinocytes and fibroblasts. The aim of this study was to examine the ability of CD109 to prevent skin fibrosis in a mouse model of bleomycin-induced SSc. Transgenic mice overexpressing CD109 in the epidermis and their wild-type (WT) littermates were injected with bleomycin in phosphate buffered saline (PBS) or with PBS alone every other day for 21 days or 28 days. Dermal thickness and collagen deposition were determined histologically using Masson's Trichrome and Picrosirius red staining. In addition, Collagen and Fibronectin content was analyzed using Western blotting, and activation of TGFβ signaling was examined by determining phospho-Smad2 and phospho-Smad3 levels using Western blotting and immunohistochemistry. Transgenic mice overexpressing CD109 in the epidermis showed resistance to Bleomycin-induced skin fibrosis, as evidenced by a significant decrease in dermal thickness, collagen crosslinking, collagen and fibronectin content, and phospho-Smad2/3 levels, as compared to their WT littermates suggesting that CD109 inhibits TGFβ signaling and fibrotic responses in experimental murine scleroderma and that CD109 regulates dermal-epidermal interactions to decrease extracellular matrix synthesis in the dermis. Thus, CD109 can be a potential molecular biomarker for therapeutic intervention in scleroderma.

Idiopathic intermediate uveitis (IIU) is a potentially sight-threatening inflammatory disorder with well-defined anatomic diagnostic criteria. It is associated with MS, and both conditions are linked to HLA-DRB1*15. Atan et al. (2013) showed that non-infectious uveitis (NIU) is associated with IL-10 polymorphisms, IL10-2849A (rs6703630), IL10+434T (rs2222202), and IL10+504G (rs3024490), while a LTA+252AA/TNFA-238GG haplotype (rs909253/rs361525) is protective. In this study, it was determined whether patients with IIU have a similar genetic profile as patients with NIU or MS. Twelve polymorphisms were genotyped, spanning the TNF and IL-10 genomic regions, in 44 patients with IIU and 92 population controls was associated with the TNFA-308A and TNFA-238A polymorphisms. The combination of TNFA-308 and -238 loci was more associated with IIU than any other loci across the major histocompatibility complex, including HLA-DRB1. TNF polymorphisms, associated with increased TNF production, were associated with IIU. These results offer the potential to ascribe therapeutic response and risk (i.e., the influence of HLA-DRB1*15 status and TNFR1 polymorphism) to anti-TNF therapy in IIU.

Recently it has been shown that Muc1, a membrane tethered glycoprotein, has an ability to suppress inflammatory responses in cultured DC. Yen et al. (2013) investigated the possible involvement of Muc1 in the development of MS using EAE in mice. (1) Muc1(-/-) mice developed greater EAE severity compared with wild type (wt) mice, which correlated with increased numbers of Th1 and Th17 cells infiltrating into the CNS; (2) upon stimulation, splenic DC from Muc1(-/-) mice produced greater amounts of IL-1β, IL-6, and IL-12 but less amounts of IL-10 compared with those from wt mice; and (3) the ability of splenic DC to differentiate antigen-specific CD4+ T cells into Th1 and Th17 cells was greater in Muc1(-/-) mice compared with wt mice suggesting that Muc1 plays an anti-inflammatory role in EAE. This was the first report demonstrating the involvement of Muc1 in the development of MS and might provide a potential target for immunotherapy.

Coquet et al. (2013) reported that T helper 17 (Th17) cells protect against infection but also promote inflammation and autoimmunity. Therefore, the factors that govern Th17 cell differentiation are of special interest. The CD27 and CD70 costimulatory pathway impeded Th17 effector cell differentiation and associated autoimmunity in a mouse model of MS. CD27 or CD70 deficiency exacerbated disease, whereas constitutive CD27 signaling reduced disease incidence and severity. CD27 signaling did not impact master regulators of T helper cell lineage but repressed transcription of the key effector molecules IL-17 and the chemokine receptor CCR6 in differentiating Th17 cells. CD27 mediated this repression via the c-Jun N-terminal kinase (JNK) pathway that restrained IL-17 and CCR6 expression in differentiating Th17 cells. CD27 signaling also resulted in epigenetic silencing of the Il17a gene. Thus, CD27 costimulation via JNK signaling, transcriptional, and epigenetic effects suppresses Th17 effector cell function and associated pathological consequences.

PET Imaging in MS The activation of microglia and the upregulation of the translocator protein (18 kDa) (TSPO) system are key features of neuroinflammation. Recent PET imaging studies using TSPO radioligands such as [^{11}C]PK11195 and [^{11}C]PBR28 indicated the usefulness of these biomarkers in patients with neuroinflammatory diseases, including MS. [^{18}F]FEDAA1106 is a recently developed PET radioligand for the *in vivo* quantification of TSPO. Takano et al. (2013) investigated the diagnostic usefulness of *[^{18}F]*FEDAA1106 in patients with MS. Nine patients (three on the interferon β therapy and six without immunomodulatory therapy; seven females/two males; with RRMS in acute relapse and with Gadolinium (Gd)-enhancing lesion(s) in the MRI and five healthy controls participated in this study. Genetic information about the TSPO binding could not be obtained because knowledge about the importance of genetic background for TSPO binding was not available at the time the study was performed. Dynamic PET measurements were performed for a total of 150 min, with a 30-min break after the injection of 153.4 ± 10.2 MBq of [^{18}F]FEDAA1106. Metabolite-corrected arterial plasma samples were used to calculate the input function. PET data were analyzed in the following ways: (1) ROI analysis for cortical and subcortical regions was performed using a two-tissue compartment kinetic model in order to estimate binding potentials (BPND) and distribution volume (VT), (2) the feasibility of the estimation of BPND and VT was investigated for MS lesions, and (3) VT parametric images by a Logan plot and SUVs were compared with the corresponding MRI, focusing on MRI-identified MS lesions. There were no significant differences in the BPND or VT values between patients with MS and healthy controls. Visual inspection of VT and SUVs did not reveal high uptake of the radioligand inside and beyond MRI-identified active MS lesions with the exception of one Gd-enhanced MS lesion in the whole patient population. [^{18}F]FEDAA1106 as a PET radioligand could neither differentiate patients with MS from healthy controls nor active plaques in the brain of MS patients. Acute disseminated encephalomyelitis (ADEM) and RRMS share overlapping clinical, radiologic and laboratory features at onset. Because autoantibodies may contribute to the pathogenesis of both diseases, autoantibody biomarkers were identified that are capable of distinguishing them. Van Haren (2013) used custom antigen arrays to profile anti-myelin-peptide autoantibodies in sera derived from individuals with pediatric ADEM, pediatric MS(Ped MS) and adult MS. Using isotype-specific secondary antibodies, both IgG and IgM reactivities were profiled. Statistical Analysis of Microarrays software was used to confirm the differences in autoantibody reactivity profiles between ADEM and MS samples. Prediction Analysis of Microarrays software was used to generate and validate prediction algorithms, based on the autoantibody reactivity profiles. ADEM was characterized by IgG autoantibodies targeting epitopes derived from myelin basic protein, proteolipid protein, myelin-associated oligodendrocyte basic glycoprotein, and α-B-crystallin. In contrast, MS was characterized by IgM autoantibodies targeting myelin basic protein, proteolipid protein, myelin-associated oligodendrocyte basic glycoprotein and oligodendrocyte-specific protein. Prediction algorithms that distinguish ADEM serum (sensitivity 62-86%; specificity 56-79%) from MS serum (sensitivity 40-87%; specificity 62-86%) on the basis of combined IgG and IgM anti-myelin autoantibody reactivity to a small number of myelin peptides were validated. Combined profiles of serum IgG and IgM autoantibodies identified myelin antigens that may be useful for distinguishing MS from ADEM.

Impaired Treg Function in MS The suppressor function of regulatory T cells (Tregs) is impaired in MS, but the mechanisms underlying this deficiency are not fully understood. As Tregs counteract the sustained elevation of $[Ca^{2+}]_i$, which is indispensable for full activation of conventional T cells (Tcons), Schwarz et al. (2013) hypothesized that interference with this pathway might prompt MS-related Treg dysfunction. Using single-cell live imaging, these investigators observed that Tregs reduce Ca^{2+} influx and downstream signals in Tcons upon cell contact, yet differ in their potency to suppress several target cells at the same time. Strikingly, individual Tregs harboring a CD4(+)CD25(+)FOXP3(+)CD45RA(+) naive phenotype suppressed more adjacent Tcons than did CD4(+)CD25(+)FOXP3(+)CD45RA(-) memory Tregs. Some constituents completely failed to dampen Tcon Ca^{2+} influx and were contained exclusively in the memory subset. In accordance with their more powerful suppressive performance, the Ca^{2+} signature was enhanced in naive Tregs in response to TCR triggering, compared with the memory counterparts. MS Tregs displayed a diminished suppression of mean Ca^{2+} influx in the sum of individual Tcons recorded. This reduced inhibitory activity was closely linked to decreased numbers of individual Tcons becoming suppressed by adjacent Tregs and correlated with a marked reduction of naive subtypes and concomitant expansion of nonsuppressive memory phenotypes. The superior achievement of naive Tregs is pivotal in maintaining Treg efficiency. As a consequence, MS Tregs become defective because they lack subtypes and are disproportionately enriched in memory cells that have lost their inherent downregulatory activity.

MIF and its Receptor, CD74 in MS MIF and its receptor, CD74, are key regulators of the immune system. Benedek et al. (2013) demonstrated that partial MHC class II constructs comprised of linked β1α1 domains with covalently attached antigenic peptides (also referred to as recombinant T-cell receptor ligands - RTLs) can inhibit MIF activity by not only blocking the binding of rhMIF to immunopurified CD74, but also downregulating CD74 cell-surface expression. This bifunctional inhibition of MIF/CD74 interactions blocked downstream MIF effects, including enhanced secretion of proinflammatory cytokines, anti-apoptotic activity, and inhibition of random migration that contribute to the reversal of clinical and histological signs of EAE. Moreover, enhanced CD74 cell-surface expression on monocytes in mice with EAE and subjects with MS can be downregulated by humanized RTLs, resulting in reduced MIF binding to the cells. Thus, binding of partial MHC complexes to CD74 blocks both the accessibility and availability of CD-74 for MIF binding and downstream inflammatory activity.

Role of LINGO-1 in MS Recent experimental data suggest a possible role of LINGO-1 in the pathogenesis of MS. In an attempt to identify genetic biomarkers related to MS susceptibility, García-Martín et al. (2013) genotyped two common SNPs in the LINGO1 gene which have been associated to other neurological conditions, in patients with MS and in healthy subjects. These SNPs are linked to several SNPs within the LINGO1 gene, especially in individuals of Oriental or Caucasian descent. These investigators analyzed the allelic and genotype frequency of two LINGO1 variants (rs9652490 and rs11856808) in 293 patients with MS and 318 healthy controls, using KASPar assays. LINGO1 rs9652490 and rs11856808 allelic and genotype frequencies did not differ between MS patients and controls. The minor allele frequencies for rs9652490 were 0.171 and 0.167 (for cases and controls respectively. For rs11856808 the minor allele frequencies were 0.317 and 0.310 for cases and controls, respectively. Allele and genotype frequencies were unrelated with the age of onset of MS, gender, and clinical course of MS. In addition, haplotype analyses did not reveal any putative risk related to haplotypes, suggesting that LINGO1 rs9652490 and rs11856808 polymorphisms are not related with risk for MS indicating that, LINGO1 SNPs could be useful risk biomarkers of developing essential tremor, but not other movement disorders.

Adhesion Molecule CD44 Adhesion Molecule in MS CD44 is expressed by multiple cell types and is implicated in various cellular and immunological processes. Flynn et al. (2013) examined the effect of global CD44 deficiency on myelin oligodendrocyte glycoprotein peptide (MOG)-induced EAE. Compared to C57BL/6 wild-type mice, CD44-deficient mice presented with greater disease severity, increased immune cell numbers in the CNS and increased anti-MOG antibody, and proinflammatory cytokine production, especially those associated with Th17 cells. Further, decreased numbers of peripheral CD4 (+) CD25 (+) FoxP3 (+) regulatory T cells (Tregs) were observed in CD44-knockout mice throughout the disease course. CD44-knockout CD4 T cells exhibited reduced TGF-β receptor type I (TGF-β RI) expression that did not impart a defect in Treg polarization *in vitro*, but correlated with enhanced Th17 polarization *in vitro*. Further, EAE in bone marrow-chimeric animals suggested CD44 expression on both circulating and noncirculating cells limited disease severity. Endothelial expression of CD-44 limited T-cell adhesion to and transmigration through murine endothelial monolayers *in vitro*. These investigators identified increased permeability of the BBB *in vivo* in CD44-deficient mice before and following immunization suggesting that CD44 has multiple protective roles in EAE, with effects on cytokine production, T-cell differentiation, T-cell-endothelial cell interactions, and BBB integrity.

Monomeric and Dimeric κ- and λ-FLC of IgG for the Diagnosis of MS In their search of new biomarkers for MS, Kaplan et al. (2013) characterized the immunoglobulin (Ig) free light chains (FLC) in patients' CSF and serum, and to evaluate the diagnostic utility of FLC monomer-dimer patterns for MS. FLC were analyzed by Western blotting and mass spectroscopy. CSF and serum samples were examined for the presence of oligoclonal Ig bands by a conventional laboratory test for MS. Three distinct pathological FLC monomer-dimer patterns, typical of MS but not of other neurological diseases, were revealed. In 31 out 56 MS patients the highly increased CSF levels of κ monomers and dimers were demonstrated. In 18 MS patients, the increased κ-FLC levels were accompanied by highly elevated λ dimers. Five MS cases showed no significant elevation in κ-FLC, but they displayed abnormally high λ dimer levels. The intensity of the immunoreactive FLC bands was measured to account for κ and λ monomer and dimer levels and their ratios in the CSF and serum. Combined usage of different FLC parameters allowed the determination of the appropriate FLC threshold values to diagnose MS. This method showed higher sensitivity and specificity as compared to those of the conventional OCB test and highlighted the role of the differential analysis of monomeric and dimeric κ- and λ-FLC for the accurate diagnosis of MS.

TNF Signaling and MS as an Autoimmune Disorder TNF receptor 1-associated periodic syndrome (TRAPS) is an autoinflammatory disorder caused by autosomal dominantly inherited mutations in the TNF receptor superfamily 1A (TNFRSF1A) gene. The D12E substitution has been described in a 4-year-old boy with fever. Havla et al. (2013) performed a for DNA sequence analysis of the TNFRSF1A gene, genomic DNA was isolated, amplified by PCR, purified, and sequenced. Three families (8 subjects) with the TNFRSF1A D12E substitution and TRAPS-related symptoms, in 4 cases associated with the autoimmune diseases MS and rheumatoid arthritis. The clinical phenotype might be associated with the TNFRSF1A D12E mutation. There is a close pathophysiological relationship between TNF signaling and autoimmune disorders.

Anti-Myelin Basic Protein (MBP) IgM in MS Annunziata et al. (2013) reported that high intrathecal levels of anti-myelin basic protein (MBP) IgM were associated with early favorable course in a cohort of patients with MS. A mAb to MBP 105-120 recognizing the 222-228 epitope of the extracellular domain of high affinity immunoglobulin gamma Fc-receptor I (CD64) was isolated from EBV(+) B cell clones of long-term stable RRMS patients. This mAb exerted immunosuppressive activity on MS-derived T cell lines through induction and release of high amounts of IL-10 and decreased levels of IL-12 from activated monocytes providing the biological basis for a new treatment of MS and other immune-mediated neurological disorders.

Biomarkers in MS Theranostics CNS disorders such as ischemic stroke, MS, or AD are characterized by the loss of BBB integrity. Adzemovic et al. (20013) demonstrated that the small tyrosine kinase inhibitor Imatinib enhances BBB integrity in EAE. Treatment was accompanied by decreased CNS inflammation and demyelination and reduced T-cell recruitment. This was supported by downregulation of the chemokine receptor (CCR) 2 in CNS and lymph nodes, and by modulation of the peripheral immune response towards an anti-inflammatory phenotype. Interestingly, Imatinib ameliorated neuroinflammation, even when the treatment was initiated after the clinical manifestation of the disease. Imatinib reduced BBB disruption and stroke volume after experimentally induced ischemic stroke by targeting platelet-derived growth factor receptor -α (PDGFR-α) signaling. PDGFR-α signaling is a central regulator of BBB integrity during neuroinflammation and therefore Imatinib should be considered as a potentially effective treatment for MS. Given the high frequency of failure of first-line therapies, there is an urgent need for second-line treatment strategies for pediatric patients with MS. Kornek et al. (2013) reported the use of Natalizumab in pediatric MS. Natalizumab, a humanized monoclonal antibody targeting α4 integrin, is effective against RRMS in adults. A total of 20 pediatric patients with MS who started treatment with Natalizumab prior to 18 years of age. These patients underwent MRI as clinically indicated, despite the fact that 19 of these 20 patients were undergoing first-line disease-modifying therapy. The mean (SD) age at initiation of Natalizumab therapy was 16.7 (1.1) years, and the mean (SD) pretreatment period was 18 (10) months. Natalizumab, was provided 300 mg every 4 weeks. Annualized relapse rates, Expanded Disability Status Scale scores, number of new T2/fluid-attenuated inversion recovery lesions and contrast-enhancing lesions on MRI, number of adverse events, the prevalence of neutralizing antibodies against Natalizumab, and serum JC virus-antibody status. Treatment with Natalizumab was associated with reductions in mean annualized relapse rates, median Expanded Disability Status Scale scores (2 without treatment vs 1 with treatment), and mean number of new T2/fluid-attenuated inversion recovery lesions per year (7.8 without treatment vs 0.5 with treatment). Two patients developed high-titer neutralizing antibodies against Natalizumab and had to stop therapy. Adverse events included headaches, asthenia, infections, and hypersensitivity. Abnormal laboratory results were found for 8 patients. JC virus antibodies were found in 5 of 13 patients. After the discontinuation of Natalizumab therapy, relapse activity occurred in 6 of 8 patients within 6 months indicating that Natalizumab may be safe and effective against MS in pediatric patients with breakthrough disease.

Natalizumab is a very effective, relatively new drug for the treatment of RRMS. Inflammatory and neurodegenerative processes in the CNS cause adverse effects during the course of this disease. To monitor the effects of Natalizumab treatment on the CSF proteome of patients, CSF samples were taken from patients before commencing treatment as well as after 1 year of treatment. Proteomics experiments using electrospray Orbitrap mass spectrometry and pair wise comparison of patients before and after 1 year of Natalizumab treatment revealed a number of candidate biomarkers that were differentially abundant between before and after treatment groups. Three proteins were validated using selected reaction monitoring (SRM) in a new, independent sample set. All three proteins, *Ig mu chain C region and haptoglobin*, both known inflammation-related proteins, as well as *Chitinase-3-like protein 1*, were confirmed by SRM to be lower abundant in CSF of MS patients after 1 year of Natalizumab treatment. The findings for Chitinase-3-like protein 1, a presumed biomarker for more rapid progression from a first clinically isolated syndrome to clinically definite MS, was confirmed by ELISA.

To report first experiences with IL-6 receptor inhibition in therapy-resistant neuromyelitis optica (NMO), Ayzenberg et al. (2013) performed a retrospective case series. Patients with an aggressive course of NMO switched to Tocilizumab after failure of anti-CD20 therapy. Annualized relapse rate and disability progression measured by the Expanded Disability Status Scale. 3 female patients with a median age of 39 years (range, 26-40 years) and Aquaporin 4-positive NMO. All patients had been treated with different immunosuppressive and immunomodulating agents, followed by 1 to 3 cycles of Rituximab. Despite complete CD20-cell depletion during Rituximab therapy, the median annualized relapse rate was 3.0. Expanded Disability Status Scale score increased from 5.0 to 6.5. After the switch to Tocilizumab, the median annualized relapse rate decreased to 0.6. A total of 2 relapses occurred; however, they were mild and there were no changes in clinical disability. IL-6 receptor-blocking therapy can be effective in therapy-resistant cases of NMO. Annunziata et al. (2013) reported that high intrathecal levels of anti-myelin basic protein (MBP) IgM were associated with early favorable course in a cohort of patients with MS. A mAb to MBP 105-120 recognizing the 222-228 epitope of the extracellular domain of high affinity immunoglobulin gamma Fc-receptor I (CD64) was isolated from EBV(+) B cell clones of long-term stable RRMS patients. This mAb exerted immunosuppressive activity on MS-derived T cell lines through induction and release of high amounts of IL-10 and decreased levels of IL-12 from activated monocytes providing the biological basis for a potential new treatment for MS and other immune-mediated neurological disorders.

Glatiramer Therapy in MS Treatment with Glatiramer acetate (GA) decreases disease activity in MS. The mechanism of action is incompletely understood and differences in the response to treatment between individuals may exist. Sellebjerg et al. (2013) performed a study to examine the activation of CD4+ T cells, monocytes and dendritic cells (DC) in relation to disease activity in MS patients treated with GA. Flow cytometry was used to study the activation of CD4+ T cells and T cell subsets (CD25 (high) and CD26(high) cells, monocytes and DCs in a cross-sectional study of 39 untreated and 29 GA-treated MS patients, the latter followed prospectively for one year. Gd-enhanced MRI studies were conducted in all patients. Disease activity was assessed as relapses. The median percentage of DCs expressing CD40 was 10% in untreated MS patients and 5.9% in GA-treated patients. The hazard ratio of relapse was 1.32 (95% confidence interval 1.05-1.64) per 1% increase in CD40+ DCs. Patients treated with GA had fewer CD4+ T cells expressing surface markers associated with T helper type 1 effector responses and more CD4+ T cells expressing surface markers associated with regulatory, naïve or central memory T cell populations, but CD4+ T cell activation was not related with relapse risk. MS patients treated with GA showed prominent changes in circulating antigen-presenting cells and CD4+ T cells. Expression of CD40 on DCs was lower and associated with relapse risk in MS patients treated with GA.

Dendritic Cell Inhibitors in MS Vorinostat, a histone deacetylase inhibitor, has been used clinically as an anticancer drug and also has immunosuppressive properties. However, the underlying mechanisms of effects of Vorinostat on CNS inflammatory diseases remain incomplete. In a study Gde et al. (2013) investigated the effects of Vorinostat on human CD14(+) monocyte-derived dendritic cells (DCs) and mouse immature DC *in vitro* and explored the therapeutic effects and cellular mechanisms of Vorinostat on animal model of MS, EAE *in vivo*. Vorinostat inhibited human CD14 (+) monocyte-derived DCs differentiation, maturation, endocytosis, and inhibited mDCs' stimulation of allogeneic T-cell proliferation. In addition, Vorinostat inhibited DC-directed Th1 and Th17-polarizing cytokine production. Furthermore, Vorinostat ameliorated Th1- and Th17-mediated EAE by reducing CNS inflammation and demyelination. Th1 and Th17 cell functions were suppressed in Vorinostat-treated EAE mice. Finally, Vorinostat suppressed expression of costimulatory molecules of DC in EAE mice suggesting therapeutic potential of Vorinostat on EAE by suppressing DCs and DCs-mediated Th1 and Th17 cell functions.

IFN-β in MS Huang et al. (2013) investigated the effect of pharmacologically relevant doses of IFN (β-1a) on B-cell expression of B7.1 and B7.2. Culture of peripheral blood mononuclear cells with IFN β-1a 100 IU/mL decreased B-cell expression of B7.1 and increased B7.2 expression. IL-10 in B cells was enhanced by IFN β-1a. Anti-CD3 and anti-CD28 monoclonal antibody-mediated T-cell proliferations were suppressed in the presence of B cells pretreated with IFN β-1a, suggesting that IFN β-1a and B cells play a beneficial role in the treatment of MS.

Isoprostanes (IsoP) in MS Isoprostanes (IsoP) are sensitive biomarkers of oxidative stress. Their CSF level is increased in several neurological conditions, including MS. In particular, in RRMS, IsoP have been proposed as an index of neurodegeneration. The mechanisms leading to neuroaxonal damage in MS are not fully understood but oxidative mechanisms play a key role. Although axonal loss is present in MS patients since their first clinical symptoms, IsoP levels at this early stage have not been evaluated yet. Sbardella et al. (2013) performed a study (a) to assess IsoP levels in CSF of patients with a first clinical attack suggestive of MS; (b) to correlate IsoP levels with MRI measures of brain damage and (c) to assess IsoP value in predicting disease. Thirty-nine patients with a first attack suggestive of MS underwent neurological examination, lumbar puncture with IsoP levels quantification and conventional/spectroscopic-MRI. Patients were followed up for 24 months. CSF IsoP levels were higher in patients than controls and inversely correlated to normalized brain volume and N-Acetylaspartate/Choline (NAA/Cho). The risk of experiencing clinical relapses differed according to IsoP level: subjects with levels higher than 95 pg/ml were more likely to relapse than patients with levels equal or lower than 95 pg/ml suggesting that IsoP might be useful biomarkers of tissue damage in MS with a predictive value of prognosis.

APRIL in MS González-Mendióroz et al. (2013) reported that APRIL (a proliferation-inducing ligand) is a member of the TNF superfamily that binds the receptors (TNFRs) TACI and BCMA. The involvement of APRIL in autoimmune diseases including SLE, rheumatoid arthritis (RA), Sjögren's syndrome (SS) and MS. In addition, an important role of APRIL has been described in tumour cell lines and in primary tumor tissues where high mRNA levels have been detected. Accordingly, the design of compounds mimicking the inhibition of APRIL by its receptors appears to be a promising way to treat autoimmune and cancer diseases. As a first step to achieve these goals and in order to better understand the interactions involved in these systems, a structural analysis of the inhibition of human and murine APRIL by its receptors TACI and BCMA obtained by molecular dynamics simulations has been reported. The interactions between human APRIL and its receptors can contribute to a better design of APRIL inhibitors.

Stem Cells Therapy in MS Experimental studies indicate that autologous bone marrow mesenchymal stem cells (BMSCs) can ameliorate EAE and potentially MS. However, the impact that the inflammatory environment present in EAE might have on the biological properties of BMSCs expanded *in vitro* for transplantation is yet to be established. Zacharaki et al. (2013) investigated whether BMSCs isolated from EAE-induced C57bl6/J mice and expanded *in vitro* preserve the properties of BMSCs isolated from healthy donors (BMSCs-control). The mesenchymal origin, the differentiation potential, and the transcriptional expression profile of six histone-modifying genes were studied in both groups of BMSCs. BMSCs-EAE exhibited distinct morphology and larger size compared to BMSCs-control, higher degree of proliferation and apoptosis, differences in the adipogenesis and the osteogenesis induction, and differential expression of stromal biomarkers and biomarkers of progenitor and mature neuronal/glial cells. Moreover, BMSCs-EAE exhibited different expression patterns on a number of histone-modifying genes compared to controls. Manifold differences of *in vitro* expanded BMSCs-EAE in comparison to their healthy donor-derived counterparts that may be attributed to the inflammatory environment they originated from were recorded. Darlington et al. (2013) defined changes in phenotype and functional responses of reconstituting T cells in patients with aggressive MS treated with ablative chemotherapy and autologous hematopoietic stem cell transplantation (HSCT). Clinical and brain MRI measures of disease activity were monitored serially in patients participating in the Canadian MS HSCT Study. Reconstitution kinetics of immune-cell subsets were determined by flow cytometry, whereas thymic function was assessed using T-cell receptor excision circle analyses as well as flow cytometry measurements of CD31+ thymic emigrants (RTEs). Functional assays were performed to track CNS -autoreactive antigen-specific T-cell responses, and the relative capacity to generate Th1, Th17, or Th1/17 T-cell responses. Complete abrogation of new clinical relapses and new focal inflammatory brain lesions throughout the 2 years of immune monitoring following treatment was associated with sustained decrease in naive T cells, in spite of restoration of both thymic function and release of RTEs during reconstitution. Re-emergence as well as *in vivo* expansion of autoreactive T cells to multiple myelin targets was evident in all patients. The reconstituted myelin-specific T cells exhibited the same Th1 and Th2 responses as preablation myelin-reactive T cells. In contrast, the post-therapy T-cell repertoire exhibited a diminished capacity for Th17 responses indicating that diminished Th17 and Th1/17 responses, rather than Th1 responses, are particularly relevant to the abrogation of new relapsing disease activity observed in these patients with aggressive MS following chemoablation and HSCT.

Iron Accumulation in MS The accumulation of Iron in some but not all MS lesions suggests a specific, disease-relevant process, however; its pathophysiological significance remains unknown. MRI phase imaging in MS patients and in autopsy tissue have demonstrated the presence of Iron depositions in white matter lesions. Mehta et al. (2013) explored the role of lesional Iron in MS using immunohistochemical examination of autoptic MS tissue, an *in vitro* model of Iron-uptake in human cultured macrophages and ultra-highfield phase imaging of highly active and of secondary progressive MS patients. Using Perls' stain and immunohistochemistry, Iron was detected in MS tissue sections predominantly in non-phagocytosing macrophages/microglia at the edge of established, demyelinated lesions. Moreover, Iron-containing macrophages but not myelin-laden macrophages expressed biomarkers of proinflammatory (M1) polarization. Similarly, in human macrophage cultures, Iron was preferentially taken up by non-phagocytosing, M1-polarized macrophages and induced M1 polarization. Iron uptake was minimal in myelin-laden macrophages and active myelin phagocytosis led to depletion of intracellular Iron. Finally, these investigators demonstrated in MS patients using GRE phase imaging with ultra-highfield MRI that phase hypointense lesions were more prevalent in patients with active relapsing than with secondary progressive MS. Iron is present in non-phagocytosing, M1-polarized microglia/macrophages at the rim of chronic active white matter demyelinating lesions. Phase imaging may therefore visualize specific, chronic pro-inflammatory activity in established MS lesions and thus provide important clinical information on disease status and treatment efficacy in MS patients.

Oligoclonal Immunoglobulin G Bands (OCBs) in MS Approximately 95% of MS patients display oligoclonal immunoglobulin G bands (OCB) in the CSF. From a cohort of 2094 MS patients, Karrenbauer et al. (2013) retrieved data from 40 OCB-negative and 60 OCB-positive patients to determine whether lesion load on brain MRI is affected by OCB status and carriage of HLA-DRB1*15 or HLA-DRB1*04. Positivity for OCB did not increase the risk of higher-lesion-load groups; nor did carrying HLA-DRB1*15 or HLA-DRB1*04. A trend was seen, however, OCB positivity conferred a two-fold risk of displaying higher lesion loads infratentorially.

α4-Integrin Inhibitor in MS Lymphocyte inhibition by antagonism of α4 integrins is a validated therapeutic approach for RMS. Wolf et al. (2013) investigated the effect of CDP323, an oral α4-integrin inhibitor, on lymphocyte biomarkers in RMS. Seventy-one RMS subjects aged 18-65 years with Expanded Disability Status Scale scores ≤6.5 were randomized to 28-day treatment with CDP323 100 mg twice daily (bid), 500 mg bid, 1000 mg once daily (qd), 1000 mg bid, or placebo. Relative to placebo, all dosages of CDP323 decreased the capacity of lymphocytes to bind vascular adhesion molecule-1 (VCAM-1) and the expression of α4-integrin on VCAM-1-binding cells. All but the 100-mg bid dosage increased total lymphocytes and naive B cells, memory B cells, and T cells in peripheral blood compared with placebo, and the dose-response relationship was shown to be linear. Marked increases were also observed in natural killer cells and hematopoietic progenitor cells, but only with the 500-mg bid and 1000-mg bid dosages. There were no changes in monocytes. CDP323 at daily doses of 1000 or 2000 mg induced increases in total lymphocyte count and suppressed VCAM-1 binding by reducing unbound late antigen-4 expression on lymphocytes. A study was performed to understand intracellular regulatory mechanisms in PBMCs, which are either common to many autoimmune diseases or specific to some of them. Tuller et al. (2013) incorporated large-scale data such as protein-protein interactions, gene expression and demographical information of hundreds of patients and healthy subjects, related to six autoimmune diseases with large-scale gene expression measurements: MS, systemic lupus erythematosus (SLE), juvenile rheumatoid arthritis (JRA), Crohn's disease (CD), ulcerative colitis (UC) and type 1 diabetes (T1D). These data were analyzed by statistical and systems biology approaches. Chemokines such as CXCL1-3, 5, 6 and the IL8 tend to be differentially expressed in PBMCs of patients with the analyzed autoimmune diseases. In addition, the anti-apoptotic gene BCL3, interferon-γ (IFNG), and the vitamin D receptor (VDR) gene physically interact with many genes that tend to be differentially expressed in PBMCs of patients with the analyzed autoimmune diseases. In general, similar cellular processes tend to be differentially expressed in PBMC in the analyzed autoimmune diseases. *Specifically, the cellular processes related to cell proliferation (i.e, epidermal growth factor, platelet-derived growth factor, nuclear factor-κB, Wnt/β-catenin signaling, stress-activated protein kinase c-Jun NH2-terminal kinase), inflammatory response (i.e, interleukins IL2 and IL6, the cytokine granulocyte-macrophage colony-stimulating factor and the B-cell receptor), general signaling cascades (i.e, mitogen-activated protein kinase, extracellular signal-regulated kinase, p38 and TRK) and apoptosis were activated in most of the analyzed autoimmune diseases.* However, in each of the analyzed diseases, apoptosis and chemotaxis were activated via different subsignaling pathways. Analyses of the expression levels of genes and the protein-protein interactions demonstrated that CD and UC have relatively similar gene expression signatures, whereas the gene expression signatures of T1D and JRA differ from the signatures of the other autoimmune diseases. These diseases are the only ones activated via the Fcε pathway. The relevant genes and pathways may be helpful in the diagnoses and understanding of autoimmunity and/or specific autoimmune diseases.

Involvement of Activated TFH-Cells in MS Pathology studies of progressive MS indicate a major role of inflammation including Th17-cells and meningeal inflammation with ectopic lymphoid follicles, B-cells, and plasma cells, indicating a possible role of the newly identified subset of follicular T-helper (TFH) cells. Although previous studies reported increased systemic inflammation in progressive MS it remains unclear whether systemic inflammation contributes to disease progression and intrathecal inflammation. Christensen et al. (2013) investigated systemic inflammation in progressive MS and its relationship with disease progression, using flow cytometry and gene expression analysis of CD4 (+) and CD8 (+) T-cells, B-cells, monocytes and dendritic cells. Furthermore, gene expression of CSF cells was studied. Flow cytometry studies revealed increased frequencies of ICOS (+) TFH-cells in peripheral blood from RRMS and secondary progressive (SPMS) MS patients. All MS subtypes had decreased frequencies of Th1 TFH-cells, while primary progressive (PPMS) MS patients had increased frequency of Th17 TFH-cells. The Th17-subset, interleukin-23-receptor (+) CD4 (+) T-cells, was increased in PPMS and SPMS. In the analysis of B-cells, a significant increase of plasmablasts and DC-SIGN (+) and CD83 (+) B-cells in SPMS. ICOS (+) TFH-cells and DC-SIGN (+) B-cells correlated with disease progression in SPMS patients. Gene expression analysis of peripheral blood cell subsets substantiated the flow cytometry findings by demonstrating increased expression of IL21, IL21R and ICOS in CD4(+)T-cells in progressive MS. CSF cells from RRMS and progressive MS (pooled SPMS and PPMS patients) had increased expression of TFH-cell and plasmablast biomarkers. This was the first study to demonstrate the involvement of activated TFH-cells in MS. The increased frequencies of Th17-cells, activated TFH- and B-cells parallel findings from pathology studies which, along with the correlation between activated TFH- and B-cells and disease progression, suggest a pathogenic role of systemic inflammation in progressive MS.

CSF sCD146 as a Potential Biomarker in MS The mechanisms whereby immune cells infiltrating the CNS in MS patients contribute to tissue injury remain to be defined. CD4 T cells are key players of this inflammatory response. Myelin-specific CD4 T cells expressing CD56, a surrogate biomarker of NK cells, were shown to be cytotoxic to human oligodendrocytes. Zaguia et al. (2013) identified NK-associated molecules expressed by human CD4 T cells that confer this oligodendrocyte-directed cytotoxicity. Myelin-reactive CD4 T cell lines, as well as short-term PHA-activated CD4 T cells, can express NKG2C, the activating receptor interacting with HLA-E, a nonclassical MHC class I molecule. These cells coexpress CD56 and NKG2D, have elevated levels of cytotoxic molecules FasL, granzyme B, and perforin compared with their NKG2C-negative counterparts, and mediate significant *in vitro* cytotoxicity toward human oligodendrocytes, which upregulated HLA-E upon inflammatory cytokine treatment. A significantly elevated proportion of ex vivo peripheral blood CD4 T cells, but not CD8 T cells or NK cells, from MS patients express NKG2C compared with controls. In addition, immunohistochemical analyses showed that MS brain tissues display HLA-E (+) oligodendrocytes and NKG2C (+) CD4 T cells. These results implicate a novel mechanism through which infiltrating CD4 T cells contribute to tissue injury in MS. Duan et al. (2013) showed that sCD146 is significantly elevated in the CSF of patients with active MS compared with that of inactive MS or patients with non-demyelinating diseases. Moreover, abnormally increased sCD146 in the CSF of active MS patients correlated with albumin quotient, MBP antibody and MOG antibody from both CSF and sera. The level of CSF sCD146 was correlated with levels of TNFα, IFNγ, IL-2, and IL-17A in the CSF. CSF sCD146 might originate from membrane-bound CD146 on inflamed BBB endothelial cells. In addition, sCD146 promotes leukocyte transmigration *in vitro*, by stimulating the expression of ICAM-1 and VCAM-1 on endothelial cells suggesting that CSF levels of sCD146 may provide a potential biomarker for monitoring disease severity in MS patients.

Remyelination of chronically demyelinated axons in MS requires the recruitment of endogenous cells or their replacement by transplanted, exogenous oligodendrocyte progenitor cells (OPCs). Piao et al. (2013) showed that an OPC line, CG4, preferentially migrates after transplantation toward focal areas of inflammatory demyelination and axon loss created by injection of zymosan in the rat spinal cord. Many transplanted CG4 cells had already migrated into the inflammatory lesion after 1 day. A large number of CG4 cells that had migrated, expressed the adhesion protein, CD44, and that CD44's main ligand, Hyaluronic acid (HA) was expressed in the inflammatory lesion. In an *in vitro* migration assay, migration declined following blocking of CD44 expression on CG4 cells. Likewise, migration of CG4 cells toward a zymosan lesion was inhibited when transplanted cells were exposed to a CD44 blocking antibody prior to transplantation suggesting that CD-44 is a key molecule in the migration of OPCs toward the focal inflammatory demyelinated lesion induced by zymosan and may be important in OPC repair in MS.

Interleukin 7 Receptor in MS IL7R Interleukin 7 receptor, IL7R, is expressed exclusively on cells of the lymphoid lineage, and its expression is crucial for the development and maintenance of T cells. Alternative splicing of IL7R exon 6 results in membrane-bound (exon 6 included) and soluble (exon 6 skipped) IL7R isoforms. Interestingly, the inclusion of exon 6 is affected by a single-nucleotide polymorphism associated with the risk of developing MS. Given the potential association of exon 6 inclusion with MS, the cis-acting elements and trans-acting factors that regulate exon 6 splicing were estimated. Evsyukova et al. (2013) identified multiple exonic and intronic cis-acting elements that impact inclusion of exon 6 and utilized RNA affinity chromatography followed by mass spectrometry to identify trans-acting protein factors that bind exon 6 and regulate its splicing. These experiments identified cleavage and polyadenylation specificity factor 1 (CPSF1) among protein-binding candidates. A consensus polyadenylation signal AAUAAA is present in intron 6 of IL7R directly downstream from the 5' splice site. Mutations to this site and CPSF1 knockdown both resulted in an increase in exon 6 inclusion. No evidence that this site is used to produce cleaved and polyadenylated mRNAs, suggesting that CPSF1 interaction with intronic IL7R pre-mRNA interferes with spliceosome binding to the exon 6 5' splice site suggesting that competing mRNA splicing and polyadenylation regulate exon 6 inclusion and consequently determine the ratios of soluble to membrane-bound IL7R. This may be relevant for both T cell ontogeny and function and development of MS.

PUFA in MS Eicosapentaenoic acid (EPA), one of the n-3 polyunsaturated fatty acids, is a neuroprotective lipid with anti-inflammatory properties. Unoda et al. (2013) investigated the potential therapeutic effect of EPA on EAE). EAE mice were fed a diet with or without EPA. The clinical EAE scores of the EPA-fed mice were lower than those of the non-EPA mice. In the EPA-treated mice, IFN-γ and IL-17 productions were remarkably inhibited and the peroxisome proliferator-activated receptors were enhanced in the CNS-infiltrating CD4T cells. Thus EPA shows promise as a potential new therapeutic agent against MS.

LRP1 as a Receptor for Endocytosis During Cellular Damage and Necrosis. In the CNS, fast neuronal signals are facilitated by the oligodendrocyte-produced myelin sheath. Oligodendrocyte turnover or injury generates myelin debris that is cleared by phagocytic cells. Failure to remove dying oligodendrocytes leads to accumulation of degraded myelin, which, if recognized by the immune system, may contribute to the development of autoimmunity in diseases such as MS. Fernandez-Castaneda et al. (2013) identified low density lipoprotein receptor-related protein-1 (LRP1) as a novel phagocytic receptor for myelin debris. The characterization of the LRP1 interactome in CNS myelin was reported. Fusion proteins were designed corresponding to the extracellular ligand-binding domains of

LRP1. LRP1 partners were isolated by affinity purification and characterized by mass spectrometry. LRP1 binds intracellular proteins via its extracellular domain and functions as a receptor for necrotic cells. Peptidyl arginine deiminase-2 and cyclic nucleotide phosphodiesterase are novel LRP1 ligands identified in screen, which interact with full-length LRP1. Furthermore, the extracellular domain of LRP1 is a target of peptidyl arginine deiminase-2-mediated deimination *in vitro*. Hence LRP1 may function as a receptor for endocytosis of intracellular components released during cellular damage and necrosis.

Fetuin as a Biomarkers in MS Fetuin-A has been recently identified as a potential biomarker in MS CSF. Fetuin-A has diverse functions, including a role in immune pathways. A study was performed to investigate whether Fetuin-A is a direct indicator of disease activity. Fetuin-A was estimated in CSF and plasma of patients with MS and correlated these findings to clinical disease activity and Natalizumab response. Fetuin-A expression was characterized in MS brain tissue and in EAE mice. The pathogenic role of Fetuin-A in EAE using Fetuin-A-deficient mice was also investigated. Elevated CSF Fetuin-A correlated with disease activity in MS. In Natalizumab-treated patients, CSF Fetuin-A levels were reduced one year post-treatment, correlating with therapeutic response. Fetuin-A was elevated in demyelinated lesions and in gray matter within MS brain tissue. Similarly, Fetuin-A was elevated in degenerating neurons around demyelinated lesions in EAE. Fetuin-A-deficient mice demonstrated delayed onset and reduced severity of EAE symptom suggesting that CSF Fetuin-A is a biomarker of disease activity and Natalizumab response in MS.

CSF and Urinary Biomarkers of MS Biomarkers with the potential for longitudinal measurements are needed in MS. Dobson et al. (2013) took 39 paired CSF and urine samples. Oligoclonal bands (OCBs) were measured in CSF. Kappa and lambda free light chain (FLC), Neopterin and Ubiquitin C-terminal hydrolase-L1 (UCHL1) were measured in CSF and urine. 16/39 samples had OCBs unique to the CSF. CSF FLC levels were higher in OCB-positive subjects, with no difference in urinary FLC. CSF and urinary FLC did not correlate. There were a significant correlation between total CSF FLC and CSF Neopterin in MS samples and a strong correlation between CSF lambda FLC and CSF Neopterin in MS samples. There was a strong correlation between urinary Neopterin/Creatinine levels and urinary total FLC/protein levels. Only three CSF samples (8%) had detectable levels of UCHL1. 18/38 (48%) (8/15 MS and 10/23 control) urine samples had detectable levels of UCLH1, confirming the relationship between CSF OCBs and CSF FLCs, and highlighting the importance of intrathecal B- and plasma-cell activation in MS. There is a relationship between CSF FLC and CSF Neopterin in MS, highlighting the multifaceted immune activation seen in MS. Correlations in the OCB-positive group highlighted the multifaceted immune activation seen in MS.

Neurofilaments and N-Acetyl Aspartate in MS Axonal damage is considered a major cause of disability in MS and may start early in the disease. Specific biomarkers for this process are of great interest. Khalil et al. (2013) determined if CSF biomarkers for axonal damage reflect and predict disease progression already in the earliest stages of the disease, in clinically isolated syndrome (CIS). These investigators assessed CSF levels of neurofilament heavy (NFH), neurofilament light (NFL) and N-Acetylaspartate (NAA) in 67 patients with CIS and 18 controls with neuropsychiatric diseases of non-inflammatory etiology (NC). Patients with CIS underwent baseline MRI at 3T, and a follow-up MRI after 1 year was obtained in 28 of them. Compared with NC, patients with CIS had higher NFH and NFL levels. No significant differences were found for NAA. Patients' NFH levels correlated with physical disability and with change in brain volume but not with change in T2 lesion load, confirming increased neurofilament levels in CIS related to the level of physical disability. The association of NFH levels with brain volume but not lesion volume changes supported the association of these biomarkers with axonal damage.

Immunoadsorption Technique in MS MS is the most common autoimmune inflammatory demyelinating disease of the CNS with a frequently relapsing or progressive course. For steroid-resistant relapse, plasma exchange (PE) has been established as guidelines-recommended treatment option. While PE is a non-selective extracorporeal blood purification process with elimination of plasma and subsequent substitution, immunoadsorption (IA) is a selective technique for the removal of autoantibodies and immune complexes with less adverse effects. So far there are only few reports on the treatment of MS by IA. Heigl et al. (2013) assessed the efficacy and safety of IA as an escalation therapy in MS patients. A total of 60 patients with steroid-refractory MS relapse were treated by IA and analyzed retrospectively. Patients received six standardized IA sessions using a non-regenerable Tryptophan immunoadsorber, at average 58 days after first indications of relapse. The treated plasma volume was two liters per IA session. Outcome was measured as improvement in relapse symptoms. From the pilot phase of the study comprising the first fourteen patients, detailed neurological examinations before and after IA such as Expanded Disability Status Scale (EDSS), Functional System Score (FS) and visual acuity were reported. In 53 of 60 patients clinically relevant improvement of the main symptom of MS relapse was noted after IA, there was no change in six patients, deterioration in one. This corresponds to a response rate of 88%. Symptomatic improvement was registered on average after the third IA. 87.5% of patients could be treated through a peripheral venous access. Only 12.5% needed a central venous catheter. In four of 396 single treatments (1%) significant complications occurred, mild side effects or discomfort were registered 16 times (4%). If peripheral venous access was chosen, missed puncture or puncture hematoma occurred in 22 cases (5.5%) suggesting that immunoadsorption for the treatment of steroid-refractory MS relapse is safe and effective. The response rate was 88% and non-inferior to previous results with plasma exchange. Due to good tolerability, the treatment with immunoadsorption, which is usually possible through a peripheral venous access, could be performed on an outpatient basis. Klingel et al. (2013) reported immediate antibody elimination, pulsed induction of antibody redistribution, and immunomodulation are major forces of efficacy of therapeutic apheresis (i.e., plasma exchange [PE] or immunoadsorption [IA]) for autoimmune neurologic disorders. Therapeutic apheresis can offer rapid response for severe acute neurologic symptoms, and stable rehabilitation in long-term clinical courses being refractory to drug based strategies or complicated by drug side effects. These investigators emphasiezed that PE or IA in these situations must be considered as part of multimodal or escalating immune treatment strategies in combination or in competition with i.v administered immunoglobulins (iv Ig), corticosteroids, the full spectrum of immunosuppressive drugs, and bioengineered antibodies. Selective IA is increasingly replacing PE due to its superior safety profile and increasing knowledge on pathogenic relevance of autoantibodies. Recent experiences in autoimmune diseases of the CNS, e.g., MS, neuromyelitis optica, and autoimmune encephalitis confirmed this concept.

Myelin-Specific CD8 (+) T Cells to Recognize Oligodendrocytes. Ji et al. (2013) reported that myelin presentation to T cells in the CNS sustains inflammation in MS. CD4(+) and CD8(+) T cells contribute to MS, but only cells that present myelin to CD4(+) T cells have been identified. These investigators showed that MHC class I-restricted myelin basic protein (MBP) was presented by oligodendrocytes and cross-presented by Tip-dendritic cells (DCs) during EAE, an animal model of MS initiated by CD4(+) T cells. Tip-DCs activated naive and effector CD8 (+) T cells ex vivo, and naive MBP-specific CD8(+) T cells were activated in the CNS during CD4(+) T cell-induced EAE suggesting that CD4(+) T cell-mediated CNS autoimmunity leads to spreading to myelin-specific CD8(+) T cells that can recognize oligodendrocytes.

Cholinergic System in MS An impairment of the cholinergic system activity has been demonstrated in MS. The correlation between the cholinergic system and the cognitive dysfunction in MS has led to studies on the use of acetylcholinesterase inhibitors (AChEI). The acetylcholinesterase (AChE), essential enzyme for the regulation of turnover of ACh, can be considered the most important biochemical indicator of cholinergic signaling in the CNS. Besides its catalytic properties, AChE has a crucial role in the regulation of the immune function. Based on the role of the AChe in the regulation of cholinergic signaling in the CNS, the aim of this study was to evaluate the activity of AChE in different pathological conditions: MS, other inflammatory neurological disorders (OIND) and non-inflammatory neurological disorders (NIND). Antonelli et al. (2013) measured AChE activity in CSF samples obtained from 34 relapsing-remitting MS patients and, as controls, 40 patients with other inflammatory neurological disorders (OIND) and 40 subjects with other non-inflammatory neurological disorders (NIND). Fluorimetric detection of the AChE in MS patients and in the controls showed no significant differences: 1.507 ± 0.403 nmol/ml/min in MS patients, 1.484 ± 0.496 nmol/ml/min in OIND and 1.305 ± 0.504 nmol/ml/min in NIND. Similar results were obtained in another recent study, using a different method. Further studies must be conducted on a larger number of patients, with different degrees of cognitive impairment. However, these authors highlighted that AChE measured in CSF can not be considered a useful biomarker for the assessment of the functional alterations of cholinergic system in pathological conditions.

Intrathecal Synthesis of IgG in MS Intrathecal synthesis of IgG is observed in patients with MS. Whereas the extent of intrathecal IgG synthesis varies largely between patients, it remains rather constant in the individual patient over time. Buck et al. (2013) performed a study to identify common genetic variants associated with the IgG index as a biomarker of intrathecal IgG synthesis in MS. These investigators performed a genome-wide association study of the IgG index in a discovery series of 229 patients. For confirmation they performed a replication in 2 independent series comprising 256 and 153 patients, respectively. The impact of associated SNPs on MS susceptibility was analyzed in an additional 1,854 cases and 5,175 controls. Significant association between the IgG index and 5 SNPs was detected in the discovery and confirmed in both replication series. All identified SNPs are clustered around the immunoglobulin heavy chain (IGHC) locus on chromosome 14q32.33 and are in linkage disequilibrium. The best associated SNP is located in an intronic region of the immunoglobulin gamma3 heavy chain gene. Additional sequencing identified the GM21* haplotype to be associated with a high IgG index. Further evaluation of the IGHC SNPs revealed no association with susceptibility to MS in this data. The extent of intrathecal IgG in MS was influenced by the IGHC locus. No association with susceptibility to MS was found, indicating that GM haplotypes might affect intrathecal IgG synthesis independently of the underlying disease.

CSF Metal Ions in MS **Roos et al. (2013)** analyzed metal concentrations in CSF and blood plasma in ALS patients diagnosed with quantitative electromyography. Metal analyses were performed with high-resolution inductively coupled plasma mass spectrometry (ICP-MS). Statistically significant higher concentrations of Manganese, Aluminium, Cadmium, Cobalt, Copper, Zinc, Lead, Vanadium and Uranium were found in ALS CSF compared to control CSF. Higher concentrations of these metals in ALS CSF than in ALS blood plasma, indicated mechanisms of accumulation, e.g., inward directed transport. A pattern of multiple toxic metals was seen in ALS CSF, supporting the hypothesis that metals with neurotoxic effects are involved in the pathogenesis of ALS.

Fingolimod (FTY-720) is a Sphingosine-1-Phosphate Receptor Modulator in MS Dinkin et al. (2013) evaluated patients with MS, optical coherence tomography (OCT) is gaining traction as a tool to assess thinning of the retinal nerve fiber layer (RNFL) and, more recently, for looking at total macular volume (TMV) thickness, with both measures used as potential biomarkers for progression of disease. In medicine, it is not uncommon for structural changes to be presumed to reflect a certain physiologic process, when in fact, an alternative mechanism is at play. Fingolimod (FTY-720) is a Sphingosine-1-phosphate receptor modulator that is an approved oral treatment for MS and leads to reduced cortical volume loss in patients with MS.(1) Similar to other disease-modifying agents, it is likely to be judged in part by its ability to slow loss of the RNFL and TMV.

GF As a Localized Form of IgG4-RD GF might represent a localized form of IgG4-RD The pathogenesis of granuloma faciale (GF), framed in the group of cutaneous vasculopathic dermatitis, is poorly understood. Cesinaro et al. (2013) investigated whether GF might be part of the spectrum of IgG4-related sclerosing diseases (IgG4-RD) and erythema elevatum diutinum (EED), believed to belong to the same group of disorders as GF, for comparison. Thirty-one biopsies of GF obtained from 25 patients (18 men, 7 women) and 5 cases of EED (4 women and 1 man) were analyzed morphologically and for the expression of IgG and IgG4 by immunohistochemistry. The distribution of Th1, T regulatory and Th2 T-cell subsets, respectively, identified by anti-T-bet, anti-FoxP3, and anti-GATA-3 antibodies, was also evaluated. The dermal inflammatory infiltrate in GF contained eosinophils and plasma cells in variable proportions. Obliterative venulitis was found in 16 cases, and storiform fibrosis, a typical feature of IgG4-RD, was observed in 8 cases and was prominent in 3 of them. On immunohistochemical analysis 7 of 31 biopsies (22.6%) from 6 GF patients fulfilled the criteria for IgG4-RD (IgG4/IgG ratio >40%, and absolute number of IgG4 per high-power field >50). Interestingly, the 6 patients were male, and 4 showed recurrent and/or multiple lesions. In an additional 5 cases, only the IgG4/IgG ratio was abnormal. None of the 5 EED cases fulfilled the criteria for IgG4-RD. The T-cell subsets in GF were quite variable in number, GATA-3 lymphocytes were generally more abundant, but no relationship with the number of IgG4 plasma cells was found, indicating that a significant number of GF cases are associated with an abnormal content of IgG4 plasma cells; this association was particularly obvious in male patients and in cases presenting with multiple or recurrent lesions. As morphologic changes typically found in IgG4-RD, such as obliterative vascular inflammation and storiform sclerosis, are found in GF, suggesting that GF might represent a localized form of IgG4-RD.

Circadian Rhythm in MS Inflammatory serum parameters have been investigated in the search of biomarkers for disease activity and treatment response in MS. A reason for contradictory results might be the timing of blood collection for analyzing serum concentrations of inflammatory parameters which are subject to diurnal changes. Wipfler et al. (2013) included 34 untreated patients with RRMS and 34 age- and sex-matched healthy controls. 12 MS patients showed acute disease activity in corresponding MRI scans. Blood samples were obtained at 7.00, 11.00 am, 2.30, 6.00 and 9.30 pm within 1 day. These investigators determined serum levels of Cortisol and inflammatory markers including *soluble tumor necrosis factor-beta (sTNF-β), soluble TNF-Receptor-1 (sTNF-R1) and -2 (sTNF-2), soluble vascular adhesion molecule-1 (sVCAM-1) and soluble intercellular adhesion molecule-1 (sICAM-1) by ELISA*. Significantly higher serum levels of sTNF-R1 and sTNF-R2 were observed in the morning and a significant decline of sICAM-1 and sVCAM-1 was observed in the afternoon in both, MS patients and healthy controls. Comparison of diurnal serum levels between MS patients with active versus with non-active disease revealed significantly higher serum levels of sVCAM-1 around noon and in the early afternoon in MS patients with active disease. A significant decline of sICAM-1 in the afternoon was seen in MS patients with active and non-active disease indicating that increased awareness of potential diurnal serum fluctuations of biomarkers can eliminate one major cause of biased data as they occur in most of the immunological parameters.

Benign Multiple Sclerosis (BMS) Benign multiple sclerosis (BMS) is a controversial concept which is still debated. However identification of this kind of patients is crucial to prevent them from unnecessary exposure to aggressive and/or long term medical treatments. Leray et al. (2013) assessed two definitions of 'clinically definite benign multiple sclerosis' (CDBMS) using long-term follow-up data, and to look for prognostic factors of CDBMS. In 874 patients with definite RRMS, followed up for at least 10 years, disability was assessed using the Disability Status Scale (DSS). CDBMS was defined by either DSS score$\leq$2 (CDBMS1 group) or DSS score$\leq$ 3 (CDBMS2 group) at 10 years. They estimated the proportion of patients who were still benign at 20 and 30 years after clinical onset. CDBMS frequency estimates were 57.7% and 73.9% when using CDBMS1 and CDBMS2 definitions, respectively. In the CDBMS1 group, only 41.7% (105/252) of cases were still benign 10 years later, and 41.1% (23/56) after an additional decade, while there were 53.8% (162/301) and 59.5% (44/74) respectively in the CDBMS2 group. This 30-year observational study indicated that favorable 10-year disability scores of DSS 2 or 3 fail to ensure a long-term benign course of multiple sclerosis. After every decade almost half of the CDBMS were no longer benign. CDBMS, as currently defined, is an unwarranted conceptual hodgepodge. Other criteria using new biomarkers (genetic, biologic or MRI) should be found to detect benign cases of MS.

Neuropsychological Biomakers in MS Attachment style and temperament could influence a stress-relapse relationship in MS. Fazekas et al. (2013) aimed to probe for an association of these personality-related variables with disease activity in patients with clinically isolated syndrome and early MS. Study participants completed following psychometric instruments: Adult Attachment Scale (AAS), Temperament and Character Inventory (TCI-125), Hospital Anxiety and Depression Scale (HADS). Clinical data encompassed the expanded disability status scale (EDSS), annualized relapse rate, disease duration and therapy. Relapses and MRI data were recorded at regular outpatient visits. Study participants (n=84), 38 with a clinically isolated syndrome suggestive of MS (CIS) and 46 with RRMS, were assessed with a low EDSS. No significant differences concerning personality-related variables were revealed by group comparisons between CIS and RRMS and within the RRMS subgroup based on clinical measures (EDSS/year; within RRMS subgroup: annualized relapse rate). However, a higher lesion load per years of disease duration within the RRMS subgroup was associated with higher values in the temperament trait harm avoidance. Although harm avoidance may be related to subclinical disease activity in early RRMS adult attachment and temperament do not seem to contribute to differences between CIS and RRMS or clinical variability in early MS.

Pediatric-Onset Multiple Sclerosis (pMS) Pediatric-onset multiple sclerosis (pMS) is MS occurring before the age of 18 years and may present and develop differently from adult-onset MS (aMS). Whether there are also differences regarding the accrual of brain changes remain unknown. Pichler et al. (2013) compared the evolution of the T2- and T1-lesion load (LL), the black hole ratio (BHR), and annualised brain volume change (aBVC) between 21 pMS patients (age at onset: 14.4 ± 2.3 years) and 21 aMS patients (age at onset: 29.4 ± 6.5 years) matched for disease duration (pMS: 1.0 ± 1.8 years; aMS: 1.6 ± 1.7 years, p=0.27). Follow-up was for 4.2 ± 3.7 years in pMS and 3.1 ± 0.6 years in aMS. Clinical comparisons included the course of disability assessed with the Expanded Disability Status Scale (EDSS) score and annualised relapse rate (ARR). At baseline, pMS and aMS had similar EDSS, T1-LL, BHR, whereas T2-LL was higher in aMS (aMS: 9.2 ± 11.6 ccm; pMS: 4.1 ± 6.2 ccm, p = 0.02). The change of T2-LL and T1-LL during the observation period was similar in both groups. At follow-up, disability was lower in pMS (EDSS score in pMS: 0.9 ± 0.9; aMS: 1.7 ± 1.3, p = 0.04), despite a significantly higher accrual of destructive brain lesions (BHR in pMS: 23.7 ± 23.7%; aMS: 5.9 ± 4.0%, p=0.02) and a similar rate of brain volume loss. This observation of a morphologically more aggressive disease evolution paralleled by less disability in pMS than in aMS (defined using EDSS) suggests a higher compensatory capacity in pMS. This fact may obscure the need for treatment of pMS patients with disease modifying treatments (DMTs) based solely on clinical observation.

Memory Biomarkers in MS Patients with MS suffer memory impairment but the link between MS-related neuroanatomical changes (brain atrophy) and memory is relatively weak. Sumowski et al. (2013) performed a study to use fMRI to investigate task-induced default network (DN) deactivation as a neurophysiologic biomarker of memory functioning in MS. Twenty-eight MS patients underwent high-resolution MRIs to measure brain atrophy (third ventricle width, cerebral gray matter, cerebral white matter, parenchymal fraction, and thalamic, caudate, hippocampal, and amygdala volumes), and fMRI blood oxygen level dependent (BOLD) signal to measure DN deactivation during sustained attention relative to rest. Neuropsychological assessment of episodic memory was performed on a separate day. These researchers used hierarchical regression to predict memory, with age, education, and depression in step one, brain atrophy within step two, DN activity within step three, and the interaction between brain atrophy and DN activity in step four. Brain atrophy predicted worse memory but DN activity independently predicted memory over-and-above measurements of brain atrophy (R (2) =0.108), with greater DN activity (lesser deactivation) linked to better memory. A significant brain atrophy by DN activity interaction indicated a stronger relationship between memory and DN activity among patients with more advanced disease, at which point higher DN activity protects patients from disease/atrophy-related memory impairment. To establish specificity, these investigators showed no relationship between DN activity and non-memory cognition, and no relationship between non-DN brain activity and memory. Maintenance of DN activity during sustained attention was supported as a sensitive and specific neurophysiologic biomarker of episodic memory functioning in MS, even when controlling for neuroanatomical changes (brain atrophy).

Neuroaxonal Degeneration and Plasticity in Early MS The extent of irreversible neuroaxonal damage is the key determinant of permanent disability in traumatic and inflammatory conditions of the CNS. Structural damage is nevertheless in part compensated by neuroplastic events. However, it is unknown whether the same kinetics and mechanisms of neuroaxonal de- and regeneration take place in inflammatory and traumatic conditions. Schirmer e t al (2013) analyzed neuroaxonal degeneration and plasticity in early MS lesions and traumatic brain injury (TBI). Neuroaxonal degeneration identified by the presence of SMI31+ chromatolytic neurons and SMI32+ axonal profiles were characteristic features of leukocortical TBI lesions. Axonal transport disturbances as determined by Amyloid Precursor Protein (APP) + spheroids were present in both TBI and MS lesions to a similar degree. Neurons expressing growth-associated protein 43 (GAP43) and synaptophysin (Syn) were found under both pathological conditions. However, axonal swellings immunopositive for GAP43 and Syn clearly prevailed in subcortical MS lesions, suggesting a higher regenerative potential in MS. In this context, GAP43+/APP+ axonal spheroid ratios correlated with macrophage infiltration in TBI and MS lesions, supporting the idea that phagocyte activation might promote neuroplastic events. Furthermore, axonal GAP43+ and Syn+ swellings correlated with prolonged survival after TBI, indicating a sustained regenerative response.

Novel IL17/IL-17R Antibodies in Autoimmune Diseases. The role of T cell subpopulations in human disease is in a transition phase due to continuous discovery of new subsets of T cell, one of which is Th17, characterized by the production of signature cytokine IL-17. In the last couple of years, many articles are coming out on the role of Th17 and its signature cytokine IL-17 in different autoimmune diseases like rheumatoid arthritis, psoriasis, psoriatic arthritis (PsA), SLE and MS. Raychaudhuri (2013) reported that psoriasis and PsA are immune-mediated diseases, affecting the skin and joints, respectively. Initially, it was thought that psoriasis and PsA were Th1-mediated diseases; however, studies in knockout animal models (IL-17 knockout mice) as well as human experimental data indicate that Th17 and its signature cytokine IL-17 have a critical role in the pathogenesis of psoriatic disease. Th17 cells were identified from the dermal extracts of psoriatic lesions. Subsequently, this research group substantiated that Th17 cells are enriched in the papillary dermis of psoriatic plaques and in freshly isolated effector T lymphocytes from the synovial fluid of PsA patients, and reported that the majority of these CD4 + IL-17+ T cells are of memory phenotype (CD4RO(+)CD45RA(-)CD11a(+)). Recent reports also suggested that the synovial tissue in psoriatic arthritis is enriched with IL-17R, and its receptor IL-17RA is functionally active in psoriatic arthritis. These researchers discussed the role of IL-17 in psoriatic disease and narrated about the novel IL17/IL-17R antibodies for its therapeutic uses in autoimmune diseases.

Miscellaneous Biomarkers in MS: Various diversified biomarkers that can also be used for the clinical management of MS, are presented in Figure 50. *For example, β-1,4-GalT-I as an inflammatory mediator regulating adhesion and migration of inflammatory cells in EAE, Oxidative Stress Biomarker, Isoprostanes (IsoP) are sensitive biomarkers of oxidative stress, PET Biomarkers, TSPO (18 KD Proteins), [18]FdG Imaging, Modification of galactosylated carbohydrate chains to modulate selectin-ligand biosynthesis, In-Vivo Gd-enhancement MRI to determine BBB integrity, interaction with E-Selectin. NFL, GFAP and β-Tub II proteins are increased in MS patients. CD70: therapeutic target in human MS. In addition, CD70, MRS biomarker (Reduced NAA), invasive investigations, noninvasive investigations, MTs, α-Synuclein index (SI), and the existence of Charnoly Body (CB) can be used as biomarkers of* *neurodegeneration/regeneration in MS. α-Synuclein index (SI) is the ratio of nitrated α-Synuclein vs native α-Synuclein (Sharma et al., 2003); MTs are neuroprotective anti-inflammatory, low molecular weight, metal (Zn^{2+})-binding, -SH rich antioxidant proteins, which prevent various neurodegenerative α-synucleinopathies by preventing CB formation and by acting as free radical scavengers. CBs are formed due to mitochondrial degeneration as a consequence of free radical overproduction as the researchers have reported in our recent publications* (Sharma et al., 2013a; Sharma et al., 2013b).

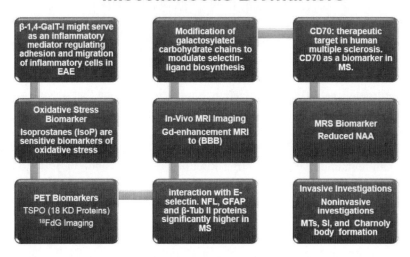

Figure 50. *Miscellaneous Biomarkers in MS:* This flow diagram illustrates various diversified biomarkers that can be used for the clinical management of MS. For example, β-1,4-GalT-I as an inflammatory mediator regulating adhesion and migration of inflammatory cells in EAE, Oxidative Stress Biomarker, Isoprostanes (IsoP) are sensitive biomarkers of oxidative stress, PET Biomarkers, TSPO (18 KD Proteins), [18]FdG Imaging, Modification of galactosylated carbohydrate chains to modulate selectin-ligand biosynthesis, *In-Vivo* Gd-enhancement MRI to determine BBB integrity, interaction with E-Selectin. NFL, GFAP and β-Tub II proteins are significantly increased in MS patients. CD70: therapeutic target in human MS. In addition, CD70, MRS Biomarker (Reduced NAA), invasive Investigations, noninvasive investigations, MTs, α-Synuclein index (SI), and the existence of Charnoly body can be used as biomarkers of neurodegeneration/regeneration in MS. α-Synuclein index (SI) is the ratio of nitrated α-Synuclein vs native α-Synuclein (Sharma et al., 2003); MTs are neuroprotective anti-inflammatory, low molecular weight, metal (Zn^{2+})-binding, -SH rich antioxidant proteins, which prevent various neurodegenerative α-Synucleinopathies by preventing Charnoly body formation and by acting as free radical scavengers. Charnoly bodies are formed due to mitochondrial degeneration as a consequence of free radical overproduction as the researchers have reported in our recent publications (Sharma et al., 2013a; Sharma et al., 2013b).

PERSONALIZED THERANOSTICS OF MS

Evidence-Based Personalized Treatment of MS The advent of a large number of new therapies for MS warrants the development of tools that enable selection of the best treatment option for each new patient with MS. Evidence from clinical trials supports the efficacy of

IFN-β for the treatment of MS, but few factors that predict a response to this drug in individual patients have emerged. This deficit could be due to the lack of definition of the clinical outcomes that signify improvement or worsening of the disease. MRI biomarkers and clinical relapses have been widely studied factors to predict long-term response to IFN-β, although the results are conflicting. Recently Sormani and Stefano (2013) provided MRI and clinical biomarkers as a useful approach for the management of patients with MS. These investigators focused on the definitions of clinical response to IFN-β and explored the biomarkers that can be used to predict response and highlighted the advantages and limitations of the scoring systems in light of biomarkers and other classes of emerging therapies for MS. A French multicentric phase IV study of Natalizumab (NTZ)-treated RRMS patients collected clinical, radiological and biological data on 1204 patients starting NTZ, and evaluated the clinical/radiological response to NTZ after 2 years of treatment. Patients starting NTZ at 18 French MS centres since June 2007 were included. Good response to NTZ was defined by the absence of clinical and radiological activity. Data focussed on patients who started NTZ at least 2 years ago. The proportion of patients without combined disease activity was 45.59% during the first two successive years of treatment. Systematic dosage of anti-NTZ antibodies (Abs) detected only two supplementary patients with anti-NTZ Abs compared with strict application of recommendations. A decrease of IgG, M concentrations at 2 years of treatment was found. The efficacy of NTZ therapy on RRMS was confirmed in the BIONAT cohort, suggesting that the identification of biomarkers predicting response to NTZ therapy and adverse events is very important.

Endogenous Retroviruses of the HERV-W Family, as Biomarkers Several viruses have been reported as co-factors triggering the pathogenesis of MS, including the endogenous retroviruses of the HERV-W family, that were also proposed as biomarkers of disease progression and therapy outcome. Arru et al. (2013) performed a study to clarify whether in MS patients treatment with Natalizumab has effects on MSRV/Syncytin-1/HERV-W expression and the possible relationship with disease outcome. Peripheral blood mononuclear cells were collected from 22 patients with RRMS, at entry and after 3, 6, and 12 months of treatment with Natalizumab. The cell subpopulations and the expression of MSRVenv/syncytin-1/HERV-Wenv were analyzed by flow cytometry and by discriminatory env-specific RT-PCR assays. By flow cytometry the relative amounts of T, NK and monocyte subpopulations remained fairly constant. A relative increase of B lymphocytes was observed at 3 to 6 months. The MSRVenv and Syncitin-1 transcripts were reduced at six to 12 months of therapy. Accordingly, the plasma-membrane levels of the HERV-Wenv protein were reduced. B cells, NK and monocytes but not T cells expressing the HERV-Wenv protein. None of the patients relapsed during therapy suggesting that Natalizumab treatment downregulates MSRV/Syncytin-1/HERV-W expression.

IFN-β Treatment in MS Neutralizing antibodies (NAb) affect efficacy of Interferon-β (IFN-β) treatment in MS patients. NAbs evolve in up to 44% of treated patients, between 6-18 months on therapy. To investigate whether early binding antibody (BAb) titers or different IFN-β biomarkers predict NAb evolution, Hegen et al. (2013) included patients with MS or clinically isolated syndrome (CIS) receiving IFN-β treatment. Blood samples were collected at baseline, before and after the first IFN-β administration, and again after 3, 12 and 24 months for the determination of NAbs, BAbs, gene expression of MxA, and protein concentrations of MMP-9, TIMP-1, sTRAIL, CXCL-10 and CCL-2. 22 of 164 patients developed NAbs during a median time of 23.8 months on IFN-b treatment. Of these patients,

78.9% were BAb-positive after 3 months. BAb titers ≥ 1:2400 predicted NAb evolution with a sensitivity of 74.7% and a specificity of 98.5%. MxA levels were diminished in the BAb/NAb-positive samples; similarly, CXCL-10 and sTRAIL concentrations in BAb/NAb-positive and BAb-positive/NAb-negative samples were also diminished compared to BAb/NAb-negative samples. Hence BAb titers can reliably predict NAbs. CXCL-10 is a sensitive biomarker for IFN-β response and its abrogation by anti-IFN-β antibodies. Fernandez et al. (2013) prepared Post-ECTRIMS review which discusses the biology of recovery and remyelination in MS as well as the different repair and endogenous and exogenous remyelination strategies being evaluated based on the fact that resident microglia and oligodendroglial progenitor cells (OPC) were implicated in the remyelination process. These authors also discussed the current state and future use of biomarkers in MS and proposed as markers of neurodegeneration the following: *T2 lesion volume and brain atrophy using MRI and the loss of the ganglion cell layer as assessed by optical coherence tomography*. Future utility for double inversion recovery (DIR) sequences was proposed to correlate cognitive impairment with MS impairment, given its higher diagnostic yield in locating and defining cortical lesions.

Alemtuzumab for RRMS Treatment Alemtuzumab (previously known as Campath (®)) is a humanized monoclonal antibody directed against the CD52 antigen on mature lymphocytes that results in lymphopenia and subsequent modification of the immune repertoire. Brown and Coles (2013) explored evidence for its efficacy and safety in RRMS. One Phase II and two Phase III trials of Alemtuzumab versus active comparator (Interferon β-1a) have been reported. Two of these rater-blinded randomized studies assessed clinical and radiological outcomes in treatment-naïve patients; one explored patients who had relapsed despite first-line therapy. Compared to interferon β-1a, Alemtuzumab reduced the relapse rate by 49%-74%, and in two studies it reduced the risk of sustained disability accumulation by 42%-71%. In one study there was no significant difference compared to interferon, perhaps reflecting the surprisingly low frequency of disability events in the comparator group. After Alemtuzumab, the Expanded Disability Status Scale score improved by 0.14-1.2 points, culminating in a net advantage with Alemtuzumab of 0.41-0.77 points over interferon in the CAMMS223 and CARE-MS2 trials. Radiological biomarkers of new lesion formation and brain atrophy following Alemtuzumab were improved when compared to interferon in all studies. Adverse events were more common following Alemtuzumab than Interferon β-1a (7.2-8.66 versus 4.9-5.7 events per person-year). While infusion reactions are the most common, autoimmunity is the most concerning; within Phase III studies, thyroid disorders (17%-18% versus 5%-6%) and immune thrombocytopenic purpura (1% versus 0%) were reported in patients taking Alemtuzumab and Interferon β-1a, respectively. All patients responded to conventional therapy. One patient taking Alemtuzumab in the Phase II study suffered a fatal intracranial hemorrhage following immune thrombocytopenic purpura, heralding assiduous monitoring of all patients thereafter.

Mesenchymal Stem Cells Treatment in MS Kassis et al. (2013) reported that several animal studies and few pilot clinical trials have tested the therapeutic potential of mesenchymal stem cells (MSC) in EAE and in MS. In almost all of the preclinical studies, healthy animals (or humans) served as donors of the MSCs which does not accurately simulate the clinical situation of autologous transplantation in patients with MS. These researchers used MSC isolated from mice with EAE in order to mimic human autologous transplantation and to test if the inflammatory process affects the functional properties of

MSC. MSCEAE retained their mesodermal features (*as evidenced by the expression of surface cell biomarkers and their ability to differentiate toward cells of the mesodermal lineage*). Moreover, MSCEAE were able to support neurite outgrowth in the N2A cell line and to suppress the proliferation of lymphocytes induced by the mitogen phytohaemagglutinin (PHA). I.V administration of MSCEAE suppressed the clinical course of EAE (*0% mortality, disease score vs. mortality and EAE score in saline-treated controls*), paralleled by a strong reduction of CNS inflammation and demyelination. These beneficial effects were indistinguishable from the effects induced by MSC obtained from healthy syngeneic donors demonstrating that the inflammatory process in EAE does not exert any deleterious effect on the functional/biological properties of the MSC and provide additional support for the use of autologous MSC that are obtained from MS-patients, in future clinical applications.

Natalizumab is a monoclonal antibody used to treat MS. Tasset et al. (2013) determined whether the protective action of Natalizumab involved a reduction in oxidative damage. Twenty-two MS patients fulfilling the revised McDonald criteria were assigned to treatment with 300 mg Natalizumab i. v. once monthly in accordance with Spanish guidelines. *Carbonylated proteins, 8-hydroxy-2'-deoxyguanosine, total Glutathione, reduced Glutathione, superoxide dismutase, Glutathione peroxidase, and myeloperoxidase levels were measured at baseline and after 14 months' treatment, and the antioxidant gap was calculated.* Natalizumab reduced oxidative-damage biomarker levels, together with a reduction in myeloperoxidase levels and in the myeloperoxidase/neutrophil granulocyte ratio. Natalizumab also induced nuclear translocation of Nrf2 and a fall in serum vascular cell adhesion molecule-1 levels suggesting that it has a beneficial effect on oxidative damage observed in MS patients. In addition, Fingolimod (FTY720) is an orally available sphingosine-1-phosphate (S1P) receptor modulator reducing relapse frequency in patients with RRMS. In addition to immunosuppression, neuronal protection by FTY720 has also been suggested, but remains controversial. Wang et al. (2013) employed axial and radial diffusivities derived from DTI as noninvasive biomarkers of axonal injury and demyelination to assess axonal protection by FTY720 in EAE mice. EAE was induced through active immunization of C57BL/6 mice using myelin oligodendrocyte glycoprotein peptide (MOG35-55). These investigators evaluated both the prophylactic and therapeutic treatment effect of FTY720 at doses of 3 and 10 mg/kg on EAE mice by daily clinical scoring and end-point *in vivo* DTI. Prophylactic administration of FTY720 suppressed the disease onset and prevented axon and myelin damage when compared with EAE mice without treatment. Therapeutic treatment by FTY720 did not prevent EAE onset, but reduced disease severity, improving axial and radial diffusivity towards the control values. *In vivo* DTI-derived axial and radial diffusivity correlated with clinical scores in EAE mice supporting the use of DTI as an effective biomarker for drug development. Schwab et al. (2013) performed a study to find biomarkers for patients at risk to develop progressive multifocal leukoencephalopathy (PML) during Natalizumab treatment. Patients were recruited from 10 European and US cohorts. Of 289 patients with MS, 224 had been treated with Natalizumab (18-80 months), 21 received other immune-modulatory treatments, and 28 were untreated. Eight of Natalizumab PML patients had given blood before the diagnosis of PML. These investigators also analyzed non-Natalizumab-treated patients who developed PML and age- and sex-matched healthy donors. Flow cytometric assessment was done on previously cryopreserved, viable peripheral blood mononuclear cells. The percentage of l-selectin-expressing CD4+ T cells was lower in patients treated with Natalizumab (when compared with patients not receiving Natalizumab or healthy controls. Lower percentage was correlated with the risk of developing PML in the patient group with available pre-PML samples when compared with non-PML Natalizumab-treated patients. Samples were gathered between 4 and 26 months before PML diagnosis. The cell-based assessment of the percentage of l-selectin-expressing CD4 T cells could provide a biomarker for PML risk assessment.

Therapeutic Response to Eculizumab in MS Complement activation after binding of an IgG autoantibody to aquaporin 4 (AQP4) is thought to be a major determinant of CNS inflammation and astrocytic injury in neuromyelitis optica. Pittock et al. (2013) investigated the use of Eculizumab--a therapeutic monoclonal IgG that neutralizes the complement protein C5--in neuromyelitis optica spectrum disorders. These investigators recruited patients from two US centres into an open-label trial. Patients were AQP4-IgG-seropositive, aged at least 18 years, had a neuromyelitis optica spectrum disorder, and had at least two attacks in the preceding 6 months or three in the previous 12 months. Patients received meningococcal vaccine at a screening visit and 2 weeks later began Eculizumab treatment. They received 600 mg intravenous Eculizumab weekly for 4 weeks, 900 mg in the fifth week, and then 900 mg every 2 weeks for 48 weeks. The primary endpoints were efficacy and safety. Secondary endpoints were disability (measured by expanded disability status scale), ambulation (Hauser score), and visual acuity. At follow-up visits, complete neurological examination was undertaken and an adverse event questionnaire completed. 14 women patients were enrolled. After 12 months of Eculizumab treatment, 12 patients were relapse free; two had had possible attacks. The median number of attacks per year fell from three before treatment to zero during treatment. No patient had worsened disability by any outcome measure. Median score on the expanded disability status scale improved from 4·3 before treatment to 3·5 during treatment. Two patients improved by two points and three improved by one point on the Hauser score; no change was recorded for the other patients. Visual acuity had improved in at least one eye by one point in four patients, and by two points in one patient; no change was recorded for other patients. One patient had meningococcal sepsis and sterile meningitis about 2 months after the first Eculizumab infusion, but resumed treatment after full recovery. No other drug-related serious adverse events occurred. Eight attacks in five patients were reported within 12 months of Eculizumab withdrawal. Eculizumab was well tolerated, significantly reduced attack frequency, and stabilized or improved neurological disability measures in patients with aggressive neuromyelitis optica spectrum disorders.

Ferreira et al. (2013) reviewed studies on Glutathione, one of the most important agents of the endogenous antioxidant defense system, protecting cells from damage caused by oxidative stress. It evaluated Glutathione and the enzymes Glutathione peroxidase and Glutathione reductase in various forms and stages of the disease. It is imperative to achieve a consensus on the pathogenesis responsible for severe disability, and explore sensitive biomarkers of its progression and indicators of oxidative stress. It is also important to promote the development of new therapies, with more studies on other substances such as Acrolein, Lipoic acid and Dimethyl Fumarate. Clarification of the mechanisms involved in oxidative stress, in different forms of MS, could result in improvements in the prognosis of the disease, with increase in a patient's quality of life. In the last few years, studies have expanded our understanding of demographic and presenting features for optic neuritis in the pediatric population. Collinge and Sprunger (2013) reported that pediatric optic neuritis is a rare disorder with significant distinctions from its adult counterpart. Recognizing the features of this disorder and the potential association with progressive demyelinating processes is important for patients' evaluation and prognosis. Emerging research on biomarkers and optical coherence tomography offers potential prognostic value in patient management. In addition, research data have allowed for better understanding of the risks factors for progression from isolated optic neuritis to systemic demyelinating processes, such as MS. Although definitive evidence is lacking, corticosteroids remain the cornerstone of treatment. Various other immunosuppressive therapy studies have also reported success, particularly in refractory cases. Furthermore, Fialova et al. (2013) examined CSF and serum NFL levels and IgG antibodies against NFL in 19 patients with a clinically isolated syndrome (CIS) early converted into MS, 20 CIS-non-converters, 23 MS patients and 32 controls. CSF NFL levels were higher in all patient groups. The highest CSF or intrathecally synthesized anti-NFL antibodies and CSF/serum ratios of anti-NFL antibodies were observed in CIS-converters suggesting that CSF NFL and/or IT anti-NFL antibodies could be biomarkers of axonal injury in early MS.

Munoz et al. (2013) performed a study to correlate body mass index (BMI) or biomarkers with the frequency of common adverse events (AEs) with subcutaneous IFN β-1a during treatment in patients with RRMS previously naïve to IFN β. Eighty-four patients were followed up during 8 weeks, 25.3% were overweight and 14.5% were obese. Biomarkers steadily increased during all study period by 45.3% for β2-Microglobulin, 262.8% for Oligoadenylate synthetase-1, and 92.8% for Neopterin. Overall AE reporting did not vary with the dose or treatment duration. BMI was not predictive of increased risk for AEs. Biomarkers did not discriminate on the frequency of any AE either.

Fluorescent pigments are the end-products of reactions involving free radical attack on biological molecules and can be formed, for example, in reactions between lipid peroxidation products, mainly unsaturated aldehydes, with free amino groups. Their emission maximum was found to be at 420-470 nm after being excited at 340-390 nm. The mechanism of their formation and chemical identity has been revealed in in-vitro studies, in which reactive aldehydes were incubated with amino group-containing molecules. Owing to their intrinsic fluorescent properties and molecular stability these products are easily measured by means of spectrofluorimetry and are used as biomarkers of oxidative stress. It has been found that the fluorescent products are formed with increased free radical production, such as atherosclerosis, AD and MS. Ivica et al. (2013) searched the literature using "MEDLINE" and "Web of Science" in order to get an overview of the state of knowledge about fluorescent products of free radicals, that is, their analysis from *in vitro* studies, animal and human studies and their use as biomarkers of oxidative damage. Although their chemical structure may not have been elucidated, the fluorophores formed in this way have found application as biomarkers of oxidative stress. *In vitro* experiments using model reactions have given some clues as to how certain fluorescent pigments arise during oxidative reactions *in vivo*. Advances in analytical techniques should lead the chemical characterization of pigments of different origin to completeness.

Hirsch et al. (2013) reported that JC polyomavirus (JCPyV) was the first of now 12 PyVs detected in humans, when in 1964, PyV particles were revealed by E.M in progressive multifocal leukoencephalopathy (PML) tissues. JCPyV infection is common in 35-70% of the general population, and the virus thereafter persists in the renourinary tract. One third of healthy adults asymptomatically shed JCPyV at ~50,000 copies/mL urine. PML is rare having an incidence of <0.3 per 100,000 person years in the general population. This increased to 2.4

per 1000 person years in HIV-AIDS patients without combination antiretroviral therapy (cART). Recently, PML emerged in MS patients treated with Natalizumab to 2.13 cases per 1000 patients. Natalizumab blocks α4-integrin-dependent lymphocyte homing to the brain suggesting that not the overall cellular immunodeficiency but local failure of brain immune surveillance is a pivotal factor for PML. Recovering JCPyV-specific immune control, e.g., by starting cART or discontinuing Natalizumab, improves PML survival, but is challenged by the immune reconstitution inflammatory syndrome. Important steps of PML pathogenesis are undefined, and antiviral therapies are lacking. New clues might come from molecular and functional profiling of JCPyV and PML pathology and comparison with other replicative pathologies such as granule cell neuronopathy and meningoencephalitis, and non-replicative JCPyV pathology possibly contributing to some malignancies.

CONCLUSION

Biomarkers capable of predicting the clinical course and the rate of disease progression in MS are currently unavailable. Of treatable inflammatory CNS disorders, neurofilaments are promising candidates to fulfil this task. There is no single test that is diagnostic for MS, and existing diagnostic criteria are inadequate which can lead to diagnostic delay. Some patients require multiple (sometimes invasive) investigations, and extensive clinical follow-up to confirm or exclude a diagnosis of MS. There is an urgent need for biomarkers in MS that can reliably determine ongoing disease activity relative to *inflammation, neurodegeneration, and demyelination/remyelination.* Myelin basic proteins in MS. α4 integrin, is effective against active RRMS. CD44 deficiency, HLA-DRB1 polymorphisms, oligoclonal bands, vitamin D, and conventional and nonconventional imaging techniques. Moreover, TOB-1 polymorphisms, cytotoxic NKG2C+ CD4 T cells, spinal PKCγ on regulating pain sensitivity, impaired locomotor function, and idiopathic intermediate uveitis (IIU) are inflammatory disorders noticed in RRMS patients. The detection of monomeric and dimeric κ- and λ-FLC facilitate in the precise diagnosis of MS as urinary metabolites. In addition, oligoclonal protein bands (OCBs) can be measured in CSF. Kappa and lambda free light chain (FLC), Neopterin, Fetuin-A, and ubiquitin C-terminal hydrolase-L1 (UCHL1) can be measured in CSF and urine of MS patients. OCBs unique to the CSF are used in the diagnosis of MS. Myelin basic proteins and α4 integrin are effective against active RRMS. CD44 deficiency, HLA-DRB1 polymorphisms, vitamin D, and conventional and nonconventional imaging techniques can be used as biomarkers for the EBPT of RRMS. Moreover, recently characterized TOB-1 polymorphisms, cytotoxic NKG2C+ CD4 T cells, spinal PKCγ on regulating pain sensitivity have a significant role in locomotor function. In addition, CD20, elevated sCD146. CD44 is a key molecule in the migration of OPCs. Overactivation of CD4(+) T cells, especially the Th1 and Th17 subpopulations. Low density lipoprotein receptor-related protein-1 (LRP1), Muc1 plays an anti-inflammatory role in EAE. Muc1 is a membrane tethered glycoprotein. MRI-based brain volumetry, differential lymphocyte reconstitution after Alemtuzumab treatment may be a biomarker for RRMS. Increased synthesis of IgG and APRIL (a proliferation-inducing ligand) are frequently observed in patients with MS. MC-deficient Kit/Kit mice display increased neurodegeneration in the lesion area after brain trauma. Epigenetic changes to DNA influence gene expression without altering the underlying DNA sequence. *DNA methylation, histone modification, and miRNA-associated silencing are the most important epigenetic mechanisms that influence gene expression.* Gd-enhanced MRI can be used to determine the stuctural and functional intectness of BBB in MS. CSF-SOD, abnormal myelin hypercitrullination, even in normal-appearing white matter, by peptidylarginine deiminases (PADs) correlate with disease severity and might have an important role in MS progression.

MicroRNA let-7e. CD226 Gly307Ser (rs763361) is associated with the risk of autoimmune diseases. Reduced CSF levels of Aβ and soluble APP (sAPP) fragments are reported in inflammatory diseases, including MS; but the precise pathway of APP metabolism and whether it can be affected by disease-modifying treatments remains unclear. 24S-Hydroxycholesterol in plasma and FasL expression of astrocytes plays an important role in the control and elimination of autoimmune T cells from the CNS, thereby determining recovery from EAE. Response gene to complement (RGC)-32, BDNF in MS. Enhanced mB7-H3 expression and reduced sB7-H3 levels in MS patients. Translocator protein 18 kDa (TSPO) expression is enhanced in MS patients. Isoprostanes (IsoP) are sensitive biomarkers of oxidative stress. CSF IsoP might be useful biomarkers of tissue damage in MS. A reduction of angiotensin II and angiotensin converting enzyme (ACE) 2 levels, and an increase in ACE level in CSF from patients with MS. β-1,4-GalT-I might serve as an inflammatory mediator regulating adhesion and migration of inflammatory cells in EAE, possibly through influencing the modification of galactosylated carbohydrate chains to modulate selectin-ligand biosynthesis and interaction with E-selectin. NFL, GFAP and β-Tub II proteins are significantly higher in MS. CD70: being a therapeutic target in human MS, can be used as a theranostic biomarker in MS.

A theranostic biomarker that is pathologically specific for the inflammatory demyelination in MS could overhaul current diagnostic algorithms. To prospectively assess the diagnostic value of visualizing central veins in brain lesions with MRI for patients with possible MS for whom the diagnosis is uncertain. MS is a classic multifactorial disease in which etiology interaction of external factors and structural features of a large number of genes plays an important role. Identifying risk factors for MS and creating an integrated model of pathogenesis are urgent tasks of neurology. Revealing true risk factors is possible only in studies with sufficient statistical power with a large amount of samples.

In summary; *(a) a definitive diagnostic biomarker for MS is direly needed; (b) a combination of biomarkers may facilitate personalized MS diagnosis and treatment; (c) clinical significance of B7-H3 in MS remains unknown; (d) HLA-DRB1 polymorphisms, OCBs, and MBPs are conventional biomarkers of MS; (e) neuroimaging with specific PET radioligands may facilitate MS diagnosis; and (f) α-synuclein index (SI) and Charnoly body may be used as emerging biomarkers of MS.*

REFERENCES

Adzemovic, M. Z., Zeitelhofer, M., Eriksson, U., Olsson, T. & Nilsson, I. (2013). Imatinib ameliorates neuroinflammation in a rat model of multiple sclerosis by enhancing blood-brain barrier integrity and by modulating the peripheral immune response. *PLoS One.*, *8*(2), e56586.

Agrawal, S. M., Williamson, J., Sharma, R., Kebir, H., Patel, K., Prat, A. & Yong, V. W. (2013). Extracellular MMPs inducer shows active perivascular cuffs in multiple sclerosis. *Brain.*, *136*, 1760-1777.

Annunziata, P., Cioni, C., Cantalupo, L., Di Genova, G., Savellini, G. G. & Cusi, G. (2013). Immunosuppressive monoclonal antibody to CD64 from patients with long-term stable multiple sclerosis. *J. Neuroimmunol.*, *256*, 62-70.

Annunziata, P., Cioni, C., Cantalupo, L., Di Genova, G., Savellini, G. G. & Cusi, G. (2013). Immunosuppressive monoclonal antibody to CD64 from patients with long-term stable multiple sclerosis. *J. Neuroimmunol.*, *256*, 62-70.

Antonelli, T., Tomasini, M. C., Castellazzi, M., Sola, P., Tamborino, C., Ferraro, D., Ferraro, L. & Granieri, E. (2013). Biological markers in cerebrospinal fluid for axonal impairment in multiple sclerosis: acetylcholinesterase activity cannot be considered a useful biomarker. *Neurol Sci.*, *34*, 769-71.

Arru, G., Leoni, S., Pugliatti, M., Mei, A., Serra, C., Delogu, L. G., Manetti, R., Dolei, A., Sotgiu, S. & Mameli, G. (2013). Natalizumab inhibits the expression of human endogenous retroviruses of the W family in multiple sclerosis patients: a longitudinal cohort study. *Mult Scler.*, Jul 22.

Ashbaugh, J. J., Brambilla, R., Karmally, S. A., Cabello, C., Malek, T. R. & Bethea, J. R. (2013). IL7Rα contributes to experimental autoimmune encephalomyelitis through altered T cell responses and nonhematopoietic cell lineages. *J Immunol.*, *190*(9), 4525-434.

Atan, D., Heissigerova, J., Kuffová, L., Hogan, A., Kilmartin, D. J., Forrester, J. V., Bidwell, J. L., Dick, A. D. & Churchill, A. J. (2013). Tumor necrosis factor polymorphisms associated with tumor necrosis factor production influence the risk of idiopathic intermediate uveitis. *Mol Vis.*, *19*, 184-195.

Augutis, K., Axelsson, M., Portelius, E., Brinkmalm, G., Andreasson, U., Gustavsson, M. K., Malmeström, C., Lycke, J., Blennow, K., Zetterberg, H. & Mattsson, N. (2013). Cerebrospinal fluid biomarkers of β-amyloid metabolism in multiple sclerosis. *Mult. Scler.*, *19*, 543-52.

Axelsson, M., Malmeström, C., Gunnarsson, M., Zetterberg, H., Sundström, P., Lycke, J. & Svenningsson, A. (2013). Immunosuppressive therapy reduces axonal damage in progressive multiple sclerosis. *Mult. Scler.*, May 23.

Ayoglu, B., Häggmark, A., Khademi, M., Olsson, T., Uhlén, M., Schwenk, J. M. & Nilsson, P. (2013). Autoantibody profiling in multiple sclerosis using arrays of human protein fragments. *Mol. Cell Proteomics.*, *12*(9), 2657-2672.

Ayzenberg, I., Kleiter, I., Schröder, A., Hellwig, K., Chan, A., Yamamura, T. & Gold, R. (2013). Interleukin 6 receptor blockade in patients with neuromyelitis optica nonresponsive to anti-CD20 therapy. *JAMA Neurol.*, *70*, 394-397.

Benedek, G., Meza-Romero, R., Andrew, S., Leng, L., Burrows, G. G., Bourdette, D., Offner, H., Bucala, R., Vandenbark, A. A. & Partial, (2013). M.H.C. class II constructs inhibit MIF/CD74 binding and downstream effects. *Eur. J. Immunol.*, *43*, 1309-1321.

Brown, J. W. & Coles, A. J. (2013). Alemtuzumab: evidence for its potential in relapsing-remitting multiple sclerosis. *Drug Des Devel Ther.*, *7*, 131-138.

Buck, D., Albrecht, E., Aslam, M., Goris, A., Hauenstein, N. & Jochim, A. (2013). International Multiple Sclerosis Genetics Consortium; Wellcome Trust Case Control Consortium, Cepok S, Grummel V, Dubois B, Berthele A, Lichtner P, Gieger C,

Winkelmann J, Hemmer B. Genetic variants in the immunoglobulin heavy chain locus are associated with the IgG index in multiple sclerosis. *Ann Neurol.*, *73*(1), 86-94.

Cesinaro, A. M., Lonardi, S. & Facchetti, F. (2013). Granuloma faciale: a cutaneous lesion sharing features with IgG4-associated sclerosing diseases. *Am. J. Surg. Pathol.*, *37*, 66-73.

Chanson, J. B., de Seze, J., Eliaou, J. F. & Vincent, T. (2013). Immunological follow-up of patients with neuromyelitis optica: is there a good biomarker? *Lupus.*, *22*, 229-232.

Coen, M., Menegatti, E., Salvi, F., Mascoli, F., Zamboni, P., Gabbiani, G. & Bochaton-Piallat, M. L. (2013). Altered collagen expression in jugular veins in multiple sclerosis. *Cardiovasc Pathol.*, *22*, 33-38.

Collinge, J. E. & Sprunger, D. T. (2013). Update in pediatric optic neuritis. *Curr Opin Ophthalmol.*, *24*, 448-452.

Comabella, M., Caminero, A. B., Malhotra, S., Agulló, L., Fernández, O., Reverter, F., Vandenbroeck, K., Rodríguez-Antigüedad, A., Matesanz, F., Izquierdo, G., Urcelay, E., López-Larios, A., Sánchez, A., Otero, S., Tintoré, M. & Montalban, X. (2013). TNFRSF1A polymorphisms rs1800693 and rs4149584 in patients with multiple sclerosis. *Neurology.*, *80*, 2010-2016.

Coquet, J. M., Middendorp, S., van der Horst, G., Kind, J., Veraar, E. A., Xiao, Y., Jacobs, H. & Borst, J. (2013). The CD27 and CD70 costimulatory pathway inhibits effector function of T helper 17 cells and attenuates associated autoimmunity. *Immunity.*, *38*, 53-65.

Cossburn, M. D., Harding, K., Ingram, G., El-Shanawany, T., Heaps, A., Pickersgill, T. P., Jolles, S. & Robertson, N. P. (2013). Clinical relevance of differential lymphocyte recovery after Alemtuzumab therapy for multiple sclerosis. *Neurology.*, *80*, 55-61.

Cyranoski, D. (2013). China drugs head fired over article row. *Nature.*, *498*, 283-284.

D'Amico, E., Factor-Litvak, P., Santella, R. M. & Mitsumoto, H. (2013). Clinical perspective on oxidative stress in sporadic amyotrophic lateral sclerosis. *Free Radic Biol Med.*, *655*, 509-527.

Darlington, P. J., Touil, T., Doucet, J. S., Gaucher, D., Zeidan, J., Gauchat, D., Corsini, R., Kim, H. J., Duddy, M., Jalili, F., Arbour, N., Kebir, H., Chen, J., Arnold, D. L., Bowman, M., Antel, J., Prat, A., Freedman, M. S., Atkins, H., Sekaly, R., Cheynier, R. & Bar-Or, A. (2013). Canadian MS/BMT Study Group. Diminished Th17 (not Th1) responses underlie multiple sclerosis disease abrogation after hematopoietic stem cell transplantation. *Ann Neurol.*, *73*(3), 341-354.

Deboux, C., Ladraa, S., Cazaubon, S., Ghribi-Mallah, S., Weiss, N., Chaverot, N., Couraud, P. O. & Baron-Van Evercooren, A. (2013). Overexpression of CD44 in neural precursor cells improves trans-endothelial migration and facilitates their invasion of perivascular tissues *in vivo*. *PLoS One.*, *8*, e57430.

Dhib-Jalbut, S., Sumandeep, S., Valenzuela, R., Ito, K., Patel, P. & Rametta, M. (2013). Immune response during interferon beta-1b treatment in patients with multiple sclerosis who experienced relapses and those who were relapse-free in the START study. *J. Neuroimmunol.*, *254*, 131-140.

Dinkin, M. & Paul, F. (2013). Higher macular volume in patients with MS receiving fingolimod: positive outcome or side effect? *Neurology.*, *80*, 128-129.

Dobson, R., Ramagopalan, S., Davis, A. & Giovannoni, G. (2013). Cerebrospinal fluid oligoclonal bands in multiple sclerosis and clinically isolated syndromes: a meta-analysis of prevalence, prognosis and effect of latitude. *J Neurol Neurosurg Psychiatry.*, *84*, 909-914.

Dobson, R., Topping, J., Davis, A., Thompson, E. & Giovannoni, G. (2013). Cerebrospinal fluid and urinary biomarkers in multiple sclerosis. *Acta Neurol Scand.*, *128*(5), 321-327.

Duan, H., Luo, Y., Hao, H., Feng, L., Zhang, Y., Lu, D., Xing, S., Feng, J., Yang, D., Song, L. & Yan, X. (2013). Soluble CD146 in cerebrospinal fluid of active multiple sclerosis. *Neuroscience.*, *235*, 16-26.

Evsyukova, I., Bradrick, S. S., Gregory, S. G. & Garcia-Blanco, M. A. (2013). Cleavage and polyadenylation specificity factor 1 (CPSF1) regulates alternative splicing of interleukin 7 receptor (IL7R) exon 6. *RNA.*, *19*(1), 103-115.

Fazekas, C., Khalil, M., Enzinger, C., Matzer, F., Fuchs, S. & Fazekas, F. (2013). No impact of adult attachment and temperament on clinical variability in patients with clinically isolated syndrome and early multiple sclerosis. *Clin Neurol Neurosurg.*, *115*(3), 293-297.

Fernández Carbonell, C. & Chitnis, T. (2013). Inflammatory demyelinating diseases in children: an update. *Minerva Pediatr.*, *65*(3), 307-323.

Fernandez, O., Arnal-Garcia, C., Arroyo-Gonzalez, R., Brieva, L., Calles-Hernandez, MC., et al., (2013). Review of the novelties presented at the 28th Congress of the European Committee for Treatment and Research in Multiple Sclerosis (ECTRIMS) (II). *Rev Neurol.*, *57*(6), 269-281.

Fernández, Ó., Arroyo-González, R., Rodríguez-Antigüedad, A., García-Merino, J. A., Comabella, M., Villar, L. M., Izquierdo, G., Tintoré, M., Oreja-Guevara, C., Álvarez-Cermeño, J. C., Meca-Lallana, J. E., Prieto, J. M., Ramió-Torrentà, L., Martínez-Yélamos, S. & Montalban, X. (2013). [Biomarkers in multiple sclerosis]. *Rev Neurol.*, *56*(7), 375-390.

Fernández, O. (2013). Integrating the tools for an individualized prognosis in multiple sclerosis. *J Neurol Sci.*, *331*, 10-13.

Fernandez-Castaneda, A., Arandjelovic, S., Stiles, T. L., Schlobach, R. K., Mowen, K. A., Gonias, S. L. & Gaultier, A. (2013). Identification of the low density lipoprotein (LDL) receptor-related protein-1 interactome in central nervous system myelin suggests a role in the clearance of necrotic cell debris. *J. Biol. Chem.*, *288*, 4538-4548.

Ferraro, D., Simone, A. M., Bedin, R., Galli, V., Vitetta, F., Federzoni, L., D'Amico, R., Merelli, E., Nichelli, P. F. & Sola, P. (2013). Cerebrospinal fluid oligoclonal IgM bands predict early conversion to clinically definite multiple sclerosis in patients with clinically isolated syndrome. *J Neuroimmunol.*, *257*, 76-81.

Ferreira, B., Mendes, F., Osório, N., Caseiro, A., Gabriel, A. & Valado, A. (2013). Glutathione in multiple sclerosis. *Br. J. Biomed. Sci.*, *70*(2), 75-79.

Fialová, L., Bartos, A., Svarcová, J., Zimova, D., Kotoucova, J. & Malbohan, I. (2013). Serum and cerebrospinal fluid light neurofilaments and antibodies against them in clinically isolated syndrome and multiple sclerosis. *J. Neuroimmunol.*, *262*(1-2), 113-120.

Filippi, M., Absinta, M. & Rocca, M. A. (2013). Future MRI tools in multiple sclerosis. *J. Neurol. Sci.*, *331*, 14-18.

Filippi, M., Agosta, F., Spinelli, E. G. & Rocca, M. A. (2013). Imaging resting state brain function in multiple sclerosis. *J. Neurol.*, *260*(7), 1709-1713.

Filippi, M., Evangelou, N., Kangarlu, A., Inglese, M., Mainero, C., Horsfield, M. A. & Rocca, M. A. (2014). Ultra-high-field MR imaging in multiple sclerosis. *J Neurol Neurosurg Psychiatry.*, *85*(1), 60-66.

Flynn, K. M., Michaud, M. & Madri, J. A. CD44 deficiency contributes to enhanced experimental autoimmune encephalomyelitis: a role in immune cells and vascular cells of the blood-brain barrier. *Am. J. Pathol.*, 2013 Apr, *182*(4), 1322-1336.

Gajofatto, A., Bongianni, M., Zanusso, G., Bianchi, M. R., Turatti, M., Benedetti, M. D. & Monaco, S. (2013). Clinical and biomarker assessment of demyelinating events suggesting multiple sclerosis. *Acta Neurol Scand.*, 2013 Apr 1.

García-Martín, E., Lorenzo-Betancor, O., Martínez, C., Pastor, P., Benito-León, J., Millán-Pascual, J., Calleja, P., Díaz-Sánchez, M., Pisa, D., Turpín-Fenoll, L., Alonso-Navarro, H, Ayuso-Peralta, L., Torrecillas, D., Lorenzo, E., Plaza-Nieto, J. F., Agúndez, J. A. & Jiménez-Jiménez, F. J. (2013). LINGO1 rs9652490 and rs11856808 polymorphisms are not associated with risk for multiple sclerosis. *BMC Neurol.*, *13*, 34.

Gardner, R. C., Valcour, V. & Yaffe, K. (2013). Dementia in the oldest old: a multi-factorial and growing public health issue. *Alzheimers Res Ther.*, *5*(4), 27.

Ge, Z., Da, Y., Xue, Z., Zhang, K., Zhuang, H., Peng, M., Li, Y., Li, W., Simard, A., Hao, J., Yao, Z. & Zhang, R. (2013). Vorinostat, a histone deacetylase inhibitor, suppresses dendritic cell function and ameliorates experimental autoimmune encephalomyelitis. *Exp Neurol.*, *241*, 56-66.

Gebregiworgis, T., Massilamany, C., Gangaplara, A., Thulasingam, S., Kolli, V., Werth, M. T., Dodds, E. D., Steffen, D., Reddy, J. & Powers, R. (2013). Potential of urinary metabolites for diagnosing multiple sclerosis. *ACS Chem Biol.*, *8*(4), 684-690.

Giorgio, A. & De Stefano, N. (2013). Clinical use of brain volumetry. *J. Magn. Reson. Imaging.*, *37*(1), 1-14.

GIroni, M., Saresella, M., Rovaris, M., Vaghi, M., Nemni, R., Clerici, M. & Grossi, E. (2013). A novel data mining system points out hidden relationships between immunological markers in multiple sclerosis. *Immun Ageing.*, *10*(1), 1.

González-Mendióroz, M., Alvarez-Vázquez, A. B. & Rubio-Martinez, J. (2013). Structural analysis of the inhibition of APRIL by TACI and BCMA through molecular dynamics simulations. *J Mol Graph Model.*, *39*, 13-22.

Gourraud, P. A., Sdika, M., Khankhanian, P., Henry, R. G., Beheshtian, A., Matthews, P. M., Hauser, S. L., Oksenberg, J. R., Pelletier, D. & Baranzini, S. E. (2013). A genome-wide association study of brain lesion distribution in multiple sclerosis. *Brain.*, *136*(Pt 4), 1012-1024.

Griffith, J. W. & Luster, A. D. (2013). Targeting cells in motion: migrating toward improved therapies. *Eur. J. Immunol.*, *43*(6), 1430-1235.

Guan, H., Fan, D., Mrelashvili, D., Hao, H., Singh, N. P., Singh, U. P., Nagarkatti, P. S. & Nagarkatti, M. (2013). MicroRNA let-7e is associated with the pathogenesis of experimental autoimmune encephalomyelitis. *Eur. J. Immunol.*, *43*(1), 104-114.

Guedes, J., Cardoso, A. L. & Pedroso de Lima, M. C. (2013). Involvement of microRNA in microglia-mediated immune response. *Clin. Dev. Immunol.*, 2013, 186872.

Hamann, I., Dörr, J., Glumm, R., Chanvillard, C., Janssen, A., Millward, J. M., Paul, F., Ransohoff, R. M. & Infante-Duarte, C. (2013). Characterization of natural killer cells in paired CSF and blood samples during neuroinflammation. *J. Neuroimmunol.*, *254*(1-2), 165-169.

Harberts, E., Datta, D., Chen, S., Wohler, J. E., Oh, U. & Jacobson, S. (2013). Translocator protein 18 kDa (TSPO) expression in multiple sclerosis patients. *J. Neuroimmune Pharmacol.*, *8*(1), 51-57.

Harris, V. K., Donelan, N., Yan, Q. J., Clark, K., Touray, A., Rammal, M. & Sadiq, S. A. (2013). Cerebrospinal fluid Fetuin-A is a biomarker of active multiple sclerosis. *Mult. Scler.*, *19*(11), 1462-1472.

Harrison, D. M., Shiee, N., Bazin, P. L., Newsome, S. D., Ratchford, J. N., Pham, D., Calabresi, P. A. & Reich, D. S. (2013). Tract-specific quantitative MRI better correlates with disability than conventional MRI in multiple sclerosis. *J Neurol.*, *260*(2), 397-406.

Havla, J., Lohse, P., Gerdes, L. A., Hohlfeld, R. & Kümpfel, T. (2013). Symptoms related to tumor necrosis factor receptor 1-associated periodic syndrome, multiple sclerosis, and severe rheumatoid arthritis in patients carrying the TNF receptor superfamily 1A D12E/p.Asp41Glu mutation. *J. Rheumatol.*, *40*(3), 261- 264.

Hegen, H., Millonig, A., Bertolotto, A., Comabella, M., Giovanonni, G., Guger, M., et al., (2014). Early detection of neutralizing antibodies to interferon-beta in multiple sclerosis patients: binding antibodies predict neutralizing antibody development. *Mult Scler.*, *20*(5), 577-587.

Heigl, F., Hettich, R., Arendt, R., Durner, J., Koehler, J. & Mauch, E. (2013). Immunoadsorption in steroid-refractory multiple sclerosis: clinical experience in 60 patients. *Atheroscler Suppl.*, *14*(1), 167-173.

Hendrickx, D. A., Koning, N., Schuurman, K. G., van Strien, M. E., van Eden, C. G., Hamann, J. & Huitinga, I. (2013). Selective upregulation of scavenger receptors in and around demyelinating areas in multiple sclerosis. *J. Neuropathol Exp. Neurol.*, *72*(2), 106-118.

Hendrix, S., Kramer, P., Pehl, D., Warnke, K., Boato, F., Nelissen, S., Lemmens, E., Pejler, G., Metz, M., Siebenhaar, F. & Maurer, M. (2013). Mast cells protect from post-traumatic brain inflammation by the mast cell-specific chymase mouse mast cell protease-4. *FASEB J.*, *27*(3), 920-929.

Hirsch, H. H., Kardas, P., Kranz, D. & Leboeuf, C. (2013). The human JC polyomavirus (JCPyV): virological background and clinical implications. *APMIS.*, *121*(8), 685-727.

Hong, G. U., Kim, N. G., Jeoung, D. & Ro, J. Y. (2013). Anti-CD40 Ab- or 8-oxo-dG-enhanced Treg cells reduce development of experimental autoimmune encephalomyelitis via down-regulating migration and activation of mast cells. *J. Neuroimmunol.*, *260*(1-2), 60-73.

Huang, H., Ito, K., Dangond, F. & Dhib-Jalbut, S. (2013). Effect of interferon beta-1a on B7.1 and B7.2 B-cell expression and its impact on T-cell proliferation. *J Neuroimmunol.*, *258*(1-2), 27-31.

Ilhan-Mutlu, A., Wagner, L., Widhalm, G., Wöhrer, A., Bartsch, S., Czech, T., Heinzl, H., Leutmezer, F., Prayer, D., Marosi, C., Base, W. & Preusser, M. (2013). Exploratory investigation of eight circulating plasma markers in brain tumor patients. *Neurosurg. Rev.*, *36*(1), 45-55.

Iñarrea, P., Alarcia, R., Alava, M. A., Capablo, J. L., Casanova, A., Iñiguez, C., Iturralde, M., Larrodé, P., Martín, J., Mostacero, E. & Ara, J. R. (2014). Mitochondrial Complex Enzyme Activities and Cytochrome c Expression Changes in Multiple Sclerosis. *Mol Neurobiol.*, *49*(1), 1-9.

Ivica, J. & Wilhelm, J. (2014). Lipophilic fluorescent products of free radicals. *Biomed Pap Med Fac Univ Palacky Olomouc Czech Repub.*, *158*(3), 365-372

Ji, Q., Castelli, L. & Goverman, J. M. (2013). MHC class I-restricted myelin epitopes are cross-presented by Tip-DCs that promote determinant spreading to CD8⁺ T cells. *Nat. Immunol.*, *14*(3), 254-261.

Jiang, J., Jiang, J., Liu, C., Zhang, G., Gao, L., Chen, Y., Zhu, R., Wang, T., Wang, F., Zhang, X. & Xue, Q. (2013). Enhancement of membrane B7-H3 costimulatory molecule but reduction of its soluble form in multiple sclerosis. *J Clin Immunol.*, *33*, 118-126.

Jin, X. F., Wu, N., Wang, L. & Li, J. (2013). Circulating microRNAs: a novel class of potential biomarkers for diagnosing and prognosing central nervous system diseases. *Cell Mol. Neurobiol.*, *33*(5), 601-613.

Kanekiyo, K., Inamori, K., Kitazume, S., Sato, K., Maeda, J., Higuchi, M., Kizuka, Y., Korekane, H., Matsuo, I., Honke, K. & Taniguchi, N. (2013). Loss of branched O-mannosyl glycans in astrocytes accelerates remyelination. *J. Neurosci.*, *33*(24), 10037-10047.

Kaplan, B., Golderman, S., Yahalom, G., Yeskaraev, R., Ziv, T., Aizenbud, B. M., Sela, B. A. & Livneh, A. (2013). Free light chain monomer-dimer patterns in the diagnosis of multiple sclerosis. *J Immunol Methods.*, *390*, 74-80.

Karlström, S., Nordvall, G., Sohn, D., Hettman, A., Turek, D., Åhlin, K., Kers, A., Claesson, M., Slivo, C., Lo-Alfredsson, Y., Petersson, C., Bessidskaia, G., Svensson, P. H., Rein, T., Jerning, E., Malmberg, Å., Ahlgen, C., Ray, C., Vares, L., Ivanov, V. & Johansson, R. (2013). Substituted 7-amino-5-thio-thiazolo[4,5-d]pyrimidines as potent and selective antagonists of the fractalkine receptor (CX3CR1). *J Med Chem.*, *56*(8), 3177-3190.

Karrenbauer, V. D., Prejs, R., Masterman, T., Hillert, J., Glaser, A. & Imrell, K. (2013). Impact of cerebrospinal-fluid oligoclonal immunoglobulin bands and HLA-DRB1 risk alleles on brain magnetic-resonance-imaging lesion load in Swedish multiple sclerosis patients. *J Neuroimmunol.*, *254*(1-2), 170-173.

Kassis, I., Petrou, P., Halimi, M. & Karussis, D. (2013). Mesenchymal stem cells (MSC) derived from mice with experimental autoimmune encephalomyelitis (EAE) suppress EAE and have similar biological properties with MSC from healthy donors. *Immunol Lett.*, *154*(1-2), 70-76.

Katsavos, S. (2013). Anagnostouli M. Biomarkers in Multiple Sclerosis: An Up-to-Date Overview. *Mult Scler Int.*, 2013, 340508.

Keller, A., Leidinger, P., Steinmeyer, F., Stähler, C., Franke, A., Hemmrich-Stanisak, G., et al., (2013). Comprehensive analysis of microRNA profiles in multiple sclerosis including next-generation sequencing. *Mult Scler.*, *20*(3), 295-303.

Khademi, M., Dring, A. M., Gilthorpe, J. D., Wuolikainen, A., Al Nimer, F., Harris, R. A., Andersson, M., Brundin, L., Piehl, F., Olsson, T. & Svenningsson, A. (2013). Intense inflammation and nerve damage in early multiple sclerosis subsides at older age: a reflection by cerebrospinal fluid biomarkers. *PLoS One.*, *8*(5), e63172.

Khalil, M., Enzinger, C., Langkammer, C., Ropele, S., Mader, A., Trentini, A., Vane, M. L., Wallner-Blazek, M., Bachmaier, G., Archelos, J. J. & Koel-Simmelink, M. J. (2013). Blankenstein MA, Fuchs S, Fazekas F, Teunissen CE. CSF neurofilament and N-acetylaspartate related brain changes in clinically isolated syndrome. *Mult Scler.*, *19*(4), 436-442.

Kinnunen, T., Chamberlain, N., Morbach, H., Cantaert, T., Lynch, M., Preston-Hurlburt, P., Herold, K. C., Hafler, D. A., O'Connor, K. C. & Meffre, E. (2013). Specific peripheral B cell tolerance defects in patients with multiple sclerosis. *J. Clin. Invest.*, *123*(6), 2737-2741.

Kishitani, T., Matsunaga, A. & Yoneda, M. (2013). [The biomarker and treatment in Hashimoto's encephalopahty]. *Nihon Rinsho.*, *71*(5), 893-897.

Kivisäkk, P., Healy, B. C., Francois, K., Gandhi, R., Gholipour, T., Egorova, S., Sevdalinova, V., Quintana, F., Chitnis, T., Weiner, H. L. & Khoury, S. J. (2014). Evaluation of circulating Osteopontin levels in an unselected cohort of patients with multiple sclerosis: relevance for biomarker development. *Mult Scler.*, *20*(4), 438-444.

Klingel, R., Heibges, A. & Fassbender, C. (2013). Neurologic diseases of the central nervous system with pathophysiologically relevant autoantibodies--perspectives for immunoadsorption. *Atheroscler Suppl.*, *14*(1)161-165.

Koch, M. W., Metz, L. M. & Kovalchuk, O. (2013). Epigenetics and miRNAs in the diagnosis and treatment of multiple sclerosis. *Trends Mol Med.*, *19*(1), 23-30.

Kornek, B., Aboul-Enein, F., Rostasy, K., Milos, R. I., Steiner, I., Penzien, J., Hellwig, K., Pitarokoili, K., Storm van's Gravesande, K., Karenfort, M., Blaschek, A., Meyer, A., Seid, 1 R., Debelic, D., Vass, K., Prayer, D., Kristoferitsch, W. & Bayas, A. (2013). Natalizumab therapy for highly active pediatric multiple sclerosis. *JAMA Neurol.*, *70*(4), 469-475.

Korobko, D. S., Malkova, N. A., Bulatova, E. V., Babenko, L. A., Sazonov, D. V., Sokolova, E. A. & Filipenko, M. L. (2013). [The effect of genetic factors on the phenotypic expression of multiple sclerosis]. *Zh Nevrol Psikhiatr Im S S Korsakova.*, *113*(2 Pt 2), 10-16.

Koziolek, M. J., Kitze, B., Mühlhausen, J. & Müller, G. A. (2013). Immunoadsorption in steroid-refractory multiple sclerosis. *Atheroscler Suppl.*, *14*(1), 175-178.

Kroksveen, A. C., Aasebø, E., Vethe, H., Van Pesch, V., Franciotta, D., Teunissen, C. E., Ulvik, R. J., Vedeler, C., Myhr, K. M., Barsnes, H. & Berven, F. S. (2013). Discovery and initial verification of differentially abundant proteins between multiple sclerosis patients and controls using iTRAQ and SID-SRM. *J Proteomics.*, *78*, 312-325.

Kuhle, J., Malmeström, C., Axelsson, M., Plattner, K., Yaldizli, O., Derfuss, T., Giovannoni, G., Kappos, L. & Lycke, J. (2013). Neurofilament light and heavy subunits compared as therapeutic biomarkers in multiple sclerosis. *Acta Neurol Scand.*, *128*(6), e33-6.

Kuhle, J., Plattner, K., Bestwick, J. P., Lindberg, R. L., Ramagopalan, S. V., Norgren, N., Nissim, A., Malaspina, A., Leppert, D., Giovannoni, G. & Kappos, L. (2013). A comparative study of CSF neurofilament light and heavy chain protein in MS. *Mult Scler.*, *19*(12), 1597-1603.

Leidinger, P., Backes, C., Deutscher, S., Schmitt, K., Muller, S. C., Frese, K., Haas, J., Ruprecht, K., Paul, F., Stahler, C., Lang, C. J., Meder, B., Bartfai, T., Meese, E. & Keller, A. (2013). A blood based 12-miRNA signature of Alzheimer disease patients. *Genome Biol.*, *14*(7), R78.

Leoni, V. & Caccia, C. (2013). 24S-hydroxycholesterol in plasma: a marker of cholesterol turnover in neurodegenerative diseases. *Biochimie.*, *95*(3), 595-612.

Leray, E., Coustans, M., Le, Page, E., Yaouanq, J., Oger, J. & Edan, G. (2013). 'Clinically definite benign multiple sclerosis', an unwarranted conceptual hodgepodge: evidence from a 30-year observational study. *Mult Scler.*, *19*(4), 458-465.

Li, C. F., Zhou, R. W., Mkhikian, H., Newton, B. L., Yu, Z. & Demetriou, M. (2013). Hypomorphic MGAT5 polymorphisms promote multiple sclerosis cooperatively with MGAT1 and interleukin-2 and 7 receptor variants. *J. Neuroimmunol.*, *256*(1-2), 71-76.

Li, H., Gonnella, P., Safavi, F., Vessal, G., Nourbakhsh, B., Zhou, F., Zhang, G. X. & Rostami, A. (2013). Low dose zymosan ameliorates both chronic and relapsing experimental autoimmune encephalomyelitis. *J. Neuroimmunol.*, *254*, 28-38.

Li, Z., Li, K., Zhu, L., Kan, Q., Yan, Y., Kumar, P., Xu, H., Rostami, A. & Zhang, G. (2013). Inhibitory effect of IL-17 on neural stem cell proliferation and neural cell differentiation. *BMC Immunol.*, *23*, 14, 20.

Lieu, A., Tenorio, G. & Kerr, B. J. (2013). Protein kinase C gamma (PKCγ) as a novel marker to assess the functional status of the corticospinal tract in experimental autoimmune encephalomyelitis (EAE). *J Neuroimmunol.*, *256*(1-2), 43-48.

Lill, C. M., Schjeide, B. M., Graetz, C., Ban, M., Alcina, A., Ortiz, M. A., et al., (2013). International Multiple Sclerosis Genetics Consortium, MANBA, CXCR5, SOX8, RPS6KB1 and ZBTB46 are genetic risk loci for multiple sclerosis. *Brain.*, *136*(Pt 6), 1778-82.

Lim, M. (2013). A glimpse at the cerebrospinal fluid immunoglobulins in neurological conditions. Does it help the clinician? *Dev Med Child Neurol.*, *55*(1), 10-2.

Lundström, W., Highfill, S., Walsh, S. T., Beq, S., Morse, E., Kockum, I., Alfredsson, L., Olsson, T., Hillert, J. & Mackall, C. L. (2013). Soluble IL7Rα potentiates IL-7 bioactivity and promotes autoimmunity. *Proc Natl Acad Sci U S A.*, *110*(19), E1761-770.

Madeddu, R., Farace, C., Tolu, P., Solinas, G., Asara, Y., Sotgiu, M. A., Delogu, L. G., Prados, J. C., Sotgiu, S. & Montella, A. (2013). Cytoskeletal proteins in the cerebrospinal fluid as biomarker of multiple sclerosis. *Neurol Sci.*, *34*(2), 181-186.

Malekzadeh, A. & Teunissen, C. (2013). Recent progress in omics-driven analysis of MS to unravel pathological mechanisms. *Expert Rev Neurother.*, (9), 1001-1016.

Marignier, R., Bernard-Valnet, R., Giraudon, P., Collongues, N., Papeix, C., Zéphir, H., Cavillon, G., Rogemond, V., Casey, R., Frangoulis, B., De Sèze, J., Vukusic, S., Honnorat, J. & Confavreux, C. NOMADMUS Study Group. Aquaporin-4 antibody-negative neuromyelitis optica: distinct assay sensitivity-dependent entity. *Neurology.*, *80*(24), 2194-2000

Marschallinger, R., Golaszewski, S. M., Kunz, A. B., Kronbichler, M., Ladurner, G., Hofmann, P., Trinka, E., McCoy, M. & Kraus, J. (2013). Usability and Potential of Geostatistics for Spatial Discrimination of Multiple Sclerosis Lesion Patterns. *J. Neuroimaging.*, *24*(3), 278-86.

Mehta, V., Pei, W., Yang, G., Li, S., Swamy, E., Boster, A., Schmalbrock, P. & Pitt, D. (2013). Iron is a sensitive biomarker for inflammation in multiple sclerosis lesions. *PLoS One.*, *8*(3), e57573.

Methner, A. & Zipp, F. (2013). Multiple sclerosis in 2012: Novel therapeutic options and drug targets in MS. *Nat Rev Neurol.*, *9*(2), 72-73.

Mistry, N., Dixon, J., Tallantyre, E., Tench, C., Abdel-Fahim, R., Jaspan, T., Morgan, P. S., Morris, P. & Evangelou, N. (2013). Central veins in brain lesions visualized with high-field magnetic resonance imaging: a pathologically specific diagnostic biomarker for inflammatory demyelination in the brain. *JAMA Neurol.*, *70*(5), 623-628.

Mogi, M. & Horiuchi, M. (2013). Effect of angiotensin II type 2 receptor on stroke, cognitive impairment and neurodegenerative diseases. *Geriatr Gerontol Int.*, *13*(1), 13-18.

Moscarello, M. A., Lei, H., Mastronardi, F. G., Winer, S., Tsui, H., Li, Z., Ackerley, C., Zhang, L., Raijmakers, R. & Wood, D. D. Inhibition of peptidyl-arginine deiminases reverses protein-hypercitrullination and disease in mouse models of multiple sclerosis. *Dis. Model Mech.*, 2013 (2), 467-478.

Moyano, A. L., Pituch, K., Li, G., van Breemen, R., Mansson, J. E. & Givogri, M. I. (2013). Levels of plasma sulfatides C18: 0 and C24: 1 correlate with disease status in relapsing-remitting multiple sclerosis. *J. Neurochem.*, *127*, 600-42013.

Muñoz, D., Escartín, A., Dapena, D., Coret, F., Fernández-Uría, D., Pérez, D., Casanova, B., Guijarro-Castro, C., Munteis, E., del-Campo Amigo, M., Pego, R., Calles, C., García-Rey, C., Monsalve, N. & Sánchez-Matienzo, D. (2013). Adverse events during the titration phase of interferon-beta in remitting-relapsing multiple sclerosis are not predicted by body mass index nor by pharmacodynamic biomarkers. *BMC Neurol.*, *13*, 82.

Nielsen, A. S., Kinkel, R. P., Madigan, N., Tinelli, E., Benner, T. & Mainero, C. (2013). Contribution of cortical lesion subtypes at 7T MRI to physical and cognitive performance in MS. *Neurology.*, *81*(7), 641-649.

Ohayon, J., Oh, U., Richert, N., Martin, J., Vortmeyer, A., McFarland, H. & Bielekova, B. (2013). CNS vasculitis in a patient with MS on Dacluzimab monotherapy. *Neurology.*, *80*(5), 453-457.

Ohyama, K., Koike, H., Iijima, M., Hashimoto, R., Tomita, M., Kawagashira, Y., Satou, A., Nakamura, S. & Sobue, G. (2013). IgG4-related neuropathy: a case report. *JAMA Neurol.*, *70*(4), 502-505.

Orbach, R., Gurevich, M. & AchIron, A. (2014). Interleukin-12p40 in the spinal fluid as a biomarker for clinically isolated syndrome. *Mult Scler.*, *20*(1), 35-42.

Ortiz-Pérez, S., Martínez-Lapiscina, E. H., Gabilondo, I., Fraga-Pumar, E., Martínez-Heras, E., Saiz, A., Sanchez-Dalmau, B. & Villoslada, P. (2013). Retinal periphlebitis is associated with multiple sclerosis severity. *Neurology.*, *81*(10), 877-881.

Osnes, L. T., Nakken, B., Bodolay, E. & Szodoray, P. (2013). Assessment of intracellular cytokines and regulatory cells in patients with autoimmune diseases and primary immunodeficiencies - novel tool for diagnostics and patient follow-up. *Autoimmun Rev.*, *12*(10), 967-971.

Ouallet, J. C., Bodiguel, E., Bensa, C., Blanc, F., Brassat, D., Laplaud, D., Zephir, H., de Seze, J. & Magy, L. (2013). Groupe de Re´flexion sur la Scle´rose en Plaques: GRESE. Recommendations for useful serum testing with suspected multiple sclerosis. *Rev Neurol (Paris).*, *169*(1), 37-46.

Outteryck, O., Ongagna, J. C., Brochet, B., Rumbach, L., Lebrun-Frenay, C., Debouverie, M., Zéphir, H., Ouallet, J. C., Berger, E., Cohen, M., Pittion, S., et al. (2014). BIONAT network, and CFSEP. A prospective observational post-marketing study of Natalizumab-treated multiple sclerosis patients: clinical, radiological and biological features and adverse events. The BIONAT cohort. *Eur J Neurol.*, *21*(1), 40-48.

Oyebamiji, A. I., Finlay, T. M., Hough, R. M., Hoghooghi, V., Lim, E. M., Wong, C. H. & Ousman, S. S. (2013). Characterization of migration parameters on peripheral and central nervous system T cells following treatment of experimental allergic encephalomyelitis with CRYAB. *J Neuroimmunol.*, *259*, 66-74.

Paul, F. (2013). Hope for a rare disease: Eculizumab in neuromyelitis optica. *Lancet Neurol.*, *12*(6), 529-531.

Petković, F., Blaževski, J., Momčilović, M., Timotijević, G., Zocca, M. B., Mijatović, S., Maksimović-Ivanić, D., Mangano, K., Fagone, P., Stošić-Grujičić, S., Nicoletti, F. & Miljković, D. (2013). Saquinavir-NO inhibits S6 kinase activity, impairs secretion of the encephalytogenic cytokines interleukin-17 and interferon-gamma and ameliorates experimental autoimmune encephalomyelitis. *J Neuroimmunol.*, *259*, 55-65.

Piao, J. H., Wang, Y. & Duncan, I. D. (2013). CD44 is required for the migration of transplanted oligodendrocyte progenitor cells to focal inflammatory demyelinating lesions in the spinal cord. *Glia.*, *61*(3), 361- 367.

Piazza, F., Greenberg, S. M., Savoiardo, M., Gardinetti, M., Chiapparini, L., Raicher, I., Nitrini, R., Sakaguchi, H., Brioschi, M., Billo, G., Colombo, A., Lanzani, F., Piscosquito, G., Carriero, M. R., Giaccone, G., Tagliavini, F., Ferrarese, C. & Difrancesco, J. C. (2013). Anti-amyloid β autoantibodies in cerebral amyloid angiopathy-related inflammation: Implications for Amyloid-Modifying Therapies. *Ann Neurol.*, *73*(4), 449-458.

Pichler, A., Enzinger, C., Fuchs, S., Plecko-Startinig, B., Gruber-Sedlmayr, U., Linortner, P., Langkammer, C., Khalil, M., Ebner, F., Ropele, S. & Fazekas, F. (2013). Differences and similarities in the evolution of morphologic brain abnormalities between paediatric and adult-onset multiple sclerosis. *Mult Scler.*, *19*(2), 167-172.

Piqué-Duran, E., Eguía, P. & García-Vázquez, O. (2013). Acquired perforating dermatosis associated with Natalizumab. *J Am Acad Dermatol.*, *68*(6), e185-7.

Pittock, S. J., Lennon, V. A., McKeon, A., Mandrekar, J., Weinshenker, B. G., Lucchinetti, C. F., O'Toole, O. & Wingerchuk, D. M. (2013). Eculizumab in AQP4-IgG-positive relapsing neuromyelitis optica spectrum disorders: an open-label pilot study. *Lancet Neurol.*, *12*(6), 554-562.

Podojil, J. R. & Miller, S. D. (2013). Targeting the B7 family of co-stimulatory molecules: successes and challenges. *BioDrugs.*, *27*(1), 1-13.

Pravica, V., Markovic, M., Cupic, M., Savic, E., Popadic, D., Drulovic, J. & Mostarica-Stojkovic, M. (2013). Multiple sclerosis: individualized disease susceptibility and therapy response. *Biomark Med*, *7*(1), 59-71.

Qin, B., Huang, F., Liang, Y., Yang, Z. & Zhong, R. (2013). Analysis of altered microRNA expression profiles in peripheral blood mononuclear cells from patients with primary biliary cirrhosis. *J Gastroenterol Hepatol.*, *28*(3), 543-550.

Qiu, Z. X., Zhang, K., Qiu, X. S., Zhou, M. & Li, W. M. (2013). CD226 Gly307Ser association with multiple autoimmune diseases: a meta-analysis. *Hum Immunol.*, *74*(2), 249-255.

Raychaudhuri, S. P. (2013). Role of IL-17 in psoriasis and psoriatic arthritis. *Clin Rev Allergy Immunol.*, *44*(2), 183-193.

Raz, E., Bester, M., Sigmund, E. E., Tabesh, A., Babb, J. S., Jaggi, H., Helpern, J., Mitnick, R. J. & Inglese, M. (2013). A better characterization of spinal cord damage in multiple sclerosis: a diffusional kurtosis imaging study. AJNR. *Am. J. Neuroradiol.*, *34*(9), 1846-1852.

Riddell, C. A., Zhao, Y. & Petkau, J. (2013). An adaptive clinical trials procedure for a sensitive subgroup examined in the multiple sclerosis context. *Stat Methods Med Res.* (in press).

Rimkus, Cde M., Junqueira, Tde F., Callegaro. D., Otaduy, M. C. & Leite, Cda C. (2013). Segmented corpus callosum diffusivity correlates with the Expanded Disability Status

Scale score in the early stages of relapsing-remitting multiple sclerosis. *Clinics (Sao Paulo).*, *68*(8), 1115-1120.

Romme Christensen, J., Börnsen, L., Ratzer, R., Piehl, F., Khademi, M., Olsson, T., Sørensen, P. S. & Sellebjerg, F. (2013). Systemic inflammation in progressive multiple sclerosis involves follicular T-helper, Th17- and activated B-cells and correlates with progression. *PLoS One.*, *8*(3), e57820.

Roos, P. M., Vesterberg, O., Syversen, T., Flaten, T. P. & Nordberg, M. (2013). Metal concentrations in cerebrospinal fluid and blood plasma from patients with amyotrophic lateral sclerosis. *Biol Trace Elem Res.*, *151*(2), 159-170.

Rudick, R. A. & Cutter, G. (2013). MRI lesions: a surrogate for relapses in multiple sclerosis? *Lancet Neurol.*, *12*(7), 628-630.

Sato, D. K., Nakashima, I., Takahashi, T., Misu, T., Waters, P., Kuroda, H., Nishiyama, S., Suzuki, C., Takai, Y., Fujihara, K., Itoyama, Y. & Aoki, M. (2013). Aquaporin-4 antibody-positive cases beyond current diagnostic criteria for NMO spectrum disorders. *Neurology.*, *80*(24), 2210-2216.

Sbardella, E., Greco, A., Stromillo, M. L., Prosperini, L., Puopolo, M., Cefaro, L. A., Pantano, P., De Stefano, N., Minghetti, L. & Pozzilli, C. (2013). Isoprostanes in clinically isolated syndrome and early multiple sclerosis as biomarkers of tissue damage and predictors of clinical course. *Mult Scler.*, *19*(4), 411-417.

Schirmer, L., Merkler, D., König, F. B., Brück, W. & Stadelmann, C. (2013). Neuroaxonal regeneration is more pronounced in early multiple sclerosis than in traumatic brain injury lesions. *Brain Pathol.*, *23*(1), 2-12.

Schirmer, L., Rothhammer, V., Hemmer, B., Korn, T. & Enriched, (2013). CD161high CCR6+ γδ T cells in the cerebrospinal fluid of patients with multiple sclerosis. *JAMA Neurol.*, *70*(3), 345-351.

Schneider, H., Weber, C. E., Hellwig, K., Schroten, H. & Tenenbaum, T. (2013). Natalizumab treatment during pregnancy - effects on the neonatal immune system. *Acta Neurol Scand.*, *127*(1), e1-4.

Schulze-Topphoff, U., Casazza, S., Varrin-Doyer, M., Michel, K., Sobel, R. A., Hauser, S. L., Oksenberg, J. R., Zamvil, S. S. & Baranzini, S. E. (2013). Tob1 plays a critical role in the activation of encephalitogenic T cells in CNS autoimmunity. *J Exp Med.*, *210*(7), 1301-139.

Schwab, N., Schneider-Hohendorf, T., Posevitz, V., Breuer, J., Göbel, K., Windhagen, S., Brochet, B., et al., (2013). L-Selectin is a possible biomarker for individual PML risk in Natalizumab-treated MS patients. *Neurology.*, *81*, 865-871.

Schwarz, A., Schumacher, M., Pfaff, D., Schumacher, K., Jarius, S, Balint, B., Wiendl, H., Haas, J. & Wildemann, B. (2013). Fine-tuning of regulatory T cell function: the role of calcium signals and naive regulatory T cells for regulatory T cell deficiency in multiple sclerosis. *J Immunol.*, *190*(10), 4965-4970.

Sellebjerg, F., Hesse, D., Limborg, S, Lund, H., Søndergaard, H. B., Krakauer, M. & Sørensen, P. S. (2013). Dendritic cell, monocyte and T cell activation and response to Glatiramer acetate in multiple sclerosis. *Mult Scler.*, *19*(2), 179-187.

Serafini, B., Muzio, L., Rosicarelli, B. & Aloisi, F. (2013). Radioactive *in situ* hybridization for Epstein-Barr virus-encoded small RNA supports presence of Epstein-Barr virus in the multiple sclerosis brain. *Brain.*, *136*(Pt 7), e233.

Shamim, Z., Spellman, S., Haagenson, M., Wang, T., Lee, S. J., Ryder, L. P. & Müller, K. (2013). Polymorphism in the interleukin-7 receptor-alpha and outcome after allogeneic hematopoietic cell transplantation with matched unrelated donor. *Scand J Immunol.*, *78*(2), 214-220.

Sharma, S., Moon, C. S., Khogali, A., Haidous, A., Chabenne, A., Ojo, C., Jelebinkov, M., Kurdi, Y. & Ebadi, M. (2013). Biomarkers in Parkinson's disease (recent update). *Neurochem Int.*, *63*(3), 201-229.

Sinclair, A. J., Wienholt, L., Tantsis, E., Brilot, F. & Dale, R. C. (2013). Clinical association of intrathecal and mirrored oligoclonal bands in paediatric neurology. *Dev Med Child Neurol.*, *55*(1), 71-75.

Sokolova, E. A., Malkova, N. A., Korobko, D. S., Rozhdestvenskiĭ, A. S., Kakulia, A. V., Khanokh, E. V., Delov, R. A., et al., (2013). [The first results of a combined all-Russian study on clinical genetics of multiple sclerosis]. *Zh Nevrol Psikhiatr Im S S Korsakova.*, *113*, 6-9.

Søndergaard, H. B., Hesse, D., Krakauer, M., Sørensen, P. S. & Sellebjerg, F. (2013). Differential microRNA expression in blood in multiple sclerosis. *Mult Scler.*, *19*(14), 1849-1857.

Sormani, M. P. & Bruzzi, P. (2013). MRI lesions as a surrogate for relapses in multiple sclerosis: a meta-analysis of randomised trials. *Lancet Neurol.*, *12*(7), 669-676.

Sormani, M. P. & De Stefano, N. (2013). Defining and scoring response to IFN-β in multiple sclerosis. *Nat Rev Neurol.*, *9*(9), 504-512.

Stangel, M., Fredrikson, S., Meinl, E., Petzold, A., Stüve, O. & Tumani, H. (2013). The utility of cerebrospinal fluid analysis in patients with multiple sclerosis. *Nat Rev Neurol.*, *9*(5), 267-276.

Stoop, M. P., Singh, V., Stingl, C., Martin, R., Khademi, M., Olsson, T., Hintzen, R. Q. & Luider, T. M. (2013). Effects of Natalizumab treatment on the cerebrospinal fluid proteome of multiple sclerosis patients. *J Proteome Res.*, *12*(3), 1101-1107.

Sumowski, J. F., Wylie, G. R., Leavitt, V. M., Chiaravalloti, N. D. & DeLuca, J. (2013). Default network activity is a sensitive and specific biomarker of memory in multiple sclerosis. *Mult Scler.*, *19*(2), 199-208.

Sunwoo, L., Choi, S. H., Park, C. K., Kim, J. W., Yi, K. S., Lee, W. J., et al. (2013). Correlation of apparent diffusion coefficient values measured by diffusion MRI and MGMT promoter methylation semiquantitatively analyzed with MS-MLPA in patients with glioblastoma multiforme. *J Magn Reson Imaging.*, *37*(2), 351-358.

Szalardy, L., Zadori, D., Simu, M., Bencsik, K., Vecsei, L. & Klivenyi, P. (2013). Evaluating biomarkers of neuronal degeneration and neuroinflammation in CSF of patients with multiple sclerosis-Osteopontin as a potential marker of clinical severity. *J Neurol Sci.*, *331*, 38-42.

Takano, A., Piehl, F., Hillert, J., Varrone, A., Nag, S., Gulyás, B., Stenkrona, P., et al. *In vivo* TSPO imaging in patients with multiple sclerosis: a brain PET study with [^{18}F]FEDAA1106. *EJNMMI Res.*, *3*(1), 30.

Tasset, I., Bahamonde, C., Agüera, E., Conde, C., Cruz, A. H., Pérez-Herrera, A., Gascón, F, Giraldo, A. I., Ruiz, M. C., Lillo, R., Sánchez-López, F. & Túnez, I. (2013). Effect of Natalizumab on oxidative damage biomarkers in relapsing-remitting multiple sclerosis. *Pharmacol Rep.*, *65*(3), 634-641.

Tegla, C. A., Cudrici, C. D., Azimzadeh, P., Singh, A. K., Trippe, R3rd, Khan, A., Chen, H., Andrian-Albescu, M., Royal, W3rd., Bever, C., Rus, V. & Rus, H. (2013). Dual role of Response gene to complement-32 in multiple sclerosis. *Exp Mol Pathol.*, *94*, 17-28.

Tenembaum, S. N. (2013). Acute disseminated encephalomyelitis. *Handb Clin Neurol.*, *112*, 1253-1262.

Tenorio-Laranga, J., Peltonen, I., Keskitalo, S., Duran-Torres, G., Natarajan, R., Männistö, P. T., Nurmi, A., Vartiainen, N., Airas, L., Elovaara, I. & García-Horsman, J. A. (2013). Alteration of prolyl oligopeptidase and activated α-2-macroglobulin in multiple sclerosis subtypes and in the clinically isolated syndrome. *Biochem Pharmacol.*, *85*, 1783-1794.

Teunissen, C., Menge, T., Altintas, A., Alvarez-Cermeño, J. C., Bertolotto, A., et al., (2013). A Consensus definitions and application guidelines for control groups in cerebrospinal fluid biomarker studies in multiple sclerosis. *Mult Scler.*, *19*(13), 1802-1809

Tourdias, T. & Dousset, V. (2013). Neuroinflammatory imaging biomarkers: relevance to multiple sclerosis and its therapy. *Neurotherapeutics.*, *10*(1), 111-123.

Tuller, T., Atar, S., Ruppin, E., Gurevich, M. & AchIron, A. (2013). Common and specific signatures of gene expression and protein-protein interactions in autoimmune diseases. *Genes Immun.*, *14*(2), 67-82.

Turner, M. R., Bowser, R., Bruijn, L., Dupuis, L., Ludolph, A., McGrath, M., et al., (2013). Mechanisms, models and biomarkers in amyotrophic lateral sclerosis. *Amyotroph Lateral Scler Frontotemporal Degener.*, 14 Suppl 1, 19-32.

Unoda, K., Doi, Y., Nakajima, H., Yamane, K., Hosokawa, T., Ishida, S., Kimura, F. & Hanafusa, T. (2013). Eicosapentaenoic acid (EPA) induces peroxisome proliferator-activated receptors and ameliorates experimental autoimmune encephalomyelitis. *J Neuroimmunol.*, *256*(1-2), 7-12.

Van Haren, K., Tomooka, B. H., Kidd, B. A., Banwell, B., Bar-Or, A., Chitnis, T., Tenembaum, S. N., et al., (2013). Serum autoantibodies to myelin peptides distinguish acute disseminated encephalomyelitis from relapsing- remitting multiple sclerosis. *Mult Scler.*, *19*, 1726-1733.

Vingara, L. K., Yu, H. J., Wagshul, M. E., Serafin, D., Christodoulou, C., Pelczer, I., Krupp, L. B. & Maletić-Savatić, M. (2013). Metabolomic approach to human brain spectroscopy identifies associations between clinical features and the frontal lobe metabolome in multiple sclerosis. *Neuroimage.*, *82*, 586-594.

Vorstenbosch, J., Al-Ajmi, H., Winocour, S., Trzeciak, A., Lessard, L. & Philip, A. (2013). CD109 overexpression ameliorates skin fibrosis in a mouse model of bleomycin-induced scleroderma. *Arthritis Rheum.*, *65*(5), 1378-1383.

Wagner, M., Wiśniewski, A., Bilińska, M., Pokryszko-Dragan, A., Nowak, I., Kuśnierczyk, P. & Jasek, M. (2013). ALCAM--novel multiple sclerosis locus interfering with HLA-DRB1*1501. *J Neuroimmunol.*, *258*, 71-76.

Wang, B., Higgs, B. W., Chang, L., Vainshtein, I., Liu, Z., Streicher, K., Liang, M., White. W. I., Yoo, S., Richman, L., Jallal, B., Roskos, L. & Yao, Y. (2013). Pharmacogenomics and translational simulations to bridge indications for an anti-interferon-α receptor antibody. *Clin Pharmacol Ther.*, *93*(6), 483-492.

Wang, X., Brieland, J. K., Kim, J. H., Chen, Y. J., O'Neal, J., O'Neil, S. P., Tu, T. W., Trinkaus, K. & Song, S. K. (2013). Diffusion tensor imaging detects treatment effects of FTY720 in experimental autoimmune encephalomyelitis mice. *NMR Biomed.*, *26*(12), 1742-1750.

Wang, X. & Dong, C. (2013). The CD70-CD27 axis, a new brake in the T helper 17 cell response. *Immunity.*, *38*(1), 1-3

Wang, X., Haroon, F., Karray, S., Deckert, M. & Schlüter, D. (2013). Astrocytic Fas ligand expression is required to induce T-cell apoptosis and recovery from experimental autoimmune encephalomyelitis. *Eur J Immunol.*, *43*(1), 115-124.

Wang, Y., Thomson, C. A., Allan, L. L., Jackson, L. M., Olson, M., Hercus, T. R., et al., (2013). Characterization of pathogenic human monoclonal autoantibodies against GM-CSF. *Proc Natl Acad Sci U S A.*, *110*(19), 7832-7837.

Wangdong, X. (2013). CD70: probably being a therapeutic target in human multiple sclerosis. *Rheumatol Int.*, *33*(3), 815.

Wei, L. (2013). Wasilewski E, Chakka SK, Bello AM, Moscarello MA, Kotra LP. Novel inhibitors of protein arginine deiminase with potential activity in multiple sclerosis animal model. *J Med Chem.*, *56*(4), 1715-1722.

Weinshenker, B. & Tienari, P. J. (2013). TNFRSF1A polymorphisms and MS: statistical signals transform into pathogenetic mechanisms. *Neurology.*, *80*(22), 2002-2003.

Wheway, J., Obeid, S., Couraud, P. O., Combes, V. & Grau, G. E. (2013). The brain microvascular endothelium supports T cell proliferation and has potential for alloantigen presentation. *PLoS One.*, *8*(1), e52586.

Wimmer, D. B., Ro, J. Y., Lewis, A., Schwartz, M. R., Caplan, R., Schwarz, P. & Ayala, A. G. (2013). Extranodal rosai-dorfman disease associated with increased numbers of immunoglobulin g4 plasma cells involving the colon: case report with literature review. *Arch Pathol Lab Med.*, *137*, 999-1004.

Winer, L, Srinivasan, D., Chun, S., Lacomis, D., Jaffa, M., Fagan, A., Holtzman, D. M., Wancewicz, E., Bennett, C. F., Bowser, R., Cudkowicz, M. & Miller, T. M. (2013). SOD1 in cerebral spinal fluid as a pharmacodynamic marker for antisense oligonucleotide therapy. *JAMA Neurol.*, *70*(2), 201-207.

Wipfler, P., Heikkinen, A., Harrer, A., Pilz, G., Kunz, A., Golaszewski, S. M., Reuss, R., Oschmann, P. & Kraus, J. (2013). Circadian rhythmicity of inflammatory serum parameters: a neglected issue in the search of biomarkers in multiple sclerosis. *J Neurol.*, *260*(1), 221-227.

Wolf, C., Sidhu, J., Otoul, C., Morris, D. L., Cnops, J., Taubel, J. & Bennett, B. (2013). Pharmacodynamic consequences of administration of VLA-4 antagonist CDP323 to multiple sclerosis subjects: a randomized, double-blind phase 1/2 study. *PLoS One.*, *8*(3), e58438.

Yen, J. H., Xu, S., Park, Y. S., Ganea, D. & Kim, K. C. (2013). Higher susceptibility to experimental autoimmune encephalomyelitis in Muc1-deficient mice is associated with increased Th1/Th17 responses. *Brain Behav Immun.*, *29*, 70-81.

Young, E. E., Vichaya, E. G., Reusser, N. M., Cook, J. L., Steelman, A. J., Welsh, C. J. & Meagher, M. W. (2-13). Chronic social stress impairs virus specific adaptive immunity during acute Theiler's virus infection. *J Neuroimmunol.*, *254*, 19-27.

Zacharaki, D., Lagoudaki, R., Touloumi, O., Kotta, K., Voultsiadou, A., Poulatsidou, K. N., Lourbopoulos, A., Hadjigeorgiou, G., Dardiotis, E., Karacostas, D. & Grigoriadis, N. (2013). Characterization of *in vitro* expanded bone marrow-derived mesenchymal stem cells isolated from experimental autoimmune encephalomyelitis mice. *J Mol Neurosci.*, *51*(2), 282-297.

Zaguia, F., Saikali, P., Ludwin, S., Newcombe, J., Beauseigle, D., McCrea, E., Duquette, P., Prat, A., Antel, J. P. & Arbour, N. (2013). Cytotoxic NKG2C+ CD4 T cells target oligodendrocytes in multiple sclerosis. *J Immunol.*, *190*(6), 2510-2518.

Zare-Shahabadi, A., Renaudineau, Y. & Rezaei, N. (2013). MicroRNAs and multiple sclerosis: from physiopathology toward therapy. *Expert Opin Ther Targets.*, *17*(12), 1497-1507.

Zhang, F., Wei, W., Chai, H. & Xie, X. (2013). Aurintricarboxylic acid ameliorates experimental autoimmune encephalomyelitis by blocking chemokine-mediated pathogenic cell migration and infiltration. *J Immunol.*, *190*(3), 1017-1025.

Zhao, J., Gao, Y., Cheng, C., Yan, M. & Wang, J. (2013). Upregulation of β-1,4-galactosyltransferase I in rat spinal cord with experimental autoimmune encephalomyelitis. *J Mol Neurosci.*, *49*, 437-445.

Zhou, H. L., Wang, Y. T., Gao, T., Wang, W. G. & Wang, Y. S. (2013). Distribution and expression of fibroblast-specific protein chemokine CCL21 and chemokine receptor CCR7 in renal allografts. *Transplant Proc.*, *45*(2), 538-545.

Zhu, H., Luo, H. & Zuo, X. (2013). MicroRNAs: their involvement in fibrosis pathogenesis and use as diagnostic biomarkers in scleroderma. *Exp Mol Med.*, *45*, e41.

INDEX

G

H

I

L

M

N

O

P